Intraocular Pressure and Ocular Hypertension

Intraocular Pressure and Ocular Hypertension

Editors

Paolo Brusini
Maria Letizia Salvetat
Marco Zeppieri

MDPI • Basel • Beijing • Wuhan • Barcelona • Belgrade • Manchester • Tokyo • Cluj • Tianjin

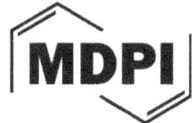

Editors

Paolo Brusini
Department of
Ophthalmology
Policlinico "Città di Udine"
Udine
Italy

Maria Letizia Salvetat
Department of
Ophthalmology
Azienda Sanitaria Friuli
Occidentale
Pordenone
Italy

Marco Zeppieri
Department of
Ophthalmology
University Hospital of Udine
Udine
Italy

Editorial Office
MDPI
St. Alban-Anlage 66
4052 Basel, Switzerland

This is a reprint of articles from the Special Issue published online in the open access journal *Journal of Clinical Medicine* (ISSN 2077-0383) (available at: www.mdpi.com/journal/jcm/special_issues/Ocular_Hypertension).

For citation purposes, cite each article independently as indicated on the article page online and as indicated below:

LastName, A.A.; LastName, B.B.; LastName, C.C. Article Title. *Journal Name* **Year**, *Volume Number*, Page Range.

ISBN 978-3-0365-5100-5 (Hbk)
ISBN 978-3-0365-5099-2 (PDF)

Contents

About the Editors ix

Paolo Brusini, Maria Letizia Salvetat and Marco Zeppieri
It Is All about Pressure
Reprinted from: *J. Clin. Med.* **2022**, *11*, 3640, doi:10.3390/jcm11133640 . . . . **1**

Paolo Brusini, Maria Letizia Salvetat and Marco Zeppieri
How to Measure Intraocular Pressure: An Updated Review of Various Tonometers
Reprinted from: *J. Clin. Med.* **2021**, *10*, 3860, doi:10.3390/jcm10173860 . . . . **7**

Ban Luo, Wei Wang, Xinyu Li, Hong Zhang, Yaoli Zhang and Weikun Hu
Correlation Analysis between Intraocular Pressure and Extraocular Muscles Based on Orbital
Magnetic Resonance T2 Mapping in Thyroid-Associated Ophthalmopathy Patients
Reprinted from: *J. Clin. Med.* **2022**, *11*, 3981, doi:10.3390/jcm11143981 . . . . **31**

Tomislav Sarenac, Anela Bečić Turkanović, Peter Ferme and Tomaž Gračner
A Review of Selective Laser Trabeculoplasty: "The Hype Is Real"
Reprinted from: *J. Clin. Med.* **2022**, *11*, 3879, doi:10.3390/jcm11133879 . . . . **41**

**Agnieszka Jóźwik, Joanna Przeździecka-Dołyk, Ewa Wałek, Magdalena Czerniak and
Magdalena Asejczyk**
Corneal Behavior during Tonometer Measurement during the Water Drinking Test in Eyes with
XEN GelStent in Comparison to Non-Implanted Eyes
Reprinted from: *J. Clin. Med.* **2022**, *11*, 2962, doi:10.3390/jcm11112962 . . . . **57**

Patrick Murtagh and Colm O'Brien
Corneal Hysteresis, Intraocular Pressure, and Progression of Glaucoma: Time for a "Hyst-Oric"
Change in Clinical Practice?
Reprinted from: *J. Clin. Med.* **2022**, *11*, 2895, doi:10.3390/jcm11102895 . . . . **69**

**Alicja Strzalkowska, Nina Pirlich, Julia V. Stingl, Alexander K. Schuster, Jasmin Rezapour
and Felix M. Wagner et al.**
Intraocular Pressure Measurement in Childhood Glaucoma under Standardized General
Anaesthesia: The Prospective EyeBIS Study
Reprinted from: *J. Clin. Med.* **2022**, *11*, 2846, doi:10.3390/jcm11102846 . . . . **83**

Rong Du, Chen Xin, Jingjiang Xu, Jianping Hu, Huaizhou Wang and Ningli Wang et al.
Pulsatile Trabecular Meshwork Motion: An Indicator of Intraocular Pressure Control in Primary
Open-Angle Glaucoma
Reprinted from: *J. Clin. Med.* **2022**, *11*, 2696, doi:10.3390/jcm11102696 . . . . **93**

Paolo Brusini, Veronica Papa and Marco Zeppieri
Canaloplasty in Pseudoexfoliation Glaucoma. Can It Still Be Considered a Good Choice?
Reprinted from: *J. Clin. Med.* **2022**, *11*, 2532, doi:10.3390/jcm11092532 . . . . **103**

Dries Wijnants, Ingeborg Stalmans and Evelien Vandewalle
The Effects of Intranasal, Inhaled and Systemic Glucocorticoids on Intraocular Pressure: A
Literature Review
Reprinted from: *J. Clin. Med.* **2022**, *11*, 2007, doi:10.3390/jcm11072007 . . . . **113**

María Dolores Díaz-Barreda, Ignacio Sánchez-Marín, Ana Boned-Murillo, Itziar
Pérez-Navarro, Juana Martínez and Elena Pardina-Claver et al.
Modification of Corneal Biomechanics and Intraocular Pressure Following Non-Penetrating
Deep Sclerectomy
Reprinted from: *J. Clin. Med.* **2022**, *11*, 1216, doi:10.3390/jcm11051216 . . . . **127**

Anne-Sophie Simons, Ingele Casteels, John Grigg, Ingeborg Stalmans, Evelien Vandewalle
and Sophie Lemmens
Management of Childhood Glaucoma Following Cataract Surgery
Reprinted from: *J. Clin. Med.* **2022**, *11*, 1041, doi:10.3390/jcm11041041 . . . . **137**

Juliette Buffault, Françoise Brignole-Baudouin, Élodie Reboussin, Karima Kessal, Antoine
Labbé and Stéphane Mélik Parsadaniantz et al.
The Dual Effect of Rho-Kinase Inhibition on Trabecular Meshwork Cells Cytoskeleton and
Extracellular Matrix in an In Vitro Model of Glaucoma
Reprinted from: *J. Clin. Med.* **2022**, *11*, 1001, doi:10.3390/jcm11041001 . . . . **163**

Marc-Antoine Hannappe, Florian Baudin, Anne-Sophie Mariet, Pierre-Henri Gabrielle,
Louis Arnould and Alain M. Bron et al.
Mid-Term Impact of Anti-Vascular Endothelial Growth Factor Agents on Intraocular Pressure
Reprinted from: *J. Clin. Med.* **2022**, *11*, 946, doi:10.3390/jcm11040946 . . . . **177**

Rupalatha Maddala, Leona T. Y. Ho, Shruthi Karnam, Iris Navarro, Anja Osterwald and
Sandra S. Stinnett et al.
Elevated Levels of Growth/Differentiation Factor-15 in the Aqueous Humor and Serum of
Glaucoma Patients
Reprinted from: *J. Clin. Med.* **2022**, *11*, 744, doi:10.3390/jcm11030744 . . . . **187**

Giacomo Toneatto, Marco Zeppieri, Veronica Papa, Laura Rizzi, Carlo Salati and Andrea
Gabai et al.
360° Ab-Interno Schlemm's Canal Viscodilation with OMNI Viscosurgical Systems for
Open-Angle Glaucoma—Midterm Results
Reprinted from: *J. Clin. Med.* **2022**, *11*, 259, doi:10.3390/jcm11010259 . . . . **199**

Kazunobu Sugihara and Masaki Tanito
Different Effects of Aging on Intraocular Pressures Measured by Three Different Tonometers
Reprinted from: *J. Clin. Med.* **2021**, *10*, 4202, doi:10.3390/jcm10184202 . . . . **215**

Hiromitsu Onoe, Kazuyuki Hirooka, Hideaki Okumichi, Yumiko Murakami and Yoshiaki
Kiuchi
Corneal Higher-Order Aberrations after Microhook ab Interno Trabeculotomy and Goniotomy
with the Kahook Dual Blade: Preliminary Early 3-Month Results
Reprinted from: *J. Clin. Med.* **2021**, *10*, 4115, doi:10.3390/jcm10184115 . . . . **223**

Silvia Mendez-Martinez, Teresa Martínez-Rincón, Manuel Subias, Luis E. Pablo, David
García-Herranz and Julian García Feijoo et al.
Influence of Chronic Ocular Hypertension on Emmetropia: Refractive, Structural and
Functional Study in Two Rat Models
Reprinted from: *J. Clin. Med.* **2021**, *10*, 3697, doi:10.3390/jcm10163697 . . . . **231**

Do-Young Park and Soon-Cheol Cha
Factors Associated with Increased Neuroretinal Rim Thickness Measured Based on Bruch's
Membrane Opening-Minimum Rim Width after Trabeculectomy
Reprinted from: *J. Clin. Med.* **2021**, *10*, 3646, doi:10.3390/jcm10163646 . . . . **251**

Naoki Okada, Kazuyuki Hirooka, Hiromitsu Onoe, Yumiko Murakami, Hideaki Okumichi and Yoshiaki Kiuchi
Comparison of Efficacy between 120° and 180° Schlemm's Canal Incision Microhook Ab Interno Trabeculotomy
Reprinted from: *J. Clin. Med.* **2021**, *10*, 3181, doi:10.3390/jcm10143181 . . . . **259**

Yu-Min Chang, Jiann-Torng Chen, Ming-Cheng Tai, Wei-Liang Chen and Ying-Jen Chen
Serum Calcium Level as a Useful Surrogate for Risk of Elevated Intraocular Pressure
Reprinted from: *J. Clin. Med.* **2021**, *10*, 1839, doi:10.3390/jcm10091839 . . . . **267**

proposed. The manuscript highlights advantages and drawbacks of the various devices, emphasizing the concept that the continuous monitoring of IOP, which is still under evaluation, will be an important step in the diagnosis and management of the glaucomatous patients.

In the article entitled "Intraocular pressure measurement in childhood glaucoma under standardized general anesthesia: the prospective EyeBIS study", Alicja Strzalkowska et al. [12] addresses the important topic of the IOP measurement in children. The authors compared the IOP measurements taken with the iCare PRO rebound tonometer and Perkins applanation tonometer in glaucomatous and healthy children (mean age of 45 ± 30 months) under general anesthesia. The results of the study demonstrated that the IOP values taken with both tonometers appeared inversely related to the anesthesia depth, and that iCare IOP values were significantly higher than those obtained with Perkins tonometer in both glaucomatous and healthy children.

Several studies have compared the performances of different tonometers, and how different variables can affect the accuracy. Sugihara and Tanito [13] analyze the effects of aging on IOP measured by three different tonometers. Corneal biomechanical properties change with age, which can differently influence the IOP measurement obtained with different devices. Comparing the IOP measurements taken with GAT, non-contact tonometer, and rebound tonometer, the authors found that age appeared negatively correlated with the IOP values measured with non-contact and rebound tonometers, whereas GAT IOP measurements were not influenced by age.

The Ocular Response Analyzer (ORA) was used by Jóźnik et al. [14] to assess the biomechanical behavior of the cornea after a water drinking test in patients with or without a previous XEN Gel implant. They found a significant difference between the two groups in various analyzed parameters, results indicating that ORA could be useful in postoperative glaucoma diagnostics. Moreover, Diaz-Barreda et al. [15] reported significant modifications in corneal biomechanical parameters measured with ORA in patients that underwent a deep sclerectomy with Esnoper V2000 implant. Corneal hysteresis remained above preoperative values at 3 months of follow-up, whereas corneal resistance factor was at a lower level. The clinical relevance of this information, however, needs to be confirmed with further studies.

Another paper regarding the correlation between glaucoma surgery and corneal properties was written by Onoe et al. [16]. These authors found a significant increase in corneal higher-order aberrations after ab interno trabeculotomy or goniotomy performed with the Kahook Dual Blade combined with phacoemulsification. These findings should be considered when planning this type of surgical procedures. Moreover, patients should be informed about this possible complication prior to surgery.

In a further study, Okada et al. [17] did not find any significant difference in the outcomes in patients operated with phacoemulsification associated either with a 120° or 180° incision of the Schlemm's canal performed by means of an ab-interno trabeculotomy. Given that the same group in the study cited above found an increase of corneal aberrations following an extensive incision of Schlemm's canal, the authors suggest to preferably perform a 120° incision during an ab-interno trabeculotomy.

The effects of treatment on anatomic structures can be helpful in better understanding physiologic pathways and in the discovery of new mechanisms to treat diseases. The paper entitled "The dual effect of Rho-kinase inhibition on trabecular meshwork cells cytoskeleton and extracellular matrix in an in vitro model of glaucoma" [18] shows that Rho-kinase inhibitor can have an effect on the cytoskeleton organization and extracellular matrix of the TM, thus providing new insights to TM outflow pathway mechanisms involved in glaucoma that can be of clinical interest in the development of treatments for elevated IOP.

The causes of glaucoma are multifactorial and in part still unknown. Several risk factors like family history, thin cornea, African American race, ocular hypertension, etc. are known; however, factors associated with the manifestation of the disease have yet to be discovered. Maddala et al. addressed this lacuna by looking at the levels of growth/differential factor-15 (GDF15) in the AH and serum samples in patients with glaucoma and age- and

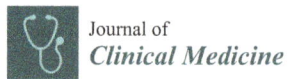

Journal of
Clinical Medicine

MDPI

Editorial

It Is All about Pressure

Paolo Brusini [1], Maria Letizia Salvetat [2] and Marco Zeppieri [3,*]

1   Department of Ophthalmology, Policlinico "Città di Udine", 33100 Udine, Italy; brusini@libero.it
2   Department of Ophthalmology, Azienda Sanitaria Friuli Occidentale, 33170 Pordenone, Italy;
    mlsalvetat@hotmail.it
3   Department of Ophthalmology, University Hospital of Udine, 33100 Udine, Italy
*   Correspondence: markzeppieri@hotmail.com; Tel.: +39-0432-552-743

Glaucoma is an ocular disease caused by elevated intraocular pressure that leads to progressive optic neuropathy. The irreversible morphologic and functional damage is characterized by progressive visual field loss and retinal ganglion cell degeneration. Glaucoma tends to be a silent disease, in which central visual acuity is only affected at late stages; if left untreated, it can lead to blindness. The prevalence of this disease worldwide is more than 70 million, which is thought to increase to over 100 million by the year 2040 [1,2]. The main risk factor for primary open-angle glaucoma (POAG) and other forms of glaucoma, which is also the target for therapy, is elevated intraocular pressure [3,4]. Local medical therapy, laser, and surgical treatments are all geared to lowering IOP to reduce the incidence and progression of glaucoma [5,6]. Thus, it is of the utmost importance that all patients, especially those with risk factors, undergo periodic ophthalmic examinations that include tonometry. The primary goal of this Special Issue entitled "Intraocular Pressure and Ocular Hypertension" is to provide a collection of pertinent topics and highlight the importance of IOP, tonometry, aqueous humor (AH) dynamics, trabecular meshwork (TM) outflow pathways, and treatment options in glaucoma and ocular hypertension (OHT).

Aqueous production and outflow are both involved in IOP regulation; however, most glaucomatous conditions, such as POAG, are characterized by reduced outflow. The TM plays an important role in the disease process. IOP homeostasis is influenced by aqueous humor outflow, which is characterized by a pulsatile flow pattern evident in Schlemm's canal and in the TM pathway [7]. Du et al. [8] reported that phase-sensitive optical coherence tomography demonstrates that pulsatile movement of the TM tends to be reduced in POAG patients, especially those with greater diurnal IOP fluctuations. TM has shown to be more rigid and less flexible in glaucomatous patients. This type of innovative diagnostic testing method has the potential of being of clinical use when deciding on treatment options in those glaucoma patients that do not reach IOP target levels and show progression of disease, which may require more aggressive treatment and/or prompt surgery.

Given that the IOP measurement is a fundamental part of any complete ophthalmological examination, numerous instruments, known as tonometers, have been proposed in order to obtain IOP measurements [9,10]. The measurement of the true IOP value in vivo requires invasive intraocular manometry. All tonometric methods available on the market just provide an estimation of IOP. The evaluation of the precision and accuracy of the different tonometers and the identification of the variables that can influence a correct IOP measurement represent an important field of research.

Our Review article, entitled "How to measure intraocular pressure: an update review of various tonometers" [11], describes the different instruments used to measure the IOP through the ages. Even if the Goldmann applanation tonometer (GAT) is still considered the gold standard technique in measuring IOP, several other instruments based on different operating principles (indentation, applanation, rebound, contour matching) have been

Citation: Brusini, P.; Salvetat, M.L.; Zeppieri, M. It Is All about Pressure. *J. Clin. Med.* **2022**, *11*, 3640. https://doi.org/10.3390/jcm11133640

Received: 20 June 2022
Accepted: 22 June 2022
Published: 23 June 2022

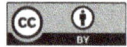

About the Editors

Paolo Brusini

Dr. Paolo Brusini was born in Udine, Italy. He obtained his medical degree from the University of Trieste in 1975, and a specialization in ophthalmology at the University of Messina in 1979. He was Head of the Ophthalmic Unit at the Hospital of San Donà di Piave, then Chief of the Department of Ophthalmology at Santa Maria della Misericordia Hospital of Udine, and has been Chief of the Department of Ophthalmology at "Città di Udine" Health Center from 1 November 2015 to date. A reviewer for numerous scientific journals, he has been a guest speaker at lectures and delivered invited presentations at more than 200 meetings, conducted more than 350 clinical courses on computerized perimetry, glaucoma, and cataract surgery, and is the first author and/or co-author of more than 250 published scientific articles. Dr. Brusini has vast experience in the fields of cataract and glaucoma surgery and cornea transplantation.

Maria Letizia Salvetat

Dr. Maria Letizia Salvetat was born in Pordenone, Italy. She achieved her medical degree at the University of Trieste in 1990 and a specialization in ophthalmology at the University of Trieste in 1994. She worked at the Departments of Ophthalmology at Trieste, Udine, and is currently working in Pordenone at Azienda Sanitaria Friuli Occidentale. She has been a reviewer for many scientific journals, and guest speaker at numerous national and international congresses. Her topics of interest include perimetry, glaucoma, cornea, pediatric ophthalmology, and cataract surgery. She has published more than 70 scientific articles and book chapters.

Marco Zeppieri

Dr. Marco Zeppieri was born in Ontario, Canada, and currently lives in Udine, Italy. He obtained a degree in biology from the University of Toronto in1992. He obtained his medical degree at the University of Milan-Bicocca, Italy in 2003. He then obtained his specialization in ophthalmology at the University of Udine in 2007. In 2012, he completed his Ph.D. at the University of Udine. He also completed a Post Doctoral Glaucoma Research Fellowship at the Discoveries in Sight, Devers Eye Institute in Portland, Oregon, USA in 2006. He obtained his national qualifications as a 2 °level university professor in 2018. Since January 2008 to date, he has worked as an ophthalmologist at the Department of Ophthalmology at Santa Maria Della Misericordia Hospital in Udine, Italy. He has won several awards, such as the Best Video SOI (2004), AIGS Travel Grant (2007), and ARVO GB Bietti Foundation for Ophthalmology Travel Grant (2007). His scientific interests include new techniques for the morphological and functional diagnosis of ocular hypertension and glaucoma, the use of stem cells for corneal wound lesions, ocular surface and lid diagnostics and treatments, and community-based screening procedures. He has participated as an invited speaker at numerous national and international ophthalmology conferences. He is a reviewer for numerous international peer-reviewed journals. He is the author of over 70 indexed scientific publications in international scientific journals and book chapters.

gender- matched controls [19]. The study showed significant and important serum and AH levels of GDF15 in patients with POAG when compared to controls. The paper entitled "Serum Calcium Level as a Useful Surrogate for Risk of Elevated Intraocular Pressure" [20] also looked at possible factors associated with glaucoma, and found that high serum total calcium levels were significantly associated with elevated IOP in a large cohort of Asians. Studies like the ones reported here can help find potential biomarkers for the diagnosis, management and prognosis of glaucoma, in addition to providing better understanding of the physiological pathway mechanisms involved in the disease process and in identifying future specific targets in the development of new treatments for glaucoma.

The identification of risk factors is of the utmost importance in the diagnosis and management of any disease. Unlike genetics, race, and other non-modifiable factors, the use of certain medications that may cause or worsen the pathology can be considered and modified accordingly based on a case-to-case situation of the patient. Wijnants et al., reported an interesting literature review based on the effects of glucocorticoids on IOP [21]. It is well known that about one third of patients are responders, showing elevated IOP after the use of corticosteroids. This literature review showed that most studies reported no significant effects on IOP with the use of intranasal and inhaled glucocorticoids (unless high doses are used). Four out of five studies, however, found elevated IOP levels caused by systemic glucocorticoids, with a possible dose-response relationship. The findings of the current literature regarding use of corticosteroids in patients with either ocular hypertension or glaucoma or patients with risk factors must be kept in mind when managing these patients. If possible, therapy with corticosteroids, especially administered systemically, should be either avoided or limited for brief intervals of time. Patients that do not have alternatives and must continue systemic glucocorticoids for other pathologies need more stringent follow-ups to prevent or promptly treat corticosteroid-induced IOP elevations.

The identification of markers helping in the early glaucoma diagnosis and detection of subtle signs of disease progression is a fascinating field of investigation. In the review article, Murtagh and O'Brien [22] summarize the current knowledge about corneal hysteresis (CH). CH is a relatively new ocular parameter provided by two devices available on the market, which include the Ocular Response Analyzer tonometer (ORA) and the Corneal Visualization Scheimpflug Technology tonometer (Corvis ST). The CH parameter can be defined as the capacity of shock absorption of the cornea, which can be considered as a marker for the ocular compliance. Previous studies have demonstrated that low CH values are a risk factor for the development of glaucoma and marker of its progression, indicating that the CH parameter could play an important role in glaucoma diagnosis and treatment. In the conclusions, the authors suggest that the CH values should be included in an algorithm incorporating IOP, central corneal thickness, and visual field test results, in order to establish the different risk rate for glaucoma development and progression.

The use of intravitreal injections of anti-vascular endothelial growth factor (anti-VEGF) agents to treat various retinal diseases, such as choroidal neovascularization in age-related macular degeneration or high myopia, or macular edema in diabetic retinopathy or retinal vein occlusion, has dramatically increased in the last years. The evaluation of efficacy and safety of the different anti-VEGF agents has been addressed by several authors. Hannape et al. [23] report the clinical results on mid-term impact of anti-VGEF agents on IOP. The Authors retrospectively evaluated the data of 750 patients who were unilaterally injected with anti-VEGF agents; the fellow untreated eye was used as control. An overall slightly significantly increase in IOP between treated and untreated eyes was noticed at 6 months. The comparison amongst different anti-VEGF agents showed that Ranibizumab was associated with a higher rate of clinically significant IOP increase ($\geq$6 mmHg from baseline) at 6 months.

Studies on animal models are of great importance in understanding the impact of ocular hypertension on the ocular structure and function. Mendez-Martinez et al. [24] investigate the influence of chronic ocular hypertension (OHT) on emmetropia in rats. The authors analyzed the effect of an induced mild-moderate chronic OHT on refraction and neuroretina in 260 eyes of young-adult rats over 24 weeks by using optical coherence tomography and electroretinography. The study results clearly show that the OHT accelerates emmetropia in rat eyes towards slowly progressive myopia; OHT also seems to induce an initial increase in structure and function of the neuroretina, which reversed over time.

Glaucoma is more prevalent in adults; however, IOP elevation can also be found in younger age groups. The study entitled "Management of childhood glaucoma following cataract surgery" is a review that evaluates the different treatment options and clinical management strategies reported in current literature for children with glaucoma following cataract surgery [25]. The various therapeutic approaches include medical therapy, angle surgery, glaucoma drainage device implantation, trabeculectomy, and cyclodestructive procedures. A useful flowchart has been provided to guide clinicians in the management of children with glaucoma after cataract surgery.

Two other studies report results obtained with different surgical approaches. Brusini et al. [26] present the results obtained with canaloplasty in a rather large cohort of patients affected with pseudoexfoliation glaucoma with a follow-up period of up to 14 years. Even if this surgical procedure appears to be effective on average, an acute IOP rise was observed in more than 60% of eyes after a long period of satisfactory control. For this reason, the authors conclude that canaloplasty should be either avoided or performed very cautiously in these kinds of patients.

Minimally invasive glaucoma surgery (MIGS) is gaining an increasingly important place in the surgical armamentarium for the treatment of glaucoma. Amongst various MIGS techniques, ab-interno procedures that aims to enlarge Schlemm's canal facilitating the outflow of aqueous humor through the physiological pathways, are of particular interest. Toneatto et al. [27] show the results of OMNI surgical system alone or in combination with phacoemulsification in 73 patients with open-angle glaucoma. According to this study, this procedure seems to be safe and relatively effective, with a rate of success ranging between 40 and 67.9%.

Another very intriguing topic concerns the possibility of reverseing the structural damage in glaucoma. It is really possible? Park et al. [28] present an interesting study regarding neuroretinal rim recovery after a successful trabeculectomy. This improvement was associated with young age and the amount of IOP reduction obtained, demonstrating that at least a part of neural tissue can undergo a regression of structural damage in the presence of adequate control of IOP.

As guest editors for this Special Issue, we hope you find the manuscripts prepared by our esteemed international colleagues innovative, practical, interesting, and of clinical value.

Author Contributions: P.B., M.L.S. and M.Z. contributed equally to this Editorial. All authors have read and agreed to the published version of the manuscript.

Funding: This research received no external funding.

Conflicts of Interest: The authors declare no conflict of interest.

References

1. Allison, K.; Patel, D.; Alabi, O. Epidemiology of Glaucoma: The Past, Present, and Predictions for the Future. *Cureus* **2020**, *12*, e11686. [CrossRef] [PubMed]
2. Quigley, H.A.; Broman, A.T. The number of people with glaucoma worldwide in 2010 and 2020. *Br. J. Ophthalmol.* **2006**, *90*, 262–267. [CrossRef]
3. Tham, Y.-C.; Li, X.; Wong, T.Y.; Quigley, H.A.; Aung, T.; Cheng, C.-Y. Global Prevalence of Glaucoma and Projections of Glaucoma Burden through 2040: A systematic review and meta-analysis. *Ophthalmology* **2014**, *121*, 2081–2090. [CrossRef]
4. Bahrami, H. Causal Inference in Primary Open Angle Glaucoma: Specific Discussion on Intraocular Pressure. *Ophthalm. Epidemiol.* **2006**, *13*, 283–289. [CrossRef]
5. Kass, M.A.; Heuer, D.K.; Higginbotham, E.J.; Johnson, C.A.; Keltner, J.L.; Miller, J.P.; Parrish, R.K., 2nd; Wilson, M.R.; Gordon, M.O. The Ocular Hypertension Treatment Study: A randomized trial determines that topical ocular hypotensive medication delays or prevents the onset of primary open-angle glaucoma. *Arch. Ophthalmol.* **2002**, *120*, 701–713; discussion 829–830. [CrossRef] [PubMed]

6. Heijl, A.; Leske, M.C.; Bengtsson, B.; Hyman, L.; Bengtsson, B.; Hussein, M.; Early Manifest Glaucoma Trial Group. Reduction of intraocular pressure and glaucoma progression: Results from the Early Manifest Glaucoma Trial. *Arch. Ophthalmol.* **2002**, *120*, 1268–1279. [CrossRef] [PubMed]
7. Xin, C.; Wang, R.K.; Song, S.; Shen, T.; Wen, J.; Martin, E.; Jiang, Y.; Padilla, S.; Johnstone, M. Aqueous outflow regulation: Optical coherence tomography implicates pressure-dependent tissue motion. *Exp. Eye Res.* **2017**, *158*, 171–186. [CrossRef] [PubMed]
8. Du, R.; Xin, C.; Xu, J.; Hu, J.; Wang, H.; Wang, N.; Johnstone, M. Pulsatile Trabecular Meshwork Motion: An Indicator of Intraocular Pressure Control in Primary Open-Angle Glaucoma. *J. Clin. Med.* **2022**, *11*, 2696. [CrossRef]
9. Kniestedt, C.; Punjabi, O.; Lin, S.; Stamper, R.L. Tonometry though the Ages. *Surv. Ophthalmol.* **2008**, *53*, 568–591. [CrossRef]
10. Brusini, P. Intraocular Pressure and Its Measurement. In *Atlas of Glucoma*, 3rd ed.; Choplin, N.T., Traverso, C.E., Eds.; CRC Press: Boca Raton, FL, USA, 2014; pp. 29–36.
11. Brusini, P.; Salvetat, M.L.; Zeppieri, M. How to Measure Intraocular Pressure: An Updated Review of Various Tonometers. *J. Clin. Med.* **2021**, *10*, 3860. [CrossRef]
12. Strzalkowska, A.; Pirlich, N.; Stingl, J.; Schuster, A.; Rezapour, J.; Wagner, F.; Buse, J.; Hoffmann, E. Intraocular Pressure Measurement in Childhood Glaucoma under Standardized General Anaesthesia: The Prospective EyeBIS Study. *J. Clin. Med.* **2022**, *11*, 2846. [CrossRef] [PubMed]
13. Sugihara, K.; Tanito, M. Different Effects of Aging on Intraocular Pressures Measured by Three Different Tonometers. *J. Clin. Med.* **2021**, *10*, 4202. [CrossRef]
14. Jóźwik, A.; Przeździecka-Dołyk, J.; Wałek, E.; Czerniak, M.; Asejczyk, M. Corneal Behavior during Tonometer Measurement during the Water Drinking Test in Eyes with XEN GelStent in Comparison to Non-Implanted Eyes. *J. Clin. Med.* **2022**, *11*, 2962. [CrossRef]
15. Díaz-Barreda, M.D.; Sánchez-Marín, I.; Boned-Murillo, A.; Pérez-Navarro, I.; Martínez, J.; Pardina-Claver, E.; Pérez, D.; Ascaso, F.J.; Ibáñez, J. Modification of Corneal Biomechanics and Intraocular Pressure following Non-Penetrating Deep Sclerectomy. *J. Clin. Med.* **2022**, *11*, 1216. [CrossRef]
16. Onoe, H.; Hirooka, K.; Okumichi, H.; Murakami, Y.; Kiuchi, Y. Corneal Higher-Order Aberrations after Microhook ab Interno Trabeculotomy and Goniotomy with the Kahook Dual Blade: Preliminary Early 3-Month Results. *J. Clin. Med.* **2021**, *10*, 4115. [CrossRef]
17. Okada, N.; Hirooka, K.; Onoe, H.; Murakami, Y.; Okumichi, H.; Kiuchi, Y. Comparison of Efficacy between 120° and 180° Schlemm's Canal Incision Microhook Ab Interno Trabeculotomy. *J. Clin. Med.* **2021**, *10*, 3181. [CrossRef]
18. Buffault, J.; Brignole-Baudouin, F.; Reboussin, É.; Kessal, K.; Labbé, A.; Mélik Parsadaniantz, S.; Baudouin, C. The Dual Effect of Rho-Kinase Inhibition on Trabecular Meshwork Cells Cytoskeleton and Extracellular Matrix in an In Vitro Model of Glaucoma. *J. Clin. Med.* **2022**, *11*, 1001. [CrossRef]
19. Maddala, R.; Ho, L.; Karnam, S.; Navarro, I.; Osterwald, A.; Stinnett, S.; Ullmer, C.; Vann, R.; Challa, P.; Rao, P. Elevated Levels of Growth/Differentiation Factor-15 in the Aqueous Humor and Serum of Glaucoma Patients. *J. Clin. Med.* **2022**, *11*, 744. [CrossRef]
20. Chang, Y.; Chen, J.; Tai, M.; Chen, W.; Chen, Y. Serum Calcium Level as a Useful Surrogate for Risk of Elevated Intraocular Pressure. *J. Clin. Med.* **2021**, *10*, 1839. [CrossRef]
21. Wijnants, D.; Stalmans, I.; Vandewalle, E. The Effects of Intranasal, Inhaled and Systemic Glucocorticoids on Intraocular Pressure: A Literature Review. *J. Clin. Med.* **2022**, *11*, 2007. [CrossRef]
22. Murtagh, P.; O'Brien, C. Corneal Hysteresis, Intraocular Pressure, and Progression of Glaucoma: Time for a "Hyst-Oric" Change in Clinical Practice? *J. Clin. Med.* **2022**, *11*, 2895. [CrossRef] [PubMed]
23. Hannappe, M.; Baudin, F.; Mariet, A.; Gabrielle, P.; Arnould, L.; Bron, A.; Creuzot-Garcher, C. Mid-Term Impact of Anti-Vascular Endothelial Growth Factor Agents on Intraocular Pressure. *J. Clin. Med.* **2022**, *11*, 946. [CrossRef]
24. Mendez-Martinez, S.; Martínez-Rincón, T.; Subias, M.; Pablo, L.; García-Herranz, D.; Feijoo, J.; Bravo-Osuna, I.; Herrero-Vanrell, R.; Garcia-Martin, E.; Rodrigo, M. Influence of Chronic Ocular Hypertension on Emmetropia: Refractive, Structural and Functional Study in Two Rat Models. *J. Clin. Med.* **2021**, *10*, 3697. [CrossRef]
25. Simons, A.; Casteels, I.; Grigg, J.; Stalmans, I.; Vandewalle, E.; Lemmens, S. Management of Childhood Glaucoma following Cataract Surgery. *J. Clin. Med.* **2022**, *11*, 1041. [CrossRef]
26. Brusini, P.; Papa, V.; Zeppieri, M. Canaloplasty in Pseudoexfoliation Glaucoma. Can It Still Be Considered a Good Choice? *J. Clin. Med.* **2022**, *11*, 2532. [CrossRef]
27. Toneatto, G.; Zeppieri, M.; Papa, V.; Rizzi, L.; Salati, C.; Gabai, G.; Brusini, P. 360° Ab-Interno Schlemm's Canal Viscodilation with OMNI Viscosurgical Systems for Open-Angle Glaucoma—Midterm Results. *J. Clin. Med.* **2022**, *11*, 259. [CrossRef]
28. Park, D.-Y.; Cha, S.-C. Factors Associated with Increased Neuroretinal Rim Thickness Measured Based on Bruch's Membrane Opening-Minimum Rim Width after Trabeculectomy. *J. Clin. Med.* **2021**, *10*, 3646. [CrossRef]

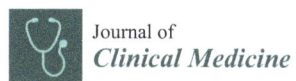

Journal of
Clinical Medicine

Review

How to Measure Intraocular Pressure: An Updated Review of Various Tonometers

Paolo Brusini [1], Maria Letizia Salvetat [2] and Marco Zeppieri [3,*]

[1] Department of Ophthalmology, Policlinico "Città di Udine", 33100 Udine, Italy; brusini@libero.it
[2] Department of Ophthalmology, Azienda Sanitaria Friuli Occidentale, 33170 Pordenone, Italy; mlsalvetat@hotmail.it
[3] Department of Ophthalmology, University Hospital of Udine, 33100 Udine, Italy
* Correspondence: markzeppieri@hotmail.com; Tel.: +39-0432-552743

Abstract: Intraocular pressure (IOP) is an important measurement that needs to be taken during ophthalmic examinations, especially in ocular hypertension subjects, glaucoma patients and in patients with risk factors for developing glaucoma. The gold standard technique in measuring IOP is still Goldmann applanation tonometry (GAT); however, this procedure requires local anesthetics, can be difficult in patients with scarce compliance, surgical patients and children, and is influenced by several corneal parameters. Numerous tonometers have been proposed in the past to address the problems related to GAT. The authors review the various devices currently in use for the measurement of intraocular pressure (IOP), highlighting the main advantages and limits of the various tools. The continuous monitoring of IOP, which is still under evaluation, will be an important step for a more complete and reliable management of patients affected by glaucoma.

Keywords: intraocular pressure (IOP); tonometry; Goldmann applanation tonometer (GAT); central corneal thickness (CCT); ocular hypertension; glaucoma

Citation: Brusini, P.; Salvetat, M.L.; Zeppieri, M. How to Measure Intraocular Pressure: An Updated Review of Various Tonometers. *J. Clin. Med.* **2021**, *10*, 3860. https://doi.org/10.3390/jcm10173860

Academic Editors: Bryan J. Winn and Tunde Peto

Received: 13 May 2021
Accepted: 23 August 2021
Published: 27 August 2021

Publisher's Note: MDPI stays neutral with regard to jurisdictional claims in published maps and institutional affiliations.

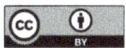
1. Introduction

Intraocular pressure (IOP) is an important measurement, which should be taken in every patient over the age of 40 that undergoes a complete ophthalmic examination and in all patients with ocular hypertension (OHT) or with risk factors for developing primary open-angle glaucoma (POAG) (i.e., family history, myopia, increased cup-to-disc ratio, etc.). IOP measurement is obviously a fundamental tool in subjects with diagnosed ocular hypertension or glaucoma. Even if the IOP measurement in vivo is only an estimate of the true IOP (which is only possible with invasive manometry), this value, rightly or wrongly, is often taken as an indicator of the efficacy of any treatment for glaucoma and to assess glaucoma severity and progression in patient management. It is thus of great importance to acquire accurate and precise IOP measurements in clinical practice.

Numerous instruments, called tonometers, have been proposed since the 19th century to obtain IOP measurements [1–3]. Based on the operating principle, these instruments can be differentiated into two main groups: (1) indentation tonometers; (2) applanation tonometers.

2. Indentation Tonometry

The prototype of the indentation tonometers is the Schiøtz tonometer that was introduced many years ago [4] and is no longer currently used (Figure 1).

Using this instrument, the cornea is indented by a plunger loaded with different weights. The IOP is based on the depth of indentation. The values are shown on a scale ranging from 0 to 20 units, in which the protrusion of the plunger of 0.05 mm represents each unit of measurement. The value indicated on the handle needs to be converted in mmHg using a conversion scale. The coefficient of ocular rigidity, which can differ amongst eyes, should be taken into consideration to obtain corrected measurements of

IOP. The Schiøtz tonometer is a simple and relatively inexpensive instrument. It is still sometimes used in developing countries [5,6] and in children under general anesthesia [7]. This tonometer, however, is subject to several sources of error, which include improper positioning on the eye, defective or dirty instruments, high variability in comparison with other devices and measurements influenced by individual ocular rigidity [8]. Moreover, patients must be in a supine position when taking measurements with this tonometer.

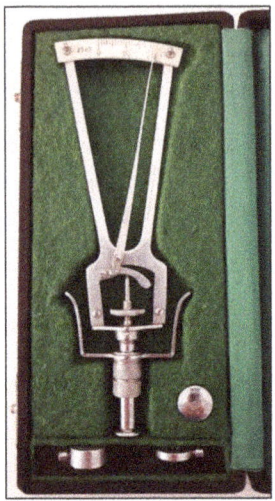

Figure 1. Schiøtz tonometer with different weights.

3. Applanation Tonometry

Applanation tonometers are currently considered the most reliable instruments for an accurate IOP measurement. Such tonometers use the Imbert–Fick law: $P = F/S$, in which P is pressure, S represents the surface of the flattened area, and F is the force needed to flatten a fixed corneal area. Apart from the tonometer by Maklakoff and several other instruments that are no longer currently in use, in which the force is provided by the weight of the tonometer itself, applanation tonometry is based on the area of flattened cornea that is calculated and converted in mmHg [2]. In almost all instruments of this type, the F value is varied to get the proper corneal applanation for a predetermined area. The Goldmann applanation tonometer (GAT) was first invented in 1948 by Hans Goldmann [9] and is still considered the gold standard to date. The tonometer needs to be positioned on a slit lamp.

A truncated cone, with a 7.35 mm^2 surface area and a dimeter of 3.06 mm, illuminated by a blue light, is pushed on the center of the anaesthetized cornea. A doubling prism embedded in the cone divides the circular meniscus on the surface of the flattened cornea e into two arcs, which need to be aligned in order to obtain a precise and standardized applanation (Figure 2).

The force used needed to flatten the corresponding surface of the cornea is directly proportional to the IOP, expressed in mmHg that can be directly read in the scale of the measuring drum or in the posterior window for the digital version (Figure 3A,B).

Contrary to what Hans Goldmann believed, corneal thickness may show a significant effect on IOP measurements. Thin corneas can give rise to an underestimation of the IOP and vice versa. Several authors have tried to address this problem by proposing a number of correction formulae [10–14]; however, none have been shown to be of widespread use. Several corneal biomechanical properties, which are not all completely known, may be involved, thus rendering the proposed correction factors misleading and limiting their clinical use [15–17]. Studies have reported that a thin cornea can be a factor of risk for developing glaucoma [18], in addition to the underestimated IOP with GAT.

A 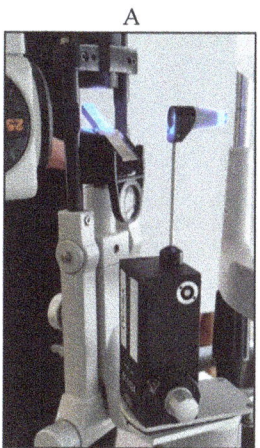   B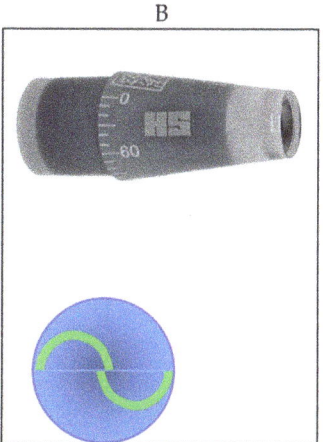

Figure 2. Goldmann applanation tonometer positioned on the slit lamp (**A**) with its cone prism (**B**) (on the top right); the two arcs appear correctly aligned (**B**) (on the bottom right).

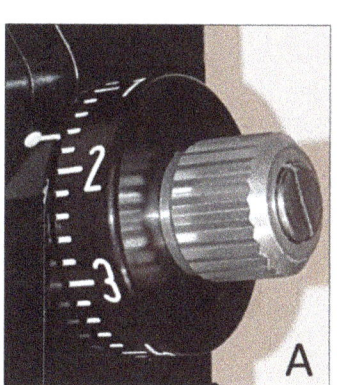 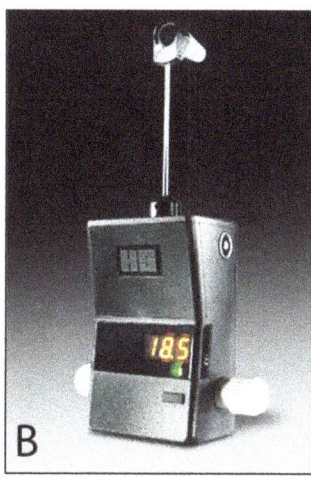

Figure 3. (**A**) Scale with IOP values in the Goldmann tonometer; (**B**) digital Goldmann tonometer (posterior view).

GAT it is still the tonometer most commonly used in clinics, thanks to the ease of use, accuracy, reproducibility and affordability. There are, however, several drawbacks that should be kept in mind, as recently reported by Gazzard et al. [19]. GAT is affected by parameters of the cornea, which include central corneal thickness when this is far from the average (540 microns) [14,15], in addition to corneal curvature, axial length, hysteresis, etc. Moreover, GAT measurements are subjective and can depend on the physician experience. Studies have reported that even for the same physician, clinically significant differences can be found with a 95% repeatability coefficient of ± 2 mmHg [20]. Other possible errors and drawbacks are due to the tear film with too little or too much fluorescein or an irregular or scarred cornea. GAT needs to be positioned on a slit lamp, and the subject must be in an upright position [21]. It is also important to remember that topic anesthesia is needed and that GAT should be periodically calibrated to provide good precision [22].

Portable handheld versions, such as the Perkins and Draeger tonometers (Figure 4), allow for measurements of IOP to also be taken supine and can be particularly useful in bedridden subjects and patients under general anesthesia.

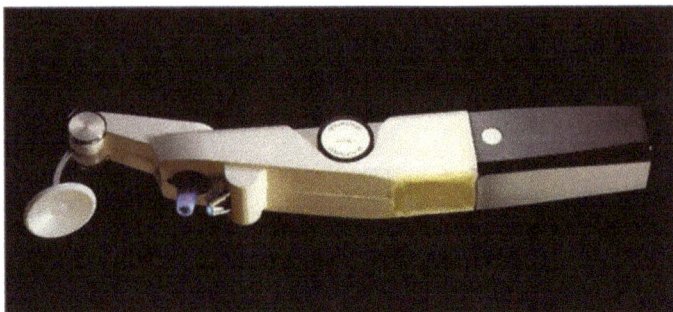

Figure 4. Handheld Perkins tonometer.

Other applanation instruments that use the same principle have been introduced several years ago. The Tono-Pen and the more recent Tono-Pen Avia (Reichert Ophthalmic Instruments, Depew, NY, USA) are portable lightweight battery-powered devices, which use the principles of applanation and indentation (Figure 5A,B). The reliability of each measurement is reported on a small display based on the standard deviation of the average of 10 readings. A disposable latex cap is used for each patient, which helps to reduces the risk of infection between patients.

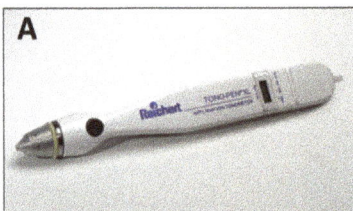 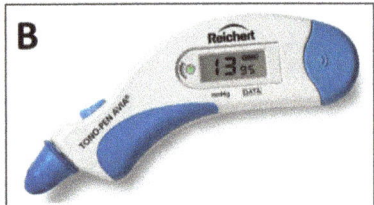

Figure 5. (**A**) Tono-Pen; (**B**) Tono-Pen Avia.

Numerous studies have reported the usefulness of these devices in clinics in comparison with GAT [23–26], but the repeatability coefficients for intra-session repeated measurement have been shown to be quite high (±4.3 mmHg) [27]. Clinical studies have shown that Tono-Pen can be significantly affected by CCT [28]. This tonometry, however, seems to provide better accuracy in edematous corneas in comparison with GAT and dynamic contour tonometry [29]. It is important to note that different tonometers cannot be used interchangeably [30,31].

The advantages of Tono-Pen include portability and instrumentation that does not require a slit lamp or electricity. IOP readings can be measured in both supine and upright positions. Topo-Pen can be especially useful in patients with eye scarring or irregular corneas, and in children and bedridden subjects.

Studies have shown the clinical limits of this instrument. Tono-pen was found to consistently underestimate IOP, with a significant error for IOP values >30 mmHg [32]. Several concerns still remain regarding the reproducibility of measurements when used in a routine clinical setting, considering that significant variations from Goldmann readings may occur in some patients.

4. Non-Contact Tonometry (Air-Puff Tonometry)

Non-contact tonometry (NCT) was first designed by Zeiss and developed by Grolman in 1972 [33]. Several models have been proposed in the past few decades that use a pulse of air to flatten the cornea without the need for touching the eye (Figure 6); such models, therefore, do not require anesthesia or fluorescein drops. In the Pulsair tonometer, a light beam is used in combination with a sensor that stops the production of air and measures the force used at the moment of corneal flattening.

A

B

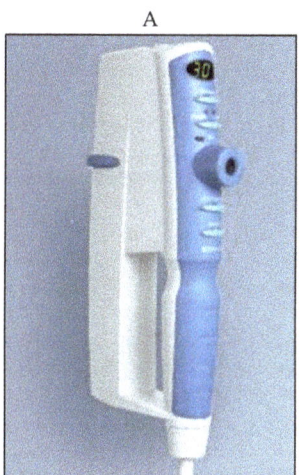
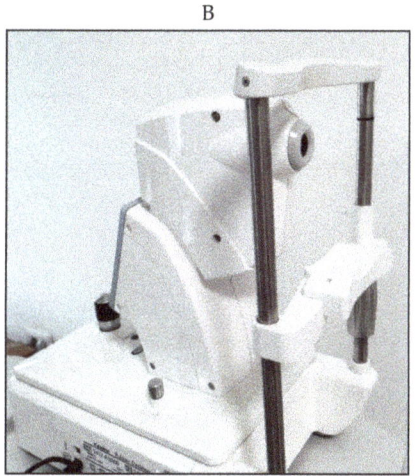

Figure 6. Pulsair EasyEye handheld (**A**) and Pulsair desktop (**B**) non-contact tonometers.

Numerous studies have examined the differences in IOP measured with various types of NCT instruments and other non-conventional tonometers compared to GAT [34,35]. Demirci et al. showed that IOP measurements with NCT were significantly higher than those obtained with both GAT and rebound tonometry, with significant differences ($p < 0.001$) in all age groups [36]. A recent study confirmed that NCT tends to overestimate IOP GAT measurements in patients with IOP > 16 mmHg, which was more evident when IOP > 20 mmHg [37], showing a decrease in accuracy at higher values.

Early studies in 1989 based on the comparisons with GAT, showed that up to 70% of NCT measurements fell within ± 3 mmHg of readings taken with GAT. When using a screening criteria of IOP > 21 mmHg, NCT showed a sensitivity of 85% and a specificity of 95% [38].

Similar to GAT and other instruments, NCT is influenced by corneal parameters. Kyei et al. showed a significant association between CCT and NCT, which is greater than that reported with GAT [39]. These finding were confirmed in a recent study, which concluded that GAT measurements are not equivalent and cannot be interchanged with those obtained by NCT [40].

The pros of NCT are mostly based on the ease of use, non-contact nature and portability of several devices. Measurements can be taken by non-medical staff and patient compliance is relatively good in most casesNCT does not require slit-lamp positioning; thus, it is easily used in cases with elderly individuals, children, disabled patients and patients with limited collaboration. NCT can be considered for patients that may not tolerate topical anesthetics, patients with limited collaboration or those at greater risk of infection.

The disadvantages of NCT include the fact that NCT is less accurate when IOP > 20 mmHg. Studies have shown that NCT results depend on the instrument brand, unit and model of the device used [41]. Comparison studies between three NTC devices showed that, when taking GAT as the gold standard and aiming to detect IOP > 21 mmHg, sensitivities greatly differed from 40%, 48% and 80%, which showed that NCT readings are device dependent and that devices require regular calibration [38]. Although NCT offers a non-contact mode of measuring that limits the risk of infection due to contaminated drops or Goldmann prisms, the risk of air-borne infection could be greater considering the air-puff nature, which should be considered in the midst of the recent COVID era [42–45].

NCT could be helpful in a day-to-day clinical setting that involves dealing mostly with normal patients undergoing routine checkups. This type of tonometry can be ideal as a screening tool, which can easily be performed by non-medical staff. Although studies have shown that NCT tends to overestimate GAT measurements, NCT can prove to be useful for post-operative patients with lid edema, limited collaboration, ocular pain, discomfort and increased tear film meniscus size, which are all factors that influence proper GAT measurements. NCT can be a useful screening tool, but should never replace or be interchanged with GAT, especially in the management of patients with risk factors, ocular hypertension, suspect patients and glaucoma.

Other types of non-contact tonometers, with new interesting features, have recently been introduced. In addition to the traditional tonometers, these devices show IOP values that take CCT and corneal biomechanics into account, claiming to provide more accurate IOP measurements [19,46].

The Ocular Response Analyzer (Reichert Technologies, Depew, NY, USA) or ORA, developed in 2005 by Luce et al. [46], is a non-contact air-puff tonometer that provides an optical electrical device to measure the deformation of the cornea caused by the impact of the air (Figure 7).

The force of the air makes the cornea move in an inward fashion in a first applanation state, causing it to take on a slight concave shape, to then move outward in a further applanation state, and finally to take on a normal configuration state. The electro-optical applanation detection system registers the curvature of the cornea in a diameter of 3 mm in the center for 20 msec. The two inward and outward applanation events, which are delayed by the viscoelastic corneal damping, allow for the calculations of two different IOP values based on the applanation principle. The instruments provide an average of these two pressure measurements and supply the so-called Goldmann-correlated IOP value (IOPg); the corneal hysteresis (CH) parameter is based on the difference between these two measurements of pressure. The instrument also provides a corneal-compensated IOP (IOPcc), which is based on the biomechanical properties of the cornea (elasticity and viscosity), to compensate for the measured IOP values [46,47].

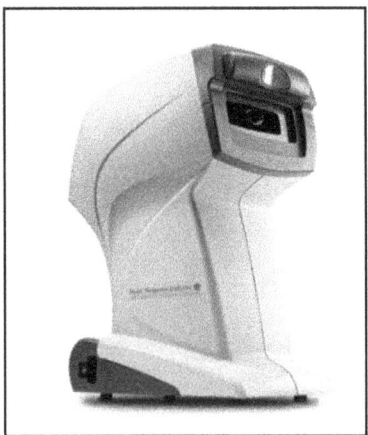

Figure 7. Ocular Response Analyzer (ORA) mod.G3.

There are several pros and cons to this device. The ORA is a relatively expensive device, but it is easy to handle, and topical anesthesia and fluorescein are not needed. In comparison with GAT, ORA has been demonstrated to significantly overestimate the IOP values, especially at high IOP levels [47,48]. Several authors have demonstrated that the IOPcc is less affected by corneal properties [48–51] and may better reflect the true IOP after refractive surgery of the cornea when compared to GAT IOP values [52].

Recent studies have shown that the ORA IOPcc values were superior to the GAT IOP measurements in predicting rates of glaucoma progression [53,54]. The CH parameter has been associated with other parameters of damage due to glaucoma, such as high cup-to-disc ratio and defects in the visual field. Several studies have shown a low CH value to be an independent predictor of functional damage occurrence or progression in the visual field in patients affected by ocular hypertension or glaucoma [55–58]. Moreover, the CH value can help in detecting patients with pathologies of the cornea such as keratoconus [59]. It may also be a useful parameter for patients at risk of developing corneal ectasia after refractive LASIK surgery [60].

The Corvis ST (Oculus, Wezlar, Germany), a novel non-contact instrument, released in 2011 [61], is based on the system that causes indentation of the cornea by a jet of air. The tonometer has a built-in Scheimpflug ultra-high-speed device (Figure 8).

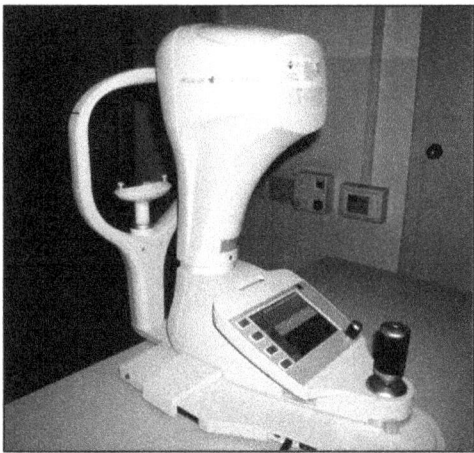

Figure 8. Corvis tonometer.

This instrument provides IOP measurements based on the indentation principle, in addition to pachymetry taken by on optical device and other biomechanical parameters of the cornea obtained by registering the surface deformation due to an applied air pulse, similar to an ORA device. A Scheimpflug camera visualizes an 8.5 mm diameter of the center of the surface of the cornea and precisely records the corneal deformation induced by the air-jet and its return to its normal shape with a high resolution and more than 4300 frames per second. A biomechanically corrected IOP value (bIOP), which takes the individual corneal deformation parameters into account, is also provided by the device.

The Corvis ST precision for the CCT and IOP values has been shown to be excellent; however, it is moderate for the corneal deformation parameters [62–64]. Previous studies demonstrated that Corvis ST tends to underestimate IOP readings obtained with GAT [61,62,65,66]. The Corvis ST biomechanically corrected IOP values (bIOP) have been shown to be less influenced by the CCT and corneal biomechanics and to be more effective in measuring the IOP in subjects who underwent refractive surgery [67]. Moreover, the Corvis ST corneal deformation parameters have been shown to be effective in discriminating between normal and keratoconic eyes [68].

5. Pneumotonometry

Pneumotonometers are devices based on the applanation principle, which use a different technology [69,70]: the tonometer probe consists of a hollow central tube flanked by a side exhaust, and the sensor is air pressure, which is dependent on the resistance of the exhaust. During the cornea applanation, the pressure within the central tubes increases to match the force generated by the IOP. A pneumatic electronic transducer converts the air pressure to a tracer on a strip of paper (Figure 9).

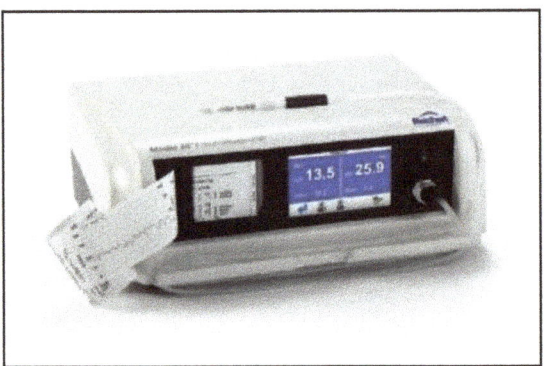

Figure 9. Pneumotonometer.

In several studies, pneumotonometry proved to be quite accurate and reliable in glaucoma screening and showed a greater reliability compared to GAT after PRK and LASIK [71–73]. Pneumotonometers such as the Pulsatile Ocular Blood Flow (OBF, Figure 10) have been used in the past to measure the pulse fluctuation and thereby give indirect information regarding the ocular blood pulse [74–77]. OBF measurements, however, appear to be more influenced by CCT and more variable than GAT readings, with a significant overestimation [78–80]. The clinical usefulness of this instrument in clinics still remains controversial.

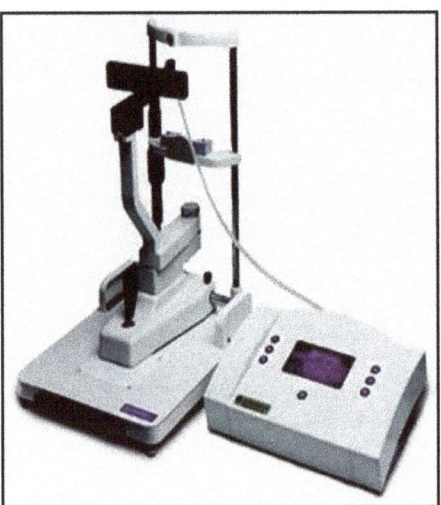

Figure 10. Langham Ocular Blood Flow pneumotonometer.

6. Rebound Tonometry

From a clinical point of view, the iCare rebound tonometer, introduced in 2000 by Kontiola [81], is currently one of the most interesting and widespread instruments used in practice (Figure 11).

A subtle probe impacts onto the cornea and then rebounds from the eye with a different velocity, which varies according to the IOP (Figure 12).

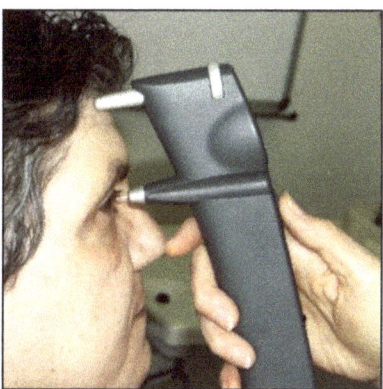

Figure 11. iCare rebound tonometer.

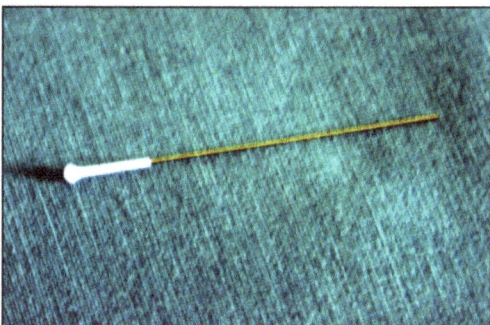

Figure 12. Disposable iCare probe.

The movement of the probe causes a voltage in the internal solenoid that is then amplified and digitally changed by a microprocessor. The IOP value is averaged from six consecutive measurements. The reliability of the final value is also displayed. The iCare tonometer is a reliable and precise instrument. It is rapid and easy to use, which is particularly helpful in busy clinics and with children, considering that there is no need for topic anesthesia [82–85]. The small surface contact makes it suitable to measure IOP after keratoplasty and in damaged corneas [85,86]. The iCare PRO version released in 2011 uses a shorter probe, which can also be used to measure IOP in a supine position. The most recent versions of this instrument, which are updated versions of the iCare PRO with a long probe (iCare IC100 and IC200) (Figure 13A,B), provide new features, such as a red or green light to show if the position of the probe is correct, in addition to providing the possibility of measuring IOP in a supine position [87,88].

A simplified version (iCare One, replaced at first by the iCare Home and, recently, by the iCare Home2 (Figure 14A–C)), which can autonomously be used by patients, has recently been introduced for at-home auto-tonometry. It can be helpful for detecting IOP peaks, especially in suspect glaucoma and in normal tension glaucoma subjects, when IOP measurements appear to be normal during office hours [89–92].

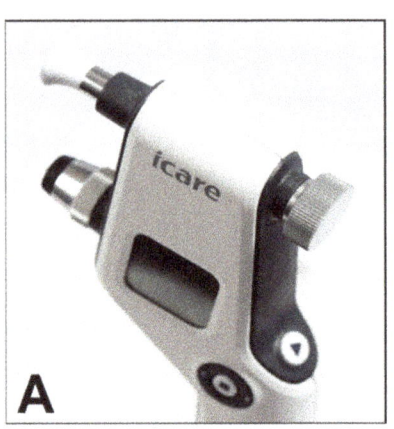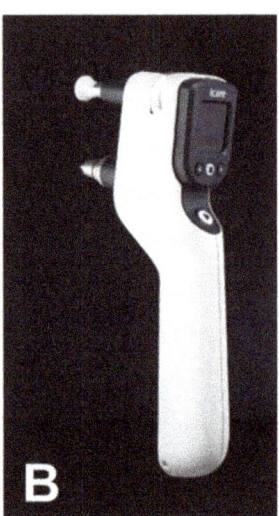

Figure 13. (**A**) iCare 100; (**B**) iCare 200 version.

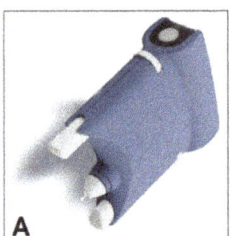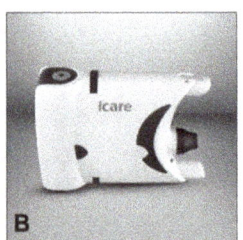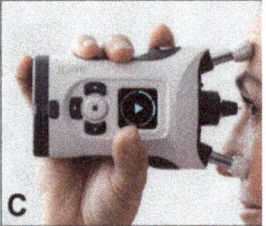

Figure 14. (**A**) iCare One; (**B**) iCare Home; (**C**) iCare Home2.

Numerous studies have compared the different versions of iCare with GAT and other non-conventional tonometers. When compared to gold standard GAT, clinical results report a good correlation of tonometry readings, with r values greater than 0.8 for low-to-moderate GAT readings [93]. A recent study showed agreement between GAT readings and iCare to be good, with a <2 mmHg mean difference for all ranges of IOP [87]. For IOP > 23 mmHg, rebound tonometry tends to underestimate IOP compared to GAT, showing readings that are significantly lower [93].

Considering that rebound tonometry may be less traumatic on the cornea compared to GAT, it could offer a better alternative in post-operative patients to provide information regarding IOP. It is important to note that GAT measurements tend to be lower than iCare for post-operative patients with corneal edema [84,94]. The agreement between iCare and GAT has been reported to be acceptable in lamellar keratoplasty subjects; yet, it has been reported to be poor for patients with penetrating keratoplasty [84]. Rebound tonometry surely cannot replace GAT. However, it may prove to be clinically useful in post-operative eyes with fragile anterior segments, or eyes with increased risk of infection, in which GAT is impractical or not indicated.

In comparing the reliability and reproducibility of IOP values with iCare tonometry, air tonometry and GAT, Valero et al. reported ICC > 0.85 and low differences with GAT [95]. Several studies have reported that iCare provides reproducible and reliability measurements when compared to other tonometers, although it appears to slightly underestimate GAT readings [88,95–101]. The repeatability of iCare has been shown to be excellent, with ICC > 0.9 [88,99]. Reliability results with iCare compared to GAT have been shown to be good (ICC > 0.87) for patients with IOP with low-to-moderate measurements; however, such results are moderate (ICC = 0.52) for IOP < 16 mmHg and >23 mmHg [88]. Studies have reported sensitivity and specificity rates greater than 0.90 for rebound tonometry [98,99].

IOP readings taken with iCare do not appear to be affected by axial length, refractive error, age and gender [87,100]. GAT and rebound tonometry, however, are influenced by corneal characteristics. IOP tends to be overestimated for central corneal thicknesses greater than 520 microns [82,93,96,99–101]. Rebound tonometry also appears to be affected by corneal curvature, corneal hysteresis and disease [96,100,101]. Tonometer measurements tend to be more accurate with iCare for middle levels of IOP, ranging 16–23 mmHg [100].

Rebound tonometry has several advantages, which include having a short learning curve, being user friendly in nature, being well tolerated, and being safe for staff and patients. The instruments are portable, self-calibrated, affordable and do not require a slit lamp, topical anesthesia or fluorescein dye. These iCare instruments can also be used by trained non-medical staff. Multiple readings can be taken if needed without the fear of corneal abrasion or other complications [88]. Unlike GAT that uses a prism in contact with the cornea, the minimal contact and duration with the disposable iCare tips limits the risk of iatrogenic damage and cross-infection, which is of great importance in the recent COVID era [101]. Moreover, iCare does not induce IOP reduction caused by ocular massaging that can be observed in GAT [102]. The iCare home version can be useful in self-twenty-four-hour measurements of IOP to monitor diurnal variations in IOP, which may assist in treatment decision making and surgical timing, especially in patients at greater risks of IOP spikes such as pigment dispersion glaucoma, angle-closure suspects and pseudoexfoliation glaucoma [100].

The rebound tonometers offer numerous advantages; however, several cons should be noted. A recent study comparing iCare with GAT in 1000 eyes showed larger mean differences between tonometers in eyes with IOP > 22 mmHg and in the group of glaucoma patients with medications [103]. The precision and accuracy of iCare can be influenced by peripheral measurements of the cornea as opposed to proper central positioning of the tip [104]. Based on the good agreement with GAT for IOP values <21 mmHg, iCare can be a time-saving and wise alternative in a routine busy clinical screening setting, in which the majority of healthy patients show low-to-moderate IOP. These instruments can offer additional helpful information in a community-based setting when used together with other pertinent screening tools. High IOP readings taken with iCare tonometers need to be checked and confirmed with gold standard GAT. Rebound tonometry applies minimal pressure on the cornea; thus, it can be used to provide indicative IOP readings in first-day post-operative patients, keeping in mind the good, yet limiting, agreement with GAT readings. The ease of use, portability, rapidity, and use in supine positions make it an excellent tool for examining children, disabled and/or bedridden patients and patients with limited collaboration, in which GAT cannot be performed or is impractical.

7. Dynamic Contour Tonometry

The Dynamic Contour Tonometer (PASCAL, DCT) (SMT Swiss Microtechnology AG, Port, Switzerland) is a relatively new device developed by Kaufmann et al. in 2003 [105] and implemented by Kanngiesser et al. in 2005 [106]. The DCT, which is not based on the applanation principle, calculates the IOP using the Pascal principle, according to which the pressure change is applied to all parts of a fluid in a contained enclosed space. The tonometer is positioned on the slit-lamp, requires the use of anesthetic drops (no fluorescein) and is automatically calibrated. It uses a concave contour tip that is equipped with a tiny sensor in the center of the contact surface (Figure 15).

A

B

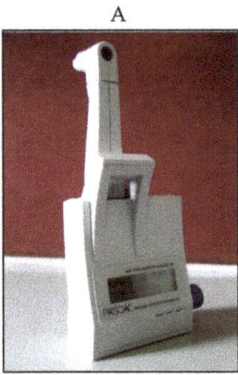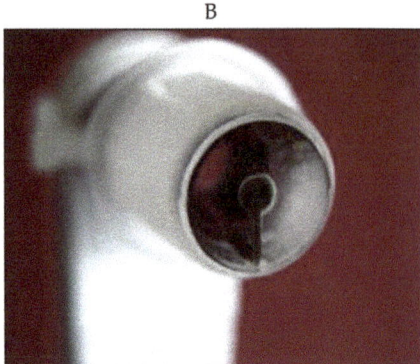

Figure 15. Dynamic Contour Pascal (**A**) with its sensor tip (**B**).

When the "contour matching" between the surface of the cornea and the tip of the instrument is reached, the tangential forces of the cornea are cancelled, and the embedded pressure sensor directly measures the IOP without any cornea deformation and bias related to corneal factors, at least theoretically [107–110]. The pressure sensor tip is protected with a thin silicone membrane covered by disposable sensor caps in order to avoid the risk of infection. The DCT requires about 8-10 s of corneal contact in order to provide IOP measurements, which are shown on an LCD screen. Quality scores and ocular pulse amplitude (OPA) values are also provided. The DCT IOP is based on the diastolic IOP, which should be considered when comparing DCT and GAT IOP measurements. The OPA provides indirect information regarding perfusion of the choroid, which has been demonstrated to be important in the onset and progression of glaucoma [111].

The DCT has been shown to be less influenced by the properties of the cornea and can be therefore helpful in taking IOP readings in subjects with previous photorefractive surgeries [112–116]. The DCT has shown high precision, with higher reproducibility than GAT [109,117]. In comparison with GAT, however, the DCT IOP measurements, although highly correlated, tend to be significantly higher [26].

The principal drawbacks of the DCT include: the need for a slit lamp, anesthetic and corneal contact; the need for trained staff and highly cooperative patients that can keep a good head and eye position for at least 8 s, meaning that this tonometer may prove to be difficult to use and not rapid in busy clinics [118]; and reduced accuracy in the presence of irregular corneas [119].

8. Applanation Resonance Tonometry

The Applanation Resonance Tonometer (ART), known in the current commercial version as BioResonator ART⋉ (BioResonator AB, Umea, Sweden) (Figure 16), was developed by Eklund et al. in 2003 [120]. It was released as both a manual and automatic version in 2012 [121]. This tonometer uses the applanation tonometry principle combined with the resonance technique. The device needs must be mounted on a slit lamp, requires the use of local anesthetic drops before IOP measurement and uses a concave surface sensor tip, which is positioned on the cornea. The sensor tip is manually pushed towards the cornea in the manual version of the instrument, whereas the automatic version provides a tiny motor for movement of the tip. A resonance piezoelectric device is found in the tip of the sensor that generates a shift in frequency which is proportional to the area of contact. The IOP is based on the contact area and force measurement parameters, which are taken continuously throughout the test [120,121].

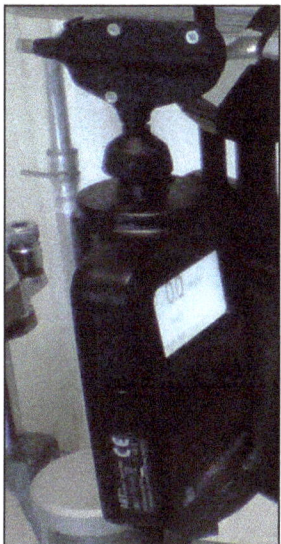

Figure 16. The BioResonator ART tonometer.

The ART probe must be carefully disinfected before each subject. This tonometer is self-calibrated and gives the repeated IOP measurement median and a quality index reflecting the standard deviation of the IOP values. The IOP measurement provided by the BioResonator ART is claimed to be more accurate than that of GAT considering that it represents the median of repeated measures; however, the precision of the instrument has been questioned [122–124].

Previous studies have reported that this tonometer can provide an overestimate in IOP values when compared to GAT [123–125]. Furthermore, it seems to be affected by CCT and corneal biomechanics [120,123,126]. Despite some advantages (repeatable and reliable measurements, no fluorescein is needed), the BioResonator ART has some drawbacks that may reduce its clinical usefulness, including: the need for a slit lamp, anesthetic and corneal contact, with sterilization issues; can be affected by various artifacts and measurement errors; moreover, its accuracy is influenced by the thickness and biomechanics of the cornea.

9. Continuous IOP Monitoring

All the aforementioned devices can be usefully employed for taking spot IOP measurements during office time. This can be acceptable in a screening setting, but, unfortunately, undetected elevated IOP spikes tend to occur during the night in many glaucomatous patients [127]. IOP readings during clinical office hours fail to detect these peaks in more than 50% of cases with a significant underestimation of IOP [128–131]. Hughes et al. reported that data obtained with continuous monitoring in IOP using a 24 h device had an influence in therapeutic decisions in 79.3% of enrolled subjects [132]. Keeping these data in mind, it can be inferred that our current standards in clinics with regard to taking IOP measurements may not suffice and thus need to be modified [133].

An important step towards a more precise management of patients affected by ocular hypertension and chronic glaucoma would be the possibility of continuously monitoring IOP values not only during the day but also in the night, as occurs with the 24 h blood pressure Holter. This information could be particularly useful in the so-called normal tension glaucoma patients, which show significant damage progression despite an apparently normalized IOP. In these cases, an elevated IOP can sometimes be found during the night, especially early in the morning, outside office hours [134,135]. A number of devices, most of them only experimental, have been proposed for this purpose over the past 20 years [136–138].

Some of them need to be surgically inserted into the eye, either during a cataract extraction procedure, usually embedded in an intraocular lens [139–141], or positioned in the anterior chamber [142,143], or in the suprachoroidal space [144]. A non-invasive continuous IOP measurement is also possible using special contact lenses with different types of miniaturized sensors and a wireless power transmission of data to a recorder.

The contact lens sensor Sensimed Triggerfish (Triggerfish CLS, Sensimed AG, Lausanne, Switzerland) is a miniaturized electromechanical system with a microprocessor embedded in a disposable silicon contact lens, which transmits a signal to an external wireless antenna located in the periocular surface (Figures 17 and 18). The data are then transferred to a portable recorder, for a total of 288 data sets in 24 h. This device can measure small modifications in the curvature of the cornea believed to be due to variations of IOP [145–149].

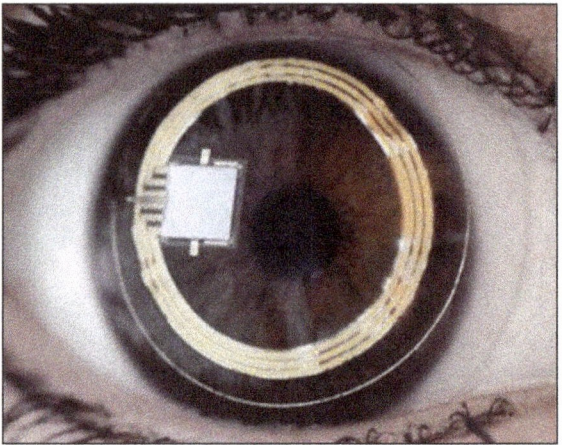

Figure 17. Sensimed Triggerfish.

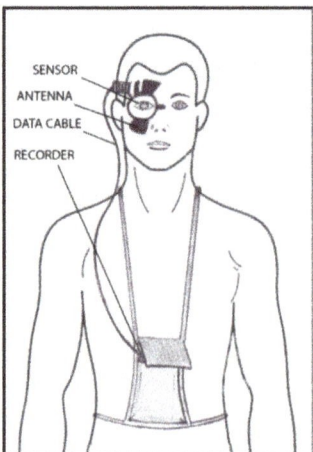

Figure 18. Schematic view of Triggerfish, wireless antenna and portable recorder.

Triggerfish CLS is usually well tolerated [150–152] and has also been shown to have high reproducibility [150–155]. The information obtained with these device parameters might be useful in assessing changes and IOP fluctuations in subjects with pseudoexfoliation syndrome, pigment dispersion, and in predicting the visual field loss progression rate [156,157]. Several studies have shown the usefulness of this contact lens sensor for assessment of the risk of glaucoma, which may prove to be important in subjects with NTG, in which IOP tends to be normal with diurnal readings [158–161].

The main problem with this device is that there is no direct correlation between corneal changes, expressed in millivolt equivalent (mVeq), and IOP values. Studies have shown that IOP measurements taken with GAT and Triggerfish values tend to have a high correlation at the beginning, after the insertion of CLS [148]; however, the correlation becomes poor after 24 h [153,154].

CLS is advantageous because it is not invasive, can be easily removed and dismantled [155], readily available [155], accepted and tolerated by patients [150–152], and provides good reproducibility [151,153,154]. The validity (i.e., considering the estimation accuracy of IOP readings) and relatively costly equipment of CLS are important drawbacks, which render the clinical usefulness of this instrument still debatable in literature [153,154].

Other types of devices able to measure IOP, either implantable or non-invasive [162–173], have been proposed, but almost all are still experimental and need further studies before being introduced into clinical practice.

10. Conclusions

As shown in Table 1, numerous tonometers have been proposed in the past. It is important to note that in managing and treating glaucoma patients, it is preferable and more reliable to measure IOP every time with the same type of equipment for each individual glaucoma patient. Several instruments have provided specific advantages compared to Goldmann tonometry. Alternative systems reported in literature, either non-invasive or implantable, remain experimental. Despite promising preliminary results, none have obtained widespread use and are adaptable in a routine clinal setting. New is not always better. The Goldmann tonometer, despite its limitations and a lack of innovative and novel advancements in the past 70 years, continues to be theoretically more precise and considered the gold standard tonometer to diagnose and manage patients with ocular hypertension and glaucoma.

J. Clin. Med. **2021**, 10, 3860

Table 1. Summary of the characteristics of the various available tonometers.

Tonometer Type	Production Year	Working Principle	Contact/ Noncontact	Advantages	Disadvantages	Clinical Suitability	Cost *
Schioetz tonometer	1905	indentation	contact	Simple Inexpensive No need of slit-lam, electricity or charging batteries	High variability Can be used in a supine position only Affected by various sources of error Topical anesthesia is needed	still used only in developing countries	feasible
Goldmann applanation tonometer (GAT)	1955	applanation	contact	Quite simple to use Accurate and reproducible measurements It is currently considered as the gold standard in IOP measurement	Affected by corneal thickness and other corneal parameters The accuracy depends on the clinician's experience Needs to be used with a slit-lamp Can be used in the upright position only Topical anesthesia and fluorescein are needed	good	feasible
Perkins tonometer	1965	applanation	contact	Can be used in a supine position too	Affected by corneal thickness and other corneal parameters Topical anesthesia and fluorescein are needed	good	feasible
TonoPen	1989	indentation/ applanation	contact	Lightweight and portable Quick and simple to use Can be used in any position No need of slit-lamp or electricity Self-calibration, provides quality index	Hight variability and quite poor repeatability Can underestimate IOP values Topical anesthesia is needed Influenced by corneal parameters	moderate	feasible
Air-puff tonometers	1973	applanation	noncontact	Easy and fast to use No need to touch the cornea No need of topical anesthesia and fluorescein Can be used by paramedical staff	Need of regular calibration Readings are device-dependent Possible germs aerosol Influenced by corneal parameters Less accurate when IOP > 20 mmHg	ideal as a screening tool	medium
Ocular Response Analyzer	2005	applanation	noncontact	Simple to use, self-calibration, provides quality index No need of topical anesthesia and fluorescein Can be used by paramedical staff Provides additional information (corneal central thickness and biomechanics) IOP correction for corneal biomechanical parameters Useful after corneal refractive surgery Detection of corneal diseases	Possible germs aerosol	good	expensive

Table 1. *Conts.*

Tonometer Type	Production Year	Working Principle	Contact/ Noncontact	Advantages	Disadvantages	Clinical Suitability	Cost *
Corvis ST	2011	indentation/ applanation	noncontact	Simple to use, self-calibration, provides quality index / No need of fluorescein and topical anesthesia / Can be used by paramedical staff / Provides additional information (corneal central thickness and biomechanics) / IOP correction for corneal biomechanical parameters / Useful after corneal refractive surgery / Detection of corneal diseases	Tends to underestimate the GAT IOP values	good	expensive
Pneumotonometers	1969	applanation	contact	OBF provides information on the ocular blood pulse	Affected by corneal thickness / Overestimates IOP values	controversial	expensive
iCare tonometer	1997	ballistic probe (rebound)	contact	Ease of use with a short learning curve / Portable and self-calibrated / No slit-lamp or topical anesthesia or fluorescein dye required / Can be used by trained non-medical staff / Can be used in supine positions / (iCare PRO and iCare 200) / Minimal corneal trauma / (useful in post-operative patients) / The home version can be useful in self-twenty-four-hour monitoring of IOP	Needs a proper central positioning of the tip / Influenced by corneal thickness	excellent	feasible
Dynamic contour tonometer (DCT, PASCAL)	2005	contour matching	contact	No need of fluorescein, disposable probes / Self-calibration, provides quality index / Independent from corneal properties / Useful after corneal refractive surgery / High precision / Additional information (ocular pulse amplitude)	Need of slit lamp and topical anesthesia / Difficult to use / Need of highly cooperative patients	poor	medium
BioResonator ART	2003	applanation	contact	No need of fluorescein / Self-calibration, provides quality index / High reliability / (median of repeated IOP measurements)	Need of slitlamp and local anesthetic / Need of probe disinfection / Required training to use / Affected by corneal properties	moderate	medium
Sensimed Triggerfish	2004	corneal curvature monitoring	contact	Continuous measurements over a 24-hour period / Good tolerability / High reproducibility	It does not provide direct IOP values / IOP estimation accuracy not known	moderate	feasible

* feasible: 0–5000 euros; medium range 5000–10,000 euros; expensive: >10,000 euros.

Author Contributions: All authors (P.B., M.L.S. and M.Z.) contributed equally to all aspects of the manuscript, including conceptualization, methodology, validation, formal analysis, investigation, resources, writing and preparation of all drafts, editing, visualization, supervision, and project administration. All authors have read and agreed to the published version of the manuscript.

Funding: This research received no external funding.

Institutional Review Board Statement: Not applicable.

Informed Consent Statement: Not applicable.

Conflicts of Interest: The authors declare no conflict of interest.

References

1. Kniestedt, C.; Punjabi, O.; Lin, S.; Stamper, R.L. Tonometry through the Ages. *Surv. Ophthalmol.* **2008**, *53*, 568–591. [CrossRef]
2. Stamper, R.L. A History of Intraocular Pressure and Its Measurement. *Optom. Vis. Sci.* **2011**, *88*, E16–E28. [CrossRef] [PubMed]
3. Brusini, P. Intraocular Pressure and Its Measurement. In *Atlas of Glaucoma*, 3rd ed.; Choplin, N.T., Traverso, C.E., Eds.; CRC Press: Boca Raton, FL, USA, 2014; pp. 29–36.
4. Albert, D.M.; Keeler, R. The Pressure: Before and after Schiøtz. *Ophthalmol. Glaucoma* **2020**, *3*, 409–413. [CrossRef]
5. Kyari, F.; Nolan, W.; Gilbert, C. Ophthalmologists' practice patterns and challenges in achieving optimal management for glaucoma in Nigeria: Results from a nationwide survey. *BMJ Open.* **2016**, *6*, e012230. [CrossRef]
6. Nagarajan, S.; Velayutham, V.; Ezhumalai, G. Comparative evaluation of applanation and indentation tonometers in a community ophthalmology setting in Southern India. *Saudi. J. Ophthalmol.* **2016**, *30*, 83–87. [CrossRef]
7. Lasseck, J.; Jehle, T.; Feltgen, N.; Lagrèze, W.A. Comparison of intraocular tonometry using three different non-invasive tonometers in children. *Graefe's Arch. Clin. Exp. Ophthalmol.* **2008**, *246*, 1463–1466. [CrossRef] [PubMed]
8. Ohana, O.; Varssano, D.; Shemesh, G. Comparison of intraocular pressure measurements using Goldmann tonometer, I-care pro, Tonopen XL, and Schiotz tonometer in patients after Descemet stripping endothelial keratoplasty. *Indian J. Ophthalmol.* **2017**, *65*, 579–583. [CrossRef] [PubMed]
9. Goldmann, H.; Schmidt, T. Über Applanationstonometrie. *Acta. Ophthalmol.* **1957**, *134*, 221–242. [CrossRef]
10. Ehlers, N.; Bramsen, T.; Sperling, S. Applanation tonometry and central corneal thickness. *Acta. Ophthalmol.* **2009**, *53*, 34–43. [CrossRef] [PubMed]
11. Whitacre, M.M.; Stein, R.A.; Hassanein, K. The Effect of Corneal Thickness on Applanation Tonometry. *Am. J. Ophthalmol.* **1993**, *115*, 592–596. [CrossRef]
12. Herndon, L.W.; Choudhri, S.A.; Cox, T.; Damji, K.F.; Shields, M.B.; Allingham, R.R. Central Corneal Thickness in Normal, Glaucomatous, and Ocular Hypertensive Eyes. *Arch. Ophthalmol.* **1997**, *115*, 1137–1141. [CrossRef]
13. Wolfs, R.C.; Klaver, C.; Vingerling, J.R.; Grobbee, D.E.; Hofman, A.; de Jong, P.T. Distribution of Central Corneal Thickness and Its Association With Intraocular Pressure: The Rotterdam Study. *Am. J. Ophthalmol.* **1997**, *123*, 767–772. [CrossRef]
14. Doughty, M.J.; Zaman, M.L. Human Corneal Thickness and Its Impact on Intraocular Pressure Measures: A Review and Meta-analysis Approach. *Surv. Ophthalmol.* **2000**, *44*, 367–408. [CrossRef]
15. Park, S.J.; Ang, G.S.; Nicholas, S.; Wells, A.P. The Effect of Thin, Thick, and Normal Corneas on Goldmann Intraocular Pressure Measurements and Correction Formulae in Individual Eyes. *Ophthalmology* **2012**, *119*, 443–449. [CrossRef] [PubMed]
16. Brandt, J.D.; Gordon, M.O.; Gao, F.; Beiser, J.A.; Miller, J.P.; Kass, M. Adjusting Intraocular Pressure for Central Corneal Thickness Does Not Improve Prediction Models for Primary Open-Angle Glaucoma. *Ophthalmology* **2012**, *119*, 437–442. [CrossRef] [PubMed]
17. Gunvant, P.; O'Leary, D.J.; Baskaran, M.; Broadway, D.C.; Watkins, R.J.; Vijaya, L. Evaluation of Tonometric Correction Factors. *J. Glaucoma* **2005**, *14*, 337–343. [CrossRef] [PubMed]
18. Brandt, J.D.; Beiser, J.A.; Kass, M.; Gordon, M.O. Central corneal thickness in the ocular hypertension treatment study (OHTS). *Ophthalmology* **2001**, *108*, 1779–1788. [CrossRef]
19. Gazzard, G.; Jayaram, H.; Roldan, A.M.; Friedman, D.S. When gold standards change: Time to move on from Goldmann tonometry? *Br. J. Ophthalmol.* **2021**, *105*, 1–2. [CrossRef]
20. Kotecha, A.; White, E.; Schlottmann, P.G.; Garway-Heath, D. Intraocular Pressure Measurement Precision with the Goldmann Applanation, Dynamic Contour, and Ocular Response Analyzer Tonometers. *Ophthalmology* **2010**, *117*, 730–737. [CrossRef]
21. Whitacre, M.M.; Stein, R. Sources of error with use of Goldmann-type tonometers. *Surv. Ophthalmol.* **1993**, *38*, 1–30. [CrossRef]
22. Choudhari, N.S.; Rao, H.L.; Ramavath, S.; Rekha, G.; Rao, A.; Senthil, S.; Garudadri, C.S. How Often the Goldmann Applanation Tonometer Should be Checked for Calibration Error? *J. Glaucoma* **2016**, *25*, 908–913. [CrossRef] [PubMed]
23. Frenkel, R.E.P.; Hong, Y.J.; Shin, D.H. Comparison of the Tono-Pen to the Goldmann Applanation Tonometer. *Arch. Ophthalmol.* **1988**, *106*, 750–753. [CrossRef] [PubMed]
24. Iester, M.; Mermoud, A.; Achache, F.; Roy, S. New TonoPen XL: Comparison with the Goldmann tonometer. *Eye* **2001**, *15*, 52–58. [CrossRef] [PubMed]
25. Blumberg, M.J.; Varikuti, V.N.V.; Weiner, A. Real-world comparison between the Tonopen and Goldmann applanation tonometry in a university glaucoma clinic. *Int. Ophthalmol.* **2021**, *41*, 1815–1825. [CrossRef]

26. Salvetat, M.L.; Zeppieri, M.; Tosoni, C.; Brusini, P. Comparisons between Pascal dynamic contour tonometry, the TonoPen, and Goldmann applanation tonometry in patients with glaucoma. *Acta. Ophthalmol. Scand.* **2006**, *85*, 272–279. [CrossRef] [PubMed]
27. Tonnu, P.-A.; Ho, T.; Sharma, K.; White, E.; Bunce, C.; Garway-Heath, D. A comparison of four methods of tonometry: Method agreement and interobserver variability. *Br. J. Ophthalmol.* **2005**, *89*, 847–850. [CrossRef]
28. Tonnu, P.-A.; Ho, T.; Newson, T.; El Sheikh, A.; Sharma, K.; White, E.; Bunce, C.; Garway-Heath, D. The influence of central corneal thickness and age on intraocular pressure measured by pneumotonometry, non-contact tonometry, the Tono-Pen XL, and Goldmann applanation tonometry. *Br. J. Ophthalmol.* **2005**, *89*, 851–854. [CrossRef]
29. Kontadakis, G.A.; Pennos, A.; Pentari, I.; Kymionis, G.D.; Pallikaris, I.G.; Ginis, H. Accuracy of dynamic contour tonometry, Goldmann applanation tonometry, and Tono-Pen XL in edematous corneas. *Ther. Adv. Ophthalmol.* **2020**, *12*. [CrossRef]
30. Cronemberger, S.; Veloso, A.W. Comparison of Tono-Pen Avia and Handheld Applanation Tonometry in Primary Congenital Glaucoma. *J. Glaucoma* **2021**, *30*, e227–e230. [CrossRef]
31. Deuter, C.M.E.; Schlote, T.; Hahn, G.A.; Bende, T.; Derse, M. Messung des Augeninnendrucks mit dem Tono-Pen im Vergleich zum Applanationstonometer nach Goldmann—eine klinische Studie an 100 Augen. *Klin. Mon. Für Augenheilkd.* **2002**, *219*, 138–142. [CrossRef] [PubMed]
32. Gopesh, T.; Camp, A.; Unanian, M.; Friend, J.; Weinreb, R.N. Rapid and Accurate Pressure Sensing Device for Direct Measurement of Intraocular Pressure. *Transl. Vis. Sci. Technol.* **2020**, *9*, 28. [CrossRef]
33. Grolman, B. A new tonometer system. *Optom. Vis. Sci.* **1972**, *49*, 646–660. [CrossRef]
34. Hansen, M.K. Clinical comparison of the XPERT non-contact tonometer and the conventional Goldmann applanation tonometer. *Acta. Ophtahlmol. Scand.* **1995**, *73*, 176–180. [CrossRef]
35. Vincent, S.; Vincent, R.A.; Shields, D.; Lee, G.A. Comparison of intraocular pressure measurement between rebound, non-contact and Goldmann applanation tonometry in treated glaucoma patients. *Clin. Exp. Ophthalmol.* **2011**, *40*, e163–e170. [CrossRef] [PubMed]
36. Demirci, G.; Erdur, S.K.; Tanriverdi, C.; Gulkilik, G.; Ozsutcu, M. Comparison of rebound tonometry and non-contact airpuff tonometry to Goldmann applanation tonometry. *Ther. Adv. Ophthalmol.* **2019**, *11*. [CrossRef] [PubMed]
37. Stock, R.A.; Ströher, C.; Sampaio, R.R.; Mergener, R.A.; Bonamigo, E.L. A Comparative Study between the Goldmann Applanation Tonometer and the Non-Contact Air-Puff Tonometer (Huvitz HNT 7000) in Normal Eyes. *Clin. Ophthalmol.* **2021**, *15*, 445–451. [CrossRef]
38. Moseley, M.J.; Evans, N.M.; Fielder, A.R. Comparison of a new non-contact tonometer with Goldmann applanation. *Eye* **1989**, *3*, 332–337. [CrossRef] [PubMed]
39. Kyei, S.; Assiamah, F.; Kwarteng, M.A.; Gboglu, C.P. The Association of Central Corneal Thickness and Intraocular Pressure Measures by Non-Contact Tonometry and Goldmann Applanation Tonometry among Glaucoma Patients. *Ethiop. J. Health Sci.* **2020**, *30*, 999–1004. [CrossRef]
40. Rebours, A.K.; Kouassi, F.; Soumahoro, M.; Ellalie, C.K.C.; Siméon, K.A.N.; Agbohoun, R. Comparaison de la tonomérie de Goldmann à la tonométrie à air pulsé à propos de 159 patients à Abidjan. *J. Français D'Ophtalmol.* **2021**, *44*, 41–47. [CrossRef]
41. Atkinson, P.L.; Wishart, P.K.; James, J.N.; Vernon, S.A.; Reid, F. Deterioration in the accuracy of the Pulsair non-contact tonometer with use: Need for regular calibration. *Eye* **1992**, *6*, 530–534. [CrossRef]
42. Britt, J.M. Microaerosol Formation in Noncontact 'Air-Puff' Tonometry. *Arch. Ophthalmol.* **1991**, *109*, 225–228. [CrossRef]
43. Lai, T.H.T.; Tang, E.W.; Chau, S.K.Y.; Fung, K.S.C.; Li, K.K.W. Stepping up infection control measures in ophthalmology during the novel coronavirus outbreak: An experience from Hong Kong. *Graefe's Arch. Clin. Exp. Ophthalmol.* **2020**, *258*, 1049–1055. [CrossRef]
44. Almazyad, E.M.; Ameen, S.; Khan, M.A.; Malik, R. Guidelines and recommendations for tonometry use during the COVID-19 era. *Middle East Afr. J. Ophthalmol.* **2020**, *27*, 73–78. [CrossRef]
45. Mostafa, I.; Bianchi, E.; Brown, L.; Tatham, A.J. What is the best way to measure intraocular pressure (IOP) in a virtual clinic? *Eye* **2021**, *35*, 448–454. [CrossRef]
46. Luce, D.A. Determining in vivo biomechanical properties of the cornea with an ocular response analyzer. *J. Cataract. Refract. Surg.* **2005**, *31*, 156–162. [CrossRef]
47. Kynigopoulos, M.; Schlote, T.; Kotecha, A.; Tzamalis, A.; Pajic, B.; Haefliger, I. Repeatability of Intraocular Pressure and Corneal Biomechanical Properties Measurements by the Ocular Response Analyser. *Klin. Mon. Für Augenheilkd.* **2008**, *225*, 357–360. [CrossRef]
48. Martinez-De-La-Casa, J.M.; García-Feijóo, J.; Fernández-Vidal, A.; Mendez-Hernandez, C.; Garcia-Sanchez, J. Ocular Response Analyzer versus Goldmann Applanation Tonometry for Intraocular Pressure Measurements. *Investig. Opthalmol. Vis. Sci.* **2006**, *47*, 4410–4414. [CrossRef]
49. Medeiros, F.A.; Weinreb, R.N. Evaluation of the Influence of Corneal Biomechanical Properties on Intraocular Pressure Measurements Using the Ocular Response Analyzer. *J. Glaucoma* **2006**, *15*, 364–370. [CrossRef] [PubMed]
50. Touboul, D.; Roberts, C.; Kérautret, J.; Garra, C.; Maurice-Tison, S.; Saubusse, E.; Colin, J. Correlations between corneal hysteresis, intraocular pressure, and corneal central pachymetry. *J. Cataract. Refract. Surg.* **2008**, *34*, 616–622. [CrossRef]
51. Bayoumi, N.H.L.; Bessa, A.S.; El Massry, A.A.K. Ocular Response Analyzer and Goldmann Applanation Tonometry. *J. Glaucoma* **2010**, *19*, 627–631. [CrossRef]
52. Zhang, H.; Sun, Z.; Li, L.; Sun, R.; Zhang, H. Comparison of intraocular pressure measured by ocular response analyzer and Goldmann applanation tonometer after corneal refractive surgery: A systematic review and meta-analysis. *BMC Ophthalmol.* **2020**, *20*, 23–29. [CrossRef]

53. Lascaratos, G.; Garway-Heath, D.F.; Russell, R.A.; Crabb, D.P.; Zhu, H.; Hirn, C.; Kotecha, A.; Suzuki, K.; UKGTS Investigators. Intraocular pressure (IOP) measured with the ocular response ana-lyser is a better predictor of glaucoma progression than Goldmann IOP in the United Kingdom Glaucoma Treatment study (UKGTS). *Investig. Ophthalmol. Vis. Sci.* **2014**, *55*, 128–138.
54. Susanna, B.N.; Ogata, N.G.; Daga, F.B.; Susanna, C.N.; Diniz-Filho, A.; Medeiros, F.A. Association between Rates of Visual Field Progression and Intraocular Pressure Measurements Obtained by Different Tonometers. *Ophthalmology* **2019**, *126*, 49–54. [CrossRef] [PubMed]
55. Congdon, N.G.; Broman, A.T.; Bandeen-Roche, K.; Grover, D.; Quigley, H.A. Central Corneal Thickness and Corneal Hysteresis Associated With Glaucoma Damage. *Am. J. Ophthalmol.* **2006**, *141*, 868–875. [CrossRef]
56. Medeiros, F.A.; Meira-Freitas, D.; Lisboa, R.; Kuang, T.-M.; Zangwill, L.M.; Weinreb, R.N. Corneal Hysteresis as a Risk Factor for Glaucoma Progression: A Prospective Longitudinal Study. *Ophthalmology* **2013**, *120*, 1533–1540. [CrossRef]
57. Susanna, B.N.; Ogata, N.G.; Jammal, A.A.; Susanna, C.N.; Berchuck, S.I.; Medeiros, F.A. Corneal Biomechanics and Visual Field Progression in Eyes with Seemingly Well-Controlled Intraocular Pressure. *Ophthalmology* **2019**, *126*, 1640–1646. [CrossRef] [PubMed]
58. Fujino, Y.; Murata, H.; Matsuura, M.; Nakakura, S.; Shoji, N.; Nakao, Y.; Kiuchi, Y.; Asaoka, R. The Relationship between Corneal Hysteresis and Progression of Glaucoma After Trabeculectomy. *J. Glaucoma* **2020**, *29*, 912–917. [CrossRef]
59. Kirgiz, A.; Erdur, S.K.; Atalay, K.; Gurez, C. The Role of Ocular Response Analyzer in Differentiation of Forme Fruste Keratoconus from Corneal Astigmatism. *Eye Contact Lens. Sci. Clin. Pr.* **2019**, *45*, 83–87. [CrossRef] [PubMed]
60. Randleman, J.B. Post-laser in-situ keratomileusis ectasia: Current understanding and future directions. *Curr. Opin. Ophthalmol.* **2006**, *17*, 406–412. [CrossRef]
61. Reznicek, L.; Muth, D.; Kampik, A.; Neubauer, A.S.; Hirneiss, C. Evaluation of a novel Scheimpflug-based non-contact tonometer in healthy subjects and patients with ocular hypertension and glaucoma. *Br. J. Ophthalmol.* **2013**, *97*, 1410–1414. [CrossRef]
62. Salvetat, M.L.; Zeppieri, M.; Tosoni, C.; Felletti, M.; Grasso, L.; Brusini, P. Corneal Deformation Parameters Provided by the Corvis-ST Pachy-Tonometer in Healthy Subjects and Glaucoma Patients. *J. Glaucoma* **2015**, *24*, 568–574. [CrossRef]
63. Lopes, B.T.; Roberts, C.J.; Elsheikh, A.; Vinciguerra, R.; Vinciguerra, P.; Reisdorf, S.; Berger, S.; Koprowski, R.; Ambrósio, R. Repeatability and Reproducibility of Intraocular Pressure and Dynamic Corneal Response Parameters Assessed by the Corvis ST. *J. Ophthalmol.* **2017**, *2017*, 8515742. [CrossRef]
64. Serbecic, N.; Beutelspacher, S.; Markovic, L.; Roy, A.S.; Shetty, R. Repeatability and reproducibility of corneal biomechanical parameters derived from Corvis ST. *Eur. J. Ophthalmol.* **2020**, *30*, 1287–1294. [CrossRef]
65. Luebke, J.; Bryniok, L.; Neuburger, M.; Jordan, J.F.; Boehringer, D.; Reinhard, T.; Wecker, T.; Anton, A. Intraocular pressure measurement with Corvis ST in comparison with applanation tonometry and Tomey non-contact tonometry. *Int. Ophthalmol.* **2019**, *39*, 2517–2521. [CrossRef] [PubMed]
66. Nakao, Y.; Kiuchi, Y.; Okumichi, H. Evaluation of biomechanically corrected intraocular pressure using Corvis ST and comparison of the Corvis ST, noncontact tonometer, and Goldmann applanation tonometer in patients with glaucoma. *PLoS ONE* **2020**, *15*, e0238395. [CrossRef]
67. Bao, F.; Huang, W.; Zhu, R.; Lu, N.; Wang, Y.; Li, H.; Wu, S.; Lin, H.; Wang, J.; Zheng, X.; et al. Effectiveness of the Goldmann Applanation Tonometer, the Dynamic Contour Tonometer, the Ocular Response Analyzer and the Corvis ST in Measuring Intraocular Pressure following FS-LASIK. *Curr. Eye Res.* **2019**, *45*, 144–152. [CrossRef]
68. Yang, K.; Xu, L.; Fan, Q.; Gu, Y.; Song, P.; Zhang, B.; Zhao, D.; Pang, C.; Ren, S. Evaluation of new Corvis ST parameters in normal, Post-LASIK, Post-LASIK keratectasia and keratoconus eyes. *Sci. Rep.* **2020**, *10*, 5676. [CrossRef] [PubMed]
69. Durham, D.G.; Bigliano, R.P.; Masino, J.A. Pneumatic applanation tonometer. *Trans. Am. Acad. Ophthalmol. Otolaryngol. Am. Acad. Ophthalmol. Otolaryngol.* **1965**, *69*, 1029–1047.
70. West, C.E.; Capella, J.A.; Kaufman, H.E. Measurement of Intraocular Pressure with a Pneumatic Applanation Tonometer. *Am. J. Ophthalmol.* **1972**, *74*, 505–509. [CrossRef]
71. Guildford, J.; O'day, D.M. Applanation Pneumotonometry in Screening for Glaucoma. *South. Med. J.* **1985**, *78*, 1081–1083. [CrossRef] [PubMed]
72. Abbasoglu Özlem, E.; Bowman, R.; Cavanagh, H.; McCulley, J.P. Reliability of intraocular pressure measurements after myopic excimer photorefractive keratectomy. *Ophthalmology* **1998**, *105*, 2193–2196. [CrossRef]
73. Zadok, D.; Tran, D.B.; Twa, M.; Carpenter, M.; Schanzlin, D.J. Pneumotonometry versus Goldmann tonometry after laser in situ keratomileusis for myopia. *J. Cataract. Refract. Surg.* **1999**, *25*, 1344–1348. [CrossRef]
74. Langham, M.E. Discussion on pneumatic applanation tonometer. *Tr. Am. Acad. Ophth. Otolaryng.* **1965**, *69*, 1042.
75. Langham, M.E.; McCarthy, E. A Rapid Pneumatic Applanation Tonometer. *Arch. Ophthalmol.* **1968**, *79*, 389–399. [CrossRef]
76. Silver, D.M.; Farrell, R.A. Validity of pulsatile ocular blood flow measurements. *Surv. Ophthalmol.* **1994**, *38*, S72–S80. [CrossRef]
77. Esgin, H.; Alimgil, M.; Erda, S. Clinical comparison of the ocular blood flow tonograph and the Goldmann applanation tonometer. *Eur. J. Ophthalmol.* **1998**, *8*, 162–166. [CrossRef]
78. Gunvant, P.; Baskaran, M.; Vijaya, L.; Joseph, I.S.; Watkins, R.J.; Nallapothula, M.; Broadway, D.C.; O'Leary, D.J. Effect of corneal parameters on measurements using the pulsatile ocular blood flow tonograph and Goldmann applanation tonometer. *Br. J. Ophthalmol.* **2004**, *88*, 518–522. [CrossRef]
79. Bhan, A.; Bhargava, J.; Vernon, S.A.; Armstrong, S.; Bhan, K.; Tong, L.; Sung, V. Repeatability of ocular blood flow pneumotonom-etry. *Ophthalmology* **2003**, *110*, 1551–1554. [CrossRef]

80. Spraul, C.W.; Lang, G.E.; Ronzani, M.; Högel, J.; Lang, G.K. Reproducibility of measurements with a new slit lamp-mounted ocular blood flow tonograph. *Graefe's Arch. Clin. Exp. Ophthalmol.* **1998**, *236*, 274–279. [CrossRef]
81. Kontiola, A.I. A new induction-based impact method for measuring intraocular pressure. *Acta. Ophthalmol. Scand.* **2000**, *78*, 142–145. [CrossRef]
82. Brusini, P.; Salvetat, M.L.; Zeppieri, M.; Tosoni, C.; Parisi, L. Comparison of ICare Tonometer with Goldmann Applanation Tonometer in Glaucoma Patients. *J. Glaucoma* **2006**, *15*, 213–217. [CrossRef]
83. Kageyama, M.; Hirooka, K.; Baba, T.; Shiraga, F. Comparison of ICare Rebound Tonometer with Noncontact Tonometer in Healthy Children. *J. Glaucoma* **2011**, *20*, 63–66. [CrossRef]
84. Salvetat, M.L.; Zeppieri, M.; Miani, F.; Tosoni, C.; Parisi, L.; Brusini, P. Comparison of iCare tonometer and Goldmann applanation tonometry in normal corneas and in eyes with automated lamellar and penetrating keratoplasty. *Eye* **2011**, *25*, 642–650. [CrossRef] [PubMed]
85. Realini, T.; McMillan, B.; Gross, R.L.; Devience, E.; Balasubramani, G.K. Assessing the Reliability of Intraocular Pressure Measurements Using Rebound Tonometry. *J. Glaucoma* **2021**, *30*, 629–633. [CrossRef] [PubMed]
86. Rosentreter, A.; Athanasopoulos, A.; Schild, A.M.; Lappas, A.; Cursiefen, C.; Dietlein, T.S. Rebound, Applanation, and Dynamic Contour Tonometry in Pathologic Corneas. *Cornea* **2013**, *32*, 313–318. [CrossRef] [PubMed]
87. Badakere, S.V.; Chary, R.; Choudhari, N.S.; Rao, H.L.; Garudadri, C.; Senthil, S. Agreement of Intraocular Pressure Measurement of Icare ic200 with Goldmann Applanation Tonometer in Adult Eyes with Normal Cornea. *Ophthalmol. Glaucoma* **2021**, *4*, 89–94. [CrossRef] [PubMed]
88. Ve, R.S.; Jose, J.; Pai, H.V.; Biswas, S.; Parimi, V.; Poojary, P.; Nagarajan, T. Agreement and repeatability of Icare ic100 tonometer. *Indian J. Ophthalmol.* **2020**, *68*, 2122–2125. [CrossRef]
89. Halkiadakis, I.; Stratos, A.; Stergiopoulos, G.; Patsea, E.; Skouriotis, S.; Mitropoulos, P.; Papaconstantinou, D.; Georgopoulos, G. Evaluation of the Icare-ONE rebound tonometer as a self-measuring intraocular pressure device in normal subjects. *Graefe's Arch. Clin. Exp. Ophthalmol.* **2012**, *250*, 1207–1211. [CrossRef]
90. Rosenfeld, E.; Barequet, D.; Mimouni, M.; Fischer, N.; Kurtz, S. Role of home monitoring with iCare ONE rebound tonometer in glaucoma patients management. *Int. J. Ophthalmol.* **2021**, *14*, 405–408. [CrossRef]
91. Cvenkel, B.; Velkovska, M.A.; Jordanova, V.D. Self-measurement with Icare HOME tonometer, patients' feasibility and acceptability. *Eur. J. Ophthalmol.* **2019**, *30*, 258–263. [CrossRef]
92. Quérat, L.; Chen, E. Clinical Use of iC are Home® tonometer. *Acta. Ophthalmol.* **2020**, *98*, e131–e132. [CrossRef]
93. Gao, F.; Liu, X.; Zhao, Q.; Pan, Y. Comparison of the iCare rebound tonometer and the Goldmann applanation tonometer. *Exp. Ther. Med.* **2017**, *13*, 1912–1916. [CrossRef]
94. Kiddee, W.; Tanjana, A. Variations of Intraocular Pressure Measured by Goldmann Applanation Tonometer, Tono-Pen, iCare Rebound Tonometer, and Pascal Dynamic Contour Tonometer in Patients With Corneal Edema After Phacoemulsification. *J. Glaucoma* **2021**, *30*, 317–324. [CrossRef]
95. Valero, B.; Fénolland, J.-R.; Rosenberg, R.; Sendon, D.; Mesnard, C.; Sigaux, M.; Giraud, J.-M.; Renard, J.-P. Fiabilité et reproductibilité des mesures de la pression intraoculaire par le tonomètre Icare ®Home (modèle TA022) et comparaison avec les mesures au tonomètre à aplanation de Goldmann chez des patients glaucomateux. *J. Français D'Ophtalmol.* **2017**, *40*, 865–875. [CrossRef]
96. Nakakura, S.; Mori, E.; Fujio, Y.; Fujisawa, Y.; Matsuya, K.; Kobayashi, Y.; Tabuchi, H.; Asaoka, R.; Kiuchi, Y. Comparison of the Intraocular Pressure Measured Using the New Rebound Tonometer Icare ic100 and Icare TA01i or Goldmann Applanation Tonometer. *J. Glaucoma* **2019**, *28*, 172–177. [CrossRef]
97. Kato, Y.; Nakakura, S.; Matsuo, N.; Yoshitomi, K.; Handa, M.; Tabuchi, H.; Kiuchi, Y. Agreement among Goldmann applanation tonometer, iCare, and Icare PRO rebound tonometers; non-contact tonometer; and Tonopen XL in healthy elderly subjects. *Int. Ophthalmol.* **2017**, *38*, 687–696. [CrossRef] [PubMed]
98. Scuderi, G.; Cascone, N.C.; Regine, F.; Perdicchi, A.; Cerulli, A.; Recupero, S.M. Validity and Limits of the Rebound Tonometer (ICare®): Clinical Study. *Eur. J. Ophthalmol.* **2011**, *21*, 251–257. [CrossRef]
99. Nakakura, S.; Asaoka, R.; Terao, E.; Nagata, Y.; Fukuma, Y.; Oogi, S.; Shiraishi, M.; Kiuchi, Y. Evaluation of rebound tonometer iCare IC200 as compared with IcarePRO and Goldmann applanation tonometer in patients with glaucoma. *Eye Vis.* **2021**, *8*, 25. [CrossRef]
100. Liu, J.; De Francesco, T.; Schlenker, M.; Ahmed, I.I. Icare Home Tonometer: A Review of Characteristics and Clinical Utility. *Clin. Ophthalmol.* **2020**, *14*, 4031–4045. [CrossRef] [PubMed]
101. Chen, M.; Zhang, L.; Xu, J.; Chen, X.; Gu, Y.; Ren, Y.; Wang, K. Comparability of three intraocular pressure measurement: iCare pro rebound, non-contact and Goldmann applanation tonometry in different IOP group. *BMC Ophthalmol.* **2019**, *19*, 225. [CrossRef] [PubMed]
102. Ting, S.L.; Lim, L.T.; Ooi, C.Y.; Rahman, M. Comparison of Icare Rebound Tonometer and Perkins Applanation Tonometer in Community Eye Screening. *Asia-Pac. J. Ophthalmol.* **2019**, *8*, 229–232. [CrossRef]
103. Subramaniam, A.G.; Allen, P.; Toh, T. Comparison of the Icare ic100 rebound tonometer and the Goldmann applanation tonometer in 1000 eyes. *Ophthalmic Res.* **2020**, *64*, 321–326. [CrossRef]
104. Muttuvelu, D.V.; Baggesen, K.; Ehlers, N. Precision and accuracy of the ICare tonometer—Peripheral and central IOP measurements by rebound tonometry. *Acta. Ophthalmol.* **2010**, *90*, 322–326. [CrossRef] [PubMed]

105. Kaufmann, C.; Bachmann, L.M.; Thiel, M.A. Intraocular Pressure Measurements Using Dynamic Contour Tonometry after Laser In Situ Keratomileusis. *Investig. Opthalmol. Vis. Sci.* **2003**, *44*, 3790–3794. [CrossRef] [PubMed]
106. Kanngiesser, H.E.; Kniestedt, C.; Robert, Y.C.A. Dynamic Contour Tonometry. *J. Glaucoma* **2005**, *14*, 344–350. [CrossRef] [PubMed]
107. Kamppeter, B.A.; Jonas, J.B. Dynamic Contour Tonometry for Intraocular Pressure Measurement. *Am. J. Ophthalmol.* **2005**, *140*, 318–320. [CrossRef] [PubMed]
108. Ceruti, P.; Morbio, R.; Marraffa, M.; Marchini, G. Comparison of Goldmann applanation tonometry and dynamic contour tonometry in healthy and glaucomatous eyes. *Eye* **2008**, *23*, 262–269. [CrossRef] [PubMed]
109. Fogagnolo, P.; Figus, M.; Frezzotti, P.; Iester, M.; Oddone, F.; Zeppieri, M.; Ferreras, A.; Brusini, P.; Rossetti, L.; Orzalesi, N. Test-retest variability of intraocular pressure and ocular pulse amplitude for dynamic contour tonometry: A multicentre study. *Br. J. Ophthalmol.* **2009**, *94*, 419–423. [CrossRef] [PubMed]
110. Katsimpris, J.M.; Theoulakis, P.E.; Vasilopoulos, K.; Skourtis, G.; Papadopoulos, G.E.; Petropoulos, I.K. Correlation between Central Corneal Thickness and Intraocular Pressure Measured by Goldmann Applanation Tonometry or Pascal Dynamic Contour Tonometry. *Klin. Mon. Für Augenheilkd.* **2015**, *232*, 414–418. [CrossRef]
111. Schwenn, O. Ocular pulse amplitude in patients with open angle glaucoma, normal tension glaucoma, and ocular hypertension. *Br. J. Ophthalmol.* **2002**, *86*, 981–984. [CrossRef]
112. Kniestedt, C.; Kanngiesser, H.; Stamper, R.L. Assessment of Pascal dynamic contour tonometer in monitoring IOP after LASIK. *J. Cataract. Refract. Surg.* **2005**, *31*, 458–459. [CrossRef]
113. Siganos, D.S.; Papastergiou, G.I.; Moedas, C. Assessment of the Pascal dynamic contour tonometer in monitoring intraocular pressure in unoperated eyes and eyes after LASIK. *J. Cataract. Refract. Surg.* **2004**, *30*, 746–751. [CrossRef]
114. Lee, S.Y.; Kim, E.W.; Choi, W.; Park, C.K.; Kim, S.; Bae, H.W.; Seong, G.J.; Kim, C.Y. Significance of dynamic contour tonometry in evaluation of progression of glaucoma in patients with a history of laser refractive surgery. *Br. J. Ophthalmol.* **2019**, *104*, 276–281. [CrossRef]
115. Kandarakis, A.; Soumplis, V.; Pitsas, C.; Kandarakis, S.; Halikias, J.; Karagiannis, D. Comparison of dynamic contour tonometry and Goldmann applanation tonometry following penetrating keratoplasty. *Can. J. Ophthalmol.* **2010**, *45*, 489–493. [CrossRef]
116. Sales-Sanz, M.; Arranz-Marquez, E.; Arruabarrena, C.; Teus, M.A. Influence of LASEK on Schiøtz, Goldmann and dynamic contour Tonometry. *Graefe's Arch. Clin. Exp. Ophthalmol.* **2017**, *256*, 173–179. [CrossRef] [PubMed]
117. Wang, A.S.; Alencar, L.; Weinreb, R.N.; Tafreshi, A.; Deokule, S.; Vizzeri, G.; Medeiros, F.A. Repeatability and Reproducibility of Goldmann Applanation, Dynamic Contour, and Ocular Response Analyzer Tonometry. *J. Glaucoma* **2013**, *22*, 127–132. [CrossRef] [PubMed]
118. Bochmann, F.; Kaufmann, C.; Theil, M.A. Dynamic contour tonometry versus Goldmann applanation tonometry: Challenging the gold standard. *Expert. Rev. Ophthalmol.* **2015**, *5*, 743–749. [CrossRef]
119. Okafor, K.C.; Brandt, J.D. Measuring intraocular pressure. *Curr. Opin. Ophthalmol.* **2015**, *26*, 103–109. [CrossRef] [PubMed]
120. Eklund, A.; Hallberg, P.; Linden, C.; Lindahl, O.A. An Applanation Resonator Sensor for Measuring Intraocular Pressure Using Combined Continuous Force and Area Measurement. *Investig. Opthalmol. Vis. Sci.* **2003**, *44*, 3017–3024. [CrossRef]
121. Jóhannesson, G.; Hallberg, P.; Eklund, A.; Lindén, C. Introduction and clinical evaluation of servo-controlled applanation resonance tonometry. *Acta. Ophthalmol.* **2011**, *90*, 677–682. [CrossRef]
122. Hallberg, P.; Eklund, A.; Bäcklund, T.; Lindén, C. Clinical Evaluation of Applanation Resonance Tonometry. *J. Glaucoma* **2007**, *16*, 88–93. [CrossRef] [PubMed]
123. Salvetat, M.L.; Zeppieri, M.; Tosoni, C.; Brusini, P. Repeatability and accuracy of applanation resonance tonometry in healthy subjects and patients with glaucoma. *Acta. Ophthalmol.* **2013**, *92*, e66–e73. [CrossRef] [PubMed]
124. Ottobelli, L.; Fogagnolo, P.; Frezzotti, P.; De Cillà, S.; Vallenzasca, E.; Digiuni, M.; Paderni, R.; Motolese, I.; Bagaglia, S.A.; Motolese, E.; et al. Repeatability and reproducibility of applanation resonance tonometry: A cross-sectional study. *BMC Ophthalmol.* **2015**, *15*, 36. [CrossRef] [PubMed]
125. Mulak, M.; Czak, W.A.; Mimier, M.; Kaczmarek, R. A comparison of intraocular pressure values obtained using a Goldmann applanation tonometer and a handheld version of applanation resonance tonometer: A preliminary report. *Adv. Clin. Exp. Med.* **2018**, *27*, 481–485. [CrossRef] [PubMed]
126. Jóhannesson, G.; Hallberg, P.; Eklund, A.; Koskela, T.; Lindén, C. Change in Intraocular Pressure Measurement After Myopic LASEK. *J. Glaucoma* **2012**, *21*, 255–259. [CrossRef] [PubMed]
127. Liu, J.H.; Kripke, D.F.; Hoffman, R.E.; Twa, M.; Loving, R.T.; Rex, K.M.; Gupta, N.; Weinreb, R.N. Nocturnal elevation of intraocular pressure in young adults. *Investig. Ophthalmol. Vis. Sci.* **1998**, *39*, 2707–2712.
128. Konstas, A.G.P.; Mantziris, D.A.; Stewart, W.C. Diurnal Intraocular Pressure in Untreated Exfoliation and Primary Open-angle Glaucoma. *Arch. Ophthalmol.* **1997**, *115*, 182–185. [CrossRef]
129. Asrani, S.; Zeimer, R.; Wilensky, J.; Gieser, D.; Vitale, S.; Lindenmuth, K. Large Diurnal Fluctuations in Intraocular Pressure Are an Independent Risk Factor in Patients With Glaucoma. *J. Glaucoma* **2000**, *9*, 134–142. [CrossRef]
130. Tan, S.; Baig, N.; Hansapinyo, L.; Jhanji, V.; Wei, S.; Tham, C.Y.C. Comparison of self-measured diurnal intraocular pressure profiles using rebound tonometry between primary angle closure glaucoma and primary open angle glaucoma patients. *PLoS ONE* **2017**, *12*, e0173905. [CrossRef]
131. Barkana, Y.; Anis, S.; Liebmann, J.; Tello, C.; Ritch, R. Clinical Utility of Intraocular Pressure Monitoring Outside of Normal Office Hours in Patients With Glaucoma. *Arch. Ophthalmol.* **2006**, *124*, 793–797. [CrossRef]

132. Hughes, E.; Spry, P.; Diamond, J. 24-Hour Monitoring of Intraocular Pressure in Glaucoma Management: A Retrospective Review. *J. Glaucoma* **2003**, *12*, 232–236. [CrossRef] [PubMed]
133. Konstas, A.G.P.; Quaranta, L.; Bozkurt, B.; Katsanos, A.; Feijoo, J.G.; Rossetti, L.; Shaarawy, T.; Pfeiffer, N.; Miglior, S. 24-h Efficacy of Glaucoma Treatment Options. *Adv. Ther.* **2016**, *33*, 481–517. [CrossRef]
134. Ho, C.H.; Wong, J.K.W. Role of 24-Hour Intraocular Pressure Monitoring in Glaucoma Management. *J. Ophthalmol.* **2019**, *2019*, 3632197–3632213. [CrossRef] [PubMed]
135. Mcmonnies, C.W. The importance of and potential for continuous monitoring of intraocular pressure. *Clin. Exp. Optom.* **2017**, *100*, 203–207. [CrossRef]
136. Ittoop, S.M.; SooHoo, J.R.; Seibold, L.K.; Mansouri, K.; Kahook, M.Y. Systematic Review of Current Devices for 24-h Intraocular Pressure Monitoring. *Adv. Ther.* **2016**, *33*, 1679–1690. [CrossRef] [PubMed]
137. Molaei, A.; Karamzadeh, V.; Safi, S.; Esfandiari, H.; Dargahi, J.; Khosravi, M. Upcoming methods and specifications of continuous intraocular pressure monitoring systems for glaucoma. *J. Ophthalmic Vis. Res.* **2018**, *13*, 66–71. [CrossRef]
138. Dick, H.B.; Schultz, T.; Gerste, R.D. Miniaturization in Glaucoma Monitoring and Treatment: A Review of New Technologies That Require a Minimal Surgical Approach. *Ophthalmol. Ther.* **2019**, *8*, 19–30. [CrossRef]
139. Lee, J.O.; Park, H.; Du, J.; Balakrishna, A.; Chen, O.; Sretavan, D.; Choo, H. A microscale optical implant for continuous in vivo monitoring of intraocular pressure. *Microsyst. Nanoeng.* **2017**, *3*, 17057. [CrossRef]
140. Koutsonas, A.; Walter, P.; Roessler, G.; Plange, N. Implantation of a Novel Telemetric Intraocular Pressure Sensor in Patients with Glaucoma (ARGOS Study): 1-Year Results. *Investig. Opthalmol. Vis. Sci.* **2015**, *56*, 1063–1069. [CrossRef] [PubMed]
141. Choritz, L.; Mansouri, K.; Bosch, J.V.D.; Weigel, M.; Dick, H.B.; Wagner, M.; Thieme, H.; Rüfer, F.; Szurmann, P.; Wehner, W.; et al. Telemetric Measurement of Intraocular Pressure via an Implantable Pressure Sensor—12-Month Results from the ARGOS-02 Trial. *Am. J. Ophthalmol.* **2020**, *209*, 187–196. [CrossRef] [PubMed]
142. Chen, P.-J.; Rodger, D.; Humayun, M.S.; Tai, Y.-C. Unpowered spiral-tube parylene pressure sensor for intraocular pressure sensing. *Sens. Actuators A Phys.* **2006**, *127*, 276–282. [CrossRef]
143. Demeng, L.; Niansong, M.; Zhaofeng, Z. An ultralow power wireless intraocular pressure monitoring system. *J. Semicond.* **2014**, *35*, 105014.
144. Mariacher, S.; Ebner, M.; Januschowski, K.; Hurst, J.; Schnichels, S.; Szurman, P. Investigation of a novel implantable suprachoroidal pressure transducer for telemetric intraocular pressure monitoring. *Exp. Eye Res.* **2016**, *151*, 54–60. [CrossRef] [PubMed]
145. Leonardi, M.; Leuenberger, P.; Bertrand, D.; Bertsch, A.; Renaud, P. First Steps toward Noninvasive Intraocular Pressure Monitoring with a Sensing Contact Lens. *Investig. Opthalmol. Vis. Sci.* **2004**, *45*, 3113–3117. [CrossRef] [PubMed]
146. Hediger, A.; Kniestedt, C.; Zweifel, S.; Knecht, P.; Funk, J.; Kanngiesser, H. Kontinuierliche Augeninnendruckmessung. *Der. Ophthalmol.* **2009**, *106*, 1111–1115. [CrossRef]
147. Twa, M.; Roberts, C.J.; Karol, H.J.; Mahmoud, A.M.; Weber, P.A.; Small, R.H. Evaluation of a Contact Lens-Embedded Sensor for Intraocular Pressure Measurement. *J. Glaucoma* **2010**, *19*, 382–390. [CrossRef] [PubMed]
148. Mansouri, K.; Shaarawy, T. Continuous intraocular pressure monitoring with a wireless ocular telemetry sensor: Initial clinical experience in patients with open angle glaucoma. *Br. J. Ophthalmol.* **2011**, *95*, 627–629. [CrossRef]
149. Mansouri, K.; Weinreb, R.N.; Liu, J.H.K. Efficacy of a Contact Lens Sensor for Monitoring 24-H Intraocular Pressure Related Patterns. *PLoS ONE* **2015**, *10*, e0125530. [CrossRef] [PubMed]
150. Mansouri, K.; Medeiros, F.A.; Tafreshi, A.; Weinreb, R.N. Error in PubMed in: Global Burden of Visual Impairment and Blindness. *Arch. Ophthalmol.* **2012**, *130*, 1559. [CrossRef]
151. Lorenz, K.; Korb, C.; Herzog, N.; Vetter, J.M.; Elflein, H.; Keilani, M.M.; Pfeiffer, N. Tolerability of 24-Hour Intraocular Pressure Monitoring of a Pressure-sensitive Contact Lens. *J. Glaucoma* **2013**, *22*, 311–316. [CrossRef]
152. Dunbar, G.E.; Shen, B.Y.; Aref, A.A. The Sensimed Triggerfish contact lens sensor: Efficacy, safety, and patient perspectives. *Clin. Ophthalmol.* **2017**, *11*, 875–882. [CrossRef]
153. Mottet, B.; Aptel, F.; Romanet, J.-P.; Hubanova, R.; Pépin, J.-L.; Chiquet, C. 24-Hour Intraocular Pressure Rhythm in Young Healthy Subjects Evaluated With Continuous Monitoring Using a Contact Lens Sensor. *JAMA Ophthalmol.* **2013**, *131*, 1507–1516. [CrossRef]
154. Holló, G.; Kóthy, P.; Vargha, P. Evaluation of Continuous 24-Hour Intraocular Pressure Monitoring for Assessment of Prostaglandin-induced Pressure Reduction in Glaucoma. *J. Glaucoma* **2014**, *23*, e6–e12. [CrossRef]
155. Mansouri, K. The Road Ahead to Continuous 24-Hour Intraocular Pressure Monitoring in Glaucoma. *J. Ophthalmic Vis. Res.* **2014**, *9*, 260–268.
156. Tojo, N.; Hayashi, A.; Otsuka, M. Correlation between 24-h continuous intraocular pressure measurement with a contact lens sensor and visual field progression. *Graefe's Arch. Clin. Exp. Ophthalmol.* **2020**, *258*, 175–182. [CrossRef] [PubMed]
157. Tojo, N.; Hayashi, A.; Otsuka, M.; Miyakoshi, A. Fluctuations of the Intraocular Pressure in Pseudoexfoliation Syndrome and Normal Eyes Measured by a Contact Lens Sensor. *J. Glaucoma* **2016**, *25*, e463–e468. [CrossRef]
158. Pajic, B.; Pajic-Eggspuehler, B.; Haefliger, I. Continuous IOP Fluctuation Recording in Normal Tension Glaucoma Patients. *Curr. Eye Res.* **2011**, *36*, 1129–1138. [CrossRef]
159. Agnifili, L.; Mastropasqua, R.; Frezzotti, P.; Fasanella, V.; Motolese, I.; Pedrotti, E.; Di Iorio, A.; Mattei, P.A.; Motolese, E.; Mastropasqua, L. Circadian intraocular pressure patterns in healthy subjects, primary open angle and normal tension glaucoma patients with a contact lens sensor. *Acta. Ophthalmol.* **2014**, *93*, e14–e21. [CrossRef] [PubMed]

160. Tojo, N.; Abe, S.; Ishida, M.; Yagou, T.; Hayashi, A. The Fluctuation of Intraocular Pressure Measured by a Contact Lens Sensor in Normal-Tension Glaucoma Patients and Nonglaucoma Subjects. *J. Glaucoma* **2017**, *26*, 195–200. [CrossRef]
161. Kim, Y.W.; Kim, J.-S.; Lee, S.Y.; Ha, A.; Lee, J.; Park, Y.J.; Kim, Y.K.; Jeoung, J.W.; Park, K.H. Twenty-four–Hour Intraocular Pressure–Related Patterns from Contact Lens Sensors in Normal-Tension Glaucoma and Healthy Eyes. *Ophthalmology* **2020**, *127*, 1487–1497. [CrossRef] [PubMed]
162. Kim, Y.W.; Kim, M.J.; Park, K.H.; Jeoung, J.W.; Kim, S.H.; Jang, C.I.; Lee, S.H.; Kim, J.H.; Lee, S.; Kang, J.Y. Preliminary study on implantable inductive-type sensor for continuous monitoring of intraocular pressure. *Clin. Exp. Ophthalmol.* **2015**, *43*, 830–837. [CrossRef]
163. Mansouri, K.; Rao, H.L.; Weinreb, R.N. Short-Term and Long-Term Variability of Intraocular Pressure Measured with an Intraocular Telemetry Sensor in Patients with Glaucoma. *Ophthalmology* **2021**, *128*, 227–233. [CrossRef]
164. Xu, S.C.; Gauthier, A.C.; Liu, J. The Application of a Contact Lens Sensor in Detecting 24-Hour Intraocular Pressure-Related Patterns. *J. Ophthalmol.* **2016**, *2016*, 4727423. [CrossRef]
165. Kouhani, M.H.M.; Wu, J.; Tavakoli, A.; Weber, A.J.; Li, W. Wireless, passive strain sensor in a doughnut-shaped contact lens for continuous non-invasive self-monitoring of intraocular pressure. *Lab. Chip.* **2020**, *20*, 332–342. [CrossRef]
166. Xu, J.; Cui, T.; Hirtz, T.; Qiao, Y.; Li, X.; Zhong, F.; Han, X.; Yang, Y.; Zhang, S.; Ren, T.-L. Highly Transparent and Sensitive Graphene Sensors for Continuous and Non-invasive Intraocular Pressure Monitoring. *ACS Appl. Mater. Interfaces* **2020**, *12*, 18375–18384. [CrossRef] [PubMed]
167. Maeng, B.; Chang, H.-K.; Park, J. Photonic crystal-based smart contact lens for continuous intraocular pressure monitoring. *Lab. Chip.* **2020**, *20*, 1740–1750. [CrossRef] [PubMed]
168. Wasilewicz, R.; Varidel, T.; Simon-Zoula, S.; Schlund, M.; Cerboni, S.; Mansouri, K. First-in-human continuous 24-hour measurement of intraocular pressure and ocular pulsation using a novel contact lens sensor. *Br. J. Ophthalmol.* **2020**, *104*, 1519–1523. [CrossRef]
169. Agaoglu, S.; Diep, P.; Martini, M.; Kt, S.; Baday, M.; Araci, I.E. Ultra-sensitive microfluidic wearable strain sensor for intraocular pressure monitoring. *Lab. Chip.* **2018**, *18*, 3471–3483. [CrossRef]
170. Campigotto, A.; Leahy, S.; Zhao, G.; Campbell, R.J.; Lai, Y. Non-invasive Intraocular pressure monitoring with contact lens. *Br. J. Ophthalmol.* **2019**, *104*, 1324–1328. [CrossRef] [PubMed]
171. Fan, Y.; Tu, H.; Zhao, H.; Wei, F.; Yang, Y.; Ren, T. A wearable contact lens sensor for noninvasive in-situ monitoring of intraocular pressure. *Nanotechnology* **2021**, *32*, 095106. [CrossRef]
172. Dou, Z.; Tang, J.; Liu, Z.; Sun, Q.; Wang, Y.; Li, Y.; Yuan, M.; Wu, H.; Wang, Y.; Pei, W.; et al. Wearable Contact Lens Sensor for Non-invasive Continuous Monitoring of Intraocular Pressure. *Micromachines* **2021**, *12*, 108. [CrossRef] [PubMed]
173. Gillmann, K.; Wasilewicz, R.; Hoskens, K.; Simon-Zoula, S.; Mansouri, K. Continuous 24-hour measurement of intraocular pressure in millimeters of mercury (mmHg) using a novel contact lens sensor: Comparison with pneumatonometry. *PLoS ONE* **2021**, *16*, e0248211. [CrossRef] [PubMed]

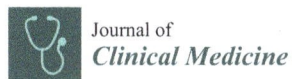

Journal of
Clinical Medicine

Article

Correlation Analysis between Intraocular Pressure and Extraocular Muscles Based on Orbital Magnetic Resonance T2 Mapping in Thyroid-Associated Ophthalmopathy Patients

Ban Luo [1] , Wei Wang [1], Xinyu Li [1], Hong Zhang [1], Yaoli Zhang [1,*] and Weikun Hu [1,2,*]

[1] Department of Ophthalmology, Tongji Hospital, Tongji Medical College, Huazhong University of Science and Technology, Wuhan 430074, China; banluoeye@hust.edu.cn (B.L.); wwnissan@163.com (W.W.); lixy07@126.com (X.L.); sgy804408@gmail.com (H.Z.)

[2] Department of Ophthalmology, Tianyou Hospital/Tongji Hospital, Wuhan University of Science and Technology, Wuhan 430072, China

* Correspondence: zhangyaoli1126@163.com (Y.Z.); huweikun1@163.com (W.H.); Tel.: +86-027-8366-3411 (W.H.)

Abstract: Background: The correlation between intraocular pressure (IOP) and the magnetic resonance imaging (MRI) parameters in thyroid-associated ophthalmopathy (TAO) patients was explored. Methods: This study included 82 eyes in 41 TAO patients who had a large difference in the IOP between each eye. We measured the T2 relaxation time (T2RT) of the extraocular muscles (EOMs), the orbital fat, and the area of the EOMs. Results: There was a positive correlation between IOP and exophthalmos, the clinical activity score (CAS), the T2RT (of the medial rectus (MR)), the area of the MR, inferior rectus (IR) and lateral rectus, and the mean area. We established a regression model with IOP as the dependent variable, and the area of the IR was statistically significant. Conclusions: High IOP in TAO patients was positively correlated with the degree of exophthalmos and EOM inflammation (especially the inferior rectus). The state of the EOMs in an orbital MRI may partially explain high IOP and provide the necessary clinical information for subsequent high IOP treatment.

Keywords: thyroid-associated ophthalmopathy; extraocular muscle; magnetic resonance imaging; intraocular pressure; T2 relaxation time

Citation: Luo, B.; Wang, W.; Li, X.; Zhang, H.; Zhang, Y.; Hu, W. Correlation Analysis between Intraocular Pressure and Extraocular Muscles Based on Orbital Magnetic Resonance T2 Mapping in Thyroid-Associated Ophthalmopathy Patients. *J. Clin. Med.* **2022**, *11*, 3981. https://doi.org/10.3390/jcm11143981

Academic Editors: Maria Letizia Salvetat, Marco Zeppieri, Paolo Brusini and Cosimo Mazzotta

Received: 2 May 2022
Accepted: 5 July 2022
Published: 8 July 2022

Publisher's Note: MDPI stays neutral with regard to jurisdictional claims in published maps and institutional affiliations.

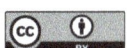

1. Introduction

Thyroid-associated ophthalmopathy (TAO) is a chronic autoimmune inflammatory disease that affects the orbital fat (OF), extraocular muscles (EOMs), eyeball, and eye appendages, and is related to thyroid autoimmune pathology [1]. Clinical signs include widened palpebral fissure, eyelid retraction, conjunctival hyperemia, exophthalmos, corneal exposure, restrictive myopathy, optic neuropathy, and other symptoms [2]. In most patients, the effects on the eye appear mild, and the severe form of the disease affects 3% to 5% of individuals [3].

Many studies have shown that people with thyroid disease have a higher risk of high intraocular pressure (IOP) and glaucoma [4,5]. However, there have also been studies that were skeptical of these findings. A study by Cockerham showed that, while a quarter of TAO patients developed ocular hypertension, glaucoma damage was rare and even lower than the relative risk for glaucoma visual field defects in healthy people [5]. There are also differing opinions on the treatments for lowering the IOP in TAO patients with ocular hypertension. Despite the various theories so far, the relationship between ocular hypertension, open-angle glaucoma, and TAO is still a mystery. The increase in IOP in TAO may be caused by inflammation that causes swelling of the EOMs, which restricts and compresses the eyeball [6]; a decrease in orbital venous drainage leads to an increase in episcleral venous pressure [7], or an increase in mucopolysaccharide deposition in the trabecular meshwork, which thereby reduces the outflow of aqueous humor [8].

A study by Stoyanova et al. showed that a group of TAO patients with a larger thickness sum in the EOMs, as shown by orbital computed tomography, had higher IOP [9]. Studies have also found a negative correlation between IOP and the flow velocity of the supraocular vein in TAO patients [7]. Some studies have proposed that inflammation-induced EOM edema and inflammation-activated fibroblasts differentiate into adipocytes in TAO patients, leading to crowding of the orbital tissue and then increased IOP. However, there have been no studies to quantify this relationship.

By using the T2 relaxation time (T2RT), orbital magnetic resonance imaging (MRI) not only detects the presence or absence of swollen tissue, but also objectively and quantitatively evaluates the inflammatory activity of the orbital tissue in TAO patients [10,11]. The increase of T2 signal intensity in MRI may indicate edema changes which caused by autoimmune inflammation and/or vascular congestion, as the T2RT reflects the water content of the tissue. Orbital MRI can provide a more comprehensive assessment of TAO patients. [10].

Studies have found a variety of systemic and ocular risk factors associated with TAO combining with open-angle glaucoma, including old age, female gender, a family history of glaucoma, myopia, diabetes, hypertension, the presence of pseudoexfoliation and thyroxine treatment [12]. There are also many factors affecting the IOP of TAO patients. The current study included patients with high IOP in a unilateral eye and compared the differences in parameters, such as the EOMs and the clinical activity score (CAS) between both eyes; it studied the factors that lead to increased IOP in patients with TAO so as to provide information for the selection of subsequent treatment options. Furthermore, this study effectively avoided the influence of confounding factors, such as age, sex, blood pressure, measurement time, medication history, thyroid hormone status, and history of other systemic diseases among the individuals with IOP.

2. Materials and Methods

2.1. Subjects

A retrospective analysis was performed on clinical data from November 2015 to December 2019 for a total of 82 eyes in 41 TAO patients who met the inclusion criteria at Tongji Hospital, Tongji Medical College of Huazhong University of Science and Technology. The age, gender, thyroid disease status, vision, IOP, CAS, exophthalmos, and orbital MRI-T2 mapping scans of the patients were collected.

Inclusion criteria: TAO was diagnosed according to the EUGOGO guidelines [13]. An IOP difference ≥ 2 mmHg between the two eyes, an IOP ≤ 21 mmHg in a unilateral eye, and an IOP > 21 mmHg in the other eye, or an IOP difference ≥ 5 between the two eyes and an IOP ≤ 21 mmHg in the bilateral eyes were included. Exclusion criteria: patients with inconsistent local corticosteroid therapy in the eyes in the past 3 months, a history of orbital decompression and EOM surgery in the past year, or intervals between the IOP measurement and orbital MRI-T2 mapping examination of greater than 1 month were excluded.

According to the IOP of the bilateral eyes, the eyeball with the lower IOP was included in the low IOP group, and the other eye with the higher IOP was included in the high IOP group. The IOP was measured with a non-contact tonometer (NIDEK). TAO activity was evaluated according to the CAS. The contents of the CAS according to EUGOGO guidelines (2021) [13] include the following points, and each positive counts as 1 point for a total of 7 points: 1. Spontaneous retrobulbar pain; 2. Pain on attempted upward or downward gaze; 3. Redness of eyelids; 4. Redness of conjunctiva; 5. Swelling of caruncle or plica; 6. Swelling of eyelids; 7. Swelling of conjunctiva (chemosis).The CAS and the degree of exophthalmos were measured by the same orbital plastic surgeon (B.L.) All data were obtained by averaging them after three measurements. The data of the cross-sectional areas of the extraocular muscles and the T2 relaxation times of the orbital tissues were mainly measured by two radiologists who had worked for more than 5 years, and the average values of the data were used. The orbital MRI-T2 mapping reports were issued by the same imaging specialist (J.Zh.) for all patients.

2.2. Measurement of Orbital MRI-T2 Mapping Parameters

An orbital MRI was performed for all participants using a 3.0 T MRI system (Signa HDxt, GE Healthcare, Pittsburgh, PA, USA). The T2RTs of the EOMs were measured using a multi-slice multi-spin echo pulse sequence with a TR of 1500 ms, 7 TE values (22, 33, 44, 55, 66, 77, and 88 ms), a 180 × 180 mm field of view, 3.0 mm slice thickness, a 256 × 256 matrix, and 1 NEX. The color-coded T2 calculation was generated by a single exponential curve fitting using T2 mapping software (ADW4.4 workstation, GE Healthcare, Pittsburgh, PA, USA) (Figure 1a). The T2RTs (ms) and the areas (mm^2) of five EOMs (inferior rectus (IR), superior rectus/levator complex (SRLCLC), medial rectus (MR), lateral rectus (LR), and superior oblique (SO)) were measured (Figure 1b). The maximum value for the T2RT or the area on the coronal section of each EOM was recorded as the final T2RT or area value.

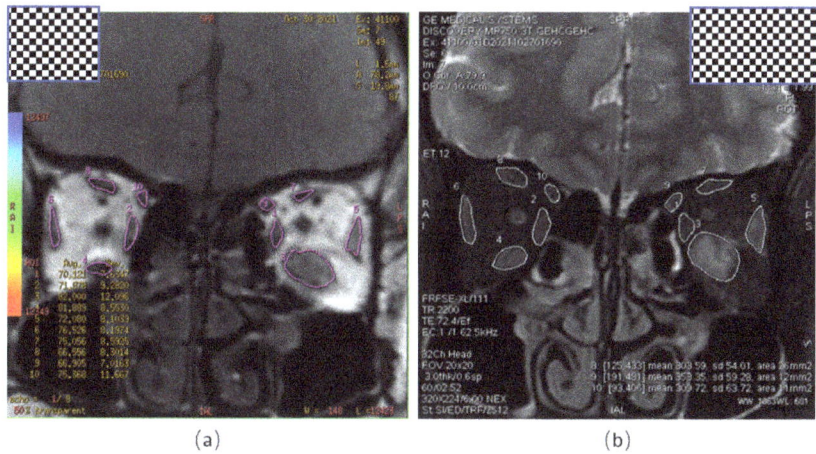

(a) (b)

Figure 1. Measurement of Orbital MRI-T2 Mapping Parameters. (**a**) Orbital coronal pseudo-color map, representing the T2RT value of the ROI in each EOM; (**b**) orbital coronal view, indicating the largest cross-sectional area of the EOM. T2RT, T2 relaxation time; ROI, region of interest; EOM, extraocular muscles.

2.3. Image Analysis

All the MR data from T2 mapping were processed using open-source software (Fire Voxel, New York University, New York, NY, USA) by two experienced neuroradiologists (approximately 4 and 7 years of clinical experience in head and neck radiology). The maximum cross-sectional area and the T2RT of the EOM were calculated for the five EOMs and orbital fat (superior, inferior, medial, lateral rectus, and superior oblique) within each orbit.

Blind to patient information, the two neuroradiologists selected the TE value that best delineated the EOM on the T2 mapping image, and carefully and independently drew a region of interest (ROI) layer by layer along the edge of the EOM, while avoiding orbital fat and air in the paranasal sinuses. Using partial volume effects to obtain the VOI (volume of interest) of the muscle, the same procedure was repeated to generate a VOI of five EOMs within each track. Due to the difficulty in separating the superior rectus and the levator superioris, they are delineated as a group of muscles called the superior rectus/levator complex. The orbital and extraocular muscles were delineated to delineate the boundary of the orbital fat, and the orbital fat VOI was obtained. The T2 relaxation time of each extraocular muscle was calculated using a single exponential T2 mapping fitting model. The value of T2 relaxation time was obtained by using S (TE) = S0 × e($-$TE/T2), where S is the signal intensity (in arbitrary units), S0 is the initial signal intensity, TE is the echo time, and T2 is the T2 relaxation time (ms). The maximum cross-sectional area of each extraocular muscle was calculated using Image J (V1.8.0.112, National Institutes of Health, Bethesda, MD, USA).

2.4. Statistical Analysis

For statistical evaluation of the data, SPSS Statistics software (ver. 26, IBM, Armonk, NY, USA) was used for the statistical analysis. A Shapiro–Wilk test was used for the normality test. A paired *t*-test was used to compare the data that satisfied the normal distribution; if they did not, a Wilcoxon signed-rank test was used. The correlation analysis used a Spearman test. Taking the IOP as the dependent variable, a single-factor regression analysis combined with clinical experience was used to screen the independent variables, and the age, gender, CAS, EOM cross-sectional area, and T2RTs of the EOMs were included as independent variables for screening to build a variable linear regression model ($p < 0.05$). $p < 0.05$ was considered statistically significant.

3. Results

The demographic characteristics of the TAO patients included in this study are shown in Table 1.

Table 1. Demographic characteristics of TAO patients.

Demographic Characteristics	
Gender (Male/Female)	21/20
Age (Year)	44.59 ± 10.77
Thyroid function (euthyroid/hyperthyroidism/hypothyroidism)	8/32/1
History of glucocorticoid use (No/Yes)	33/8

The ocular data for the low IOP (LIOP) group and the high IOP (HIOP) group are shown in Table 2 and Figure 2. It can be seen that the values for the CAS, exophthalmos, T2RT of the MR, the area of the MR, IR and LR, the average area of the five EOMs and the total area of the five EOMs were significantly higher in the HIOP group than in the LIOP group ($p = 0.001$, $p < 0.0001$, $p = 0.015$, $p = 0.002$, $p < 0.0001$, $p < 0.0001$, $p < 0.0001$, $p < 0.0001$). In order to study the clinical characteristics of TAO eyes with ocular hypertension, we performed a statistical analysis on the clinical symptoms of TAO eyes. In terms of clinical symptoms, the incidence of restricted upward movement of the eye and spontaneous retrobulbar pain (y/n) were significantly increased in the HIOP group com-pared to the LIOP group ($p = 0.0008$, $p = 0.020$).

Table 2. Ocular characteristics of TAO patients in 2 groups.

Parameters	LIOP Group (*n* = 41)	HIOP Group (*n* = 41)	*p* Value
CAS	1.90 ± 1.73	2.68 ± 1.77	0.001 [&]
Exophthalmos	17.54 ± 2.76	19.40 ± 2.74	<0.0001 [&]
T2RT (MR)	70.81 ± 11.25	74.68 ± 9.39	0.015 [&]
Area (MR)	40.24 ± 18.40	46.78 ± 21.82	0.002 [&]
T2RT (IR)	79.55 ± 7.67	79.26 ± 9.28	0.850 [$]
Area (IR)	43.05 ± 16.28	68.78 ± 27.89	<0.0001 [&]
T2RT (LR)	72.81 ± 6.52	74.38 ± 6.75	0.251 [&]
Area (LR)	48.54 ± 13.34	56.93 ± 16.52	<0.0001 [&]
T2RT (SRLC)	81.87 ± 15.38	82.96 ± 14.42	0.791 [&]
Area (SRLC)	57.15 ± 32.20	65.17 ± 37.64	0.925 [&]
T2RT (SO)	75.42 ± 6.84	75.92 ± 7.67	0.506 [$]
Area (SO)	18.10 ± 5.03	20.08 ± 6.73	0.118 [&]
T2RT (OF)	71.11 ± 14.09	70.51 ± 14.29	0.667 [&]
Average T2RT	75.26 ± 6.02	76.29 ± 5.95	0.168 [&]
Total T2RT	451.57 ± 36.13	457.71 ± 35.72	0.168 [&]
Average area	41.47 ± 13.11	51.51 ± 14.01	<0.0001 [&]
Total area	206.63 ± 66.42	257.54 ± 70.04	<0.0001 [&]
RUME (y/n)	11/30	26/15	0.0008 [#]
RDME (y/n)	9/32	10/31	0.794 [#]
RIME (y/n)	0/41	1/40	>0.999 [*]

Table 2. *Cont.*

Parameters	LIOP Group (*n* = 41)	HIOP Group (*n* = 41)	*p* Value
ROME (y/n)	6/35	9/32	0.392 [#]
Spontaneous retrobulbar pain (y/n)	9/32	19/22	0.020 [#]
Pain on attempted upward or downward gaze (y/n)	9/32	14/27	0.219 [#]
Redness of eyelids (y/n)	9/32	10/31	0.794 [#]
Redness of conjunctiva (y/n)	12/29	16/25	0.352 [#]
Swelling of eyelids (y/n)	26/15	30/11	0.343 [#]
Swelling of conjunctiva (y/n)	10/31	14/27	0.332 [#]
Swelling of caruncle or plica (y/n)	3/38	7/34	0.177 [#]

LIOP, low intraocular pressure; HIOP, high intraocular pressure; CAS, clinical activity score; T2RT, T2 relaxation time; MR, medial rectus; IR, inferior rectus; LR, lateral rectus; SRLC, superior rectus/levator complex; SO, superior oblique; OF, orbital fat; RUME, restricted upward movement of the eye; RDME, restricted downward movement of the eye; RIME, restricted inward movement of the eye; ROME, restricted outward movement of the eye; [$], paired *t*-test; [&], Wilcoxon signed-rank test; [*], Fisher test; [#], chi-square test.

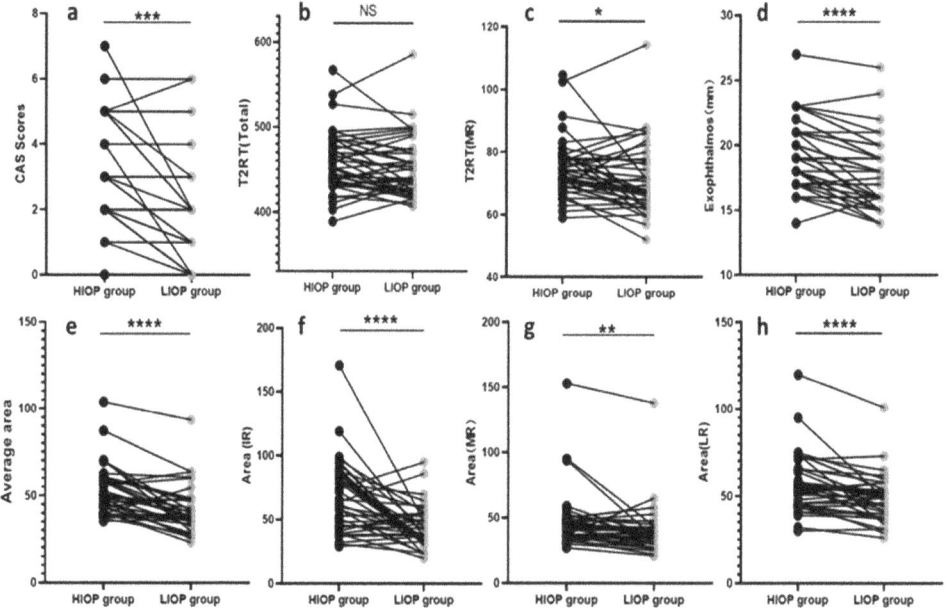

Figure 2. Wilcoxon signed-rank test charts show the differences of the CAS score (**a**), the overall orbital T2 relaxation time—T2RT (Total) (**b**), the medial rectus muscle T2 relaxation time—T2RT(MR) (**c**), exophthalmos (**d**), the average extraocular muscle cross-sectional area—average area (**e**), the inferior rectus cross-sectional area-area (IR) (**f**), the medial rectus cross-sectional area—area (MR) (**g**), and the lateral rectus cross-sectional area—area(LR) (**h**) between the HIOP and LIOP groups. CAS, clinical activity score; T2RT, T2 relaxation time; MR, medial rectus; IR, inferior rectus; LR, lateral rectus; HIOP, high intraocular pressure; LIOP, low intraocular pressure; NS, not statistically different; * $p < 0.05$; ** $p < 0.01$; *** $p < 0.001$; **** $p < 0.0001$.

3.1. Correlation Analysis

For the IOP, CAS, exophthalmos, T2RTs (ms), and the areas (mm^2) of the five EOMs, the average T2 value and the average area of the EOMs were subjected to a bivariate correlation analysis, and it was found that IOP was positively correlated with the CAS, exophthalmos, T2RTs (MR), MR, IR, and LR areas, and the average area of the five EOMs (Table 3).

Table 3. Correlation analysis between IOP and CAS, exophthalmos and OMR parameters.

Parameters	Correlation Coefficient with IOP	*p* Value
CAS	0.254	0.021
Exophthalmos	0.402	<0.001
T2RT (MR)	0.250	0.023
Area (MR)	0.257	0.020
T2RT (IR)	−0.101	0.367
Area (IR)	0.550	<0.001
T2RT (LR)	0.093	0.406
Area (LR)	0.340	0.002
T2RT (SRLC)	0.034	0.759
Area (SRLC)	0.033	0.765
T2RT (SO)	0.045	0.691
Area (SO)	0.178	0.111
T2RT(OF)	0.106	0.344
Average T2RT	0.151	0.177
Average area	0.440	<0.001

IOP, intraocular pressure; OMR, ocular magnetic resonance; CAS, clinical activity score; T2RT, T2 relaxation time; MR, medial rectus; IR, inferior rectus; LR, lateral rectus; SRLC, superior rectus/levator complex; SO, superior oblique; OF, orbital fat.

3.2. Multiple Linear Regression

Taking IOP as the dependent variable, the CAS, exophthalmos, T2RT (ms), the areas (mm^2) of the five EOMs, and the T2RT of OF were used as independent variables for variable screening ($p < 0.05$), and finally, exophthalmos, the T2RT of MR, the area of IR and LR were included in the linear regression to build a regression model (Table 4).

Table 4. Model of liner regression.

	B	P
Constant	10.426	0.061
Exophthalmos	0.345	0.153
T2RT(MR)	−0.057	0.471
Area (IR)	0.103	0.001
Area (LR)	0.050	0.307

IOP = 10.426 + 0.345 × exophthalmos—0.057 × T2RT (MR)+ 0.103 × Area (IR) + 0.050 × Area (LR). T2RT, T2 relaxation time; MR, medial rectus; IR, inferior rectus; LR, lateral rectus.

Linear regression equation:

$$IOP = 10.426 + 0.345 \times exophthalmos - 0.057 \times T2RT(MR) + 0.103 \times Area\ (IR) + 0.050 \times Area\ (LR)$$

The area of the IR muscle is statistically significant.

4. Discussion

In this study, the values for the CAS, exophthalmos, the T2RT of the MR, IR and LR areas, and the mean area in the higher IOP group were significantly higher than in the lower IOP group. The T2RTs and the areas of the EOMs were higher in the high IOP group, and there was a positive correlation between them. We suggest that there are several reasons for this. First, the thickening of the EOMs makes orbit tissue more crowded, which mechanically compresses the eyeball, resulting in increased IOP. Second, the increased volume increases the pressure of the scleral vein and affects the outflow of the aqueous humor, which also increases the IOP. A study by Seo et al. also showed that the postoperative IOP of TAO patients was significantly lower than their preoperative IOP [14], indicating that the increase in the volume of the orbital tissue did cause an increase in IOP. At the same time, some researchers have suspected that the deposition of hyaluronic acid in the trabecular meshwork of TAO patients could cause obstruction of the outflow of their aqueous humor. Studies have found that the trabecular meshwork was the target tissue of thyroid hormones and that T3 could regulate HA levels. This supports the view that thyroid hormones can regulate the levels of HA in the eyes and may affect the outflow of aqueous humor [8].

TAO is an autoimmune disease characterized by the inflammation of the orbital connective tissue. The orbital volume increases due to increased adipogenesis and the excessive production of glycosaminoglycans, as well as due to EOM fibrosis [15]. Our research found that the exophthalmos and CAS in the high IOP group were significantly higher than those in the low IOP group, and that the IOP and exophthalmos were positively correlated. We believe that high exophthalmos is one of the manifestations of hypertrophy in the intraorbital tissue because the increased tissue volume in the rigid wall of the orbit tends to push the eye forward, causing it to protrude, and the CAS can reflect the inflammation of the orbital tissue and the degree of orbital venous stasis caused by intraorbital crowding [16,17]. Therefore, more hypertrophic EOMs and greater proliferation of orbital adipose tissue will lead to greater exophthalmos and more likely cause higher IOP and CASs.

As mentioned in the introduction, the CAS is a subjective and qualitative measurement method, while an orbital MRI is an objective and quantitative measurement method. At the same time, the T2RT is more reliable in distinguishing the fibrosis expansion in the EOMs with lower disease activity from the inflammation and edema in the EOMs with higher disease activity. Our study quantitatively evaluated the EOM area and the orbital tissue T2RTs of TAO patients. We combined this with IOP measurements and used linear regression modeling to analyze the factors affecting IOP. This is more convincing than previous qualitative analyses.

In the correlation analysis, IOP had the strongest correlation with the IR area. When the regression model of the factors influencing IOP was established, the IR area became the only statistically significant EOM parameter. Previous studies have shown that the EOM most commonly affected by TAO is the IR [18]. We speculate that this may be because the most commonly involved muscle in TAO patients is the IR, which is more representative of the degree of orbital crowding than the other EOMs. At the same time, according to previous studies, the eye position while measuring IOP can also cause a temporary increase in the IOP measurement. For example, IOP is significantly higher when gazing upward than in the primary eye position, which is more pronounced in normal eyes than in TAO patients [19]. Studies on TAO IOP have shown that in a non-relaxed eye position, the infiltration and fibrosis of the EOMs can lead to an ultra-short-term increase in IOP caused by the pressure of EOMs on sclera [20]. At the same time, the study by Gomi et al. has proved that IOP can be significantly reduced by releasing the extraocular muscle restriction in TAO patients [6]. When we measured the IOP, the patients were in the primary position. Therefore, some patients with IR infiltration or fibrosis needed to resist the pulling of the IR, which will inevitably put pressure on the eyeball.

A shortcoming of our research is that a non-contact applanation tonometer was used, which could not measure the true IOP according to the patient's primary eye position as well as handheld tonometers, such as iCare. At the same time, this study found that the measured value of the non-contact applanation tonometer was higher than that of the iCare contact tonometer and the Goldman tonometer [21]. Failure to measure the central corneal thickness is another shortcoming of this study. Because of the heterogeneity between the eyes, the influence of the central corneal thickness on the IOP results needs to be considered.

Some of our research results can provide useful information for clinical use. In all cases of high IOP, clinicians should look for other signs, as elevated IOP may simply be a manifestation of TAO. For high IOP without visual field and optic nerve fiber abnormalities, the cause should be judged carefully. For patients with transient IOP increases due to changes in gaze position, they can be temporarily treated, not for lowering their IOP, but for increased IOP from the crowding of the orbital contents caused by long-term inflammatory reactions; the visual field and the thickness of the nerve fiber layer can be monitored, and the IOP can be appropriately treated according to the situation. At the same time, studies have shown that when compared with glaucoma patients, the TAO 24-h IOP rhythm pattern is closer to that of healthy subjects [22]. Therefore, for those TAO patients with high IOP, a 24-h IOP measurement can also be considered for further judgment.

5. Conclusions

The high IOP in TAO patients is positively correlated with the degree of exophthalmos and EOM inflammation. The orbital MRI EOM state can explain part of the cause of high IOP and provide necessary clinical information for subsequent high IOP treatment.

Author Contributions: Conceptualization, B.L. and X.L.; Data curation, W.W. and Y.Z.; Formal analysis, B.L. and Y.Z.; Investigation, Y.Z. and W.H.; Project administration, B.L.; Supervision, B.L.; Writing—original draft, B.L. and Y.Z.; Writing—review & editing, X.L., H.Z. and W.H. All authors have read and agreed to the published version of the manuscript.

Funding: The work was funded by Natural Science Foundation of Hubei Province (Project Number: 2019CFB494) and Scientific research project of Hubei Provincial Health Commission (Project Number WJ2021M21).

Institutional Review Board Statement: The study was conducted in accordance with the Declaration of Helsinki and approved by the Medical Ethics Committee of Tongji Hospital Affiliated to Tongji Medical College of Huazhong University of Science and Technology (protocol code TJ-IRB20190417 and 2019 April 25 of approval)" for studies involving humans.

Informed Consent Statement: Informed consent was obtained from all subjects involved in the study. Written informed consent has been obtained from the patients to publish this paper.

Data Availability Statement: Not applicable.

Conflicts of Interest: The authors declare no conflict of interest.

References

1. Hiromatsu, Y.; Eguchi, H.; Tani, J.; Kasaoka, M.; Teshima, Y. Graves' ophthalmopathy: Epidemiology and natural history. *Intern. Med.* **2014**, *53*, 353–360. [CrossRef] [PubMed]
2. Mallika, P.; Tan, A.; Aziz, S.; Alwi, S.S.; Chong, M.; Vanitha, R.; Intan, G. Thyroid associated ophthalmopathy-a review. *Malays. Fam. Physician* **2009**, *4*, 8–14. [PubMed]
3. Burch, H.B.; Wartofsky, L. Graves' ophthalmopathy: Current concepts regarding pathogenesis and management. *Endocr. Rev.* **1993**, *14*, 747–793. [PubMed]
4. Kalmann, R.; Mourits, M.P. Prevalence and management of elevated intraocular pressure in patients with Graves' orbitopathy. *Br. J. Ophthalmol.* **1998**, *82*, 754–757. [CrossRef]
5. Cockerham, K.P.; Pal, C.; Jani, B.; Wolter, A.; Kennerdell, J.S. The prevalence and implications of ocular hypertension and glaucoma in thyroid-associated orbitopathy. *Ophthalmology* **1997**, *104*, 914–917. [CrossRef]
6. Gomi, C.F.; Yates, B.; Kikkawa, D.O.; Levi, L.; Weinreb, R.N.; Granet, D.B. Effect on intraocular pressure of extraocular muscle surgery for thyroid-associated ophthalmopathy. *Am. J. Ophthalmol.* **2007**, *144*, 654–657. [CrossRef]
7. Konuk, O.; Onaran, Z.; Oktar, S.O.; Yucel, C.; Unal, M. Intraocular pressure and superior ophthalmic vein blood flow velocity in Graves' orbitopathy: Relation with the clinical features. *Graefe's Arch. Clin. Exp. Ophthalmol.* **2009**, *247*, 1555–1559. [CrossRef]
8. Duncan, K.G.; Jumper, M.D.; Ribeiro, R.C.J.; Bailey, K.R.; Yen, P.; Sugawara, A.; Patel, A.; Stern, R.; Chin, W.W.; Baxter, J.D.; et al. Human trabecular meshwork cells as a thyroid hormone target tissue: Presence of functional thyroid hormone receptors. *Graefe's Arch. Clin. Exp. Ophthalmol.* **1999**, *237*, 231–240. [CrossRef]
9. Stoyanova, N.S.; Konareva-Kostianeva, M.; Mitkova-Hristova, V.; Angelova, I. Correlation between Intraocular Pressure and Thickness of Extraocular Muscles, the Severity and Activity of Thyroid-associated Orbitopathy. *Folia Med.* **2019**, *61*, 90–96. [CrossRef]
10. Yokoyama, N.; Nagataki, S.; Uetani, M.; Ashizawa, K.; Eguchi, K. Role of magnetic resonance imaging in the assessment of disease activity in thyroid-associated ophthalmopathy. *Thyroid* **2002**, *12*, 223–227. [CrossRef]
11. Ohnishi, T.; Noguchi, S.; Murakami, N.; Tajiri, J.; Harao, M.; Kawamoto, H.; Hoshi, H.; Jinnouchi, S.; Jinnouchi, S.; Nagamachi, S. Extraocular muscles in Graves ophthalmopathy: Usefulness of T2 relaxation time measurements. *Radiology* **1994**, *190*, 857–862. [CrossRef] [PubMed]
12. Lee, A.J.; Rochtchina, E.; Wang, J.J.; Healey, P.R.; Mitchell, P. Open-angle glaucoma and systemic thyroid disease in an older population: The Blue Mountains Eye Study. *Eye* **2004**, *18*, 600–608. [CrossRef] [PubMed]
13. Bartalena, L.; Baldeschi, L.; Dickinson, A.; Eckstein, A.; Kendall-Taylor, P.; Marcocci, C.; Mourits, M.; Perros, P.; Boboridis, K.; Boschi, A.; et al. Consensus statement of the European Group on Graves' orbitopathy (EUGOGO) on management of GO. *Eur. J. Endocrinol.* **2008**, *158*, 273–285. [CrossRef] [PubMed]

14. Seo, Y.; Shin, W.B.; Bae, H.W.; Yoon, J.S. Effects of Orbital Decompression on Lamina Cribrosa Depth in Patients with Graves' Orbitopathy. *Korean J. Ophthalmol.* **2019**, *33*, 436–445. [CrossRef]

15. Eckstein, A.K.; Johnson, K.T.M.; Thanos, M.; Esser, J.; Ludgate, M.J.H. Current insights into the pathogenesis of Graves' orbitopathy. *Horm. Metab. Res.* **2009**, *41*, 456–464. [CrossRef]

16. Perros, P.; Kendall-Taylor, P. Pathogenetic mechanisms in thyroid-associated ophthalmopathy. *J. Intern. Med.* **1992**, *231*, 205–211. [CrossRef]

17. Saeed, P.; Rad, S.T.; Bisschop, P. Dysthyroid Optic Neuropathy. *Ophthalmic Plast. Reconstr. Surg.* **2018**, *34*, S60–S67. [CrossRef]

18. Currie, Z.I.; Lewis, S.; Clearkin, L.G. Dysthyroid eye disease masquerading as glaucoma. *Ophthalmic Physiol. Opt.* **1991**, *11*, 176–179. [CrossRef]

19. Takahashi, Y.; Nakamura, Y.; Ichinose, A.; Kakizaki, H. Intraocular Pressure Change with Eye Positions Before and After Orbital Decompression for Thyroid Eye Disease. *Ophthalmic Plast. Reconstr. Surg.* **2014**, *30*, 47–50. [CrossRef]

20. Haefliger, I.O.; von Arx, G.; Pimentel, A.R. Pathophysiology of intraocular pressure increase and glaucoma prevalence in thyroid eye disease: A mini-review. *Klin. Mon. Für Augenheilkd.* **2010**, *227*, 292–293. [CrossRef]

21. Kuebler, A.G.; Wiecha, C.; Reznicek, L.; Klingenstein, A.; Halfter, K.; Priglinger, S.; Hintschich, C. Comparison of different devices to measure the intraocular pressure in thyroid-associated orbitopathy. *Graefe's Arch. Clin. Exp. Ophthalmol.* **2019**, *257*, 2025–2032. [CrossRef] [PubMed]

22. Parekh, A.S.; Mansouri, K.; Weinreb, R.N.; Tafreshi, A.; Korn, B.S.; Kikkawa, D.O. Twenty-four-hour intraocular pressure patterns in patients with thyroid eye disease. *Clin. Exp. Ophthalmol.* **2015**, *43*, 108–114. [CrossRef] [PubMed]

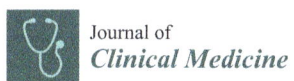

Journal of
Clinical Medicine

MDPI

Review

A Review of Selective Laser Trabeculoplasty: "The Hype Is Real"

Tomislav Sarenac [1,2] , Anela Bečić Turkanović [1], Peter Ferme [1] and Tomaž Gračner [1,2,*]

1   Department of Ophthalmology, University Medical Center Maribor, Ljubljanska 5, 2000 Maribor, Slovenia; dr.tomislav.sarenac@gmail.com (T.S.); anela.becic@gmail.com (A.B.T.); pferme@gmail.com (P.F.)
2   Faculty of Medicine, University of Maribor, Taborska Ulica 8, 2000 Maribor, Slovenia
*   Correspondence: tomaz.gracner@ukc-mb.si

Abstract: Presently, there is no efficacious treatment for glaucomatous optic neuropathy; the current treatment is focused on lowering intraocular pressure (IOP). Studies have demonstrated the safety and efficacy of selective laser trabeculoplasty (SLT) in reducing the IOP in eyes with open-angle (OAG) glaucoma or ocular hypertension (OH). Moreover, the European Glaucoma Society has instated SLT as the first-line or adjunctive treatment in OAG or OH, reiterating its clinical significance. In this review, we outline the old and the new roles of SLT, with an emphasis on clinical practice, and look further into its renewed appeal and future developments.

Keywords: glaucoma; laser treatment; trabecular meshwork; dropless treatment; intraocular pressure

Citation: Sarenac, T.; Bečić Turkanović, A.; Ferme, P.; Gračner, T. A Review of Selective Laser Trabeculoplasty: "The Hype Is Real". *J. Clin. Med.* **2022**, *11*, 3879. https://doi.org/10.3390/jcm11133879

Academic Editors: Maria Letizia Salvetat, Marco Zeppieri and Paolo Brusini

Received: 27 March 2022
Accepted: 29 June 2022
Published: 4 July 2022

Publisher's Note: MDPI stays neutral with regard to jurisdictional claims in published maps and institutional affiliations.

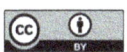
1. Introduction

Glaucoma is the third largest cause of blindness worldwide, after unaddressed refractive errors and cataracts [1]. The global prevalence in the elderly population worldwide is estimated at 3.5%. It was presumed that by 2020 there would have been 79.6 million people affected with glaucoma; this number might increase to 111.8 million globally by 2040, causing a significant decrease in the quality of life and economic burdens [2]. It is assessed that, currently, 57.5 million people are affected by primary open-angle glaucoma (POAG) [3]. The main goals of glaucoma treatment are to preserve visual functioning (adequate to individual needs), with minimal or no side effects, for the expected lifetime of the patient, without any disruption of normal activities, at a sustainable cost [4]. Glaucoma is a disease associated with optic nerve degradation (glaucomatous optic neuropathy), which causes visual field loss, and is responsible for significant visual morbidity, i.e., loss of independence. Presently, there is no proven efficacious treatment of glaucomatous optic neuropathy. Therefore, the treatment is focused on reducing intraocular pressure (IOP), which is the only risk factor linked to glaucoma progression that can be successfully influenced [5]. Reducing IOP can be achieved with medical, surgical, or laser treatments. The most common initial treatment is with hypotensive drops; however, patient adherence to a treatment regimen could be relatively low [6]. In 1998, the first successful protocol of selective laser trabeculoplasty (SLT) was established, a 532-nm Q-switched frequency-doubled Nd:YAG laser with a single pulse of short duration and low fluence was used and has become an established method for lowering the IOP in the treatment of open-angle glaucoma (OAG) and ocular hypertension (OH) [7]. It targets the trabecular meshwork (TM), which improves aqueous outflow, contributes to reducing IOP, and does not require extensive patient compliance.

Multiple studies have, to a high extent, demonstrated the safety and efficacy of SLT in reducing IOP in OAG or OH. However, most of the studies have reported on SLT as an adjunctive treatment [8–11]. This has left the role of primary SLT somewhat ambiguous; however, it appears to be vastly more important in clinical practice than ascribed in the guidelines. SLT could be considered one of the cornerstones of dropless glaucoma therapy in newly diagnosed OAG or OH [4]. This has recently been further upheld by randomized controlled trials, supporting the case for SLT as the first-line treatment of glaucoma, such as in the laser in glaucoma and ocular hypertension (LiGHT) study [12]. The European Glaucoma Society Terminology and Guidelines for Glaucoma, 5th Edition, recently listed SLT earlier in the algorithm of glaucoma treatment [13]. It was stated that SLT can be used sooner, as an alternative to failed first monotherapy, as a single glaucoma treatment, or as an adjunctive treatment later on; this has renewed the appeal of SLT to clinicians.

In the following review, we will outline some of the crucial clinical guidelines for SLT, especially in OAG and OH, and concisely provide useful data to provide more information about this topic, focusing on recent relevant studies. Our search for studies was conducted using the PubMed database; the search strategy is available in Supplementary Materials. Finally, promising future directions in this area will be introduced, with an outline of novel clinical studies.

2. Basic Principles

Although lasers have gained great popularity in glaucoma management over the last two decades, the history of laser treatment for glaucoma started back in the early 1970s with Q-switched laser goniopuncture being the first technique described [14,15]. While the technique succeeded in IOP reduction, success was short-term. A few years later, argon laser trabeculoplasty (ALT) was presented by Wise and Witter [16]. They postulated a mechanical mechanism, in which laser-induced thermal burns of the TM caused collagen shrinkage following scarring of the TM. This tightens the corresponding meshwork and reopens the adjacent, untreated intertrabecular spaces, facilitating aqueous outflow. Ultrastructural TM modifications occurred before the IOP-reducing response, suggesting the mechanism of action is more complex. The cellular theory proposes that, in response to coagulative necrosis induced by the laser, there is elevated cytokine production, causing remodeling of the juxtacanalicular extracellular matrix, a likely site for the aqueous outflow resistance, improving the outflow facility [17,18].

ALT causes IOP reduction through increased aqueous outflow, confirmed by both tonography and aqueous dynamic studies [19]. With 30% IOP reduction, ALT was presented as a first-line therapy and as a second-line therapy [20]. Adverse events related to ALT were transient acute IOP spikes following the laser, development of peripheral anterior synechiae (PAS), corneal endothelial changes, and acute anterior uveitis [21]. Although serious side effects rarely occurred, most of the authors reported falling effects over time [22,23]. Latina and Park first introduced selective laser trabeculoplasty in their in vitro study in 1995 [24]. Using Q-switched frequency-doubled 532 nm Nd:YAG laser SLT targets the pigmented TM cells selectively without damaging the adjacent non-pigmented cells or other structures of the TM [25].

3. Mechanism of Action

The mechanism by which SLT lowers IOP is not completely understood and is likely multifactorial. SLT is based on the principle of selective photothermolysis first described by Anderson and Parrish 1983, in which radiation energy applied to the TM selectively targets pigmented cells without causing thermal damage to adjunctive structures [26]. Latina and Park demonstrated the SLT effect by selectively targeting pigmented TM in their in vitro [24] study on bovine TM cell cultures, and a few years later, in their in vivo study [7]. The extent of pigmented cell depletion after SLT depends on the magnitude of the energy used and the distance from the center of the irradiated zone reported by Wood et al. in their in vitro study [27]. In 2001, Kramer and Noecker reported less structural damage to the human TM in SLT-treated eyes compared to ALT in their in vitro study [28]. In 2003, Cvenkel et al. compared histopathological changes occurring in the eyes after ALT and SLT in their in vivo study and reported a smaller extent of the damage to the TM after SLT [29]. A meta-analysis comparing ALT to SLT revealed similar efficacy in the therapeutic IOP response. However, SLT has resulted in a greater reduction in the number of glaucoma medications versus ALT [30,31]. Moreover, SLT appears to be more effective in IOP reduction in retreatment versus ALT [32]. The authors report SLT's effect in lowering IOP by increased outflow through TM [33,34] without significant differences in the aqueous humor dynamics comparing Caucasian and African races [35]. Vikas et al. discovered the IOP-lowering effect of SLT being mediated through an increase in the outflow facility using fluorophotometry and tonography in their study. They suggested higher aqueous flow and a lower outflow facility as predictive factors for better response to SLT [36]. As described, structural damage occurring to the TM in ALT is not detected in SLT patients; therefore, the mechanical and structural theories that have been suggested to explain ALT's mechanism of action do not fully apply to SLT [37]. Furthermore, the biological theory of SLT action proposes that the laser modifies cellular activity by cytokine release, facilitating aqueous outflow [38]. Lee et al. revealed that the matrix metalloproteinase release was pigment-dependent and was not detected in non-pigmented cells after SLT [39]. The biological and biochemical changes have been observed in the TM after SLT. Alvardo et al.'s in vitro study reported a substantial increase in the number of monocytes/macrophages in the TM after SLT, resulting in the outflow facility augmentation and conductivity of human Schlemm's canal endothelial cells [40].

Bradley et al. used the human anterior segment organ cultures, subjected them to laser trabeculoplasty, and detected increased stromelysin expression provoked by elevated IL-1 beta and TNF-alpha, which work synergistically [41], resulting in remodeling of the juxtacanalicular extracellular matrix and restoring normal outflow facility [17].

Izzotti et al. published a study aimed at the gene expression changes induced in TM cells by SLT using hybridization on miRNA-microarray and laser scanner analysis [42]. The study showed expression modulation of genes involved in cell motility, intercellular connections, extracellular matrix production, protein repair, DNA repair, membrane repair, reactive oxygen species production, glutamate toxicity, antioxidant activities, and inflammation. Regulation of aqueous humor outflow from the anterior chamber was reported to be modulated with SLT at the postgenomic molecular level without inducing damage at molecular or phenotypic levels.

4. Indications and Preoperative Evaluation

From a pragmatic clinical standpoint, we divide therapeutic indications for SLT into three groups.

The first group involves patients with POAG or OH without any prior glaucoma treatment, where SLT can be used as a primary (first-line) therapy. Most studies have compared SLT efficacy against topical medication and have found similar IOP-lowering efficacy. The LiGHT trial showed that 74.6% of eyes treated with primary SLT achieved drop-free disease control at the 3-year follow-up and has a comparable IOP reduction and complication profile to MIGS with smaller anatomical changes to the angle, and can therefore be recommended as an alternative or a first step treatment [43,44].

The second group involves patients with POAG or OH (with uncontrollable IOP and disease progression) who are already receiving glaucoma treatment, where SLT can be used as adjunctive therapy. Studies have shown that SLT successfully lowers IOP in (the eyes of) patients who are on hypotensive medication, have undergone previous ALT treatment, or have had glaucoma surgery [4,7,45,46]. SLT can also be repeated with an IOP reduction similar to the first treatment, or be used to delay glaucoma surgery [47–49].

The third group is patients with POAG or OH on glaucoma medication with adequate IOP control and without glaucoma progression, where SLT can be used as replacement therapy, i.e., to lessen the burden of medications. Since drops require strict daily dosing and have many side effects, adherence to medication is often poor. Treatment with SLT in patients already treated with glaucoma medication can lead to better IOP. A study by Lee et al. showed that patients treated with SLT require fewer medications to maintain their IOP goals [50]. In a study by De Keyser et al., SLT was able to completely replace medical therapy in 77% of patients' eyes after 18 months, and may severely reduce local and systemic side-effects commonly caused by medication [51].

However, in the published literature, indications for treatment are most commonly divided by glaucoma type. The majority of studies have focused on SLT treatment in POAG and OH, but it is increasingly being used in other glaucoma types. When used in patients with pseudoexfoliative glaucoma, SLT shows similar IOP reduction to POAG [38,52–55]. In pigmentary glaucoma, the results of using SLT are similar, but there seems to be an increased rate of postoperative complications, probably due to a higher TM pigmentation and greater energy absorption [56]. Normal-tension glaucoma has lower baseline IOP so the IOP reduction is proportionally smaller [50,57]. SLT has also been used in primary angle-closure glaucoma where it has shown comparable IOP reduction to POAG, but at least 180° of the TM has to be visible and patients have to have an open laser iridotomy [58,59]. SLT has also shown promising results in treating steroid-induced glaucoma [60,61].

SLT is contraindicated when the TM cannot be visualized (e.g., angle closure, anterior synechiae, corneal opacity, poor patient cooperation, etc.). Even though there is a study that suggests that it is safe to perform SLT in patients with uveitic glaucoma, it should absolutely be avoided in active uveitis and be reserved only for the most refractory cases [62]. According to mechanisms of action, SLT is not suited for neovascular and congenital glaucoma treatment, where IOP cannot be decreased by TM outflow modification, although successful cases have been reported in pediatric cases of POAG of different pathophysiologies, with normal angles [63].

5. Operative Technique

To assess if the patient is an eligible candidate for SLT, a thorough glaucoma evaluation has to be made before treatment. Special importance has to be given to gonioscopy, where the visibility and pigmentation of the TM have to be evaluated.

Studies have mostly shown that perioperative topical medications lower the risk of an IOP spike but there is no consensus on what the best prophylactic treatment is [64]. Most practitioners recommend using a topical alpha-adrenergic agonist (apraclonidine or brimonidine) 15 min to 60 min before treatment; some practitioners also use miotic drops (1% to 4% Pilocarpine). A topical anesthetic is given and a gonioscopic contact lens is selected, preferably one without a laser spot magnification. There are plenty of lenses made especially for SLT. A coupling gel should be used. A 400-micron spot size and 3 ns pulse duration are standard for SLT. The aiming beam is pointed over the entire width of the TM. The initial power is normally set at 0.8 mJ, but should be lower in heavily pigmented meshworks (e.g., 0.4 mJ), since side effects can be more severe if a higher power is used [56]. The power is then increased or decreased until the minimal power to form small cavitation bubbles is acquired (threshold power), and then decreased by 0.1 mJ to set the power used for treatment. Some practitioners prefer to treat with the threshold power though; 25–100 adjacent (but not overlapping shots) are applied over 90°–360° of the meshwork, depending on the protocol used. It is advisable to always treat the same quadrants or halves first (for example, the bottom half), so that if retreatment is performed, it can be conducted on the other (previously untreated) half. Immediately after treatment, another drop of alpha-adrenergic agonist can be given. IOP should be remeasured 30 to 60 min after treatment; if it is elevated, additional medication may be needed and a closer follow-up planned.

Many studies and meta-analyses have compared the treatment of different degrees of the TM. While some found a significant difference in the IOP-lowering effect between treating 180° and 360° of the TM in POAG [34,65], others did not [66–68], but one study showed lesser diurnal IOP fluctuations when treating 360° [69]. Most reviews have concluded that there is no significant difference when treating 180° or 360° [11,38,70], as confirmed by a recent meta-analysis [71]. Studies have also researched different power levels, mostly finding that a higher power leads to greater IOP reduction (but also more adverse effects) [72,73].

6. Postoperative Management

There is an ongoing debate regarding the best peri- and post-operative treatments, and many studies have attempted to establish the best practices, mostly with contradicting results. The main adverse effects are post-operative IOP elevation (IOP spike) and anterior chamber inflammation. Depending on the practitioner and the patient (e.g., baseline IOP, advanced glaucomatous damage), topical anti-inflammatory and IOP-lowering drops are commonly prescribed for 4–7 days but are often not needed.

IOP spikes can occur after SLT, especially in high-risk patients and they typically arise within 24 h. Zhang et al. [64] analyzed 22 randomized clinical trials (1 SLT and 21 ALT trials) and concluded that the use of perioperative IOP-lowering medications is superior to no medications in preventing IOP spikes after laser trabeculoplasty, with little to no adverse effects. Apraclonidine, brimonidine, acetazolamide, and pilocarpine are commonly used. If SLT is used as an adjunctive treatment, existing glaucoma medication is typically continued.

Another important factor is managing postoperative inflammation. Because of a typical anterior chamber inflammation seen after ALT, most practitioners routinely prescribe anti-inflammatories, especially steroids, and the practice continues with SLT. Treatment with steroids or NSAIDs has not shown a significant decrease in postoperative anterior chamber inflammation [74]. Since ALT and SLT have different mechanisms of action, questions about the long-term effects of post-SLT inflammation on the IOP-lowering effects remain.

One of the mechanisms of action in SLT is thought to be the activation of inflammatory pathways that cause TM remodeling and better functioning of the TM, with increased outflow and a reduction of IOP [33,36]; therefore, a possible contra-productiveness of using anti-inflammatory medication was proposed. On the other hand, inflammation may cause fibrosis and scarring, restricting outflow and thereby decreasing SLT efficacy, a mechanism that anti-inflammatory medications could partially prevent. Most of the studies found no benefits in postoperative treatments with anti-inflammatory drops, especially in patients with lower baseline IOP [74–77]. Surprisingly, the steroid after laser trabeculoplasty (SALT) [78] study found significantly better IOP reduction at 12 weeks in patients' eyes treated with steroid or NSAID drops after SLT (compared to the placebo) and, therefore, contradicts most previous studies.

It is therefore not possible to establish a clear protocol for postoperative management. After reviewing the available literature, our conclusion is that it should be individually tailored to the patient (baseline IOP, glaucoma risk, previous medication, or surgery) and the performed treatment (degree of trabecular meshwork treatment, energy used, etc.).

7. Outcomes

There are numerous studies that contribute to the topic of SLT and its outcomes. SLT has mainly been compared to monotherapy or is used as an adjunctive treatment in various types of glaucoma patients. Here, we concisely provide outlines of the clinically most relevant recent studies for SLT as a first-line therapy or as a means for lowering the dependence on drops or adjunctive therapy. In this section of our review, the participants were mostly patients with POAG and OH, albeit SLT could be effectively used in another OAG, such as pseudo-exfoliative or pigmentary [11].

The hype that SLT can challenge medical therapy as a first-line treatment was materialized with the LiGHT trial, which compared the cost-effectiveness, efficacy, and safety of SLT versus hypotensive medical therapy for the initial treatment of glaucoma. The authors concluded that 'SLT should be offered as a first-line treatment for open-angle glaucoma and ocular hypertension' [12]. This randomized controlled trial (RCT) was one of the largest to date and was diligently designed around putting SLT first in a real-life glaucoma practice. Another reason why this trial stands out is because of the definition of target IOP reduction from baseline. Unlike the majority of studies, where >20% reduction in IOP was targeted, a more customizable approach was taken. Target IOP was established according to each patient's glaucoma severity, and the target was modifiable during the study. In cases of glaucoma progression, despite IOP being targeted, the target IOP was further lowered, and vice versa in cases where no progression was detected. The follow-up and adjunctive treatment were similarly determined according to glaucoma progression. In our opinion, this trial setting contributes to the real-world character and subsequently provides more clinically relevant data. On the other hand, this could be considered less stringent, since "reaching the target" did not necessarily coincide with >20% reduction in IOP as strived for in most other studies reviewed. This might have contributed to the high success rate of the SLT-first group. In the trial, treatment-naïve POAG and OH patients were stratified into the medication-first group and the SLT-first group. In the SLT group, 95% of patients reached the target IOP at 36 months of this 78.2%, with no adjunctive medication, whereas in the medication group, 93.1% reached the target, with 64.6% requiring only prostaglandins, which were prescribed as a first choice. The difference was perhaps most striking in the number of trabeculectomies, where none of the 356 patients in the SLT-first group needed surgery and 11 of 362 patients in the medication-first group needed incisional glaucoma surgery. Furthermore, during the study period, less treatment escalations were observed in the SLT-first group. Transient side effects, such as discomfort and hyperemia, were common (34%); however, they were temporary in contrast to the known side effects of hypotensive medication. This trial contributed significantly to considering SLT as a first-line glaucoma treatment, with nearly no side effects, which translates to treatment efficiency, especially regarding patient compliance with medical therapy. A further post hoc analysis has shown similar results for POAG and OH patients [79], where approximately 75% of patients reached dropless IOP control at 36 months after primary or repetitive SLT, with the majority achieving the target after the first SLT. Regarding glaucoma progression (in terms of visual field testing), it has been shown that patients in the SLT- first group were less likely to have rapid visual field progression [43].

In a retrospective study by Ansari [80], with a 10-year follow-up success rate of 72% (at 10 years), with visual field loss remaining stable, 60% required retreatment in 10 years. Here, the success rate as the main outcome measure was defined as an >20% reduction in IOP and IOP < 19 mmHg. In addition, no patients in the study needed trabeculectomy at 10 years akin to results from the LiGHT trial. Albeit, the LiGHT trial has not shown significant improvements in health-related quality of life compared to medical therapy, we agree with Ansari, who stated that longer-term data from their study could imply substantial improvements in quality of life, most likely regarding medication avoidance, possible toxic effects, and costs. This matter was also studied by Ang et al. [81], where the quality of life was no different between naïve-treated SLT or topical medication; however, it was reported that a higher proportion of patients with eyelid erythema and conjunctival injection were found in the medication-only group.

One recent meta-analysis by Chi et al. [71] on SLT treatment in naïve patients versus medication with 1229 patients has reported no difference in treatments with SLT and medication-only treatments regarding the IOP reduction. Furthermore, SLT was slightly more effective when the medication-only group was taken as a reference, with 180-degree SLT performing slightly better than the rest of the trabeculoplasty methods analyzed (albeit these differences were not significant). Furthermore, Chi et al. showed that patients who underwent SLT and needed drops ultimately required less medication than the medication-only group. These findings are in accordance with other metanalyses we found [31,81,82]. In the meta-analysis by Zhou et al., where different modalities of laser trabeculoplasty were studied on 2859 eyes, they found 180-degree SLT to be somewhat more effective at reducing the number of medications needed in comparison to ALT, whereas no difference was found between five other modalities (270-degree SLT, 360-degree SLT, new laser trabeculoplasty, transscleral 360-degree SLT without gonioscopy, and low-energy 360-degree SLT). All of the above have demonstrated equal effectiveness for IOP decreases in comparison to hypotensive medications [31].

We believe that real clinical data, collected during every-day clinical practice, adds to the relevance of SLT, to some extent, when validating the results from trials and metanalyses. However, in the real world, separating the effects of SLT from the effects of coexistent hypotensive medication in patients is nearly impossible. Up until now, simultaneous use of therapies usually occurred in the average glaucoma practice. Two of such real-world data reports of retrospective studies on SLT have been published recently and have shown somewhat fewer persuasive results.

Khawaja et al. published a study that was conducted in the United Kingdom (UK); they demonstrated that 70% of eyes responded to SLT treatment at 6 months, but success by 2 years was sustained only in 27% of cases [83]. The Kaplan–Meier survival analysis has shown that 83% of eyes could fail at 36 months. The measures of failure could be considered stringent by some, e.g., an inadequate reduction in IOP (>21 mmHg or <20% reduction), an increase in the number of glaucoma medications, or a subsequent glaucoma procedure, including repeated SLT. Efficacy of SLT was higher in cases with higher baseline IOP (IOP > 21 mmHg) and was not altered by the severity of glaucoma or the coexistent use of hypotensive medication. In cases of higher baseline IOP, there was a 32% lower risk of failure compared to the (eyes of) patients with IOP ≤ 21 mmHg at baseline. It could be extrapolated that SLT is more effective in OH or high-IOP OAG than for normal-tension glaucoma. Mostly, patients were on prostaglandins and no association to SLT failure was found when compared to the rest of the hypotensive medication used. Patient selection was not as rigorous as in LiGHT and the metanalysis by Chi et al. In those publications, naïve mild glaucoma patients with no concurrent ocular diseases were included (visual field not worse than −12 dB in the better eye on the Humphrey field analyzer in the LiGHT trial).

The following study by Abe et al. [84] revolved around similar endpoints and reported significantly better results regarding SLT efficiency. SLT was studied for three common indications: uncontrolled IOP without medications, uncontrolled IOP with medications, and controlled IOP with medications for the purpose of reducing the number of hypotensive medications. Treatment failure was considered in the following cases: subsequent procedures (including SLT), IOP > 21 mmHg or IOP reduction < 20%, and an increase in the number of different glaucoma drops. A total of 54.7% failed according to these criteria during the 36-month follow-up. When the Kaplan–Meier survival analysis was stratified according to the indications listed above, SLT as a first-line treatment had 80% success at 12 months, which decreased to 46% at 36 months. The commonest scenario in the study was SLT in patients with medically well-controlled IOP, with an intention to lower the number of drops taken (55%). In this group, 49% had success with SLT at 36 months and 37% remained dropless for 36 months. This implies that SLT is a valid tool to reduce the number of hypotensive medications. Denser angle pigmentation, corticosteroid treatment following SLT, and earlier stage glaucoma were associated with lower risks of failure. The latter reiterates the concept that SLT is a valid option as a first-line treatment, especially in early, mild glaucoma compared to patients with advanced glaucoma.

8. Complications

SLT is considered a safe procedure and is well-tolerated by patients with low complication rates, ranging from 0% to 65.7% [81,85]. Complications associated with SLT are mostly transient and self-limiting, such as momentary mild redness, discomfort or mild pain, anterior chamber inflammation, or an IOP spike in the first week. The LiGHT trial reported SLT as a safe method, preserving its safety frame in the procedure's repetition [47]. Although this study reported only self-limiting adverse effects of lasers, there are some uncommon and severe complications, such as transient corneal thinning, endothelial decompensation, foveal burn, and corneal haze, as reported in the literature [11,56,86]. Significant complications, such as severe uveitis, IOP spikes that are more than 15 mmHg, etc., are contraindications for SLT repetition [87]. In this section, prevailing complications are described and case reports of sporadic serious complications are listed.

Iritis is a relatively common and mild complication occurring 2–3 days after SLT [56]. Damji et al. reported significantly lower incidences of the anterior chamber reaction in SLT compared with ALT [88]. Ayala et al. compared post-laser inflammation in the anterior chamber in patients with POAG with pseudoexfoliation (reported to be equal) [89].

Post-laser IOP elevation has been reported, ranging from 0% to 28% [38]. Latina et al. defined the IOP spike as 5 mmHg or more while Koucheki et al. defined IOP elevation as 6 mmHg or more and reported an IOP spike to be closely connected to the pigmentation extent of TM [7,56]. Harasymowycz et al. reported an IOP spike in their observational study of heavily-pigmented TMs and suggested special cautiousness with pigmentary dispersion syndrome and a heavily-pigmented TM [90].

Koktekir et al. reported severe bilateral anterior uveitis with posterior synechia, corneal haze, and endothelial loss after unilateral SLT, which proposes an autoimmune systemic response to be involved in the mechanism of action [91]. Systemic response in SLT is also supported in the findings by McIlraith et al.; they reported an IOP reduction in the untreated eye by 8% [92].

In a prospective study of 64 patients, evaluating macular thickness as measured by optical coherence tomography, the researchers did not find any significant increase in macular thickness after SLT [85]. However, there is one report of SLT-induced central macular edema and one report of worsening preexisting CME after SLT [93]. Wechsler and Wechsler reported a case of central macular edema after SLT [94]; nonetheless, it was a patient with preexisting CME and it was likely recidivant CME after topical therapy cessation rather than SLT-induced CME.

There were two cases of hyphema reported in the literature. The first case reported unilateral hyphema after bilateral SLT, which resolved spontaneously [95] and the second reported hyphema in a 77-year-old patient on topical and systemic NSAIDs [96].

In one case, choroidal effusion with narrow angles, and the other with milder previously described complications, developed after SLT, but were successfully treated and resolved [97]. While corneal edema occurs in 0.8% of cases [98], serious corneal complications, such as corneal haze and corneal melting, were reported [99,100]. An inflammatory cascade induced by SLT might reactivate herpes simplex infection, particularly in those patients on concomitant topical prostaglandin analogues [86]. An increase in central corneal thickness should also be considered in post-procedure IOP measurement [101]. There was one case of unilateral keratitis of unknown etiology after consecutive bilateral SLT [102]. Knickelbein et al. reported four cases of post-SLT corneal edema with subsequent thinning and a hyperopic shift, of which, two patients required contact lenses [103]. Special caution should be considered in treating post-LASIK patients. Holz and Pirouzian reported a case with bilateral diffuse lamellar keratitis after consecutive bilateral SLT [104].

Fortunately, severe complications are uncommon; nonetheless, they can threaten one's sight. Therefore, they should be recognized, treated promptly, and all measures should be taken to avoid them [105].

9. Other Considerations: Retreatment, Predictors of Success, Cost-Effectiveness

The definition of SLT retreatment is somewhat ambiguous, because of variable protocols of 180-degree and 360-degree TM treatments. A repeat 180-degree approach could be considered a subsequent SLT in yet untreated TM. In the following studies, the 360-degree approach was used in repeating the SLT, which might be in fact considered as retreatment. Moreover, it was demonstrated that overlapping laser spots in a 180-degree SLT are linked to lower efficacy as compared to 360-degree nonoverlapping SLT [106]. Multiple studies have shown that SLT can be effectively repeated after the initial effect wears off [49,107]. In the LiGHT trial, it was demonstrated that if SLT is repeated as needed, the Kaplan–Meier survival estimates are better than if patients were managed with a single SLT treatment [47]. Repeating SLT in treatment naïve patients would thus yield far better IOP control in the long run. This was, to some extent, confirmed in a comparable real-life study by Ang et al. [108], where 45.7% of patients who maintained IOP-reduction at 24 months were treated twice.

Another glimpse into real-world practice can be provided by a survey study by Canadian ophthalmologists on laser trabeculoplasty. A total of 87.1% of the participants thought of SLT as a repeatable procedure, mostly one or two repetitions [109]. In a retrospective study by Ansari, in the first year, 11% needed re-treatment; this increased to 40% at 5, and 58% at 10 years. Higher baseline IOP was significantly associated with an increased rate of retreatment and shorter retreatment times [80]. It was shown that repeating SLT in a timeframe shorter than one year after the initial treatment yielded a better success rate than if performed later [107]. Furthermore, the duration of success seemed longer after repeated SLT (13.1 months in comparison to 6.9 months after primary SLT) as shown by Avery et al. [110]. The notion of the added effect of second SLT was confirmed by the post hoc analysis of the SLT treatment arm in the LiGHT trial, where adjusted absolute IOP reduction was greater after SLT was repeated [47].

SLT seems to be generally accepted as effective; however, some patients in the studies performed better than others. Two recent studies [111,112] determined that pretreatment IOP was the only predictor of success after primary SLT. Hirabayashi et al. [113] stated that baseline IOP of >18 mmHg was significantly associated with increased success and that the IOP-lowering effect was greatest at 2 months and 6 months of follow-up. The effect of higher baseline IOP on success was confirmed in the real-world retrospective studies [83,84]. Khawaja et al. found that factors, such as glaucoma type or grade, TM pigmentation, or the type of topical medication, did not seem to predict SLT success. On the other hand, Abe et al. found such factors were associated with a lower risk for failure (denser angle pigmentation, corticosteroid treatment following SLT, and earlier stage glaucoma). The total energy delivered seem to have no role. The post hoc analysis of LiGHT demonstrated only two significant correlations: absolute IOP-reduction is positively predicted by higher IOP at baseline and slightly negatively by female gender [47]. It seems that patient selection based on predictors of success is yet to be fully comprehended; however, it appears that at a higher baseline, IOP could be the most significant. Recently, a retrospective study was published, examining the possibility of predicting the SLT outcome based on responsiveness to treatment with ripasudil drops. Ripasudil is one of the Rho-kinase inhibitors, which has distinct intracellular effects in the areas of tissue remodeling, fibrosis, and healing. It has a different mode of action compared to traditional medication in a way that it causes TM and Schlemm's canal changes, resulting in a higher uveoscleral outflow, lowering IOP [114]. It was shown that patients who respond well to treatment with ripasudil had significantly better SLT success ratios compared to patients who were unresponsive to ripasudil treatment [115].

Glaucoma poses a significant economic burden, specifically due to population ageing. Cost-effective care is a major public health concern. A recent study conducted in the USA reported the highest eye-related costs for patients with OAG and OHT and determined positive economic externalities from therapies that delayed disease progression [116]. SLT is known as an effective method of lowering IOP and, thus, significantly partakes in lowering the economic burden of OAG.

Dirani et al. studied the economic effects of POAG in Australia and concluded that the use of laser trabeculoplasty as primary-line treatment rather than a second-line treatment would lead to a significant decrease of healthcare system costs [117]. Lee and Hutnik projected a 6-year cost comparison of primary SLT in therapy of OAG in Canada and found SLT to be cost effective [118].

During the LiGHT trial, cost-effectiveness in the UK was analyzed. They used a lifetime model, where cost-effectiveness was calculated in regard to cost per quality adjusted life year (QALY) of the SLT-first group, compared with the medicine-first group. The economic evaluation based on this trial determined that there is a 97% probability that SLT is a treatment for OAG and OHT, which is cost-effective [119]. This furthermore underpins findings that SLT as a first-line therapy is more economical when compared to hypotensive medication as the initial glaucoma therapy.

10. Future Perspectives and Alternatives Considered

As shown here, laser trabeculoplasty is an evolving field; using different lasers for trabeculoplasty and groundbreaking SLT treatment modifications might yield improved outcomes in the future.

A study by Gandolfi et al. [120] supports the concept that a 360-degree low energy SLT (0.3 mJ, 50–60 spots) could be repeated every year independently of measured IOP. It was shown that such patients remained medical treatment-free for 6.2 years. Based on these data, the COAST trial was launched to look at low-energy SLT in terms of TM anatomy and subsequent responsivity to SLT (awaiting results) [121]. If this treatment schedule proves to deter the use of medication or incisional surgery in the long-run, this might lead to further significant modifications in the field of treatment with SLT.

Transscleral SLT was a new modality of glaucoma laser treatment, first studied in Israel [122]. In essence, it means applying energy at the limbus, delivering the energy directly on the surface of the eye and not via gonioscopy lens. A standard SLT laser with modified parameters is used here. This approach proved effective, which was further studied in a prospective trial [123]. Laser energy delivered to the surface of the eye proved as efficient as standard SLT delivered to the TM via a gonioscopy lens. This is currently further studied in a multicenter prospective study [124] with an acronym GLAUrious, which tests direct transscleral SLT, delivered ab externo in POAG. The results are yet to be published. Transscleral SLT could potentially be useful in angle-closure glaucoma, where TM is not readily visible; however, separate trials are needed for evaluation. Recently automated transscleral SLT was studied. An automated image-processing algorithm targets predetermined targets at the limbus, automatically using a video camera, delivering transscleral SLT in 7 ns pulses. It proved to be easily performed, safe, and effective with up to 27% IOP reduction at 6 months, with a significant reduction in IOP-lowering medication [123]. Low-energy SLT and transscleral SLT were also included in the meta-analysis by Zhou et al. [31], where they were proven to be equally effective in lowering IOP when compared to medications as other laser trabeculoplasty procedures.

Recently, two reviews on the micropulse diode laser trabeculoplasty were published [125,126]. The reviews were conducted in a similar manner to SLT; however, a subthreshold micropulse diode laser technique as used that split up a continuous laser beam into on-and-off pulses to enable in-between cooling, similar to the micropulse modality of retinal micropulse laser treatment. The micropulse laser trabeculoplasty had initially shown similar comparable results to SLT in POAG [127]. The precise treatment protocol and laser wavelength are yet to be determined (by future prospective trials). Albeit it might be a safer treatment modality in regard to post-procedure complications, such as IOP-spikes or inflammation since trabecular structural change is less likely to occur [128].

Pattern scanning laser trabeculoplasty is a modality where the PASCAL laser is used, where computer-guided short pulse durations are used in 100 μm spots, presumably decreasing the surrounding tissue damage. In a RCT, this modality was performed in one eye and tested against SLT in the fellow eye—no significant difference in IOP-lowering was found at 6 months [129,130].

Titanium sapphire laser trabeculoplasty was compared to standard SLT in a RCT [131]. In this technique, near-infrared energy is used, which is believed to penetrate deeper to Schlemm's canal and the ciliary body. No statistically significant differences in IOP-control or the success rate were noted, as well as no differences in the safety profiles.

11. Conclusions

More real-world studies with controls should be conducted to elucidate if the hype of SLT is real. The actual effectiveness of SLT alone was not entirely comprehended up until the LiGHT trial, where IOP-lowering was clearly demonstrated as at least equivalent to medication. In such settings, where SLT is used early in naïve patients, with higher initial IOP, it seems to be significantly more effective than when used as a later therapeutic choice. The latter supports the move of SLT up the chain of therapy in glaucoma in the new 5th edition EGS guidelines. Previously, patients might have been selected for SLT later, usually in between maximal medical therapy and surgery, at the bottom of the therapy algorithm. This might have been perceived as one of the reasons why retrospective real-world data were not as unequivocal in favor of SLT effectiveness in the long-run.

Currently, according to the available literature reviewed here and the EGS guidelines, SLT can be offered to patients as an alternative, where an initial topical therapy switch is considered or as an adjunctive therapy to the existing topical monotherapy. Be that as it may, we see SLT as a validated evidence-based alternative to medications, given as a first-line treatment in OAG and OH. This option will likely gain popularity amongst ophthalmologists in the future when more real-world data become available.

Supplementary Materials: The following supporting information can be downloaded at: https://www.mdpi.com/article/10.3390/jcm11133879/s1.

Author Contributions: Conceptualization, T.S., A.B.T., P.F. and T.G.; writing—original draft preparation, T.S., A.B.T. and P.F.; writing—review and editing, T.G. All authors have read and agreed to the published version of the manuscript.

Funding: This research received no external funding. The grant for the open-access fee was funded by the University Medical Center Maribor, Slovenia.

References

1. Vision Impairment and Blindness. Available online: https://www.who.int/news-room/fact-sheets/detail/blindness-and-visual-impairment (accessed on 15 March 2022).
2. Tham, Y.-C.; Li, X.; Wong, T.Y.; Quigley, H.A.; Aung, T.; Cheng, C.-Y. Global Prevalence of Glaucoma and Projections of Glaucoma Burden through 2040: A Systematic Review and Meta-Analysis. *Ophthalmology* **2014**, *121*, 2081–2090. [CrossRef] [PubMed]
3. Allison, K.; Patel, D.; Alabi, O. Epidemiology of Glaucoma: The Past, Present, and Predictions for the Future. *Cureus* **2020**, *12*, e11686. [CrossRef] [PubMed]
4. Gračner, T. Comparative Study of the Efficacy of Selective Laser Trabeculoplasty as Initial or Adjunctive Treatment for Primary Open-Angle Glaucoma. *Eur. J. Ophthalmol.* **2019**, *29*, 524–531. [CrossRef] [PubMed]
5. Heijl, A.; Leske, M.C.; Bengtsson, B.; Hyman, L.; Bengtsson, B.; Hussein, M. Early Manifest Glaucoma Trial Group Reduction of Intraocular Pressure and Glaucoma Progression: Results from the Early Manifest Glaucoma Trial. *Arch. Ophthalmol. Chic. Ill* **2002**, *120*, 1268–1279. [CrossRef]
6. Reardon, G.; Kotak, S.; Schwartz, G.F. Objective Assessment of Compliance and Persistence among Patients Treated for Glaucoma and Ocular Hypertension: A Systematic Review. *Patient Prefer. Adherence* **2011**, *5*, 441–463. [CrossRef] [PubMed]
7. Latina, M.A.; Sibayan, S.A.; Shin, D.H.; Noecker, R.J.; Marcellino, G. Q-Switched 532-Nm Nd:YAG Laser Trabeculoplasty (Selective Laser Trabeculoplasty): A Multicenter, Pilot, Clinical Study. *Ophthalmology* **1998**, *105*, 2082–2088; discussion 2089–2090. [CrossRef]
8. Gracner, T. Intraocular Pressure Response to Selective Laser Trabeculoplasty in the Treatment of Primary Open-Angle Glaucoma. *Ophthalmol. J. Int. Ophtalmol. Int. J. Ophthalmol. Z. Augenheilkd.* **2001**, *215*, 267–270. [CrossRef] [PubMed]
9. Kim, Y.J.; Moon, C.S. One-Year Follow-up of Laser Trabeculoplasty Using Q-Switched Frequency-Doubled Nd:YAG Laser of 523 Nm Wavelength. *Ophthalmic Surg. Lasers* **2000**, *31*, 394–399. [CrossRef]
10. Cvenkel, B. One-Year Follow-up of Selective Laser Trabeculoplasty in Open-Angle Glaucoma. *Ophthalmol. J. Int. Ophtalmol. Int. J. Ophthalmol. Z. Augenheilkd.* **2004**, *218*, 20–25. [CrossRef]
11. Garg, A.; Gazzard, G. Selective Laser Trabeculoplasty: Past, Present, and Future. *Eye Lond. Engl.* **2018**, *32*, 863–876. [CrossRef] [PubMed]
12. Gazzard, G.; Konstantakopoulou, E.; Garway-Heath, D.; Garg, A.; Vickerstaff, V.; Hunter, R.; Ambler, G.; Bunce, C.; Wormald, R.; Nathwani, N.; et al. Selective Laser Trabeculoplasty versus Eye Drops for First-Line Treatment of Ocular Hypertension and Glaucoma (LiGHT): A Multicentre Randomised Controlled Trial. *Lancet Lond. Engl.* **2019**, *393*, 1505–1516. [CrossRef]
13. European Glaucoma Society Terminology and Guidelines for Glaucoma, 5th Edition. *Br. J. Ophthalmol.* **2021**, *105*, 1–169. [CrossRef] [PubMed]
14. Krasnov, M.M. Q-Switched Laser Goniopuncture. *Arch. Ophthalmol. Chic. Ill* **1974**, *92*, 37–41. [CrossRef]
15. Krasnov, M.M. Laseropuncture of Anterior Chamber Angle in Glaucoma. *Am. J. Ophthalmol.* **1973**, *75*, 674–678. [CrossRef]
16. Wise, J.B.; Witter, S.L. Argon Laser Therapy for Open-Angle Glaucoma. A Pilot Study. *Arch. Ophthalmol. Chic. Ill* **1979**, *97*, 319–322. [CrossRef]
17. Bradley, J.M.; Anderssohn, A.; Colvis, C.; Parshley, D.E.; Zhu, X.; Ruddat, M.S.; Samples, J.; Acott, T. Mediation of Laser Trabeculoplasty-Induced Matrix Metalloproteinase Expression by IL-1beta and TNFalpha. *Investig. Ophthalmol. Vis. Sci.* **2000**, *41*, 422–430.

18. Parshley, D.E.; Bradley, J.M.; Fisk, A.; Hadaegh, A.; Samples, J.R.; Van Buskirk, E.M.; Acott, T.S. Laser Trabeculoplasty Induces Stromelysin Expression by Trabecular Juxtacanalicular Cells. *Investig. Ophthalmol. Vis. Sci.* **1996**, *37*, 795–804.
19. Ritch, R.; Podos, S. Laser Trabeculoplasty in the Exfoliation Syndrome. *Bull. N. Y. Acad. Med.* **1983**, *59*, 339.
20. Agarwal, H.C.; Sihota, R.; Das, C.; Dada, T. Role of Argon Laser Trabeculoplasty as Primary and Secondary Therapy in Open Angle Glaucoma in Indian Patients. *Br. J. Ophthalmol.* **2002**, *86*, 733. [CrossRef] [PubMed]
21. Coakes, R. Laser Trabeculoplasty. *Br. J. Ophthalmol.* **1992**, *76*, 624–626. [CrossRef] [PubMed]
22. Baez, K.A.; Spaeth, G.L. Argon Laser Trabeculoplasty Controls One Third of Patients with Progressive, Uncontrolled Open-Angle Glaucoma for Five Years. *Trans. Am. Ophthalmol. Soc.* **1991**, *89*, 47–56; discussion 56–58. [PubMed]
23. Grinich, N.P.; Van Buskirk, E.M.; Samples, J.R. Three-Year Efficacy of Argon Laser Trabeculoplasty. *Ophthalmology* **1987**, *94*, 858–861. [CrossRef]
24. Latina, M.A.; Park, C. Selective Targeting of Trabecular Meshwork Cells: In Vitro Studies of Pulsed and CW Laser Interactions. *Exp. Eye Res.* **1995**, *60*, 359–371. [CrossRef]
25. Xu, L.; Yu, R.-J.; Ding, X.-M.; Li, M.; Wu, Y.; Zhu, L.; Chen, D.; Peng, C.; Zeng, C.-J.; Guo, W.-Y. Efficacy of Low-Energy Selective Laser Trabeculoplasty on the Treatment of Primary Open Angle Glaucoma. *Int. J. Ophthalmol.* **2019**, *12*, 1432–1437. [CrossRef]
26. Anderson, R.R.; Parrish, J.A. Selective Photothermolysis: Precise Microsurgery by Selective Absorption of Pulsed Radiation. *Science* **1983**, *220*, 524–527. [CrossRef]
27. Wood, J.P.M.; Plunkett, M.; Previn, V.; Chidlow, G.; Casson, R.J. Rapid and Delayed Death of Cultured Trabecular Meshwork Cells after Selective Laser Trabeculoplasty. *Lasers Surg. Med.* **2010**, *42*, 326–337. [CrossRef]
28. Kramer, T.R.; Noecker, R.J. Comparison of the Morphologic Changes after Selective Laser Trabeculoplasty and Argon Laser Trabeculoplasty in Human Eye Bank Eyes. *Ophthalmology* **2001**, *108*, 773–779. [CrossRef]
29. Cvenkel, B.; Hvala, A.; Drnovsek-Olup, B.; Gale, N. Acute Ultrastructural Changes of the Trabecular Meshwork after Selective Laser Trabeculoplasty and Low Power Argon Laser Trabeculoplasty. *Lasers Surg. Med.* **2003**, *33*, 204–208. [CrossRef]
30. Wang, H.; Cheng, J.-W.; Wei, R.-L.; Cai, J.-P.; Li, Y.; Ma, X.-Y. Meta-Analysis of Selective Laser Trabeculoplasty with Argon Laser Trabeculoplasty in the Treatment of Open-Angle Glaucoma. *Can. J. Ophthalmol. J. Can. Ophtalmol.* **2013**, *48*, 186–192. [CrossRef]
31. Zhou, R.; Sun, Y.; Chen, H.; Sha, S.; He, M.; Wang, W. Laser Trabeculoplasty for Open-Angle Glaucoma: A Systematic Review and Network Meta-Analysis. *Am. J. Ophthalmol.* **2021**, *229*, 301–313. [CrossRef]
32. Alon, S. Selective Laser Trabeculoplasty: A Clinical Review. *J. Curr. Glaucoma Pract.* **2013**, *7*, 58–65. [CrossRef] [PubMed]
33. Beltran-Agullo, L.; Alaghband, P.; Obi, A.; Husain, R.; Lim, K.-S. The Effect of Selective Laser Trabeculoplasty on Aqueous Humor Dynamics in Patients with Ocular Hypertension and Primary Open-Angle Glaucoma. *J. Glaucoma* **2013**, *22*, 746–749. [CrossRef]
34. Goyal, S.; Beltran-Agullo, L.; Rashid, S.; Shah, S.P.; Nath, R.; Obi, A.; Lim, K.S. Effect of Primary Selective Laser Trabeculoplasty on Tonographic Outflow Facility: A Randomised Clinical Trial. *Br. J. Ophthalmol.* **2010**, *94*, 1443–1447. [CrossRef] [PubMed]
35. Beltran-Agullo, L.; Alaghband, P.; Rashid, S.; Gosselin, J.; Obi, A.; Husain, R.; Lim, K.S. Comparative Human Aqueous Dynamics Study between Black and White Subjects with Glaucoma. *Investig. Ophthalmol. Vis. Sci.* **2011**, *52*, 9425–9430. [CrossRef] [PubMed]
36. Gulati, V.; Fan, S.; Gardner, B.J.; Havens, S.J.; Schaaf, M.T.; Neely, D.G.; Toris, C.B. Mechanism of Action of Selective Laser Trabeculoplasty and Predictors of Response. *Investig. Ophthalmol. Vis. Sci.* **2017**, *58*, 1462–1468. [CrossRef]
37. Kagan, D.B.; Gorfinkel, N.S.; Hutnik, C.M.L. Mechanisms of Selective Laser Trabeculoplasty: A Review. *Clin. Exp. Ophthalmol.* **2014**, *42*, 675–681. [CrossRef]
38. Kennedy, J.B.; SooHoo, J.R.; Kahook, M.Y.; Seibold, L.K. Selective Laser Trabeculoplasty: An Update. *Asia-Pac. J. Ophthalmol. Phila. Pa* **2016**, *5*, 63–69. [CrossRef]
39. Lee, J.Y.J.; Kagan, D.B.; Roumeliotis, G.; Liu, H.; Hutnik, C.M.L. Secretion of Matrix Metalloproteinase-3 by Co-Cultured Pigmented and Non-Pigmented Human Trabecular Meshwork Cells Following Selective Laser Trabeculoplasty. *Clin. Exp. Ophthalmol.* **2016**, *44*, 33–42. [CrossRef]
40. Alvarado, J.A.; Katz, L.J.; Trivedi, S.; Shifera, A.S. Monocyte Modulation of Aqueous Outflow and Recruitment to the Trabecular Meshwork Following Selective Laser Trabeculoplasty. *Arch. Ophthalmol.* **2010**, *128*, 731–737. [CrossRef]
41. Kelley, M.J.; Rose, A.Y.; Song, K.; Chen, Y.; Bradley, J.M.; Rookhuizen, D.; Acott, T.S. Synergism of TNF and IL-1 in the Induction of Matrix Metalloproteinase-3 in Trabecular Meshwork. *Investig. Ophthalmol. Vis. Sci.* **2007**, *48*, 2634–2643. [CrossRef]
42. Izzotti, A.; Longobardi, M.; Cartiglia, C.; Rathschuler, F.; Saccà, S.C. Trabecular Meshwork Gene Expression after Selective Laser Trabeculoplasty. *PLoS ONE* **2011**, *6*, e20110. [CrossRef] [PubMed]
43. Wright, D.M.; Konstantakopoulou, E.; Montesano, G.; Nathwani, N.; Garg, A.; Garway-Heath, D.; Crabb, D.P.; Gazzard, G.; Laser in Glaucoma and Ocular Hypertension Trial (LiGHT) Study Group. Visual Field Outcomes from the Multicenter, Randomized Controlled Laser in Glaucoma and Ocular Hypertension Trial (LiGHT). *Ophthalmology* **2020**, *127*, 1313–1321. [CrossRef] [PubMed]
44. Pahlitzsch, M.; Davids, A.-M.; Winterhalter, S.; Zorn, M.; Reitemeyer, E.; Klamann, M.K.J.; Torun, N.; Bertelmann, E.; Maier, A.-K. Selective Laser Trabeculoplasty Versus MIGS: Forgotten Art or First-Step Procedure in Selected Patients with Open-Angle Glaucoma. *Ophthalmol. Ther.* **2021**, *10*, 509–524. [CrossRef] [PubMed]
45. Weinand, F.S.; Althen, F. Long-Term Clinical Results of Selective Laser Trabeculoplasty in the Treatment of Primary Open Angle Glaucoma. *Eur. J. Ophthalmol.* **2006**, *16*, 100–104. [CrossRef] [PubMed]
46. Zhang, H.; Yang, Y.; Xu, J.; Yu, M. Selective Laser Trabeculoplasty in Treating Post-Trabeculectomy Advanced Primary Open-Angle Glaucoma. *Exp. Ther. Med.* **2016**, *11*, 1090–1094. [CrossRef]

47. Garg, A.; Vickerstaff, V.; Nathwani, N.; Garway-Heath, D.; Konstantakopoulou, E.; Ambler, G.; Bunce, C.; Wormald, R.; Barton, K.; Gazzard, G. Efficacy of Repeat Selective Laser Trabeculoplasty in Medication-Naive Open-Angle Glaucoma and Ocular Hypertension during the LiGHT Trial. *Ophthalmology* **2020**, *127*, 467–476. [CrossRef]

48. Francis, B.A.; Loewen, N.; Hong, B.; Dustin, L.; Kaplowitz, K.; Kinast, R.; Bacharach, J.; Radhakrishnan, S.; Iwach, A.; Rudavska, L.; et al. Repeatability of Selective Laser Trabeculoplasty for Open-Angle Glaucoma. *BMC Ophthalmol.* **2016**, *16*, 128. [CrossRef]

49. Hong, B.K.; Winer, J.C.; Martone, J.F.; Wand, M.; Altman, B.; Shields, B. Repeat Selective Laser Trabeculoplasty. *J. Glaucoma* **2009**, *18*, 180–183. [CrossRef]

50. Lee, J.W.Y.; Shum, J.J.W.; Chan, J.C.H.; Lai, J.S.M. Two-Year Clinical Results After Selective Laser Trabeculoplasty for Normal Tension Glaucoma. *Medicine* **2015**, *94*, e984. [CrossRef]

51. De Keyser, M.; De Belder, M.; De Belder, J.; De Groot, V. Selective Laser Trabeculoplasty as Replacement Therapy in Medically Controlled Glaucoma Patients. *Acta Ophthalmol.* **2018**, *96*, e577–e581. [CrossRef]

52. Miraftabi, A.; Nilforushan, N.; Nassiri, N.; Nouri-Mahdavi, K. Selective Laser Trabeculoplasty in Patients with Pseudoexfoliative Glaucoma vs Primary Open Angle Glaucoma: A One-Year Comparative Study. *Int. J. Ophthalmol.* **2016**, *9*, 406–410. [CrossRef] [PubMed]

53. Kent, S.S.; Hutnik, C.M.L.; Birt, C.M.; Damji, K.F.; Harasymowycz, P.; Si, F.; Hodge, W.; Pan, I.; Crichton, A. A Randomized Clinical Trial of Selective Laser Trabeculoplasty versus Argon Laser Trabeculoplasty in Patients with Pseudoexfoliation. *J. Glaucoma* **2015**, *24*, 344–347. [CrossRef] [PubMed]

54. Lindegger, D.J.; Funk, J.; Jaggi, G.P. Long-Term Effect of Selective Laser Trabeculoplasty on Intraocular Pressure in Pseudoexfoliation Glaucoma. *Klin. Mon. Augenheilkd.* **2015**, *232*, 405–408. [CrossRef] [PubMed]

55. Gracner, T. Intraocular Pressure Response of Capsular Glaucoma and Primary Open-Angle Glaucoma to Selective Nd:YAG Laser Trabeculoplasty: A Prospective, Comparative Clinical Trial. *Eur. J. Ophthalmol.* **2002**, *12*, 287–292. [CrossRef]

56. Koucheki, B.; Hashemi, H. Selective Laser Trabeculoplasty in the Treatment of Open-Angle Glaucoma. *J. Glaucoma* **2012**, *21*, 65–70. [CrossRef]

57. Lee, J.W.; Ho, W.L.; Chan, J.C.; Lai, J.S. Efficacy of Selective Laser Trabeculoplasty for Normal Tension Glaucoma: 1 Year Results. *BMC Ophthalmol.* **2015**, *15*, 1. [CrossRef]

58. Narayanaswamy, A.; Leung, C.K.; Istiantoro, D.V.; Perera, S.A.; Ho, C.-L.; Nongpiur, M.E.; Baskaran, M.; Htoon, H.M.; Wong, T.T.; Goh, D.; et al. Efficacy of Selective Laser Trabeculoplasty in Primary Angle-Closure Glaucoma: A Randomized Clinical Trial. *JAMA Ophthalmol.* **2015**, *133*, 206–212. [CrossRef]

59. Ali Aljasim, L.; Owaidhah, O.; Edward, D.P. Selective Laser Trabeculoplasty in Primary Angle-Closure Glaucoma After Laser Peripheral Iridotomy: A Case-Control Study. *J. Glaucoma* **2016**, *25*, e253–e258. [CrossRef]

60. Tokuda, N.; Inoue, J.; Yamazaki, I.; Matsuzawa, A.; Munemasa, Y.; Kitaoka, Y.; Takagi, H.; Ueno, S. Effects of selective laser trabeculoplasty treatment in steroid-induced glaucoma. *Nippon. Ganka Gakkai Zasshi* **2012**, *116*, 751–757.

61. Baser, E.; Seymenoglu, R. Selective Laser Trabeculoplasty for the Treatment of Intraocular Pressure Elevation after Intravitreal Triamcinolone Injection. *Can. J. Ophthalmol. J. Can. Ophthalmol.* **2009**, *44*, e21. [CrossRef]

62. Patel, P.; Foster, C.S. Safety and Efficacy of Selective Laser Trabeculoplasty in Uveitic Glaucoma. *Investig. Ophthalmol. Vis. Sci.* **2014**, *55*, 6154.

63. Song, J.; Song, A.; Palmares, T.; Song, M. Selective Laser Trabeculoplasty Success in Pediatric Patients with Glaucoma: Two Case Reports. *J. Med. Case Rep.* **2013**, *7*, 198. [CrossRef] [PubMed]

64. Zhang, L.; Weizer, J.S.; Musch, D.C. Perioperative Medications for Preventing Temporarily Increased Intraocular Pressure after Laser Trabeculoplasty. *Cochrane Database Syst. Rev.* **2017**, *2*, CD010746. [CrossRef] [PubMed]

65. Shibata, M.; Sugiyama, T.; Ishida, O.; Ueki, M.; Kojima, S.; Okuda, T.; Ikeda, T. Clinical Results of Selective Laser Trabeculoplasty in Open-Angle Glaucoma in Japanese Eyes: Comparison of 180 Degree with 360 Degree SLT. *J. Glaucoma* **2012**, *21*, 17–21. [CrossRef] [PubMed]

66. Nirappel, A.; Klug, E.; Ye, R.; Hall, N.; Chachanidze, M.; Chang, T.C.; Solá-Del Valle, D. Effectiveness of Selective Laser Trabeculoplasty Applied to 360° vs. 180° of the Angle. *J. Ophthalmol.* **2021**, *2021*, 8860601. [CrossRef]

67. Özen, B.; Öztürk, H.; Yüce, B. Comparison of the Effects of 180° and 360° Applications of Selective Laser Trabeculoplasty on Intraocular Pressure and Cornea. *Int. Ophthalmol.* **2020**, *40*, 1103–1110. [CrossRef]

68. Woo, D.M.; Healey, P.R.; Graham, S.L.; Goldberg, I. Intraocular Pressure-Lowering Medications and Long-Term Outcomes of Selective Laser Trabeculoplasty. *Clin. Exp. Ophthalmol.* **2015**, *43*, 320–327. [CrossRef]

69. Prasad, N.; Murthy, S.; Dagianis, J.J.; Latina, M.A. A Comparison of the Intervisit Intraocular Pressure Fluctuation after 180 and 360 Degrees of Selective Laser Trabeculoplasty (SLT) as a Primary Therapy in Primary Open Angle Glaucoma and Ocular Hypertension. *J. Glaucoma* **2009**, *18*, 157–160. [CrossRef]

70. Katsanos, A.; Konstas, A.G.; Mikropoulos, D.G.; Quaranta, L.; Voudouragkaki, I.C.; Athanasopoulos, G.P.; Asproudis, I.; Teus, M.A. A Review of the Clinical Usefulness of Selective Laser Trabeculoplasty in Exfoliative Glaucoma. *Adv. Ther.* **2018**, *35*, 619–630. [CrossRef]

71. Chi, S.C.; Kang, Y.-N.; Hwang, D.-K.; Liu, C.J.-L. Selective Laser Trabeculoplasty versus Medication for Open-Angle Glaucoma: Systematic Review and Meta-Analysis of Randomised Clinical Trials. *Br. J. Ophthalmol.* **2020**, *104*, 1500–1507. [CrossRef]

72. Tang, M.; Fu, Y.; Fu, M.-S.; Fan, Y.; Zou, H.-D.; Sun, X.-D.; Xu, X. The Efficacy of Low-Energy Selective Laser Trabeculoplasty. *Ophthalmic Surg. Lasers Imaging Off. J. Int. Soc. Imaging Eye* **2011**, *42*, 59–63. [CrossRef] [PubMed]

73. Lee, J.W.Y.; Wong, M.O.M.; Liu, C.C.L.; Lai, J.S.M. Optimal Selective Laser Trabeculoplasty Energy for Maximal Intraocular Pressure Reduction in Open-Angle Glaucoma. *J. Glaucoma* **2015**, *24*, e128–e131. [CrossRef] [PubMed]

74. De Keyser, M.; De Belder, M.; De Groot, V. Randomized Prospective Study of the Use of Anti-Inflammatory Drops After Selective Laser Trabeculoplasty. *J. Glaucoma* **2017**, *26*, e22–e29. [CrossRef] [PubMed]

75. Gračner, T. Impact of Short-Term Topical Steroid Therapy on Selective Laser Trabeculoplasty Efficacy. *J. Clin. Med.* **2021**, *10*, 4249. [CrossRef]

76. Jinapriya, D.; D'Souza, M.; Hollands, H.; El-Defrawy, S.R.; Irrcher, I.; Smallman, D.; Farmer, J.P.; Cheung, J.; Urton, T.; Day, A.; et al. Anti-Inflammatory Therapy after Selective Laser Trabeculoplasty: A Randomized, Double-Masked, Placebo-Controlled Clinical Trial. *Ophthalmology* **2014**, *121*, 2356–2361. [CrossRef]

77. Rebenitsch, R.L.; Brown, E.N.; Binder, N.R.; Jani, A.; Bonham, A.J.; Krishna, R.; Pikey, K. Effect of Topical Loteprednol on Intraocular Pressure after Selective Laser Trabeculoplasty for Open-Angle Glaucoma. *Ophthalmol. Ther.* **2013**, *2*, 113–120. [CrossRef]

78. Groth, S.L.; Albeiruti, E.; Nunez, M.; Fajardo, R.; Sharpsten, L.; Loewen, N.; Schuman, J.S.; Goldberg, J.L. SALT Trial: Steroids after Laser Trabeculoplasty: Impact of Short-Term Anti-Inflammatory Treatment on Selective Laser Trabeculoplasty Efficacy. *Ophthalmology* **2019**, *126*, 1511–1516. [CrossRef]

79. Garg, A.; Vickerstaff, V.; Nathwani, N.; Garway-Heath, D.; Konstantakopoulou, E.; Ambler, G.; Bunce, C.; Wormald, R.; Barton, K.; Gazzard, G.; et al. Primary Selective Laser Trabeculoplasty for Open-Angle Glaucoma and Ocular Hypertension: Clinical Outcomes, Predictors of Success, and Safety from the Laser in Glaucoma and Ocular Hypertension Trial. *Ophthalmology* **2019**, *126*, 1238–1248. [CrossRef]

80. Ansari, E. 10-Year Outcomes of First-Line Selective Laser Trabeculoplasty (SLT) for Primary Open-Angle Glaucoma (POAG). *Graefes Arch. Clin. Exp. Ophthalmol. Albrecht Graefes Arch. Klin. Exp. Ophthalmol.* **2021**, *259*, 1597–1604. [CrossRef]

81. Wong, M.O.M.; Lee, J.W.Y.; Choy, B.N.K.; Chan, J.C.H.; Lai, J.S.M. Systematic Review and Meta-Analysis on the Efficacy of Selective Laser Trabeculoplasty in Open-Angle Glaucoma. *Surv. Ophthalmol.* **2015**, *60*, 36–50. [CrossRef]

82. Li, X.; Wang, W.; Zhang, X. Meta-Analysis of Selective Laser Trabeculoplasty versus Topical Medication in the Treatment of Open-Angle Glaucoma. *BMC Ophthalmol.* **2015**, *15*, 107. [CrossRef] [PubMed]

83. Khawaja, A.P.; Campbell, J.H.; Kirby, N.; Chandwani, H.S.; Keyzor, I.; Parekh, M.; McNaught, A.I.; Vincent, D.; Angela, K.; Nitin, A.; et al. Real-World Outcomes of Selective Laser Trabeculoplasty in the United Kingdom. *Ophthalmology* **2020**, *127*, 748–757. [CrossRef] [PubMed]

84. Abe, R.Y.; Maestrini, H.A.; Guedes, G.B.; Nascimento, M.M.; Iguma, C.I.; de Miranda Santos, H.D.; Nasr, M.G.; Lucena-Junior, R.P.; Prata, T.S. Real-World Data from Selective Laser Trabeculoplasty in Brazil. *Sci. Rep.* **2022**, *12*, 1923. [CrossRef]

85. Klamann, M.K.J.; Maier, A.-K.B.; Gonnermann, J.; Ruokonen, P.C. Adverse Effects and Short-Term Results after Selective Laser Trabeculoplasty. *J. Glaucoma* **2014**, *23*, 105–108. [CrossRef] [PubMed]

86. Song, J. Complications of Selective Laser Trabeculoplasty: A Review. *Clin. Ophthalmol.* **2016**, *10*, 137–143. [CrossRef] [PubMed]

87. Gazzard, G.; Konstantakopoulou, E.; Garway-Heath, D.; Barton, K.; Wormald, R.; Morris, S.; Hunter, R.; Rubin, G.; Buszewicz, M.; Ambler, G.; et al. Laser in Glaucoma and Ocular Hypertension (LiGHT) Trial. A Multicentre, Randomised Controlled Trial: Design and Methodology. *Br. J. Ophthalmol.* **2018**, *102*, 593–598. [CrossRef]

88. Damji, K.F.; Shah, K.C.; Rock, W.J.; Bains, H.S.; Hodge, W.G. Selective Laser Trabeculoplasty v Argon Laser Trabeculoplasty: A Prospective Randomised Clinical Trial. *Br. J. Ophthalmol.* **1999**, *83*, 718–722. [CrossRef]

89. Ayala, M.; Chen, E. Comparison of Selective Laser Trabeculoplasty (SLT) in Primary Open Angle Glaucoma and Pseudoexfoliation Glaucoma. *Clin. Ophthalmol.* **2011**, *5*, 1469–1473. [CrossRef]

90. Harasymowycz, P.J.; Papamatheakis, D.G.; Latina, M.; De Leon, M.; Lesk, M.R.; Damji, K.F. Selective Laser Trabeculoplasty (SLT) Complicated by Intraocular Pressure Elevation in Eyes with Heavily Pigmented Trabecular Meshworks. *Am. J. Ophthalmol.* **2005**, *139*, 1110–1113. [CrossRef]

91. Koktekir, B.E.; Gedik, S.; Bakbak, B. Bilateral Severe Anterior Uveitis after Unilateral Selective Laser Trabeculoplasty. *Clin. Exp. Ophthalmol.* **2013**, *41*, 305–307. [CrossRef]

92. McIlraith, I.; Strasfeld, M.; Colev, G.; Hutnik, C.M.L. Selective Laser Trabeculoplasty as Initial and Adjunctive Treatment for Open-Angle Glaucoma. *J. Glaucoma* **2006**, *15*, 124–130. [CrossRef] [PubMed]

93. Wu, Z.Q.; Huang, J.; Sadda, S. Selective Laser Trabeculoplasty Complicated by Cystoid Macular Edema: Report of Two Cases. *Eye Sci.* **2012**, *27*, 193–197. [CrossRef] [PubMed]

94. Wechsler, D.Z.; Wechsler, I.B. Cystoid Macular Oedema after Selective Laser Trabeculoplasty. *Eye Lond. Engl.* **2010**, *24*, 1113. [CrossRef] [PubMed]

95. Shihadeh, W.A.; Ritch, R.; Liebmann, J.M. Hyphema Occurring during Selective Laser Trabeculoplasty. *Ophthalmic Surg. Lasers Imaging Off. J. Int. Soc. Imaging Eye* **2006**, *37*, 432–433. [CrossRef] [PubMed]

96. Rhee, D.J.; Krad, O.; Pasquale, L.R. Hyphema Following Selective Laser Trabeculoplasty. *Ophthalmic Surg. Lasers Imaging Off. J. Int. Soc. Imaging Eye* **2009**, *40*, 493–494. [CrossRef]

97. Kim, D.Y.; Singh, A. Severe Iritis and Choroidal Effusion Following Selective Laser Trabeculoplasty. *Ophthalmic Surg. Lasers Imaging Off. J. Int. Soc. Imaging Eye* **2008**, *39*, 409–411. [CrossRef]

98. Latina, M.A.; Tumbocon, J.A.J. Selective Laser Trabeculoplasty: A New Treatment Option for Open Angle Glaucoma. *Curr. Opin. Ophthalmol.* **2002**, *13*, 94–96. [CrossRef]
99. Regina, M.; Bunya, V.Y.; Orlin, S.E.; Ansari, H. Corneal Edema and Haze after Selective Laser Trabeculoplasty. *J. Glaucoma* **2011**, *20*, 327–329. [CrossRef]
100. Moubayed, S.P.; Hamid, M.; Choremis, J.; Li, G. An Unusual Finding of Corneal Edema Complicating Selective Laser Trabeculoplasty. *Can. J. Ophthalmol. J. Can. Ophtalmol.* **2009**, *44*, 337–338. [CrossRef]
101. Guven Yilmaz, S.; Palamar, M.; Yusifov, E.; Ates, H.; Egrilmez, S.; Yagci, A. Effects of Primary Selective Laser Trabeculoplasty on Anterior Segment Parameters. *Int. J. Ophthalmol.* **2015**, *8*, 954–959. [CrossRef]
102. Keratitis and Hyperopic Refractive Shift Induced by SLT. Available online: https://glaucomatoday.com/articles/2010-sept/keratitis-and-hyperopic-refractive-shift-induced-by-slt (accessed on 20 March 2022).
103. Knickelbein, J.E.; Singh, A.; Flowers, B.E.; Nair, U.K.; Eisenberg, M.; Davis, R.; Raju, L.V.; Schuman, J.S.; Conner, I.P. Acute Corneal Edema with Subsequent Thinning and Hyperopic Shift Following Selective Laser Trabeculoplasty. *J. Cataract Refract. Surg.* **2014**, *40*, 1731–1735. [CrossRef] [PubMed]
104. Holz, H.; Pirouzian, A. Bilateral Diffuse Lamellar Keratitis Following Consecutive Selective Laser Trabeculoplasty in LASIK Patient. *J. Cataract Refract. Surg.* **2010**, *36*, 847–849. [CrossRef] [PubMed]
105. Bettis, D.I.; Whitehead, J.J.; Farhi, P.; Zabriskie, N.A. Intraocular Pressure Spike and Corneal Decompensation Following Selective Laser Trabeculoplasty in Patients With Exfoliation Glaucoma. *J. Glaucoma* **2016**, *25*, e433–e437. [CrossRef]
106. George, M.K.; Emerson, J.W.; Cheema, S.A.; McGlynn, R.; Ford, B.A.; Martone, J.F.; Shields, M.B.; Wand, M. Evaluation of a Modified Protocol for Selective Laser Trabeculoplasty. *J. Glaucoma* **2008**, *17*, 197–202. [CrossRef] [PubMed]
107. Polat, J.; Grantham, L.; Mitchell, K.; Realini, T. Repeatability of Selective Laser Trabeculoplasty. *Br. J. Ophthalmol.* **2016**, *100*, 1437–1441. [CrossRef] [PubMed]
108. Ang, G.S.; Fenwick, E.K.; Constantinou, M.; Gan, A.T.L.; Man, R.E.K.; Casson, R.J.; Finkelstein, E.A.; Goldberg, I.; Healey, P.R.; Pesudovs, K.; et al. Selective Laser Trabeculoplasty versus Topical Medication as Initial Glaucoma Treatment: The Glaucoma Initial Treatment Study Randomised Clinical Trial. *Br. J. Ophthalmol.* **2020**, *104*, 813–821. [CrossRef]
109. Lee, E.Y.; Farrokhyar, F.; Sogbesan, E. Laser Trabeculoplasty Perceptions and Practice Patterns of Canadian Ophthalmologists. *J. Curr. Glaucoma Pract.* **2020**, *14*, 81–86. [CrossRef]
110. Avery, N.; Ang, G.S.; Nicholas, S.; Wells, A. Repeatability of Primary Selective Laser Trabeculoplasty in Patients with Primary Open-Angle Glaucoma. *Int. Ophthalmol.* **2013**, *33*, 501–506. [CrossRef]
111. Kuley, B.; Zheng, C.X.; Zhang, Q.; Hamershock, R.A.; Lin, M.M.; Moster, S.J.; Murphy, J.; Moster, M.R.; Schmidt, C.; Lee, D.; et al. Predictors of Success in Selective Laser Trabeculoplasty. *Ophthalmol. Glaucoma* **2020**, *3*, 97–102. [CrossRef]
112. Alaghband, P.; Galvis, E.A.; Daas, A.; Nagar, A.; Beltran-Agulló, L.; Khawaja, A.P.; Goyal, S.; Lim, K.S. Predictors of Selective Laser Trabeculoplasty Success in Open Angle Glaucoma or Ocular Hypertension: Does Baseline Tonography Have a Predictive Role? *Br. J. Ophthalmol.* **2020**, *104*, 1390–1393. [CrossRef]
113. Hirabayashi, M.; Ponnusamy, V.; An, J. Predictive Factors for Outcomes of Selective Laser Trabeculoplasty. *Sci. Rep.* **2020**, *10*, 9428. [CrossRef] [PubMed]
114. Inoue, T.; Tanihara, H. Rho-Associated Kinase Inhibitors: A Novel Glaucoma Therapy. *Prog. Retin. Eye Res.* **2013**, *37*, 1–12. [CrossRef] [PubMed]
115. Baba, T.; Hirooka, K.; Nii, H.; Kiuchi, Y. Responsiveness to Ripasudil May Be a Potential Outcome Marker for Selective Laser Trabeculoplasty in Patients with Primary Open-Angle Glaucoma. *Sci. Rep.* **2021**, *11*, 5812. [CrossRef] [PubMed]
116. Shih, V.; Parekh, M.; Multani, J.K.; McGuiness, C.B.; Chen, C.-C.; Campbell, J.H.; Miller-Ellis, E.; Olivier, M.M.G. Clinical and Economic Burden of Glaucoma by Disease Severity: A United States Claims-Based Analysis. *Ophthalmol. Glaucoma* **2021**, *4*, 490–503. [CrossRef]
117. Dirani, M.; Crowston, J.G.; Taylor, P.S.; Moore, P.T.; Rogers, S.; Pezzullo, M.L.; Keeffe, J.E.; Taylor, H.R. Economic Impact of Primary Open-Angle Glaucoma in Australia. *Clin. Exp. Ophthalmol.* **2011**, *39*, 623–632. [CrossRef]
118. Lee, R.; Hutnik, C.M.L. Projected Cost Comparison of Selective Laser Trabeculoplasty versus Glaucoma Medication in the Ontario Health Insurance Plan. *Can. J. Ophthalmol. J. Can. Ophtalmol.* **2006**, *41*, 449–456. [CrossRef]
119. Gazzard, G.; Konstantakopoulou, E.; Garway-Heath, D.; Garg, A.; Vickerstaff, V.; Hunter, R.; Ambler, G.; Bunce, C.; Wormald, R.; Nathwani, N.; et al. *Health Economic Decision Model*; NIHR Journals Library: Southampton, UK, 2019.
120. Gandolfi, S.A.; Ungaro, N.; Varano, L.; Saccà, S. Low Power Selective Laser Trabeculoplasty (SLT) Repeated Yearly as Primary Treatment in Open Angle Glaucoma(s): Long Term Comparison with Conventional SLT and ALT. *Investig. Ophthalmol. Vis. Sci.* **2018**, *59*, 3459.
121. Realini, T.; Gazzard, G.; Latina, M.; Kass, M. Low-Energy Selective Laser Trabeculoplasty Repeated Annually: Rationale for the COAST Trial. *J. Glaucoma* **2021**, *30*, 545–551. [CrossRef]
122. Geffen, N.; Ofir, S.; Belkin, A.; Segev, F.; Barkana, Y.; Kaplan Messas, A.; Assia, E.I.; Belkin, M. Transscleral Selective Laser Trabeculoplasty Without a Gonioscopy Lens. *J. Glaucoma* **2017**, *26*, 201–207. [CrossRef]
123. Goldenfeld, M.; Belkin, M.; Dobkin-Bekman, M.; Sacks, Z.; Blum Meirovitch, S.; Geffen, N.; Leshno, A.; Skaat, A. Automated Direct Selective Laser Trabeculoplasty: First Prospective Clinical Trial. *Transl. Vis. Sci. Technol.* **2021**, *10*, 5. [CrossRef]

124. Congdon, N.; Azuara-Blanco, A.; Solberg, Y.; Traverso, C.E.; Iester, M.; Cutolo, C.A.; Bagnis, A.; Aung, T.; Fudemberg, S.J.; Lindstrom, R.; et al. Direct Selective Laser Trabeculoplasty in Open Angle Glaucoma Study Design: A Multicentre, Randomised, Controlled, Investigator-Masked Trial (GLAUrious). *Br. J. Ophthalmol.* **2021**. [CrossRef] [PubMed]

125. Gambini, G.; Carlà, M.M.; Caporossi, T.; De Vico, U.; Savastano, A.; Baldascino, A.; Rizzo, C.; Kilian, R.; Rizzo, S. Spotlight on MicroPulse Laser Trabeculoplasty in Open-Angle Glaucoma: What's on? A Review of the Literature. *Vision* **2022**, *6*, 8. [CrossRef] [PubMed]

126. Ma, A.; Yu, S.W.Y.; Wong, J.K.W. Micropulse Laser for the Treatment of Glaucoma: A Literature Review. *Surv. Ophthalmol.* **2019**, *64*, 486–497. [CrossRef] [PubMed]

127. Abramowitz, B.; Chadha, N.; Kouchouk, A.; Alhabshan, R.; Belyea, D.A.; Lamba, T. Selective Laser Trabeculoplasty vs Micropulse Laser Trabeculoplasty in Open-Angle Glaucoma. *Clin. Ophthalmol.* **2018**, *12*, 1599–1604. [CrossRef]

128. Fudemberg, S.J.; Myers, J.S.; Katz, L.J. Trabecular Meshwork Tissue Examination With Scanning Electron Microscopy: A Comparison of Micropulse Diode Laser (MLT), Selective Laser (SLT), and Argon Laser (ALT) Trabeculoplasty in Human Cadaver Tissue. *Investig. Ophthalmol. Vis. Sci.* **2008**, *49*, 1236.

129. Elahi, S.; Rao, H.L.; Paillard, A.; Mansouri, K. Outcomes of Pattern Scanning Laser Trabeculoplasty and Selective Laser Trabeculoplasty: Results from the Lausanne Laser Trabeculoplasty Registry. *Acta Ophthalmol.* **2021**, *99*, e154–e159. [CrossRef]

130. Wong, M.O.M.; Lai, I.S.; Chan, P.P.; Chan, N.C.; Chan, A.Y.; Lai, G.W.; Chiu, V.S.; Leung, C.K.-S. Efficacy and Safety of Selective Laser Trabeculoplasty and Pattern Scanning Laser Trabeculoplasty: A Randomised Clinical Trial. *Br. J. Ophthalmol.* **2021**, *105*, 514–520. [CrossRef]

131. Kaplowitz, K.; Wang, S.; Bilonick, R.; Oatts, J.T.; Grippo, T.; Loewen, N.A. Randomized Controlled Comparison of Titanium-Sapphire Versus Standard Q-Switched Nd: YAG Laser Trabeculoplasty. *J. Glaucoma* **2016**, *25*, e663–e667. [CrossRef]

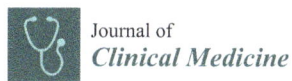
Journal of
Clinical Medicine

Article

Corneal Behavior during Tonometer Measurement during the Water Drinking Test in Eyes with XEN GelStent in Comparison to Non-Implanted Eyes

Agnieszka Jóźwik [1], Joanna Przeździecka-Dołyk [1,2,*], Ewa Wałek [2], Magdalena Czerniak [1] and Magdalena Asejczyk [1]

1 Department of Optics and Photonics, Wrocław University of Science and Technology, Wybrzeże Wyspiańskiego 27, 50-370 Wrocław, Poland; agnieszka.jozwik@pwr.edu.pl (A.J.); 236813@pwr.edu.pl (M.C.); magdalena.asejczyk@pwr.edu.pl (M.A.)
2 Department of Ophthalmology, Wroclaw Medical University, Borowska 213, 50-556 Wrocław, Poland; ewka.walek@gmail.com
* Correspondence: joanna.przezdziecka-dolyk@pwr.edu.pl

Citation: Jóźwik, A.; Przeździecka-Dołyk, J.; Wałek, E.; Czerniak, M.; Asejczyk, M. Corneal Behavior during Tonometer Measurement during the Water Drinking Test in Eyes with XEN GelStent in Comparison to Non-Implanted Eyes. *J. Clin. Med.* **2022**, *11*, 2962. https://doi.org/10.3390/jcm11112962

Academic Editors: Maria Letizia Salvetat, Marco Zeppieri and Paolo Brusini

Received: 27 March 2022
Accepted: 18 May 2022
Published: 24 May 2022

Publisher's Note: MDPI stays neutral with regard to jurisdictional claims in published maps and institutional affiliations.

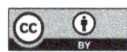
Abstract: Biomechanics of the cornea have significant influences on the non-contact measurement of the intraocular pressure. The corneal behaviour during tonometry is a fundamental factor in estimating its value. The aim of the study was to analyse the behaviour of the cornea during tonometric measurement with the forced change in intraocular pressure during the water drinking test. Ocular Response Analyser (Reichert) was used to the measurement. Besides four basic parameters connected with intraocular pressure (IOPg, IOPcc) and biomechanics (corneal hysteresis CH and corneal resistance factor (CRF), other parameters representing the behaviour of the cornea during a puff of air were analysed. There were 47 eyes included in the study, including 27 eyes with a XEN GelStent implanted and 20 without it. The eyes of people with monocular implementation were the reference group. The values of analysed parameters were compared before and after 10, 25, 40, and 55 min after drinking the water. The intraocular pressure increased by 2.4 mmHg ($p < 0.05$) for eyes with a XEN stent and 2.2 mmHg for eyes without a stent ($p < 0.05$) in the tenth minute after drinking of water. This change caused a decreasing of corneal hysteresis ($p < 0.05$) without significant changes in the corneal resistance factor ($p > 0.05$). Corneal hysteresis changed similarly in the reference group and the group with a XEN GelStent. The analysis of additional parameters showed a difference in the behaviour of the cornea in eyes with a XEN GelStent in comparison to the corneas of eyes without a stent. This was particularly visible in the analysis of the cornea's behaviour during the second applanation, when the cornea returns to its baseline state after deformation caused by air puff tonometry.

Keywords: XEN GelStent; corneal hysteresis; corneal resistance factor; open-angle glaucoma; intraocular pressure

1. Introduction

Assessment of eye biomechanics is crucial for the adequate understanding of corneal behaviour in response to mechanical actions in its structure, refractive surgery-induced tissue remodelling, or non-ablative refractive correction, as well as aspects of corneal physiology processes. Changes in its behaviour are the basic factor in estimating its value, especially during non-contact measurement. In 2001, David Luce showed that, from the signal received by the non-contact tonometer, it is possible to obtain information not only about the intraocular pressure but also about the biomechanical properties of the cornea [1]. Corneal hysteresis (CH) parameter, representing the viscoelastic nature of the cornea, became available by using a commercial device—Ocular Response Analyzer (ORA). It was shown, before, that both types of the intraocular pressure measured by ORA (Goldmann-correlated pressure IOPg and corneal-compensated pressure IOPcc) have good agreement with GAT on normal subjects [2]. IOPcc compared to GAT suggests IOPcc shows greater agreement with GAT than ORA IOPg [3].

Glaucoma, which is a disease defined primarily on the basis of changes in the optic nerve disc, also affects the biomechanics of the eyeball. One of the main factors influencing the development of glaucoma is the intraocular pressure increasing. It could cause changes in the structure of the eyeball, e.g., loss of corneal endothelial cells. This is important in primary angle closure glaucoma because, if a high IOP level remains elevated longer than 72 h, an irreversible, very large, and significant loss of endothelial cells may occur in the cornea [4]. Biomechanical parameters can be regarded as biomarkers of glaucoma susceptibility [5]. Corneal hysteresis CH in glaucomatous eyes is lower than in the healthy eyes, and this decrease is correlated with a reduction in the field of view [6]. However, the relationship between the biomechanics of the cornea and the appearance of the optic disc is still not fully known [5]. However, studies have shown that this parameter can be used to predict the progression of primary open-angle glaucoma [7–10]. The authors of the studies mentioned above reported that the progression of glaucoma is likely to be influenced by the biomechanical properties of the cornea. Researchers observed that CH measurements were significantly less in primary open-angle glaucoma and normal-tension glaucoma compared to normal subjects. Besides CH, the device gives information about corneal resistance factor (CRF). CRF is a measure of the overall resistance of the cornea related to its elastic properties. CRF is not associated with CH. Despite many researchers of this subject, there is no so clear understanding of how CRF is correlated with the occurrence of glaucoma. Some researchers show that CRF is not influenced by glaucoma [8]. However, there are results showing that CRF was significantly less in normal-tension glaucoma and maximum in primary open-angle glaucoma and ocular hypertension [9]. However, it was noted that procedures aimed at lowering the intraocular pressure, including glaucoma drainage, trabeculectomy, and trabeculectomy combined with cataract surgery, may lead to changes in CH and CRF parameters. Research conducted at the Ophthalmic Research Center in Tehran in 2014 showed that the values of CH and CRF parameters increase after successful IOP reduction and cataract removal procedures [11]. These studies analysed the results after trabeculectomy, phaco-trabeculectomy, Ahmed glaucoma valve implantation, and phacoemulsification. Refractive surgery procedures also affect the change in CH and CRF parameters, but the opposite relationship is observed compared to cases of glaucoma treatment. The values of the CH and CRF parameters decrease after these procedures [12].

One of the solutions to stop the progression of the glaucoma is the implantation of drainage microducts as a part of minimally invasive glaucoma surgery (MIGS). Such stents allow an additional path of the flow of aqueous fluid between the anterior chamber and the preconjunctival space. One of the MIGS devices is XEN GelStent (Allergan, Dublin, Ireland), which is a 6-mm long stent of collagen-derived gelatin cross-linked with glutaraldehyde. The procedure is almost always augmented with a subconjunctival or sub-Tenon injection of mitomycin C. The XEN GelStent received the CE mark approval in 2011 and the US FDA approval in 2016. The stent was inserted into the eye using a 0.4 mm diameter needle in the upper-nasal quadrant of the eyeball. The implant starts working as soon as it is placed in the eye [13]. The previous work [14] has shown if such an implementation has an impact on the biomechanics of the cornea. CRF and CH changed significantly in eyes with primary open-angle glaucoma after XEN GelStent implantation (post-XEN), in comparison to primary open-angle glaucoma control group (eyes without stent). Analysis of the basic parameters from ORA showed that the biomechanical parameters of the anterior chamber in the post-XEN group changed significantly during WDT (water drinking test).

The Ocular Response Analyzer is an air-puff tonometer. An impulse of air is released towards the cornea. It bends inward and, after reaching the maximum deflection, it returns to its initial state. During the movement both inwards and backwards, the cornea passes through the applanation state, which is equivalent to a flattening, corresponding to the one prevailing in the Goldman tonometry. Corneal deformation is recorded with an electro-optical infrared detection system, and results are presented as the applanation curve. The shape of the signal curve is obtained from ORA, and therefore, the parameters describing this curve may also reflect the biomechanical properties of the cornea, as well as the parameter CH [15]. Changes in the shape of this signal indicate various pathological deviations of the cornea, including keratoconus [16]. It was showed that the shape of this signal is also different after refractive surgery [17].

A symmetry of eyes was observed in individual patients, e.g., an astigmatic axis, IOP, higher-order aberrations, corneal curvature, and corneal thickness [18–21]. The symmetry of biomechanical parameters is purely investigated. However, symmetry of CH and CRF was proven [22,23].

The aim of the study is to investigate the influence the XEN GelStent drainage implementation on corneal biomechanical behaviour. This research is based on a comparison of the parameters, describing the deformation of the cornea, during air-puff measurement in the eyes with the stent in relation to the eyes without it.

2. Methods

The present study was registered in ClinicalTrials.gov with the number NCT03904381 and conducted at the Department of Ophthalmology, Wroclaw Medical University. Clinical data base were collected between April and May 2018. The screening phase lasts between June 2018 and August and measurements between September and December 2018. All patients were informed about the aim, benefits, and risks of all procedures of the study before screening phase. The study was performed in adherence to the Declaration of Helsinki and was approved by the local Ethics Committee (approval number: KB 563/2017).

2.1. Measurement Group

The study included 39 patients in the screening phase after XEN GelStent implantation. The 27 patients were observed in 12 months of follow-up period. Finally, 18 patients were enrolled in the research. All subjects had a XEN GelStent implant in one eye (XEN group). The other eyes without a stent were considered as a reference POAG group (Control Group). The mean age of patients was 69 ± 12 years (range: 34–81 years).

Patients with POAG after at least 3 months of post-XEN GelStent implantation were prospectively enrolled in the study between September and December 2018, and details concerning glaucoma stage, medication status, and further information are summarised in Supplementary Files–Table S1. Technical details of implantation and the perioperative period have been described previously [24]. Patients with a reduction in IOP, compared to the pre-XEN implantation measurements of at least $\geq 20\%$ baseline IOP and ≤ 21 mmHg, as well as at least 3 months post last 5-FU injection, were included to the research. With any progression (according to the EGS guidelines) within the last 3 months, any change in medication within the last month, and any systemic medication within the last 3 or more months, 5-FU injections were used as exclusion criteria. A reference group consists of POAG patients with at least 3 months on stable local anti-glaucoma medications without significant side effects and a reduction in IOP compared to the pre-medication measurements of at least $\geq 20\%$ baseline IOP and ≤ 21 mmHg. Any progression (according to the EGS guidelines) within the last 3 months, or any procedures using lasers, were criteria for excluding eyes from the research. High axial refractive errors, due to elongation of the globe (AXL > 26 mm), also excluded patients of both groups from the research. None of the included subjects took any systemic antiglaucomatous medication at least 3 months previously. Only three eyes (16%) in the XEN group required topical anti-glaucoma medications to control IOP (one patient was taking β-blocker, and two patients were taking prostaglandins eye drops). All participants underwent complete ophthalmological examination before participation to determine their refractive and health status. The detailed procedure was described previously [14].

2.2. Ocular Response Analyzer and Measurement Procedure

The biomechanical data were measured using ORA (Reichert Ophthalmic Instruments, Inc., Buffalo, NY, USA; Software version 3.0). Basically, ORA generates two separate parameters related to the intraocular pressure: Goldmann-correlated pressure (IOPg) and corneal-compensated pressure (IOPcc). In addition, using a bidirectional applanation measurement, ORA allows the determination of two parameters describing the biomechanical properties of the cornea: Corneal Hysteresis (CH) and Corneal Resistance Factor (CRF). The quality of measurement is described by the waveform score (WS) on a scale from 0 to 10, which indicates the reliability of each measurement. The deformation of the cornea is recorded with an electro-optical infrared detection system that records the intensity of light reflected from the surface of the cornea as it is deflected. There are 400 points of the light deflection that are recorded during a 25 ms period, and they form the applanation curve (black line). An exemplary applanation curve is presented in Figure 1. The applanation curve is characterized by the two characteristic peaks, which correspond to the moments of corneal flattening, when the pressure on both sides of the cornea is equalized. Additionally the air-pressure curve, representing pressure of the air flow emitted by the device, is recorded (Figure 1, grey line). Based on these two curves, the pressure during applanation states is determined. The pressure $P1$ is recorded for the first applanation, occurring as the cornea moves inward with an increasing air pulse, while $P2$ is the pressure corresponding to the second applanation when the cornea returns to its initial curvature while decreasing the stream of the air. Therefore, for corneas after intervention to its structure, the mechanical response and the entire applanation curve may be very irregular. In this case, the applanation peaks could be lower, wider, or otherwise irregular.

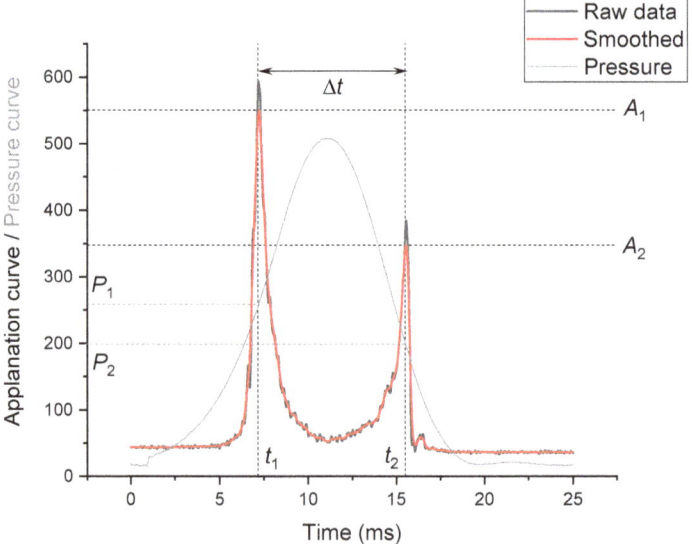

Figure 1. The applanation curve recorded by ORA (control group, before WDT, patient 11).

The ORA additionally determines 37 parameters describing the shape of the applanation curve representing the change of the curvature of the cornea during the measurement. They represent properties of corneal behaviour separately in two applanation areas, including the area under the curve (p1area, p2area), upward slope (uslope1, uslope2), downward slope (dslope1, dslope2), peak width (w1, w2), peak height (h1, h2)), length of the curve around the peaks (path1, path2), smoothness of the peaks (aindex, bindex), noise (aplhf), and six additional parameters (dive1, dive2, mslew1, mselw2, slew1, and slew2). A detailed description of the parameters is presented in the Supplementary Files–Table S2.

Additionally, the amplitudes (A_1 and A_2) and the times (t_1 and t_2) of both applanation occurrences were calculated from raw data taken from the device (Figure 1). Firstly, the applanation curve was smoothed with Gaussian estimation and with the window size 11. Smoothing was supposed to minimize sharpness of the raw data curves (Figure 1, red line). Moreover, the difference between applanation times (Δt) was calculated.

The water drinking test was used to obtain different levels of the intraocular pressure. The patient drank an amount of the water proportional to his weight, with the proportion 10 mL/kg, for 10 min. The values of parameters measured by the ORA were recorded before (reference result) and 10, 25, 40, and 55 min after stopping drinking the water. The biomechanical properties were measured, fourfold, with a waveform score higher than 5, and mean values were recorded for further analysis. All recordings were conducted on the same equipment by the same dedicated examiner. After the conduction of WDT, each patient was observed for a year, and control visits were conducted as described in the study protocol (NCT03904381).

2.3. Statistical Analysis

Statistical analyses were conducted using Statistica Software version 13.3 (TIBCO Statistica 1984–2017 TIBCO Software Inc., Palo Alto, CA, USA)) licensed by Wroclaw University of Science and Technology. The results of measurements of 4 basic parameters (IOPg, IOPcc, CH, and CRF), 37 additional parameters describing the deformation of curves signals of eyes, and 5 parameters defined in this work, in the eyes after stent implantation in relation to eyes without an implant, were compared. The Shapiro–Wilk test was used to check the normality of the sample distribution. Repeated measures analysis of variance (ANOVA and Friedmann), with the Bonferroni or Dunn adjustment for multiple comparisons, was used to determine the influence of the within-subjects factor water unload. The nonparametric Wilcoxon rank-sum or paired t-test were used to evaluate the distribution of variables between the two groups (subject groups: post-XEN and control). Results were considered statistically significant with a $p < 0.05$.

3. Results

The study included the post-XEN group with 18 eyes and 18 non-implanted eyes (control group). The group had a similar female/male ratio ($p > 0.05$). No differences in the baseline GAT, central corneal radius CCT, ACD, AXL, BCVA, MD, PSD, RNFLT, body weight, BMI, ECC, and hexagonity of endothelial cells were recorded (Table 1).

Table 1. Demographic data.

	Control Group		XEN GelStent	
	Mean ± SD	Range	Mean ± SD	Range
GAT [mm Hg]	15.9 ± 3.1	10–22	14.4 ± 3.0	9–19
CCT [μm]	534 ± 45	436–592	531 ± 39	457–589
ACD [mm]	3.05 ± 0.80	1.88–4.28	3.13 ± 0.87	1.82–4.20
AXL [mm]	23.54 ± 1.12	23.43–26.47	23.41 ± 0.83	21.67 ± 24.88

GAT–intraocular pressure (Goldmann tonometry), CCT–central corneal thickness, ACD–anterior chamber depth, AXL–eyeball axial length.

3.1. Intraocular Pressure during the WDT

According to the pre-specified criteria, WDT was positive. Results of the intraocular pressure are presented in Table 2. Before the water drinking test, the intraocular pressure of the eyes with XEN GelStent implants was lower by 2 mmHg, on average, than in the eyes in the control group. This trend continued at a similar level. However, these differences were not statistically significant. It is worth noting that values of IOPcc (corneal compensated pressure) were higher than IOPg (Goldmann-correlated pressure). It could be caused by thinner central corneal thickness, of the considered group (CCT about 530 μm), than average for healthy eyes. Independently of the group, the highest increase in intraocular pressure was observed 10 min after drinking of water. The increase after 10 min and 25 min was statistically significant ($p < 0.05$ post-hoc analysis). After this time, the IOP returned to the pre-test level in the group of eyes with the stent. This stabilisation was also observed in the control group, but it followed slower than in the XEN GelStent group.

Table 2. The WDT results on the intraocular pressure (IOPcc—corneal-compensated intraocular pressure, IOPg—Goldmann-correlated intraocular pressure) in the control and XEN GelStent groups.

	IOPg [mmHg]			IOPcc [mmHg]		
	Control	XEN GelStent	*p*-Value	Control	XEN GelStent	*p*-Value
Before	14.7 ± 4.4	12.8 ± 4.7	0.13 [I]	16.5 ± 3.9	14.6 ± 4.0	0.21 [II]
10 min	17.2 ± 3.7	14.9 ± 4.7	0.08 [I]	19.1 ± 3.6	16.8 ± 4.3	0.13 [I]
25 min	17.1 ± 3.1	14.8 ± 4.3	0.10 [II]	19.1 ± 3.1	16.8 ± 4.3	0.09 [I]
40 min	16.9 ± 4.3	13.9 ± 4.1	0.06 [I]	19.2 ± 3.8	15.9 ± 3.9	0.05 [I]
55 min	16.9 ± 5.5	13.9 ± 4.4	0.08 [II]	18.9 ± 5.4	16.0 ± 4.1	0.12 [II]
p-value	<0.005 [IV]	<0.001 [III]		<0.05 [IV]	<0.001 [III]	

[I]-*t*-test, [II]-Wilcoxon test, [III]-ANOVA test, [IV]-Friedman test.

3.2. The Biomechanical Parameters during the WDT

During the analysis of the biomechanical parameters, it was observed that CH in the control group changed significantly during WDT ($p < 0.05$), but there were not changes in CRF ($p = 0.17$). The biomechanical parameters of the anterior chamber in the XEN GelStent presented no statistical changes in WDT ($p = 0.17$ and $p = 0.41$, for CH and CRF, respectively). In the XEN GelStent, there were no statistically significant changes for CH, but the variation for CH were observed during the measurement. The corneal hysteresis decreased, both in CG and XEN GelStent groups, during particular parts of measurement, while CRF shows a similar trend to the intraocular pressure, i.e., it increased after 10 min and then decreased. Detailed results are presented in Table 3. There was not a difference between groups on each level of the measurement during the water drinking test.

Table 3. The corneal hysteresis (CH) and corneal resistance factor (CRF) during the water drinking test (WDT) in the control and XEN GelStent groups.

	CH [mmHg]			CRF [mmHg]		
	Control	XEN GelStent	*p*-Value	Control	XEN GelStent	*p*-Value
Before	9.2 ± 1.7	9.6 ± 1.7	0.27 [I]	9.2 ± 2.2	8.9 ± 2.3	0.35 [I]
10 min	8.9 ± 1.9	9.1 ± 1.8	0.52 [I]	9.6 ± 2.0	9.1 ± 2.1	0.06 [I]
25 min	8.8 ± 1.5	9.1 ± 1.6	0.31 [I]	9.5 ± 1.6	9.1 ± 1.7	0.11 [I]
40 min	8.6 ± 1.7	9.2 ± 1.7	0.10 [I]	9.3 ± 2.1	8.9 ± 1.9	0.21 [I]
55 min	8.8 ± 1.8	9.1 ± 1.5	0.31 [I]	9.5 ± 2.1	8.9 ± 1.8	0.11 [I]
p-value	<0.05 [III]	0.17 [III]		0.17 [III]	0.41 [III]	

[I]-*t*-test, [III]-ANOVA test.

3.3. Analysis of the Applanation Curve Parameters

Different behaviour of the cornea was observed in eyes with the XEN GelStent implant, in comparison to non-implanted eyes, the during the water drinking test. Exemplary applanation curves, for one patient during the water drinking test, are presented in the Figure 2. Among individuals, 50% had higher peaks in the first applanation (A1) in XEN

GelStent eyes, and 38% had peaks in the second applanation (A2). Among individuals, 45% had symmetrical behaviour in both eyes, which means there was a decrease or an increase in the peak height in both eyes simultaneously. A decrease in the maximum value, related to the first applanation, was observed in 62% of both the control and XEN GelStent eyes, but it did not occur in the same pair of eyes. During the second applanation, the lower maximum was observed in 80% of the control eyes and 38% of the XEN GelStent eyes.

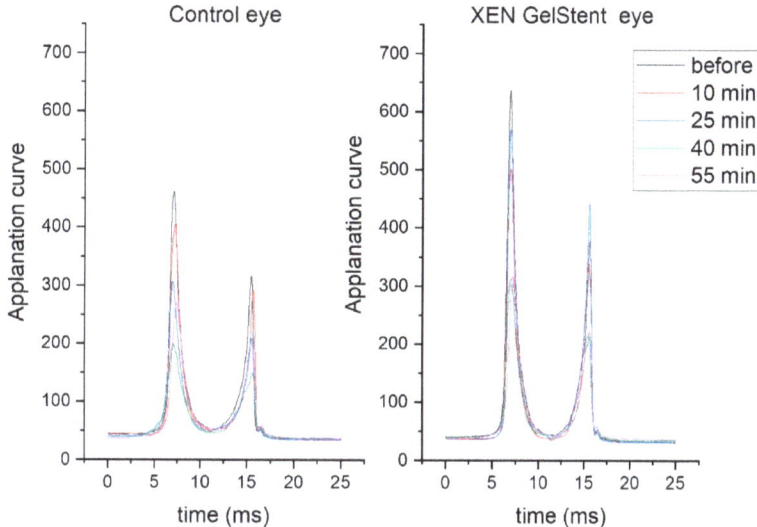

Figure 2. Exemplary applanation curves for one patient during the water drinking test.

The further analysis was divided into two parts related to the first and the second applanation. All results are present in Supplementary Files–Table S3, respectively. The only parameter that is not directly related to both applanations is aplhf, representing noise between applanations. Similarly, parameters aindex and bindex, which are correlated with the quality of the curves (during the first and the second applanation, respectively), are not susceptible to WDT. The analysis showed that changes caused by drinking water did not change the value of this parameter (Friedmann test, $p > 0.05$). Most of the analysed parameters were lower on each step of the measurement during the water drinking test. Some of them returned to the pre-WDT level after 55 min. In fact, only the width of the peaks (w1, w2, w21) behaved similarly to the tendency of the intraocular pressure or CRF. It means that there was an increase in the first 10 min after water drinking, and then, it declines, and this change was statistically significant for the control group only ($p < 0.05$).

Only a few of the analysed parameters did not change during WDT in both groups. During the first applanation, no change was observed for absolute value of path length around the peak (path1, path11) and the maximum single step increase in the rise of the peak (mslew1). During the second applanation, there were the parameters describing the area of the peak (p2area and p2area1).

Despite the lack of statistically significant differences in all analysed parameters for considered groups, some trends were observed in the parameters' values. Regardless of the applanation type, higher peaks (h1, h11, h2, h21) were obtained in the control eyes group in comparison of XEN GelStent group. There were also thicker peaks during the first (w1, w11) and wider peaks during the second (w2, w21) applanation. Analysis of slopes showed slightly lower values of the parameters describing the first applanation (uslope1, uslope11, dslope1, dslope11) in XEN GelStent group than in the control group, but it showed higher values describing the second peak (uslope2, uslope21, dslope2, dslope21). A similar tendency had the aspect ratio of the peak, calculated as dividing height by width of the peak. The aspect ratio of peak 1 (aspect 1 and aspect 11) was higher for the control group, but for peak 2 (aspect 2 and aspect 21), it was higher for the XEN GelStent group. All these changes were small and statistically insignificant.

3.4. Analysis of Parameters from Raw Data of Applanation Curve

The analysis of the maximum value of two peaks calculated from raw data is similar to previously presented h1, h11, h2, and h21 because their determination is of a similar nature (Table 4).

Table 4. Amplitudes of the first and second applanation (respectively A1 and A2) during the water drinking test (WDT) in the control and XEN GelStent groups.

	A1 [–]			A2 [–]		
	Control	XEN GelStent	*p*-Value	Control	XEN GelStent	*p*-Value
Before	570 ± 140	540 ± 170	0.56 [I]	430 ± 90	410 ± 100	0.52 [I]
10 min	530 ± 150	530 ± 120	0.83 [I]	420 ± 110	420 ± 80	0.99 [I]
25 min	510 ± 170	480 ± 160	0.48 [I]	380 ± 100	380 ± 100	0.99 [I]
40 min	430 ± 150	450 ± 140	0.66 [I]	380 ± 120	340 ± 100	<0.05 [I]
55 min	430 ± 140	440 ± 160	0.70 [II]	360 ± 110	360 ± 110	0.76 [II]
p-value	<0.001 [III]	<0.05 [IV]		<0.005 [IV]	<0.001 [III]	

[I]-*t*-test, [II]-Wilcoxon test, [III]-ANOVA test, [IV]-Friedman test.

The times of applanation occurrence differentiate for the control and XEN GelStent groups, especially when considering the interspace between applanations (Δt). The eyes with implants reacted faster to the air-puff stream than the control eyes, on particular stages of the measurement, but simultaneously when the second applanation is delayed. P-values are on the margin of the statistical significance for comparison of parameters t_1 and Δt between two groups of eyes (Table 5).

Table 5. The time of the first and second applanation (respectively t_1 and t_2) along with the interspace between applanations (Δt) during the water drinking test (WDT) in the control and XEN GelStent groups.

	t_1 [ms]			t_2 [ms]			Δt [ms]		
	Control	XEN GelStent	*p*-Value	Control	XEN GelStent	*p*-Value	Control	XEN GelStent	*p*-Value
Before	6.65 ± 0.5	6.43 ± 0.57	0.10 [I]	15.55 ± 0.17	15.62 ± 0.22	<0.05 [I]	8.90 ± 0.45	9.19 ± 0.56	<0.05 [I]
10 min	6.90 ± 0.39	6.65 ± 0.51	0.05 [I]	15.55 ± 0.17	15.59 ± 0.19	0.29 [I]	8.64 ± 0.34	8.94 ± 0.5	0.06 [I]
25 min	6.9 ± 0.4	6.6 ± 0.48	<0.05 [I]	15.52 ± 0.17	15.58 ± 0.19	0.26 [I]	8.62 ± 0.39	8.97 ± 0.5	<0.05 [I]
40 min	6.87 ± 0.51	6.58 ± 0.45	0.07 [I]	15.47 ± 0.21	15.52 ± 0.21	0.38 [I]	8.61 ± 0.56	8.94 ± 0.47	0.10 [I]
55 min	6.86 ± 0.5	6.52 ± 0.52	0.05 [I]	15.52 ± 0.22	15.54 ± 0.22	0.67 [I]	8.66 ± 0.59	9.02 ± 0.5	0.10 [I]
p-value	<0.005 [II]	<0.005 [II]		0.13 [II]	0.05 [II]		<0.05 [II]	<0.005 [II]	

[I]-*t*-test, [II]-ANOVA test.

The influence of WDT is observed in the analysis of the first applanation time. The time of the second applanation did not change significantly during WDT.

4. Conclusions

Biomechanics of the cornea are important in many diagnostic procedures. It was interesting to check whether the placement of the implant disturbs such corneal biomechanics of the eye and could influence the results of the intraocular pressure measurements. The analysis was performed based on the deflection cornea during the air-puff tonometry. The ORA, one of the most commonly used tonometers, has become a popular clinical device for evaluating biomechanical properties. CH and CRF are parameters that are important factors in understanding the biomechanical state of the cornea and the clinical diagnosis of eye diseases. ORA gives the possibility to analyse additional parameters, describing the shape of the applanation curve and being a representation of the corneal deflection, during the air-puff measurement.

The analysis is based on evaluating the behaviour of the cornea while implementing a water drinking test (WTD), with the aim being to check the influence of an increasing pressure on the biomechanical properties. The water drinking test was performed in two groups of eyes. One group included eyes with the XEN GelStent implant, and the control group consisted of the second eyes of the same patients (POAG eyes, usually with pharmacological treatment). Before WDT, there was a difference observed in the initial intraocular pressure. Higher values of IOP were observed in the control group of eyes. This means that the implant is working properly. The pressure increased 10 min after drinking water, by more than 2 mmHg, in both groups. A higher or lower increase in IOP depends, mainly, on the efficiency of the choroidal scleral outflow tract. Pressure returned to the pre-water level faster in eyes with the stent. It was especially seen in corneal compensated IOP (IOPcc). In earlier work [6,11,25], authors reported that CH parameters increase after IOP reduction. In this research, this increase is not statistically significant for comparison of the control and adequate XEN GelStent eyes. However, CH decreases after water drinking, and this change was statistically significant in the control eyes ($p < 0.05$). Subsequently, this value remained at a similar level. The lack of noticeable changes, compared to values before WDT, may be due to corneal hydration. In the XEN GelStent group, CRF was lower than in the control group, but this difference was not significant. The value of the CRF parameter did not change as a consequence of drinking water, so it can be established that the corneal resistance is a parameter that is more stable and can describe the biomechanics of the cornea more precisely. Observed higher CRF and lower CH, in 10 min after water drinking, could be indicative of a "protective effect" associated with a greater central corneal thickness in higher pressure eyes, where more force was required to induce applanation. Therefore, one would expect an overestimation of the IOP in a cornea with a higher CRF [9]. Sharifipour et al., also observed that CH and CRF changed significantly after WDT in medically or surgically (trabeculectomy) controlled glaucoma in comparison to normal individuals [26]. In this research, while CH changes after WDT were not significantly different among the groups, CRF changes in the medical group were significantly higher than the control group.

Basic parameters from Ocular Response Analyser are calculated from pressures obtained during two applanation states when the cornea deflects inwards (P1) and towards (P2). The calculated pressure depends on the time of the applanation. Our research was showing that the first applanation (t_1) was observed about 0.2–0.3 ms later, for the control, in comparison with the XEN GelStent group. It was expected since the cornea in eyes with higher intraocular pressure are more resistant to deflection. It also takes longer for the cornea in XEN GelStent eyes to return to its original shape. The second applanation (t_2) was achieved slightly later for XEN GelStent eyes, but this delay was not statistically significant. The time of the second applanation (t_2) did not change significantly during WDT in contrast to the time t_1. Based on this, it can be concluded that the second peak of the applanation curve may better reflect the corneal biomechanics, and the first peak is more related to the intraocular pressure. The most important observation is related to Δt before drinking water and shortly after there were statistically significant differences in the intervals between the applanations. After 25 min, these intervals did not differ significantly. This time was longer for the eyes with the implant.

Changes in the shape of the curves describing the intensity of light reflected from the cornea were also observed, but these differences were not statistically significant between both eyes. An analysis showed that both peaks for control eyes were higher than for XEN GelStent group, wherein the first peak was narrower, and the second peak was wider for XEN GelStent eyes. It means that the applanation area was wider for control eyes. The parameters describing the slope of the peaks, representing the rate of achieving applanation, showed that, in the XEN GelStent group, the first applanation was slower than in the control group. However, in the case of the second application, it was the other way around, and for the eyes with XEN GelStent, these speeds were higher. It could mean a slight stiffening of the cornea in eyes with the implant, or it may be caused by a change in the biomechanical properties, such as viscoelasticity of the cornea, by the stent implantation procedure. This conclusion is controversial in literature, although recent research showed that this procedure did not have to have a direct effect on the corneal endothelial cells and, thus, on its structure [27].

Most analysed parameters were sensitive to the influence of WDT in both groups. Almost all value parameters decreased in relation to the level before the drinking test. It can be effected by corneal hydration and the water absorption by the cornea near the limbus. This is due to the different packing density of the corneal stroma. The lamellas are arranged more densely in the anterior and middle parts of the stroma than in the posterior one. In addition, they are also more hydrated in the central part, as a result of which the back part of the stroma can swell easily due to the less frequent packing of these fibres [28]. Moreover, the observation of viscoelastic behaviour in the intact human cornea may be explained by the influence of corneal hydration on the stress distribution between corneal lamellae. In the swollen cornea, only the anterior corneal lamellae are able to take up tension, whereas the posterior lamellae will be slack. Clinically, this can be observed as folds in Descement's membrane. During the pressure-induced reduction in corneal volume, the posterior lamellae elongate and take up some of the corneal stress, and the stress on the anterior lamellae will decrease. Eliasson and Maurice [29], after studying the displacement of the cornea surfaces induced by corneal thinning, concluded that stress distribution across the corneal stroma is even in the normo-hydrated human cornea in vivo [30].

The statistical significance of CH and CRF parameters in glaucoma diagnosis have been reported previously [10,31–33]. However, most studies presented the comparison of ORA parameters between the healthy and glaucomatous eyes. Little work has been conducted on the postoperative diagnosis and raw data of ORA results [14,34]. The findings of the present study indicate that the analysis of ORA parameters could be utilized in postoperative and treated glaucoma diagnostics [14,35].

Supplementary Materials: The following supporting information can be downloaded at: https://www.mdpi.com/article/10.3390/jcm11112962/s1; Table S1. Demographic and clinical characteristics of the study groups (XEN group and Control group). All participants have bilateral POAG. One eye of each patient was assigned to the XEN group and the other to the Control group (the POAG group); Table S2. Variables and definitions of the corneal deformation signal parameters obtained by Ocular Response Analyzer; Table S3. Summary of parameters obtained from the corneal deformation signal parameters obtained by Ocular Response Analyzer, divided to the parameters that refers to the first and second applanation.

Author Contributions: Conceptualization, J.P.-D., A.J. and M.A.; methodology, J.P.-D., A.J., E.W. and M.A.; software, A.J.; validation, A.J., J.P.-D. and M.A.; formal analysis, A.J.; investigation, J.P.-D., E.W. and M.C.; resources, J.P.-D. and E.W.; data curation, J.P.-D.; writing—original draft preparation, A.J.; writing—review and editing, A.J. and J.P.-D.; visualization, A.J.; supervision, M.A.; project administration, J.P.-D.; funding acquisition, E.W. and J.P-D. All authors have read and agreed to the published version of the manuscript.

Funding: The study was performed with financial support of Wroclaw Medical University Grant for Young Researchers (No: STM.C240.17.037). Editorial support was funded by Wroclaw Medical University: SUB.C240.21.036. The authors maintained complete control over the content of the paper. No payment was received for authorship of the document.

Institutional Review Board Statement: The study was conducted in accordance with the Declaration of Helsinki, and approved by the Ethics Committee of Wroclaw Medical University (Approval Number KB 563/2017).

Informed Consent Statement: Informed consent was obtained from all subjects involved in the study.

Data Availability Statement: The data will be available via online access according to the Clinical Trials registration statement.

Conflicts of Interest: The authors report no conflict of interest and have no proprietary interest in any of the materials mentioned in this article.

References

1. Ambrosio, R. *Corneal Biomechanics: From Theory to Practice*; Kugler Publications: Amsterdam, The Netherlands, 2016; p. 72.
2. Lam, A.; Chen, D.; Chiu, R.; Chui, W.S. Comparison of IOP measurements between ORA and GAT in normal Chinese. *Optom. Vis. Sci.* **2007**, *84*, 909–914. [CrossRef] [PubMed]
3. McCann, P.; Hogg, R.E.; Wright, D.M.; McGuinness, B.; Young, I.S.; Kee, F.; Azuara-Blanco, A. Comparison of Goldmann applanation and Ocular Response Analyser tonometry: Intraocular pressure agreement and patient preference. *Eye* **2020**, *34*, 584–590. [CrossRef] [PubMed]
4. Salvi, S.M.; Akhtar, S.; Currie, Z. Ageing changes in the eye. *Postgrad. Med. J.* **2006**, *82*, 581–587. [CrossRef] [PubMed]
5. Roberts, C.J.; Dupps, W.J.; Downs, J.C. *Biomechanics of the Eye*; Kugler Publications: Amsterdam, The Netherlands, 2018.
6. European Glaucoma Society. *Terminology and Guidelines for Glaucoma*, 4th ed.; PubliComm: Savona, Italy, 2014.
7. Grise-Dulac, A.; Saad, A.; Abitbol, O. Assessment of corneal biomechanical properties in normal tension glaucoma and comparison with open-angle glaucoma, ocular hypertension, and normal eyes. *J. Glaucoma* **2012**, *21*, 486–489. [CrossRef] [PubMed]
8. Sullivan-Mee, M.; Billingsley, S.C.; Patel, A.D. Ocular response analyzer in subjects with and without glaucoma. *Optom. Vis. Sci.* **2008**, *85*, 463–470. [CrossRef] [PubMed]
9. Kaushik, S.; Pandav, S.S.; Banger, A. Relationship between corneal biomechanical properties, central corneal thickness, and intraocular pressure across the spectrum of glaucoma. *Am. J. Ophthalmol.* **2012**, *153*, 840–849. [CrossRef]
10. Abitbol, O.; Bouden, J.; Doan, S. Corneal hysteresis measured with the ocular response analyzer in normal and glaucomatous eyes. *Acta Ophthalmol.* **2010**, *88*, 116–119. [CrossRef]
11. Mohammad, P.; Mohsen, A.; Shahin, Y. Corneal Biomechanical Changes Following Trabeculectomy, Phaco-trabeculectomy, Ahmed Glaucoma Valve Implantation and Phacoemulsification. *J. Ophthalmic Vis. Res.* **2014**, *9*, 7–13.
12. Wu, W.; Wang, Y. The Correlation Analysis between Corneal Biomechanical Properties and the Surgically Induced Corneal High-Order Aberrations after Small Incision Lenticule Extraction and Femtosecond Laser In Situ Keratomileusis. *J.Ophthalmol.* **2015**, *7*, 1–10. [CrossRef]
13. Chaudhary, A.; Salinas, L.; Guidotti, J.; Mansouri, K.; Mermoud, A. XEN Gel Implant: A new surgical approach in glaucoma. *Expert Rev. Med. Devices* **2017**, *15*, 47–59. [CrossRef]
14. Przeździecka-Dołyk, J.; Wałek, E.; Jóźwik, A.; Helemejko, I.; Asejczyk-Widlicka, M.; Misiuk-Hojło, M. Short-Time Changes of Intraocular Pressure and Biomechanics of the Anterior Segment of the Eye during Water Drinking Test in Patients with XEN GelStent. *J. Clin. Med.* **2022**, *11*, 175. [CrossRef] [PubMed]
15. Aoki, S.; Murata, H.; Matsuura, M.; Fujino, Y.; Nakakura, S.; Nakao, Y.; Kiuchi, Y.; Asaoka, R. The Relationship between the Waveform Parameters from the Ocular Response Analyzer and the Progression of Glaucoma. *Ophthalmol. Glaucoma* **2018**, *125*, 1839–1841. [CrossRef] [PubMed]
16. Luz, A.; Lopes, B.; Hallahan, K.M. Discriminant Value of Custom Ocular Response Analyzer Waveform Derivatives in Forme Fruste Keratoconus. *Am. J. Ophthalmol.* **2016**, *164*, 14–21. [CrossRef] [PubMed]
17. Landoulsi, H.; Saad, A.; Haddad, N.N.; Guilbert, E.; Gatinel, D. Repeatability of Ocular Response Analyzer Waveform Parameters in Normal Eyes and Eyes After Refractive Surgery. *J. Refract. Surg.* **2013**, *29*, 709–714. [CrossRef]
18. McKendrick, A.M.; Brennan, N.A. The axis of astigmatism in right and left eye pairs. *Optom. Vis. Sci.* **1997**, *74*, 668–675. [CrossRef]
19. Realini, T.; Vickers, W.R. Symmetry of fellow-eye intraocular pressure responses to topical glaucoma medications. *Ophthalmology* **2005**, *112*, 599–602. [CrossRef]
20. Harris, W.F. Technical note: Accounting for anatomical symmetry in the first-order optical character of left and right eyes. *Ophthalmic Physiol. Opt.* **2007**, *27*, 412–415. [CrossRef]
21. Myrowitz, E.H.; Kouzis, A.C.; O'Brien, T.P. High interocular corneal symmetry in average simulated keratometry, central corneal thickness, and posterior elevation. *Optom. Vis. Sci.* **2005**, *82*, 428–431. [CrossRef]
22. Montard, R.; Kopito, R.; Touzeau, O.; Allouch, C.; Letaief, I.; Borderie, V.; Laroche, L. Ocular response analyzer: Feasibility study and correlation with normal eyes. *J. Fr. Ophtalmol.* **2007**, *30*, 978–984. [CrossRef]
23. Shen, M.; Wang, J.; Qu, J.; Xu, S.; Wang, X.; Fang, H.; Lu, F. Diurnal variation of ocular hysteresis, corneal thickness, and intraocular pressure. *Optom. Vis. Sci.* **2008**, *85*, 1185–1192. [CrossRef]
24. Wałek, E.; Przeździecka-Dołyk, J.; Helemejko, I.; Misiuk-Hojło, M. Efficacy of postoperative management with 5-fluorouracil injections after XEN gel stent implantation. *Int. Ophthalmol.* **2019**, *40*, 235–246. [CrossRef] [PubMed]
25. Ang, G.S.; Bochmann, F.; Townend, J.; Azuara-Blanco, A. Corneal biomechanic alproperties in primary open angle glaucoma and normal tension glaucoma. *J. Glaucoma* **2008**, *17*, 259–262. [CrossRef] [PubMed]
26. Sharifipour, F.; Malekahmadi, M.; Azimi, M.; Cheraghian, B. Intraocular pressure andcorneal biomechanical changes after water-drinking test in glaucoma patients. *J. Curr. Ophthalmol.* **2022**, *33*, 394–399. [CrossRef] [PubMed]

27. Gillmann, K.; Bravetti, G.E.; Rao, H.L.; Mermoud, A.; Mansouri, K. Impact of Combined XEN Gel Stent Implantation on Corneal Endothelial Cell Density: 2-Year Results. *J. Glaucoma* **2019**, *29*, 155–160. [CrossRef]
28. Sridhar, M.S. Anatomy of cornea and ocular Surface. *Ind. J. Ophthalmol.* **2018**, *2*, 190–194. [CrossRef]
29. Eliasson, J.; Maurice, D.M. Stress distribution across the in vivo human cornea. *Investig. Ophthalmol. Vis. Sci.* **1981**, *20*, 156.
30. Maurice, D.M. Mechanics of the cornea. In *The Cornea: Transaction of the World Congress on the Cornea III*; Cavanagh, H.D., Ed.; Raven Press Ltd.: New York, NY, USA, 1988.
31. Mangouritsas, G.; Morphis, G.; Mourtzoukos, S.; Feretis, E. Association between corneal hysteresis and central corneal thickness in glaucomatous and non-glaucomatous eyes. *Acta Ophthalmol.* **2009**, *87*, 901–905. [CrossRef]
32. Mansouri, K.; Leite, M.T.; Weinreb, R.N.; Tafreshi, A.; Zangwill, L.M.; Medeiros, F.A. Association between corneal bio-mechanical properties and glaucoma severity. *Am. J. Ophthalmol.* **2012**, *153*, 419–427.e1. [CrossRef]
33. Shah, S.; Laiquzzaman, M. Comparison of corneal biomechanics in pre and post-refractive surgery and keratoconic eyes by Ocular Response Analyser. *Cont. Lens Anterior. Eye* **2009**, *32*, 129–132. [CrossRef]
34. Jóźwik, A.; Asejczyk-Widlicka, M.; Boszczyk, A.; Kasprzak, H. Krzyżanowska-Berkowska, P. Raw data from Ocular Response Analyzer applied for differentiation of normal and glaucoma patients. *Opt. Appl.* **2020**, *50*, 147–159. [CrossRef]
35. Kotecha, A. What biomechanical properties of the cornea are relevant for the clinician? *Surv. Ophthalmol.* **2007**, *52* (Suppl. S2), S109–S114. [CrossRef] [PubMed]

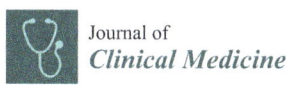

Journal of
Clinical Medicine

MDPI

Review

Corneal Hysteresis, Intraocular Pressure, and Progression of Glaucoma: Time for a "Hyst-Oric" Change in Clinical Practice?

Patrick Murtagh * and Colm O'Brien

Department of Ophthalmology, Mater Misericordiae University Hospital, Eccles Street,
D07 R2WY Dublin, Ireland; cobrien@mater.ie
* Correspondence: murtagp@tcd.ie

Abstract: It is known that as people age their tissues become less compliant and the ocular structures are no different. Corneal Hysteresis (CH) is a surrogate marker for ocular compliance. Low hysteresis values are associated with optic nerve damage and visual field loss, the structural and functional components of glaucomatous optic neuropathy. Presently, a range of parameters are measured to monitor and stratify glaucoma, including intraocular pressure (IOP), central corneal thickness (CCT), optical coherence tomography (OCT) scans of the retinal nerve fibre layer (RNFL) and the ganglion cell layer (GCL), and subjective measurement such as visual fields. The purpose of this review is to summarise the current evidence that CH values area risk factor for the development of glaucoma and are a marker for its progression. The authors will explain what precisely CH is, how it can be measured, and the influence that medication and surgery can have on its value. CH is likely to play an integral role in glaucoma care and could potentially be incorporated synergistically with IOP, CCT, and visual field testing to establish risk stratification modelling and progression algorithms in glaucoma management in the future.

Keywords: corneal hysteresis; corneal thickness; glaucoma; progression; risk stratification

Citation: Murtagh, P.; O'Brien, C. Corneal Hysteresis, Intraocular Pressure, and Progression of Glaucoma: Time for a "Hyst-Oric" Change in Clinical Practice? *J. Clin. Med.* **2022**, *11*, 2895. https:// doi.org/10.3390/jcm11102895

Academic Editors: Maria Letizia Salvetat, Marco Zeppieri and Paolo Brusini

Received: 27 March 2022
Accepted: 15 May 2022
Published: 20 May 2022

Publisher's Note: MDPI stays neutral with regard to jurisdictional claims in published maps and institutional affiliations.

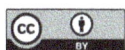

1. Introduction

The field of glaucoma is an ever-expanding one. Its intricacies and subtleties have been slowly evolving. The relationship between glaucoma and intraocular pressure (IOP) was the first association to be made but, subsequently, new and significant correlations have been discovered. The invention of the ophthalmoscope by von Helmholtz in the 1850s [1] made it possible for clinicians to document and classify optic disc appearance and correlate it to glaucoma. The advent of accurate tonometers [2] and reproducible perimetric testing [3], allowed ophthalmologists to assess the risk factors for disks and monitor disease progression. Interventions were then introduced to lower and stabilise IOP, with the introduction of surgical procedures such as the iridectomy performed by von Grafe in 1856 [4] and the use of pilocarpine in the late 1870s [5].

Glaucoma care has advanced alongside modern medicine over the past 170 years. Innovations in medications [6], the acceptance of minimally invasive glaucoma surgery (MIGS) [7], and advances in screening [8] and monitoring of the disease in terms of visual field testing and OCT scans of the RNFL and GCL, have made glaucoma a different disorder than it once was; one that is no longer "the silent thief of sight" but one that can be controlled, and the devastating visual impacts associated with it can be prevented.

Monitoring the progression and risk stratification are essential tools in glaucoma management. Additional objective markers to distinguish those with a higher probability of progression have eluded researchers and clinicians for some time but are an integral and essential part of glaucoma management. Corneal Hysteresis (CH) is a relatively new and exciting concept that could help identify those at risk of glaucoma and those who are likely to progress, and it is a property that can change with alterations in IOP. This review will explain what CH is, how it is measured, its relevance and correlation to different types of glaucoma, its significance to the progression of the disease, and the effects of changes in IOP by various methods on CH values. In this paper, we propose that it is time now to rewrite the textbooks about the value of measuring CH routinely in clinical practice.

2. Glaucoma

The term "glaucoma" is used to describe a group of optic neuropathies that are associated with progressive damage to retinal ganglion cells, and it is the second leading cause of permanent blindness in developed countries [9]. The insidious and irreversible nature of the disease makes early detection and screening paramount to avoid or halt the devastating functional, social, and economic impacts associated with it [10]. Glaucoma is more common in older age [11]. As the world's older populations grow at an unprecedented rate, so too will the burden of ocular disease, with the number of people diagnosed with glaucoma expected to double from 76 million in 2020 to almost 120 million in 2040 [12].

3. Glaucoma and IOP

Elevated IOP is a significant risk factor for the development and progression of glaucoma [13]. IOP is currently the only modifiable parameter that clinicians adapt to control or stop glaucomatous damage [14]. The correlation between raised IOP and glaucoma is not a new one. The Ancient Greeks recognised that acute blindness could be associated with an unreactive pupil and increased tension in the eye [15]. However, it was not until the mid-19th century when von Graefe developed the first tonometer to accurately measure intraocular pressure (IOP) [16], and the hypothesis arose that lowering IOP could prevent or slow down the rate of glaucomatous progression. The advent of the Goldmann applanation tonometer [17] (based on the Imbert–Fick principles) in the 1950s allowed accurate IOP measurements to come into mainstream use and permitted the clinician to make treatment decisions based on IOP values.

4. Glaucoma and Central Corneal Thickness

Objective measurements that influence glaucomatous optic neuropathy are extremely important surrogate measurements of disease. Visual field assessment is a subjective measurement of disease severity and is highly dependent on the user and can sometimes be difficult for the patient to perform, which can lead to an adverse number of false positives and negatives and a lack of reproducibility [18]. Published in 2002, The Ocular Hypertension Treatment Study [19] (OHTS) revealed the baseline factors that predicted the development of primary open-angle glaucoma (POAG) from ocular hypertension (OHT), the most significant being central corneal thickness (CCT). It was postulated that having a thicker cornea was protective against glaucomatous optic neuropathy. This finding lead to a risk stratification algorithm for patients with high IOP and no signs of optic nerve damage. These results were echoed in the European Glaucoma Prevention Study (EGPS) [20]. Subsequent work from the ocular hypertension treatment study group elucidated that for every 40 μm of corneal thinning, a twofold increase in the risk of developing GON was seen over a five-year period [21]. The underlying aetiology of this finding is still uncertain, and it is ambiguous whether it is secondary to its influence on IOP measurement, whether it is related to an intrinsic corneal characteristic and hence ocular tissue property, or a combination of both [22].

5. Age and Ocular Stiffness

Advancing age is a major risk factor for glaucoma progression [23]. Historically, the presumed mechanism of action was IOP, which resulted in mechanical stress on the optic nerve leading to ganglion cell death. Characteristic visual field loss and a cupped optic nerve head are hallmark signs of glaucomatous optic neuropathy (GON). The increase in IOP was mainly believed to be secondary to the outflow obstruction [24]. This mechanism has since been brought into question. There is a growing body of evidence that supports a decrease in the compliance of ocular structures and an increase in stiffness [25]. The structures affected include the trabecular meshwork (TM) and Schlemm's canal [26], the peripapillary sclera, and the lamina cribosa [27]. The mechanism underlying this stiffening includes extracellular matrix remodelling and fibrosis, initiated by the cytokine transforming growth factor-beta and oxidative stress [28]. The decrease in compliance of the ocular tissues leads to (1) outflow resistance in the TM due to a decrease in height, an increase in thickness [29], and (2) increased optic nerve stress due to increased rigidity in the lamina cribosa and peripapillary sclera [30]. A method to accurately measure the rigidity of these structures has been a challenge; however, a useful surrogate marker has come to the fore in recent times.

6. Hysteresis and the Cornea

Hysteresis is scientifically defined as a lag between the input and output in a system upon a change of direction [31]. It is dependent on the state of the system and its history [32]. It can reflect the intrinsic property of a material, and in biological materials, it can indicate its biomechanical qualities. The cornea can be characterised by its inherent behaviour. It has viscoelastic properties [33] and this can be reflected in the measurement of an applied force on the cornea, and its subsequent action and reaction to the said force [34]. As ophthalmologists, we are very familiar with viscoelastic materials as we routinely utilise them intraoperatively to maintain space and protect intraocular structures [35]. As the name suggests, a viscoelastic material is one that displays both viscous and elastic traits and is able to incorporate mechanical stress and disperse it sufficiently [36]. This dispersion is akin to a biological shock absorber and does not transmit force or allow it to accumulate in one specific area. It is, therefore, believed that the greater the value of this shock absorption or hysteresis, the greater the intrinsic ability of the ocular structures to deal with applied force or stress and, therefore, the lower the likelihood of nerve damage due to increased strain on the optic nerve head in the area of the lamina cribosa. Numerous studies have demonstrated that eyes with lower hysteresis values had faster rates of visual field loss than those with higher hysteresis values [37–39]. Corneal hysteresis may be a surrogate marker for hysteresis values elsewhere, specifically in the peripapillary sclera and the trabecular meshwork.

7. Corneal Hysteresis Measurement

Currently, there are two devices on the market used to measure corneal hysteresis. The first is known as the ocular response analyser (ORA; Reichert Inc., Depew, NY, USA). The ORA uses a quick jet of air to indent the cornea and an electro-optical system is used to measure the applanation pressure, once when the cornea is displaced inward, and again when it is displaced outward. The cornea has viscoelastic properties (as mentioned above) and therefore it resists inward movement caused by the air pulse and reverts to its primary position due to its elastic nature. There is a delay between these applanation events. The first inward applanation pressure is termed P1 and the second, or outward pressure event, is classified as P2. The Goldmann-correlated IOP (IOPg) is the average of these two values. The difference between P1 and P2 is known as the corneal hysteresis (CH) value [40]. Two other parameters, namely the corneal-compensated IOP (IOPcc) and a corneal resistance factor (CRF), can also be derived from the ORA data. IOPcc is a pressure measurement that utilises CH to give a pressure value that is considered to be less influenced by intrinsic corneal properties, e.g., central corneal thickness [41]. CRF is a depiction of overall corneal resistance and is algorithmically calculated [42]. Clinical use for these accessory criteria is yet to be elucidated [43].

The second device is the Corneal Visualization Scheimpflug Technology tonometer (Corvis ST; Oculus, Wetzlar, Germany). Similar to the ORA, the Corvis ST utilises an air pulse, but a high-speed Scheimpflug camera is used to calculate corneal movement. It records the cornea's reaction to the air pulse and the camera can take up to 4300 images per second. A video of 140 images taken 31 ms after the onset of the air pulse is used to provide a detailed analysis of the biomechanical properties of the cornea. A biomechanically corrected IOP (bIOP) is calculated, analogous to the IOPcc above [44]. The Corvis ST technically does not provide corneal hysteresis results, but bIOP is influenced by the effects of CH and is, therefore, a useful substitute marker. The parameters obtained by the Corvis ST are currently not directly comparable with those obtained by the ORA [45].

CH values are measured in millimetres of mercury (mmHg). The values are repeatable and vary among patients, and studies have found that CH values in non-pathological eyes have an average value of between 10.2 and 10.7 mmHg [46]. CH values display ethnic variations, with a study by Haseltine et al. [47] demonstrating that in non-glaucomatous eyes, Black, Hispanic, and Caucasian subjects have average CH values of 8.7 mmHg, 9.4 mmHg, and 9.8 mmHg, respectively. CH values are independent of other corneal measurements such as radius, refractive error, or IOP [48]. CH and CCT are positively associated [49].

8. Corneal Hysteresis and Glaucoma

Glaucoma can have devastating effects on a patient from a social, economic, and health point of view. There is a significant spectrum of diseases under the umbrella term that is glaucoma, including primary open-angle glaucoma (POAG), closed-angle glaucoma, pigment-dispersion glaucoma, pseudoexfoliative glaucoma, and normal-tension glaucoma (NTG), to name but a few. The Holy Grail of glaucoma management is to determine which patients have a greater likelihood of progressing from ocular hypertension to glaucomatous optic neuropathy and, in patients who already have glaucoma, which are more likely to deteriorate quickly. With the advent of more widespread use of CH measurement, this may soon become a reality. (Figure 1).

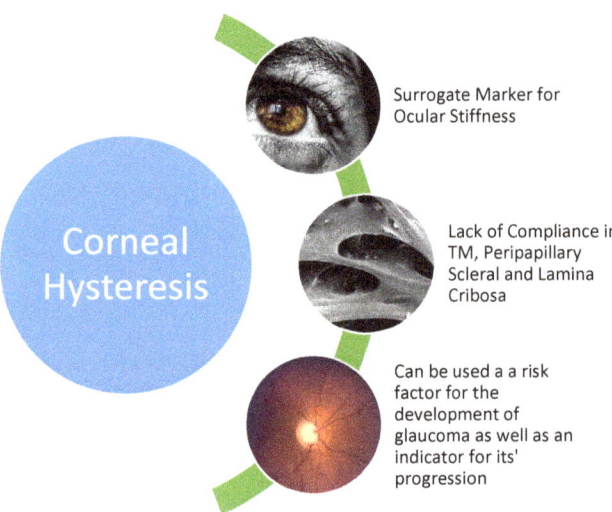

Figure 1. Corneal hysteresis is a surrogate marker for glaucoma and can be utilised to risk-stratify both those who are in danger of developing the disease and also those who are likely to progress (TM: trabecular meshwork).

9. Primary Open-Angle Glaucoma (POAG)

In simple terms, it is known that corneal hysteresis is lower in eyes with POAG than in eyes without glaucoma [50]. In a prospective cross-sectional study in 2010, Anand et al. [51] examined 117 POAG patients with asymmetric visual fields. This asymmetric POAG was associated with the corresponding asymmetry in ORA parameters but not in CCT or IOP. Lower CH was an independent risk factor for the eye with a worse visual field, irrespective of its pressure. A study by Dana et al. in 2015 [52] demonstrated a statistically significant, positive correlation between Visual Field Index (VFI) and CH, with lower CH values correlating with a lower VFI on Humphrey Visual Field testing. In a recent study published in 2021 by Jiménez-Santos et al. [53], 1573 patients from a previous cohort study with POAG were analysed in terms of glaucoma progression with respect to multiple baseline parameters including CH and CCT. It was observed that patients without progression had higher CH values and higher CCT. Using multivariate analysis, it was revealed that for every 1 mmHg reduction in CH measurement, an increase of 2.13 in terms of the hazard ratio for the risk of progression was conferred. The authors concluded that CH was considered to be a risk factor in early POAG and that CCT and CH at higher values work synergistically to slow the rate of progression. However, not all studies demonstrated this combined effect between the parameters, with Sullivan-Mee et al. [54] showing that after multivariate analysis, CH was the only factor that continued to discriminate between normal and glaucomatous eyes.

10. Angle-Closure Glaucoma (ACG)

Sun et al. [55] revealed that CH values were significantly lower in patients with chronic primary ACG as opposed to age-matched non-pathologic controls, with the presenting CH value in the glaucoma group measuring 6.83 ± 2.08 mmHg as opposed to the control eyes, which had an average CH value of 10.59 ± 1.38 mmHg. Another prospective observational study was undertaken by Narayanaswamy [56] et al., who examined 131 patients with primary ACG from a cohort of 443 Chinese patients. When confounding factors were adjusted, CH values were significantly lower in primary ACG eyes compared to normal eyes (9.4 mmHg versus 10.1 mmHg). However, other studies have found this relationship to be inconsistent, with a study by Nongpiur et al. revealing a lack of correlation between CH values and severity of disease in chronic angle-closure glaucoma [57] patients.

11. Pseudoexfoliation Glaucoma (PXFG)

A retrospective study undertaken in 2011 in Sweden [58] examined 90 patients for CH values; 30 with POAG, 30 with pseudoexfoliation glaucoma (PFXG), and 30 without glaucoma. The patients were also age matched. The results indicated that CH values were significantly lower in PFXG patients in comparison to both the POAG eyes and the non-glaucomatous eyes. Mean CH values in normal, POAG, and PXFG eyes were 9.8 ± 1.6 mmHg, 9.0 ± 1.9 mmHg, and 8.0 ± 1.5 mmHg, respectively. Yazgan et al. in 2014 [59] compared patients with pseudoexfoliation syndrome (PFXS), PFXG, and controls and revealed that CH was decreased in both PFXS and PFXG patients but to a greater degree in the PFXG patients. Yenerel et al. [60] showed that both CH and CRF values were lower in patients with both unilateral and bilateral PFXG. Interestingly, another study examining the use of the Corvis ST in measuring corneal biomarkers [61] showed no difference between eyes with PXG, POAG, and healthy controls after adjusting for IOP.

12. Normal-Tension Glaucoma (NTG)

Normal-tension glaucoma (NTG) is defined as evidence of glaucomatous optic neuropathy in eyes with an IOP of 21 mmHg or less. Studies have estimated that from a global perspective, as many as 30–50% of glaucoma patients may have IOP considered to be within the normal range [62]. Park et al. [63] analysed 95 NTG patients and evaluated them with respect to 93 patients without glaucoma. They concluded that patients with NTG had lower CH values than those in the normal group. They categorised their patients as normal, early NTG, and advanced NTG and the CH values were 10.83 ± 1.60, 10.56 ± 1.44, and 9.78 ± 1.52, respectively, with more advanced disease correlating with a lower CH value. They also determined that CH value alone remained statistically significantly associated with optic nerve head parameters (such as rim area and volume and cup-disc ratio) after adjusting for other confounding factors. They surmised that CH has a greater influence on structural biomarkers than CCT in NTG patients. The findings that NTG eyes have lower CH values than normal eyes have been echoed in numerous other studies [64–66].

Morita et al. [67] noted that IOPcc is significantly higher in eyes with NTG than in normal eyes, and Ehrlich et al. [68] noted that in comparison to eyes with POAG, there was a greater discrepancy seen between IOP measured with Goldmann Applanation Tonometry (GAT) and ccIOP with NTG eyes. A study by Hong et al. in 2016 [69] looked at the rate of progression in NTG patients and stated that eyes with a lower CH value and a higher ccIOP were likely to progress quicker than those with either higher CH values or lower ccIOP values. There was a substantial difference noted between GAT and ccIOP in these patients. They concluded that it is likely that GAT underestimates IOP in these patients and that ccIOP is a more accurate representation of actual IOP.

CCT is routinely used in NTG as a risk stratification tool. Previous studies have found that in patients with NTG, their CCT is thinner in comparison to both POAG eyes and normal eyes [70]. However, more recent studies [71] have found that CH and CRF are more robust predictors of progression in NTG than CCT.

Please see Table 1 for a summary of CH values in terms of glaucoma detection by subtype.

Table 1. Summary of main findings of CH studies in terms of glaucoma detection divided by subtype of glaucoma.

Study Lead Author and Year	Study Type	Number of Patients	Main Finding
POAG			
Sullivan-Mee et al., 2008 [54]	Retrospective	298	CH Values are useful in differentiating between patients with and without POAG.
Anand et al., 2010 [51]	Prospective	117	Asymmetric POAG was associated with asymmetry in ORA parameters. Lower CH was associated with more advanced glaucomatous disease.
Dana et al., 2015 [52]	Observational	55	Positive, statistically significant correlation between CH values and VFI. Lower CH Values are associated with lower VFI.
Jiménez-Santos et al., 2021 [53]	Cohort	1573	CH can be considered as a risk factor of progression in early-stage POAG.
ACG			
Sun et al., 2009 [55]	Prospective	80	CH was significantly lower in chronic PACG patients.
Narayanaswamy et al., 2011 [56]	Prospective	443	Corneal hysteresis was lower in eyes with glaucoma and after adjusting for confounding factors, lower CH values was found in PACG eyes.
Nongpiur et al., 2015 [57]	Prospective	204	Severity of glaucoma in PACG is *not* associated with lower CH values.
PXFG			
Ayala et al., 2011 [58]	Retrospective	90	CH was significantly lower in PXFG patients than in POAG normal patients, but no significance was found between the POAG and the normal group.
Yenerel et al., 2011 [60]	Prospective	52	CH reduces in patients with both unilateral and bilateral PEX.
Yazgan et al., 2015 [59]	Prospective	118	CH values were decreased in patients with PXFG, more so than in patients with solely PEX.
Pradhan et al., 2020 [61]	Prospective	66	After adjusting for IOP, CH values for normal eyes, POAG eyes and PEX eyes did not differ.

Table 1. *Cont.*

Study Lead Author and Year	Study Type	Number of Patients	Main Finding
NTG			
Morita et al., 2012 [67]	Prospective	166	IOPcc and CH values were significantly higher in NTG eyes than in normal eyes.
Ehrlich et al., 2012 [68]	Retrospective	614	Compared to GAT, IOPcc may be a superior test in the evaluation of glaucoma as it may account for measurement errors induced by corneal biomechanics.
Hong et al., 2016 [69]	Prospective	56	Higher IOPcc and lower CH are associated with VF progression in NTG patients.
Park et al., 2018 [63]	Retrospective	188	Lower CH values are associated with a smaller rim area and volume, thinner RNFL, and a larger cup disc ratio after adjusting for CCT, age, IOP, and disc size.

POAG = Primary Open-Angle Glaucoma, ACG = Angle-Closure Glaucoma, PACG = primary angle-closure glaucoma, CH = Corneal Hysteresis, PXFG = Pseudoexfoliative Glaucoma, PEX = Pseudoexfoliation Syndrome, NTG = Normal-Tension Glaucoma, IOPcc = corneal-compensated intraocular pressure, IOP = intraocular pressure, ORA = Ocular Response Analyser, VFI = Visual Field Index, VF = Visual Field.

13. Corneal Hysteresis and Glaucomatous Progression

The first association between CH and visual field progression was made by Congdon et al. [72] in 2006. This was an observational study which included 230 patients with either POAG (85%) or suspected glaucoma (15%). The cohort underwent routine baseline evaluations and, subsequent to multivariate generalised estimating equation modelling, a lower CH was associated with greater visual field progression, an association that was not apparent for CCT. Susanna et al. [38] performed a prospective observational study on 199 patients who were suspected of having glaucoma and were followed for an average of 3.9 years. Glaucoma progression was defined as Glaucoma Hemifield Test outside normal limits or a Pattern Standard Deviation (PSD) of <5% on three consecutive automated perimetry tests. Of the 54 eyes that developed repeatable visual field defects on follow up, their CH values were significantly lower than those whose fields remained static. They concluded that lower CH values were associated with a higher risk of developing glaucomatous visual field defects over time. De Moraes et al. [73] examined the relationship between CH, CCF, and visual field progression in terms of decibels lost per year. They deduced that eyes that have greater progression of their visual field had lower CH and CCT values and that eyes that had the greatest number of decibels lost had lower CH values. Medeiros et al. [37] examined CH values and the loss of the Visual Field Index (VFI) over time. Out of the 68 patients with known glaucoma, 114 eyes were followed for an average of 4 years. The results revealed that CH had a significant effect on progression, more so than IOP and CCT, and that for each 1 mmhg lower CH value conferred an associated risk of 0.25%/year faster rate of visual field progression over time ($p < 0.001$). In a more recent study by Estrela et al. [74], the asymmetries between glaucoma progression and the asymmetries in corneal properties were examined in a prospective study of 126 binocular glaucoma patients. Visual field progression was determined by a change in mean deviation (MD) on standard automated perimetry testing (SAP). The only corneal property of those measured (including CCT and IOP) that had a statistically significant association with an asymmetry of SAP MD rates was the difference in CH values. This remained the situation even after multivariate analysis to void confounding factors including age, race, CCT, and IOP. The authors predicted that for each 1 mmHg change in CH value in eyes of the same subject, a 34% increase in the variance of MD rates could be observed.

Subjective visual field progression was not the only parameter analysed in the studies. Zhang et al. [75] examined the relationship between CH and retinal nerve fibre layer (RNFL) thinning in a prospective follow up of 186 eyes of 133 patients. They were followed for an average of 3.8 years with a median follow up of 9 visits. Measurements of RNFL were obtained using spectral-domain optical coherence tomography and potential confounding factors were adjusted for. The authors determined that CH had a significant effect on RNFL thinning, with each 1 mmHg lower CH value being associated with a 0.13 μm/year faster rate of RNFL decline (*p* = 0.011).

A recent study by Kamalipour [76] et al. examined, in a prospective longitudinal study, CH as a risk factor for the progression of the central visual field in a cohort of glaucoma patients. Out of 143 patients, 248 eyes were examined using HVF 24-2 and 10-2 over an average of 4.8 years. Logistic regression analysis was utilised to determine the characteristics that would influence progression on a 10-2 field. The authors showed that lower CH values were associated with a statistically significant, albeit small, increased risk of central visual field progression. However, the central visual field has a huge impact on a patient's quality of life and so the paper surmised that CH should be considered by clinicians as a risk stratification parameter in glaucoma.

Table 2 summarises the main findings of the above studies with respect to CH values and glaucoma progression.

Table 2. Summary of main findings of CH studies in terms of glaucoma progression.

Study Lead Author and Year	Study Type	Number of Patients	Main Finding
Congdon et al., 2006 [72]	Observational	230	Lower CH values were associated with visual field progression.
De Moraes et al., 2012 [73]	Prospective	153	High correlation between VF progression and CH values.
Medeiros et al., 2013 [37]	Prospective	68	Eyes with lower CH had faster rates of visual field loss than those with higher CH.
Zhang et al., 2016 [75]	Prospective	133	Lower CH was significantly associated with faster rates of RNFL loss over time.
Susanna et al., 2018 [38]	Prospective	199	Baseline lower CH measurements were significantly associated with an increased risk of developing glaucomatous visual field defects over time.
Estrela et al., 2020 [74]	Prospective	126	In eyes with asymmetric CH values, there was an associated asymmetric VF progression, with lower CH values associated with greater rates of progression
Kamalipour et al., 2022 [76]	Prospective	143	Lower CH values were associated with a greater risk of progression on 10-2 VF

CH = Corneal Hysteresis, RNFL = Retinal Nerve Fibre Layer, VF = Visual Field.

14. Effect of IOP Reduction on Hysteresis

CH is a dynamic property of the cornea. As previously stated, lower CH values are associated with both an increased likelihood of developing glaucoma and a faster rate of progression. Studies have shown that by lowering the intraocular pressure, CH values can increase. In a retrospective review by Agarwal et al. in 2012 [77], 57 patients with POAG were analysed by ORA at baseline and follow up, subsequent to the commencement of a prostaglandin analogue for the treatment of their disease. It was seen that IOP was reduced by an average of 3.2 mmHg, which corresponded to an increase in the CH value of 0.5 mmHg. It was demonstrated that baseline CH, and not baseline CCT, was a significant predictor of IOP reduction, with a lower baseline CH associated with a greater reduction in IOP. The effect of topical prostaglandin analogues on CH was also demonstrated by Tsikripis et al. [78] in their study examining the influence that lower IOP had on CCT biomechanical markers including CH, CRF, and CCT. Out of the 108 eyes that were included in this study, 66 were treated with latanoprost solely and the remaining 42 eyes were treated with a combination of latanoprost and timolol. It was seen that by using topical prostaglandin analogues, the IOP values decreased with a corresponding increase in the CH and CCT values, with a range for the increase in CH values of 0.4–0.7 mmHg and 0.65–0.95 mmHg for the latanoprost and the latanoprost/timolol group, respectively.

Topical medication is not the only treatment modality for which a reduction in IOP influences CH values. A study by Pillunat [79] et al. in 2016 examined 52 eyes of 52 patients with medically uncontrolled glaucoma and performed Selective Laser Trabeculoplasty (SLT) to control IOP. They found that Goldmann-correlated IOP decreased statistically significantly from 18.0 ± 6.4 to 14.8 ± 3.8 mmHg and IOPcc from 20.2 ± 6.5 to 16.7 ± 3.4 mmHg ($p < 0.001$). CH increased from 8.53 ± 2.03 to 9.12 ± 1.83 mmHg ($p = 0.028$) and CRF decreased from 9.58 ± 2.18 to 9.1 ± 2.1 mmHg ($p = 0.037$), which was statistically significant. However, in covariance analysis, by correcting CH and CRF for the impact of IOP reduction, the CH and CRF values remained unchanged. The authors concluded that SLT may not change the corneal biomechanical properties, as these changes may solely be explained by changes in IOP. However, in 2013, Hirneiß et al. [80] analysed 68 patients with open-angle glaucoma that were insufficiently controlled by topical medications and hence underwent SLT for IOP control. They were examining the predictive values of corneal biomarkers for IOP reduction post SLT. A total of 68 patients with open-angle glaucoma (OAG) were followed for 12 months after the procedure. Linear regression analysis revealed that both CH and CRF alongside baseline IOP correlated significantly with IOP reduction. It was surmised by the authors that the original IOP, CH, and CRF values were significant predictors of the IOP-lowering effect of SLT in medically resistant OAG.

Surgery to reduce IOP has also been shown to positively impact CH values. A study by Pakravan et al. [81] examined the 89 eyes of 89 patients with ORA before and three months after either trabeculectomy and mitomycin C (MMC) (23 eyes), phacotrabeculectomy + MMC (23 eyes), Ahmed valve implantation (17 eyes), or phacoemulsification alone (26 non-glaucomatous eyes). Their findings revealed that CH was lower in glaucomatous vs. non-glaucomatous eyes. Three months post-surgery, it was shown that CH values increased in the trabeculectomy and MMC group, the phacotrabeculectomy, and the Ahmed value group by 2.16, 2.29, and 2.30 mmHg, respectively. However, an increase in CH of only 0.11 mmHg was seen in the post-phacoemulsification only eyes. The increase in CH values was most significant in the eyes where IOP was decreased by 10 mmHg or more. Fujino et al. [82] examined 24 eyes of 19 patients with POAG who underwent trabeculectomy and recorded CH values before and after surgery in conjunction with Humphrey visual field testing to assess progression. Their modelling for progression based on mean deviation on-field testing demonstrated that only CH values had a positive correlation coefficient for the rate of change. In 2019, Sorkhabi et al. [83] examined 32 eyes of 32 patients, 17 of whom had PXFG and the remaining 15 had POAG. All patients underwent trabeculectomy and MMC for uncontrolled glaucoma and ORA parameters were recorded at baseline and 3 months post procedure. The authors found that the mean CH values were lower in the PXFG group than in the POAG group at baseline. The CH values markedly increased in the PXFG group and modestly increased in the POAG group post-surgery (5.66 ± 1.13 to 6.69 ± 0.78 and 7.49 ± 0.88 to 8.23 ± 1.09). The authors also noted that there was a significant relationship between CH and IOPg changes in both the PXFG and POAG groups.

Contrary to the above studies, a recent paper by Pillunat et al. [84] demonstrated that when confounding factors were adjusted, the corneal biomechanical properties were not altered post trabeculectomy. In this study, 35 eyes of 35 patients undergoing trabeculectomy were enrolled and it was noted that the changes in CH values before and after trabeculectomy were not statistically significant.

15. Limitations

The acquisition of CH measurements in clinical practice is currently not mainstream. Not all units have access to an ORA and presently ophthalmologists are largely unfamiliar with the values and how to interpret them.

J. Clin. Med. **2022**, *11*, 2895

The precise mechanisms by which CH values affect glaucoma detection and progression are unclear apart from them being a surrogate marker for ocular stiffness. Is there a vascular or an ischaemic factor underlying these mechanisms? A recent review by Hopkins et al. [27] proposed a three-stage tissue stiffness model incorporating integrin-mediated mechanotransduction that leads to extracellular matrix remodelling and fibrosis and, in turn, to diminishing contractile ability of the lamina cribosa. Further research should be undertaken to address these obvious gaps in knowledge and elucidate the intrinsic process by which it works.

16. Conclusions

The contribution that CH will eventually have to glaucoma care has yet to be fully appreciated. This review has summarised its effects and relevance on different types of glaucoma, how its values can fluctuate with alterations in treatment, and its significance in monitoring progression. It has become apparent that corneal behaviour is a more important parameter than its thickness, but the authors believe that a combination of IOP, CCT, and CH can be utilised to create a risk stratification model for glaucoma. Undoubtedly, additional investigation is needed in this field and with it, the importance of CH in diagnosing and monitoring this potentially devastating disease will likely come to the fore.

Author Contributions: Conceptualization, C.O. and P.M.; writing—original draft preparation, P.M.; writing—review and editing, P.M.; visualization, C.O.; supervision, C.O.; project administration, C.O.; All authors have read and agreed to the published version of the manuscript.

Funding: This research received no external funding.

Institutional Review Board Statement: Not applicable.

Informed Consent Statement: Not applicable.

Conflicts of Interest: The authors declare no conflict of interest.

References

1. Keeler, C.R. The ophthalmoscope in the lifetime of Hermann von Helmholtz. *Arch. Ophthalmol.* **2002**, *120*, 194–201. [CrossRef] [PubMed]
2. Eddy, D.M.; Sanders, L.E.; Eddy, J.F. The value of screening for glaucoma with tonometry. *Surv. Ophthalmol.* **1983**, *28*, 194–205. [CrossRef]
3. Johnson, C.A.; Wall, M.; Thompson, H.S. A history of perimetry and visual field testing. *Optom. Vis. Sci.* **2011**, *88*, E8–E15. [CrossRef] [PubMed]
4. Ramakrishnan, R.; Sindhushree, R. Glaucoma Surgery. *Gems Ophthalmol. Glaucoma* **2018**, 355–474.
5. Leffler, C.T.; Schwartz, S.G.; Giliberti, F.M.; Young, M.T.; Bermudez, D. What was Glaucoma Called Before the 20th Century? *Ophthalmol. Eye Dis.* **2015**, *7*, 21–33. [CrossRef]
6. Realini, T. A history of glaucoma pharmacology. *Optom. Vis. Sci.* **2011**, *88*, 36–38. [CrossRef]
7. Brandão, L.M.; Grieshaber, M.C. Update on minimally invasive glaucoma surgery (MIGS) and new implants. *J. Ophthalmol.* **2013**, *2013*. [CrossRef]
8. Murtagh, P.; Greene, G.; O'Brien, C. Current applications of machine learning in the screening and diagnosis of glaucoma: A systematic review and meta-analysis. *Int. J. Ophthalmol.* **2020**, *13*, 149. [CrossRef]
9. Frezzotti, P.; Pescucci, C.; Papa, F.T.; Iester, M.; Mittica, V.; Motolese, I.; Peruzzi, S.; Artuso, R.; Longo, I.; Mencarelli, M.A.; et al. Association between primary open-angle glaucoma (POAG) and WDR36 sequence variance in Italian families affected by POAG. *Br. J. Ophthalmol.* **2011**, *95*, 624–626. [CrossRef]
10. Schmier, J.K.; Halpern, M.T.; Jones, M.L. The economic implications of glaucoma: A literature review. *Pharmacoeconomics* **2007**, *25*, 287–308. [CrossRef]
11. Iroku-Malize, T.; Kirsch, S. Eye Conditions in Older Adults: Open-Angle Glaucoma. *FP Essent* **2016**, *445*, 11–16. [PubMed]
12. Tham, Y.C.; Li, X.; Wong, T.Y.; Quigley, H.A.; Aung, T.; Cheng, C.Y. Global prevalence of glaucoma and projections of glaucoma burden through 2040: A systematic review and meta-analysis. *Ophthalmology* **2014**, *121*, 2081–2090. [CrossRef] [PubMed]
13. Flammer, J.; Mozaffarieh, M. What is the present pathogenetic concept of glaucomatous optic neuropathy? *Surv. Ophthalmol.* **2007**, *52* (Suppl. S2), S162–S173. [CrossRef] [PubMed]
14. Shalaby, W.S.; Ahmed, O.M.; Waisbourd, M.; Katz, L.J. A review of potential novel glaucoma therapeutic options independent of intraocular pressure. *Surv. Ophthalmol.* **2021**. [CrossRef] [PubMed]
15. Stamper, R.L. A history of intraocular pressure and its measurement. *Optom Vis Sci* **2011**, *88*, E16–E28. [CrossRef]

16. Ivanišević, M.; Stanić, R.; Ivanišević, P.; Vuković, A. Albrecht von Graefe (1828-1870) and his contributions to the development of ophthalmology. *Int. Ophthalmol.* **2020**, *40*, 1029–1033. [CrossRef]
17. Goldmann, H. A new applanation tonometer. *Bull. Mem. Soc. Fr. Ophtalmol.* **1954**, *67*, 474–477; discussion 477–478.
18. Wu, Z.; Medeiros, F.A. Recent developments in visual field testing for glaucoma. *Curr. Opin. Ophthalmol.* **2018**, *29*, 141–146. [CrossRef]
19. Gordon, M.O.; Beiser, J.A.; Brandt, J.D.; Heuer, D.K.; Higginbotham, E.J.; Johnson, C.A.; Keltner, J.L.; Miller, J.P.; Parrish, R.K., 2nd; Wilson, M.R.; et al. The Ocular Hypertension Treatment Study: Baseline factors that predict the onset of primary open-angle glaucoma. *Arch. Ophthalmol.* **2002**, *120*, 714–720; discussion 730–829. [CrossRef]
20. Miglior, S.; Pfeiffer, N.; Torri, V.; Zeyen, T.; Cunha-Vaz, J.; Adamsons, I. Predictive factors for open-angle glaucoma among patients with ocular hypertension in the European Glaucoma Prevention Study. *Ophthalmology* **2007**, *114*, 3–9. [CrossRef]
21. Gordon, M.O.; Torri, V.; Miglior, S.; Beiser, J.A.; Floriani, I.; Miller, J.P.; Gao, F.; Adamsons, I.; Poli, D.; D'Agostino, R.B.; et al. Validated prediction model for the development of primary open-angle glaucoma in individuals with ocular hypertension. *Ophthalmology* **2007**, *114*, 10–19. [CrossRef] [PubMed]
22. Iester, M.; Mete, M.; Figus, M.; Frezzotti, P. Incorporating corneal pachymetry into the management of glaucoma. *J. Cataract. Refract. Surg.* **2009**, *35*, 1623–1628. [CrossRef] [PubMed]
23. Nouri-Mahdavi, K.; Hoffman, D.; Coleman, A.L.; Liu, G.; Li, G.; Gaasterland, D.; Caprioli, J. Predictive factors for glaucomatous visual field progression in the Advanced Glaucoma Intervention Study. *Ophthalmology* **2004**, *111*, 1627–1635. [CrossRef] [PubMed]
24. Guedes, G.; Tsai, J.C.; Loewen, N.A. Glaucoma and aging. *Curr. Aging Sci.* **2011**, *4*, 110–117. [CrossRef] [PubMed]
25. Liu, B.; McNally, S.; Kilpatrick, J.I.; Jarvis, S.P.; O'Brien, C.J. Aging and ocular tissue stiffness in glaucoma. *Surv. Ophthalmol.* **2018**, *63*, 56–74. [CrossRef]
26. Wang, K.; Johnstone, M.A.; Xin, C.; Song, S.; Padilla, S.; Vranka, J.A.; Acott, T.S.; Zhou, K.; Schwaner, S.A.; Wang, R.K.; et al. Estimating Human Trabecular Meshwork Stiffness by Numerical Modeling and Advanced OCT Imaging. *Invest. Ophthalmol. Vis. Sci.* **2017**, *58*, 4809–4817. [CrossRef]
27. Hopkins, A.A.; Murphy, R.; Irnaten, M.; Wallace, D.M.; Quill, B.; O'Brien, C. The role of lamina cribrosa tissue stiffness and fibrosis as fundamental biomechanical drivers of pathological glaucoma cupping. *Am. J. Physiol. Cell Physiol.* **2020**, *319*, C611–C623. [CrossRef]
28. McElnea, E.M.; Quill, B.; Docherty, N.G.; Irnaten, M.; Siah, W.F.; Clark, A.F.; O'Brien, C.J.; Wallace, D.M. Oxidative stress, mitochondrial dysfunction and calcium overload in human lamina cribrosa cells from glaucoma donors. *Mol. Vis.* **2011**, *17*, 1182–1191.
29. Choi, W.; Bae, H.W.; Cho, H.; Kim, E.W.; Kim, C.Y.; Seong, G.J. Evaluation of the Relationship Between Age and Trabecular Meshwork Height to Predict the Risk of Glaucoma. *Sci. Rep.* **2020**, *10*, 7115. [CrossRef]
30. Albon, J.; Purslow, P.P.; Karwatowski, W.S.; Easty, D.L. Age related compliance of the lamina cribrosa in human eyes. *Br. J. Ophthalmol.* **2000**, *84*, 318–323. [CrossRef]
31. Louizos, C.; Yáñez, J.A.; Forrest, L.; Davies, N.M. Understanding the hysteresis loop conundrum in pharmacokinetic/pharmacodynamic relationships. *J. Pharm. Pharm. Sci. A Publ. Can. Soc. Pharm. Sci. Soc. Can. Des Sci. Pharm.* **2014**, *17*, 34. [CrossRef]
32. Rio-Cristobal, A.; Martin, R. Corneal assessment technologies: Current status. *Surv. Ophthalmol.* **2014**, *59*, 599–614. [CrossRef] [PubMed]
33. Boyce, B.; Jones, R.; Nguyen, T.; Grazier, J. Stress-controlled viscoelastic tensile response of bovine cornea. *J. Biomech.* **2007**, *40*, 2367–2376. [CrossRef] [PubMed]
34. Kling, S.; Bekesi, N.; Dorronsoro, C.; Pascual, D.; Marcos, S. Corneal viscoelastic properties from finite-element analysis of in vivo air-puff deformation. *PLoS ONE* **2014**, *9*, e104904. [CrossRef]
35. Hessemer, V.; Dick, B. Viscoelastic substances in cataract surgery. Principles and current overview. *Klin. Monbl. Augenheilkd.* **1996**, *209*, 55–61. [CrossRef]
36. Kobayashi, A.; Staberg, L.; Schlegel, W. Viscoelastic properties of human cornea. *Exp. Mech.* **1973**, *13*, 497–503. [CrossRef]
37. Medeiros, F.A.; Meira-Freitas, D.; Lisboa, R.; Kuang, T.M.; Zangwill, L.M.; Weinreb, R.N. Corneal hysteresis as a risk factor for glaucoma progression: A prospective longitudinal study. *Ophthalmology* **2013**, *120*, 1533–1540. [CrossRef]
38. Susanna, C.N.; Diniz-Filho, A.; Daga, F.B.; Susanna, B.N.; Zhu, F.; Ogata, N.G.; Medeiros, F.A. A Prospective Longitudinal Study to Investigate Corneal Hysteresis as a Risk Factor for Predicting Development of Glaucoma. *Am. J. Ophthalmol.* **2018**, *187*, 148–152. [CrossRef]
39. Jammal, A.A.; Medeiros, F.A. Corneal hysteresis: Ready for prime time? *Curr. Opin. Ophthalmol.* **2022**. [CrossRef]
40. Terai, N.; Raiskup, F.; Haustein, M.; Pillunat, L.E.; Spoerl, E. Identification of biomechanical properties of the cornea: The ocular response analyzer. *Curr. Eye Res.* **2012**, *37*, 553–562. [CrossRef]
41. Abd Elaziz, M.S.; Elsobky, H.M.; Zaky, A.G.; Hassan, E.A.M.; KhalafAllah, M.T. Corneal biomechanics and intraocular pressure assessment after penetrating keratoplasty for non keratoconic patients, long term results. *BMC Ophthalmol.* **2019**, *19*, 172. [CrossRef] [PubMed]
42. Luce, D.A. Determining in vivo biomechanical properties of the cornea with an ocular response analyzer. *J. Cataract Refract. Surg.* **2005**, *31*, 156–162. [CrossRef] [PubMed]

43. Lau, W.; Pye, D. A Clinical Description of Ocular Response Analyzer Measurements. *Investig. Ophthalmol. Vis. Sci.* **2011**, *52*, 2911–2916. [CrossRef] [PubMed]
44. Tian, L.; Wang, D.; Wu, Y.; Meng, X.; Chen, B.; Ge, M.; Huang, Y. Corneal biomechanical characteristics measured by the CorVis Scheimpflug technology in eyes with primary open-angle glaucoma and normal eyes. *Acta Ophthalmol.* **2016**, *94*, e317–e324. [CrossRef]
45. Fujishiro, T.; Matsuura, M.; Fujino, Y.; Murata, H.; Tokumo, K.; Nakakura, S.; Kiuchi, Y.; Asaoka, R. The Relationship Between Corvis ST Tonometry Parameters and Ocular Response Analyzer Corneal Hysteresis. *J. Glaucoma* **2020**, *29*, 479–484. [CrossRef]
46. Carbonaro, F.; Andrew, T.; Mackey, D.A.; Spector, T.D.; Hammond, C.J. The heritability of corneal hysteresis and ocular pulse amplitude: A twin study. *Ophthalmology* **2008**, *115*, 1545–1549. [CrossRef]
47. Haseltine, S.J.; Pae, J.; Ehrlich, J.R.; Shammas, M.; Radcliffe, N.M. Variation in corneal hysteresis and central corneal thickness among black, hispanic and white subjects. *Acta Ophthalmol.* **2012**, *90*, e626–e631. [CrossRef]
48. Laiquzzaman, M.; Bhojwani, R.; Cunliffe, I.; Shah, S. Diurnal variation of ocular hysteresis in normal subjects: Relevance in clinical context. *Clin. Exp. Ophthalmol.* **2006**, *34*, 114–118. [CrossRef]
49. Zhang, B.; Shweikh, Y.; Khawaja, A.P.; Gallacher, J.; Bauermeister, S.; Foster, P.J. Associations with Corneal Hysteresis in a Population Cohort: Results from 96 010 UK Biobank Participants. *Ophthalmology* **2019**, *126*, 1500–1510. [CrossRef]
50. Mangouritsas, G.; Morphis, G.; Mourtzoukos, S.; Feretis, E. Association between corneal hysteresis and central corneal thickness in glaucomatous and non-glaucomatous eyes. *Acta Ophthalmol.* **2009**, *87*, 901–905. [CrossRef]
51. Anand, A.; De Moraes, C.G.; Teng, C.C.; Tello, C.; Liebmann, J.M.; Ritch, R. Corneal hysteresis and visual field asymmetry in open angle glaucoma. *Invest. Ophthalmol. Vis. Sci.* **2010**, *51*, 6514–6518. [CrossRef] [PubMed]
52. Dana, D.; Mihaela, C.; Raluca, I.; Miruna, C.; Catalina, I.; Miruna, C.; Schmitzer, S.; Catalina, C. Corneal hysteresis and primary open angle glaucoma. *Rom. J. Ophthalmol.* **2015**, *59*, 252–254. [PubMed]
53. Jiménez-Santos, M.A.; Saénz-Francés, F.; Sánchez-Jean, R.; Martinez-de-la Casa, J.M.; García-Feijoo, J.; Jañez-Escalada, L. Synergic effect of corneal hysteresis and central corneal thickness in the risk of early-stage primary open-angle glaucoma progression. *Graefe's Arch. Clin. Exp. Ophthalmol.* **2021**, *259*, 2743–2751. [CrossRef] [PubMed]
54. Sullivan-Mee, M.; Billingsley, S.C.; Patel, A.D.; Halverson, K.D.; Alldredge, B.R.; Qualls, C. Ocular Response Analyzer in subjects with and without glaucoma. *Optom. Vis. Sci.* **2008**, *85*, 463–470. [CrossRef] [PubMed]
55. Sun, L.; Shen, M.; Wang, J.; Fang, A.; Xu, A.; Fang, H.; Lu, F. Recovery of corneal hysteresis after reduction of intraocular pressure in chronic primary angle-closure glaucoma. *Am. J. Ophthalmol.* **2009**, *147*, 1061–1066.e1062. [CrossRef]
56. Narayanaswamy, A.; Su, D.H.; Baskaran, M.; Tan, A.C.S.; Nongpiur, M.E.; Htoon, H.M.; Wong, T.Y.; Aung, T. Comparison of Ocular Response Analyzer Parameters in Chinese Subjects With Primary Angle-Closure and Primary Open-Angle Glaucoma. *Arch. Ophthalmol.* **2011**, *129*, 429–434. [CrossRef] [PubMed]
57. Nongpiur, M.E.; Png, O.; Chiew, J.W.; Fan, K.R.; Girard, M.J.; Wong, T.; Goh, D.; Perera, S.A.; Aung, T. Lack of association between corneal hysteresis and corneal resistance factor with glaucoma severity in primary angle closure glaucoma. *Investig. Ophthalmol. Vis. Sci.* **2015**, *56*, 6879–6885. [CrossRef]
58. Ayala, M. Corneal Hysteresis in Normal Subjects and in Patients with Primary Open-Angle Glaucoma and Pseudoexfoliation Glaucoma. *Ophthalmic Res.* **2011**, *46*, 187–191. [CrossRef]
59. Yazgan, S.; Celik, U.; Alagöz, N.; Taş, M. Corneal Biomechanical Comparison of Pseudoexfoliation Syndrome, Pseudoexfoliative Glaucoma and Healthy Subjects. *Curr. Eye Res.* **2015**, *40*, 470–475. [CrossRef]
60. Yenerel, N.M.; Gorgun, E.; Kucumen, R.B.; Oral, D.; Dinc, U.A.; Ciftci, F. Corneal biomechanical properties of patients with pseudoexfoliation syndrome. *Cornea* **2011**, *30*, 983–986. [CrossRef]
61. Pradhan, Z.S.; Deshmukh, S.; Dixit, S.; Sreenivasaiah, S.; Shroff, S.; Devi, S.; Webers, C.A.; Rao, H.L. A comparison of the corneal biomechanics in pseudoexfoliation glaucoma, primary open-angle glaucoma and healthy controls using Corvis ST. *PLoS ONE* **2020**, *15*, e0241296. [CrossRef] [PubMed]
62. Klein, B.E.; Klein, R.; Sponsel, W.E.; Franke, T.; Cantor, L.B.; Martone, J.; Menage, M.J. Prevalence of glaucoma. The Beaver Dam Eye Study. *Ophthalmology* **1992**, *99*, 1499–1504. [CrossRef]
63. Park, K.; Shin, J.; Lee, J. Relationship between corneal biomechanical properties and structural biomarkers in patients with normal-tension glaucoma: A retrospective study. *BMC Ophthalmol.* **2018**, *18*, 1–10. [CrossRef] [PubMed]
64. Shin, J.; Lee, J.W.; Kim, E.A.; Caprioli, J. The effect of corneal biomechanical properties on rebound tonometer in patients with normal-tension glaucoma. *Am J Ophthalmol* **2015**, *159*, 144–154. [CrossRef] [PubMed]
65. Grise-Dulac, A.; Saad, A.; Abitbol, O.; Febbraro, J.L.; Azan, E.; Moulin-Tyrode, C.; Gatinel, D. Assessment of corneal biomechanical properties in normal tension glaucoma and comparison with open-angle glaucoma, ocular hypertension, and normal eyes. *J. Glaucoma* **2012**, *21*, 486–489. [CrossRef]
66. Kaushik, S.; Pandav, S.S.; Banger, A.; Aggarwal, K.; Gupta, A. Relationship between corneal biomechanical properties, central corneal thickness, and intraocular pressure across the spectrum of glaucoma. *Am. J. Ophthalmol.* **2012**, *153*, 840–849.e842. [CrossRef]
67. Morita, T.; Shoji, N.; Kamiya, K.; Fujimura, F.; Shimizu, K. Corneal biomechanical properties in normal-tension glaucoma. *Acta Ophthalmol.* **2012**, *90*, e48–e53. [CrossRef]
68. Ehrlich, J.R.; Radcliffe, N.M.; Shimmyo, M. Goldmann applanation tonometry compared with corneal-compensated intraocular pressure in the evaluation of primary open-angle Glaucoma. *BMC Ophthalmol.* **2012**, *12*, 52. [CrossRef]

69. Hong, Y.; Shoji, N.; Morita, T.; Hirasawa, K.; Matsumura, K.; Kasahara, M.; Shimizu, K. Comparison of corneal biomechanical properties in normal tension glaucoma patients with different visual field progression speed. *Int. J. Ophthalmol.* **2016**, *9*, 973–978. [CrossRef]

70. Doyle, A.; Bensaid, A.; Lachkar, Y. Central corneal thickness and vascular risk factors in normal tension glaucoma. *Acta Ophthalmol. Scand.* **2005**, *83*, 191–195. [CrossRef]

71. Helmy, H.; Leila, M.; Zaki, A.A. Corneal biomechanics in asymmetrical normal-tension glaucoma. *Clin. Ophthalmol.* **2016**, *10*, 503–510. [CrossRef] [PubMed]

72. Congdon, N.G.; Broman, A.T.; Bandeen-Roche, K.; Grover, D.; Quigley, H.A. Central corneal thickness and corneal hysteresis associated with glaucoma damage. *Am. J. Ophthalmol.* **2006**, *141*, 868–875. [CrossRef]

73. De Moraes, C.V.G.; Hill, V.; Tello, C.; Liebmann, J.M.; Ritch, R. Lower Corneal Hysteresis is Associated with More Rapid Glaucomatous Visual Field Progression. *J. Glaucoma* **2012**, *21*, 209–213. [CrossRef] [PubMed]

74. Estrela, T.; Jammal, A.A.; Mariottoni, E.B.; Urata, C.N.; Ogata, N.G.; Berchuck, S.I.; Medeiros, F.A. The Relationship Between Asymmetries of Corneal Properties and Rates of Visual Field Progression in Glaucoma Patients. *J. Glaucoma* **2020**, *29*, 872–877. [CrossRef] [PubMed]

75. Zhang, C.; Tatham, A.J.; Abe, R.Y.; Diniz-Filho, A.; Zangwill, L.M.; Weinreb, R.N.; Medeiros, F.A. Corneal hysteresis and progressive retinal nerve fiber layer loss in glaucoma. *Am. J. Ophthalmol.* **2016**, *166*, 29–36. [CrossRef]

76. Kamalipour, A.; Moghimi, S.; Eslani, M.; Nishida, T.; Mohammadzadeh, V.; Micheletti, E.; Girkin, C.A.; Fazio, M.A.; Liebmann, J.M.; Zangwill, L.M.; et al. A Prospective Longitudinal Study to Investigate Corneal Hysteresis as a Risk Factor of Central Visual Field Progression in Glaucoma. *Am. J. Ophthalmol* **2022**. [CrossRef]

77. Agarwal, D.R.; Ehrlich, J.R.; Shimmyo, M.; Radcliffe, N.M. The relationship between corneal hysteresis and the magnitude of intraocular pressure reduction with topical prostaglandin therapy. *Br. J. Ophthalmol.* **2012**, *96*, 254–257. [CrossRef]

78. Tsikripis, P.; Papaconstantinou, D.; Koutsandrea, C.; Apostolopoulos, M.; Georgalas, I. The effect of prostaglandin analogs on the biomechanical properties and central thickness of the cornea of patients with open-angle glaucoma: A 3-year study on 108 eyes. *Drug. Des. Devel. Ther.* **2013**, *7*, 1149–1156. [CrossRef]

79. Pillunat, K.R.; Spoerl, E.; Terai, N.; Pillunat, L.E. Effect of selective laser trabeculoplasty on corneal biomechanics. *Acta Ophthalmol.* **2016**, *94*, e501–e504. [CrossRef]

80. Hirneiß, C.; Sekura, K.; Brandlhuber, U.; Kampik, A.; Kernt, M. Corneal biomechanics predict the outcome of selective laser trabeculoplasty in medically uncontrolled glaucoma. *Graefes. Arch. Clin. Exp. Ophthalmol.* **2013**, *251*, 2383–2388. [CrossRef]

81. Pakravan, M.; Afroozifar, M.; Yazdani, S. Corneal Biomechanical Changes Following Trabeculectomy, Phaco-trabeculectomy, Ahmed Glaucoma Valve Implantation and Phacoemulsification. *J. Ophthalmic Vis. Res.* **2014**, *9*, 7–13. [PubMed]

82. Fujino, Y.; Murata, H.; Matsuura, M.; Nakakura, S.; Shoji, N.; Nakao, Y.; Kiuchi, Y.; Asaoka, R. The Relationship between Corneal Hysteresis and Progression of Glaucoma After Trabeculectomy. *J. Glaucoma* **2020**, *29*, 912–917. [CrossRef] [PubMed]

83. Sorkhabi, R.; Najafzadeh, F.; Sadeghi, A.; Ahoor, M.; Mahdavifard, A. Corneal biomechanical changes after trabeculectomy with mitomycin C in primary open-angle glaucoma and pseudoexfoliation glaucoma. *Int. Ophthalmol.* **2019**, *39*, 2741–2748. [CrossRef] [PubMed]

84. Pillunat, K.R.; Spoerl, E.; Terai, N.; Pillunat, L.E. Corneal biomechanical changes after trabeculectomy and the impact on intraocular pressure measurement. *J. Glaucoma* **2017**, *26*, 278–282. [CrossRef] [PubMed]

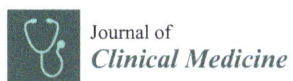

Journal of
Clinical Medicine

Article

Intraocular Pressure Measurement in Childhood Glaucoma under Standardized General Anaesthesia: The Prospective EyeBIS Study

Alicja Strzalkowska [1,†] , Nina Pirlich [2,†], Julia V. Stingl [1] , Alexander K. Schuster [1], Jasmin Rezapour [1], Felix M. Wagner [1] , Justus Buse [1] and Esther M. Hoffmann [1,*]

1   Department of Ophthalmology, University Medical Centre of the Johannes Gutenberg, University Mainz, 55131 Mainz, Germany; alicja.strzalkowska@unimedizin-mainz.de (A.S.); julia.stingl@unimedizin-mainz.de (J.V.S.); alexander.schuster@uni-mainz.de (A.K.S.); jasmin.rezapour@unimedizin-mainz.de (J.R.); felix.wagner@unimedizin-mainz.de (F.M.W.); jbuse@students.uni-mainz.de (J.B.)
2   Department of Anaesthesiology, University Medical Centre of the Johannes Gutenberg, University Mainz, 55131 Mainz, Germany; pirlich@uni-mainz.de
*   Correspondence: ehoffman@uni-mainz.de
†   These authors contributed equally to this work.

Citation: Strzalkowska, A.; Pirlich, N.; Stingl, J.V.; Schuster, A.K.; Rezapour, J.; Wagner, F.M.; Buse, J.; Hoffmann, E.M. Intraocular Pressure Measurement in Childhood Glaucoma under Standardized General Anaesthesia: The Prospective EyeBIS Study. *J. Clin. Med.* 2022, 11, 2846. https://doi.org/10.3390/jcm11102846

Academic Editors: Maria Letizia Salvetat, Marco Zeppieri and Paolo Brusini

Received: 27 March 2022
Accepted: 10 May 2022
Published: 18 May 2022

Publisher's Note: MDPI stays neutral with regard to jurisdictional claims in published maps and institutional affiliations.

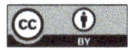
Abstract: Objective: We aimed to compare intraocular pressure (IOP) measurements using iCare® PRO rebound tonometry (iCare) and Perkins applanation tonometry (Perkins) in childhood glaucoma subjects and healthy children and the influence of anaesthesia depth, age and corneal thickness. Material: Prospective clinical, case-control study of children who underwent an ophthalmologic examination under general anaesthesia according to our protocol. Children were 45.45 ± 29.76 months old (mean ± SD (standard deviation)). Of all children, 54.05% were female. IOP was taken three times (T1–T3), according to duration and the depth of anaesthesia. The order of measurement alternated, starting with iCare. Agreement between the device measurements was evaluated using Bland–Altman analysis. Results: 53 glaucoma subjects and 22 healthy controls. Glaucoma subjects: IOP measured with iCare was at T1: 27.2 (18.1–33.8), T2: 21.6 (14.8–30.6), T3: 20.4 mmHg (14.5–27.0) and Perkins 17.5 (12.0–23.0), 15.5 (10.5–20.5), 15.0 mmHg (10.5–21.0) (median ± IQR (interquartile range)). Healthy controls: IOP with iCare: T1: 13.3 (11.1–17.0), T2: 10.6 (8.1–12.4), T3: 9.6 mmHg (7.7–11.7) and Perkins 10.3 (8.0–12.0), 7.0 (5.5–10.5), 7.0 mmHg (5.5–8.5) (median ± IQR). The median IOP was statistically significantly higher with iCare than with Perkins ($p < 0.001$) in both groups. The mean difference (iCare and Perkins) was 6.0 ± 6.1 mmHg for T1–T3, 7.3 at T1, 6.0 at T2, 4.9 mmHg at T3. Conclusion: The IOP was the highest in glaucoma subjects and healthy children at T1 (under sedation), independently of the measurement method. iCare always leads to higher IOP compared to Perkins in glaucoma and healthy subjects, regardless of the duration of anesthesia.

Keywords: childhood glaucoma; intraocular pressure measurement; iCare tonometry; Perkins tonometry; standardized anaesthesia

1. Introduction

Childhood glaucoma is a rare disease, with incidence in Europe of 1 per 20,000 live births [1]. If undiagnosed and consecutively treated too late, this disease can result in visual impairment or blindness in 1.2 to 7.1%, depending on the country of origin [2–4]. Early and accurate diagnosis in childhood glaucoma is crucial to initiate an appropriate therapy. This prevents irreversible damage to the cornea, optic nerve, as well as development of buphthalmos and myopia with vision loss [5–7].

To diagnose glaucoma in children, the ophthalmological examination with evaluation of ocular dimensions, corneal clarity, optic nerve and intraocular pressure measurement is needed [8]. However, the clinical examination can be challenging in uncooperative children [8]. Distorting factors, such as children crying, eyes squeezing or intrathoracic pressure may lead to inaccurate measurements. That is the reason why the success rate of the intraocular pressure (IOP) measurement in awake children varies between 14–60% [9,10]. To exclude these influencing factors, the necessary ophthalmological examination needs to be performed under general anaesthesia [8]. The general anaesthesia may affect the IOP itself, depending on the given sedatives, depth of anaesthesia or usage of anaesthetic techniques, such as laryngoscopy or intubation [11]. For instance, ketamine and suxamethonium increase the IOP [11–13], while remifentanil decreases IOP [14–16]. The increasing depth of anaesthesia leads to a significant reduction in the IOP [17].

Moreover, depending on the selected IOP measurement method itself, the IOP values can vary. The iCare® PRO rebound tonometry (iCare) is easy to use and does not need eye drops to carry out the measurement. However, IOP values measured with iCare, depending on device generation, are affected by corneal thickness and differ in sitting or supine position [18–20]. Age can also affect the measurement with iCare due to age-related changes in collagen fibrils in the cornea, which lead to an increase in stiffness [21,22]. To achieve reliable values with Perkins applanation tonometry (Perkins), on the other hand, some practice is required [23]. To perform the measurement with this device, fluorescein/anesthetic eye drops are needed. According to Garcia et al., the iCare measurement overestimates the IOP compared to Perkins tonometry [17]. However, Molero-Senosiaín proved that the iCare overestimates only the high IOP in comparison to Perkins [17].

Our main goal must be a precise and reliable IOP measurement in children under anaesthesia, as close as possible to the awake state without relevant changes in IOP [10,11]. To achieve that, the relationship between depth of anaesthesia and IOP has to be investigated [15,24].

In our study, the IOP and central corneal thickness (CCT) of childhood glaucoma subjects and healthy children was performed under protocol-defined standardized general anaesthesia. The protocol was established in our Childhood Glaucoma Centre at the University Medical Center in Mainz, Germany [25].

The purpose of this study was to compare IOP measurements using iCare and Perkins in childhood glaucoma subjects and healthy children at different time points of anaesthesia.

In addition, the correlation between CCT and IOP measurements, as well as between age and IOP, obtained with both devices, was analyzed.

2. Materials and Methods

2.1. Study Design

This study was approved by the local Ethics Committee of the Medical Association of the Rhineland-Palatinate state, Germany (Approval number: 2019-14207). This was a single centre, prospective cohort study of all childhood glaucoma subjects (53) who underwent an ophthalmologic examination including IOP and CCT measurement under protocol-defined standardized general anaesthesia between April 2019 and March 2021 at the University Eye Hospital Mainz, Germany. IOP was taken at three predefined time points (T1–T3) according to the depth of anaesthesia. The time of measurement was the same for each and every child. A precise description of the measurement can be found below under 'sequence of measurement'. Twenty-two children without a history of glaucoma were included as a control group. The correlation between iCare and Perkins was the primary endpoint. The IOP, the correlation between IOP and CCT, and IOP and age, were secondary endpoints.

2.2. Intraocular Pressure Measurement

IOP was measured with iCare® PRO rebound tonometry (iCare, Tiolat Oy, Helsinki, Finland) and Perkins applanation tonometry (Clement Clarke, Haag-Streit, Harlow, United Kingdom). The development of the rebound tonometry, originating from Kontiola, in 2001 led to iCare measurement. The magnetized probe launches against the eye using a solenoid. The solenoid captures the movement and impact of the probe on the eye [26].

The Perkins tonometer shares the same principle used in Goldmann tonometry. It is based on Imbert–Fick law. The force required to cover the area of a sphere to applanate is exactly the same size as the pressure inside the sphere and the applanated area [27]. Both tonometers are portable devices. The measurements were carried out by one of four ophthalmologists specialized in glaucoma in our clinic with wide experience in this field. A series of measurements was carried out on each child by the same specialist. All measurements were taken in a horizontal position.

2.3. Sequence of Measurements

IOP was measured in both eyes at three times (T1–T3). The first IOP measurement was performed immediately after the application of the propofol bolus (stage 1, T1). At this point the child was spontaneously breathing, slightly sedated, titrated with a maximum of 4 mg/kg bodyweight propofol intravenous bolus. This measurement reflects most closely the state of consciousness. The second IOP measurement was performed one minute after insertion of the laryngeal mask (stage 2, T2). At that point, a larger (anesthetic dose) bolus of propofol was given. The propofol and remifentanil were also running as perfusors. It means at this point the child was in a very deep anaesthesia. After that, the laryngeal mask was blocked according to the manufacturer's instructions and with the aid of the cuff pressure gauge to max. 60 cm H_2O. Immediately after the blocking, the third IOP measurement was acquired (stage 3, T3). At this time, the depth of anesthesia is approximately the same as at T2. At each stage, iCare measurement was followed by the measurement with Perkins, see Figure 1.

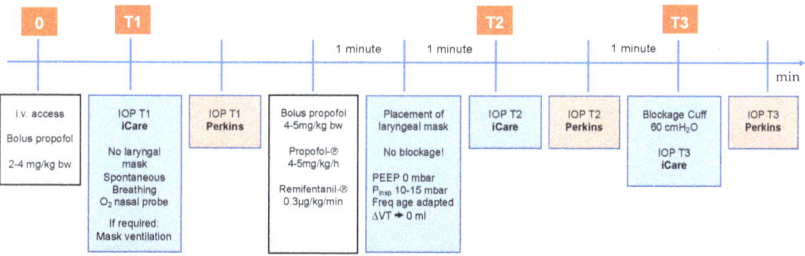

Figure 1. Sequence of measurements and procedures within EyeBIS study. Adapted from Pirlich, N.; Grehn, F.; Mohnke, K.; Maucher, K.; Schuster, A.; Wittenmeier, E.; Schmidtmann, I.; Hoffmann, E.M. Anaesthetic Protocol for Paediatric Glaucoma Examinations: The Prospective EyeBIS Study Protocol. BMJ Open 2021, 11, e045906 [25]. Abbreviation: i.v.: intravenous; bw: bodyweight; IOP: intraocular pressure; PEEP: Positive End-Expiratory Pressure; Pinsp: inspiratory pressure; Freq: frequency; VT: tidal volume.

2.4. Corneal Thickness Measurement

The corneal thickness was measured with ultrasound pachymetry (Tomey AL-3000 (Tomey, Nuremberg, Germany).

2.5. Inclusion Criteria

Children who met the following criteria were eligible for this study: indication for general anaesthesia with laryngeal mask for an operative or diagnostic intervention, age from 0.5 to 10 years, 1–3 according to the American Society of Anaesthesiologists physical status classification system (ASA classification), present written declaration of consent of the legal representatives.

2.6. Exclusion Criteria

Contraindications for the use of a laryngeal mask, known allergy to propofol or remifentanil was an exclusion criterion.

2.7. Childhood Glaucoma Subjects

To define childhood glaucoma, we used the Childhood Glaucoma Research Network criteria such as: IOP > 21 mmHg, optic disc cupping, corneal findings (Haab striae, Diameter > 11 mm in newborn, >12 mm in child < 1 year of age > 13 mm any age), progressive myopia/myopic shift, reproducible visual field defect which could not be caused by another reason. To meet the definition, at least two criteria have to be fulfilled [6].

2.8. Healthy Subjects

Those children needed an operation due to strabismus or tear duct obstruction. The children were otherwise healthy and did not require continuous local or systemic medication.

2.9. Statistical Analysis

Categorical variables were presented as frequencies with percentages, whereas median and interquartile range (IQR) or mean ± standard deviation (SD) were used to describe continuous variables. Evaluation of data normality was performed using Shapiro–Wilk test, whereas variance equality was verified by Levene's test. Normally distributed variables were compared using the *t* test. Non-normally distributed continuous variables were analysed using Friedman test, Wilcoxon test and Spearman's rank correlation coefficient. For multiple comparisons, Bonferroni correction was applied. Categorical variables were compared using the χ^2 test. Analyses were performed using R version 4.0.5 and Statistica 13.1 software for Windows. All statistical tests were two-tailed with the significance level set at $\alpha = 0.05$. Data were compared by determining interclass correlation coefficients for each tonometer and representing the differences detected as Bland–Altman plots.

3. Results

3.1. Characteristics

In this study, 150 eyes of 75 children were included; that is, 53 glaucoma subjects and 22 healthy controls. Overall age was 45.5 ± 29.8 months, glaucoma subjects 46.2 ± 29.7 and healthy children 43.8 ± 30.5 months old (mean ± SD). Of all the children, 54% were female. The mean CCT for the glaucoma subjects was statistically significantly higher than for the healthy ones, 601.6 ± 104.7 μm vs. 554.5 ± 39.7 μm, respectively ($p = 0.009$). The range of CCTs measured was 334.0–818.5 μm for glaucoma subjects and 494.0–616.5 μm for healthy children, see Figure 2. Patient 29 was excluded from the analysis because the CCT showed an extremal outlier from others, as a result of a massive corneal oedema.

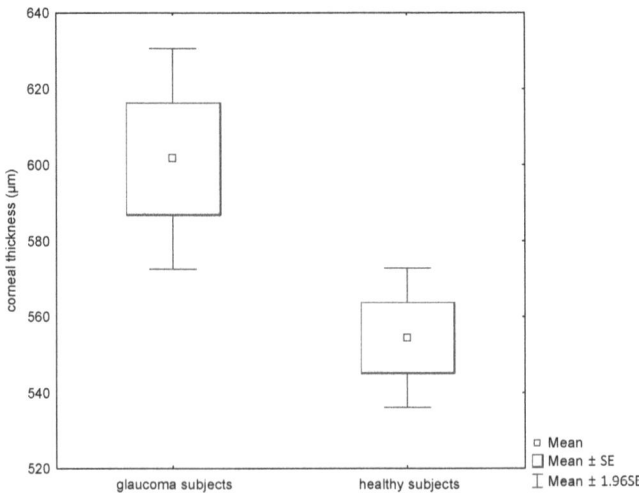

Figure 2. Corneal thickness for glaucoma vs. healthy subjects in the form of box plots.

3.2. Primary Endpoint—Correlation between iCare and Perkins

The correlation between iCare and Perkins for all children was moderate: the intraclass correlation coefficient (r) between the two methods was at T1–T3 0.63 ($p < 0.001$), at T1: 0.54 ($p < 0.001$), at T2: 0.62 ($p < 0.001$), and at T3: 0.72 ($p < 0.001$). The mean difference (iCare and Perkins) was 6.0 ± 6.1 mmHg for T1–T3, 7.3 mmHg at T1, 6.0 mmHg at T2, 4.9 mmHg at T3, see Figure 3.

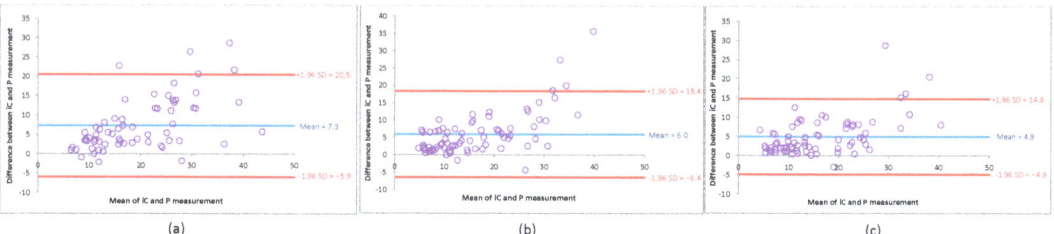

Figure 3. Difference between the measurement with iCare and Perkins in the form of Bland–Altman plot at the different time points for all children (**a**) T1, (**b**) T2, (**c**) T3. Abbreviation: IC: iCare; P: Perkins.

3.3. Secondary Endpoints

3.3.1. Median IOP with iCare and Perkins

For all children, the median IOP measured with iCare was statistically higher than measured with Perkins ($p < 0.001$). The median IOP using iCare was at T1: 20.3 (13.1–30.3), T2: 15.5 (11.0–25.2), T3: 15.7 mmHg (10.1–25.1) and for Perkins at T1: 14.5 (9.5–20.5), T2: 11.0 (7.5–19.5), T3: 11.5 mmHg (7.5–19.0) (median ± IQR). In addition, it was shown that IOP values measured with iCare and Perkins significantly decreased over time—median IOP at T1 > T2 ($p < 0.001$) and T1 > T3 ($p < 0.001$) for both devices.

For glaucoma subjects, the median IOP measured with iCare was statistically higher than measured with Perkins ($p < 0.001$). The median IOP measured with iCare was at T1: 27.2 (18.1–33.8), T2: 21.6 (14.8–30.6), T3: 20.4 mmHg (14.5–27.0) and Perkins T1: 17.5 (12.0–23.0), T2:15.5 (10.5–20.5), and T3: 15.0 mmHg (10.5–21.0) (median ± IQR). In addition, it was shown that IOP values in the iCare measurement significantly decreased over time between T1 and T2 and T1 and T3 and did not change between T2 and T3—median IOP at T1 > T2 ($p < 0.001$), T2 = T3 ($p = 0.101$), and T1 > T3 ($p < 0.001$). With Perkins, IOP values fell between T1 and T2 ($p < 0.003$). The IOP did not change significantly between T2 and T3 ($p = 0.976$) and T1 and T3 ($p < 0.022$), see Figure 4a. The IOP reduction between T1 and T2 is 21% for iCare and 11% for Perkins.

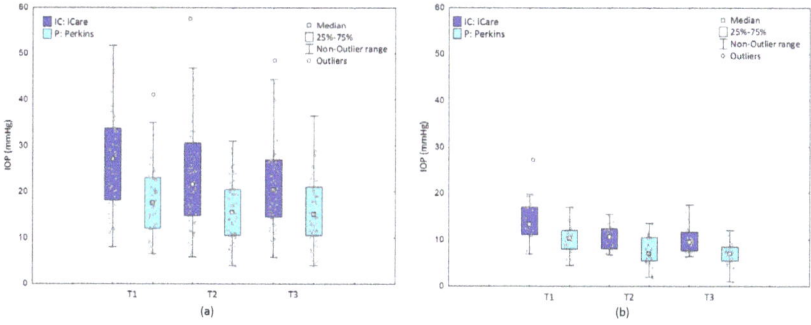

Figure 4. Median IOP at T1–T3 measured with iCare and Perkins (**a**) glaucoma subjects (**b**) healthy children. Abbreviation: IOP: intraocular pressure; IC: iCare; P: Perkins.

For healthy subjects, the median IOP measured with iCare was statistically higher than measured with Perkins ($p < 0.001$). The median IOP for iCare at T1 was: 13.3 (11.1–17.0), T2: 10.6 (8.1–12.4), T3: 9.6 mmHg (7.7–11.7) and for Perkins at T1: 10.3 (8.0–12.0), T2: 7.0 (5.5–10.5), and T3: 7.0 mmHg (5.5–8.5) (median ± IQR). In addition, it was shown that IOP values in the iCare measurement decreased significantly over time between T1 and T2 ($p < 0.001$) and T1 and T3 ($p < 0.001$) was not changed between T2 and T3—median IOP at T1 > T2 ($p < 0.001$), T2 = T3 ($p = 0.101$), and T1 > T3 ($p < 0.001$). With Perkins, IOP values fell between T1 and T2 ($p < 0.001$) and T1 and T3 ($p < 0.001$). The IOP did not change significantly between points T2 and T3—median IOP at T1 >T2 ($p < 0.001$), T2 = T3 ($p = 0.015$), and T1 > T3 ($p < 0.001$), see Figure 4b. The IOP reduction between T1 and T2 was 20% for iCare and 32% for Perkins.

3.3.2. Correlation of CCT and IOP

As for the correlation between CCT and IOP: the trend is downward in healthy children, but not statistically significant in iCare ($p = 0.837$) and not statistically significant in Perkins ($p = 0.656$). In glaucoma subjects, the trend is increasing, but is not statistically significant in iCare ($p = 0.228$) and borderline in Perkins ($p = 0.057$), see Figure 5.

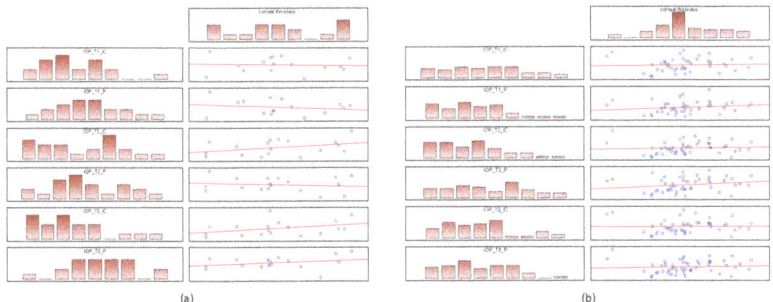

(a)   (b)

Figure 5. Correlation of CCT and IOP for iCare and Perkins (**a**) glaucoma subjects (**b**) healthy children. Abbreviation: CCT: corneal thickness; IOP: intraocular pressure; IC: iCare; P: Perkins.

3.3.3. Correlation of Age and IOP

The correlation between age and IOP with iCare at T1 was weak positive ($p = 0.009$) in glaucoma subjects and not statistically significant in healthy subject ($p = 0.243$). The correlation between age and IOP with Perkins was very weak positive ($p = 0.082$) in glaucoma subjects and not statistically significant in healthy subjects ($p = 0.263$), see Figure 6.

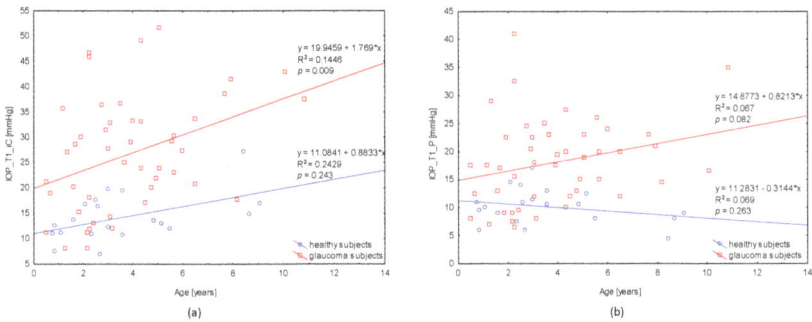

(a)   (b)

Figure 6. Correlation of age and IOP for (**a**) iCare and (**b**) Perkins at T1. Abbreviation: IOP: intraocular pressure; IC: iCare; P: Perkins; y: function; x: age; R^2: regression squared error metric; *p*: *p*-Value.

4. Discussion

In this study, we compared IOP measured with iCare and Perkins in childhood glaucoma subjects and healthy children and the influence of anaesthesia depth, age and corneal thickness.

In childhood glaucoma, a prompt and accurate diagnosis should be our main objective to avoid irreversible eye damage that can lead to blindness.

Glaucoma detection can be difficult for various reasons. It is rare that children experience the entire range of glaucoma characteristics, such as buphthalmos, corneal clouding or symptoms like epiphora, without obstruction of the tear ducts. It is common that an ophthalmological examination is not possible. In children, the vision field examination is difficult to carry out because of a lack of cooperation or refusal of eye patch [28–31].

This illustrates the importance of a precise and reliable IOP measurement in diagnosing childhood glaucoma [11]. To achieve it, it is necessary to ensure optimal test conditions. Most often, in smaller children, it is only possible under general anaesthesia.

However, until now, there has been a lack of standardized anaesthesia protocol in healthy children and children with glaucoma, which would accurately determine the type and amount of drug administered, anaesthetic procedures, such as mask application, mask blocking or intubation, depth of anaesthesia, as well as the best moment to perform the IOP measurement, as well as the optimal type of IOP measuring device must be determinate. Our study protocol was published recently [25]. In this paper, we want to present the data obtained using the described ophthalmological–anaesthetic protocol *EyeBIS*.

Our single centre, prospective, standardised cohort study, included, in total, 75 glaucoma subjects and healthy children. To the best of our knowledge, this is the first study where the IOP was measured in children during standardized general anaesthesia. Only very few studies have been published regarding IOP measurement with different devices in childhood glaucoma [32–36].

According to our study, the correlation between iCare and Perkins for all children was moderate for all three time points altogether. In the course of anaesthesia, lower IOP values were measured. The lower the IOP values, the better the correlation between the two measurement methods, T1: 0.54, T2: 0.62, and T3: 0.72. There are not many papers concerning correlation coefficients between those two devices in children, but there is even less information in this regard in glaucoma children. Martinez-de-la-Casa et al. reported a correlation coefficient of 0.87 in childhood glaucoma [20]. However, the mean IOP in this study was 22.1 ± 7.7 mm Hg for iCare and 19.1 ± 5.4 mmHg for Perkins. In our study, the IOP measured with iCare was 26.8 ± 11.2 at T1; 23.2 ± 11.4 at T2; 21.7 ± 10.3 at T3 and with Perkins 18.2 ± 7.7 at T1; 16.0 ± 7.1 at T2; 16.1 ± 7.4 at T3. Children in the study of Martinez-de-la-Casa et al. were older. They were 8.8 ± 2.9 years old, whereas in our study, the children were 45.5 ± 29.8 months old [20]. It is conceivable that the corneal characteristics and, hence, the IOP measurement in these two groups were different.

The median IOP measured with iCare was statistically higher compared with Perkins for glaucoma subjects and healthy children in our study. Our results confirm some earlier findings from the study by Borrego et al. [32]. In this study, the IOP was higher with iCare than with Perkins in the glaucoma children as well. In contrast to our study, Borrego et al. did not find a statistically significant mean IOP difference between iCare and Perkins, (0.42 ± 3.69 mmHg, $p = 0.41$) [32]. In our study, the mean difference between those two devices was statistically significant: 6.0 ± 6.1 mmHg for T1–T3, 7.3 mmHg at T1, 6.0 mmHg at T2, and 4.9 mmHg at T3. There are two explanations for it. In our study, the IOP was measured in sedation. At this time, the IOP is the highest. In higher IOP, iCare tends to overestimate IOP in comparison to Goldmann tonometry [37]. Additionally, there were many high IOP values measured within this study, maximal IOP with iCare was 33.8 vs. 29.1 mmHg compared to the Borrego et al. study. Because the mean difference between iCare and Perkins varies depending on the depth of general anaesthesia, the iCare and Perkins measurements are not interchangeable and cannot be converted directly into one another.

On the contrary, there are studies that proved that both iCare and Goldmann tonometry underestimate the real IOP. According to the study by Takagi at al., iCare tends to underestimate the IOP in comparison to Goldmann tonometry in lower IOP [38]. The reason for it was not given in this paper. The latest Messenio et al. study, concerning Goldmann tonometry, described the underestimation of IOP by Goldmann tonometry due to thinner corneas, which was already mentioned in another prior study [39,40]. We cannot support these statements with our data. Our IOP measurements were high from the beginning and the corneal thickness was normal to high.

The IOP was the highest at the measurement performed immediately after the application of propofol bolus (T1), regardless of the measurement method, for all children, glaucoma subjects and healthy children. This measurement reflects most closely the state of consciousness. After that, the deep anaesthesia was provoked and the second measurement was conducted. At this time the IOP was significantly lower in comparison to T1, once again, regardless of the measurement method for all children, glaucoma subjects and healthy children. At T3, the IOP was no different in comparison to T2 in glaucoma subjects or healthy controls. This is not surprising since the depth of general anaesthesia did not change between T2 and T3. It confirms the results of the previous study of Barclay et al. [41].

Our study confirms that the general anaesthesia reduced IOP significantly [16]. That highlights, once again, how important the cooperation and communication between anaesthesiologist and ophthalmologist are. The ophthalmologist needs to be in the operating room before the beginning of any anaesthesiologic procedures. By this and a standardized anaesthetic protocol, the measured IOP is as close to real IOP/awake IOP as possible.

In contrast to the study of Muir et al., we found differences in CCT in glaucoma subjects and healthy children [42]. It could be caused by the corneal oedema by strongly elevated IOP in our study. However, we did not find a statistically significant correlation between CCT and IOP. There are other known biomechanical properties in the cornea, which can influence the IOP, such as the corneal hysteresis [43,44], the corneal visoelastic parameter [45], which should be analysed in glaucoma children in the future.

The correlation between age and IOP with iCare and Perkins at T1 was weak positive in glaucoma subjects in our study. Therefore, we could not confirm the results of Sihota et al., where an increasing IOP with age was found [9]. It is probably caused by the small number of children who represent each age range in our study.

Strengths and Weaknesses

EyeBis has many strengths, including its prospective nature, large group of children glaucoma subjects, and standardized anaesthetic protocol for the comparison of two different IOP measurement devices. There are some limitations as well. The mean IOP was measured for both eyes of the child at each timepoint. The sequence of measuring, first iCare, then Perkins, might have, at least partly influenced the lowering of the IOP measured with Perkins. As mentioned before, the iCare probe launches against the eye using a solenoid. It could lead to aqueous massage or corneal impression. It is proven that repeated iCare readings tend to lower the IOP [36].

5. Conclusions

Under standardized general anaesthesia conditions, tonometry devices present differences in IOP. iCare leads to higher IOP compared to Perkins in glaucoma and healthy subjects, regardless of the duration of anesthesia.

The IOP changes during the course of anaesthesia and should be measured at the beginning of anaesthesia, according to our protocol, because at this point, the IOP is the highest. The knowledge of the exact anaesthesia depth during IOP measurement gives (a) more confidence in IOP values and (b) enables the glaucoma surgeon to interpret IOP results more accurately. In our study, IOP was independent of CCT.

J. Clin. Med. **2022**, *11*, 2846

Author Contributions: Conceptualization, J.B., J.V.S., A.K.S., J.R., F.M.W., N.P. and E.M.H.; Data curation, J.B.; Formal analysis, A.S.; Investigation, A.S., J.B., J.V.S., A.K.S., J.R., F.M.W., N.P. and E.M.H.; Methodology, J.B., N.P. and E.M.H.; Project administration, A.S., J.B., J.V.S., A.K.S., J.R., F.M.W., N.P. and E.M.H.; Supervision, N.P. and E.M.H.; Visualization, A.S.; Writing—original draft, A.S.; Writing—review and editing, A.S., N.P. and E.M.H. All authors have read and agreed to the published version of the manuscript.

Funding: This research received no external funding.

Institutional Review Board Statement: The study was conducted in accordance with the Declaration of Helsinki, and approved by the Ethics Committee of the Medical Association of the Rhineland-Palatinate state, Germany (Approval number: 2019-14207).

Informed Consent Statement: Informed consent was obtained from all subjects involved in the study.

Data Availability Statement: Not applicable.

Acknowledgments: We wanted to thank all the children who took part in the study and their parents who consented to participate in the study.

Conflicts of Interest: The authors declare no conflict of interest.

References

1. Genčík, A. Epidemiology and Genetics of Primary Congenital Glaucoma in Slovakia. Description of a Form of Primary Congenital Glaucoma in Gypsies with Autosomal-Recessive Inheritance and Complete Penetrance. *Dev. Ophthalmol.* **1989**, *16*, 76–115. [PubMed]
2. Lundvall, A.; Svedberg, H.; Chen, E. Application of the ICare Rebound Tonometer in Healthy Infants. *J. Glaucoma* **2011**, *20*, 7–9. [CrossRef] [PubMed]
3. Durnian, J.M.; Cheeseman, R.; Kumar, A.; Raja, V.; Newman, W.; Chandna, A. Childhood Sight Impairment: A 10-Year Picture. *Eye* **2010**, *24*, 112–117. [CrossRef]
4. Dorairaj, S.K.; Bandrakalli, P.; Shetty, C.; Vathsala, R.; Misquith, D.; Ritch, R. Childhood Blindness in a Rural Population of Southern India: Prevalence and Etiology. *Ophthalmic Epidemiol.* **2008**, *15*, 176–182. [CrossRef] [PubMed]
5. Badawi, A.H.; Al-Muhaylib, A.A.; Al Owaifeer, A.M.; Al-Essa, R.S.; Al-Shahwan, S.A. Primary Congenital Glaucoma: An Updated Review. *Saudi J. Ophthalmol.* **2019**, *33*, 382–388. [CrossRef] [PubMed]
6. Thau, A.; Lloyd, M.; Freedman, S.; Beck, A.; Grajewski, A.; Levin, A.V. New Classification System for Pediatric Glaucoma: Implications for Clinical Care and a Research Registry. *Curr. Opin. Ophthalmol.* **2018**, *29*, 385–394. [CrossRef]
7. Fung, D.S.; Roensch, M.A.; Kooner, K.S.; Cavanagh, H.D.; Whitson, J.T. Epidemiology and Characteristics of Childhood Glaucoma: Results from the Dallas Glaucoma Registry. *Clin. Ophthalmol.* **2013**, *7*, 1739–1746. [CrossRef] [PubMed]
8. Giangiacomo, A.; Beck, A. Pediatric Glaucoma: Review of Recent Literature. *Curr. Opin. Ophthalmol.* **2017**, *28*, 199–203. [CrossRef] [PubMed]
9. Sihota, R.; Tuli, D.; Dada, T.; Gupta, V.; Sachdeva, M.M. Distribution and Determinants of Intraocular Pressure in a Normal Pediatric Population. *J. Pediatr. Ophthalmol. Strabismus* **2006**, *43*, 14–18, quiz 36–37. [PubMed]
10. Oberacher-Velten, I.; Prasser, C.; Rochon, J.; Ittner, K.-P.; Helbig, H.; Lorenz, B. The Effects of Midazolam on Intraocular Pressure in Children during Examination under Sedation. *Br. J. Ophthalmol.* **2011**, *95*, 1102–1105. [CrossRef] [PubMed]
11. Dear, G.D.; Hammerton, M.; Hatch, D.J.; Taylor, D. Anaesthesia and Intra-Ocular Pressure in Young Children. A Study of Three Different Techniques of Anaesthesia. *Anaesthesia* **1987**, *42*, 259–265. [CrossRef] [PubMed]
12. Yoshikawa, E.; Murai, Y. The Effect of Ketamine on Intraocular Pressure in Children. *Surv. Anesthesiol.* **1972**, *16*, 252. [CrossRef]
13. Adams, A.K. Ketamine in Paediatric Ophthalmic Practice. *Anaesthesia* **1973**, *28*, 212–213. [CrossRef] [PubMed]
14. Alexander, R.; Hill, R.; Lipham, W.J.; Weatherwax, K.J.; El-Moalem, H.E. Remifentanil Prevents an Increase in Intraocular Pressure after Succinylcholine and Tracheal Intubation. *Br. J. Anaesth.* **1998**, *81*, 606–607. [CrossRef]
15. Hanna, S.F.; Ahmad, F.; Pappas, A.L.S.; Mikat-Stevens, M.; Jellish, W.S.; Kleinman, B.; Avramov, M.N. The Effect of Propofol/remifentanil Rapid-Induction Technique without Muscle Relaxants on Intraocular Pressure. *J. Clin. Anesth.* **2010**, *22*, 437–442. [CrossRef]
16. Termühlen, J.; Gottschalk, A.; Eter, N.; Hoffmann, E.M.; Van Aken, H.; Grenzebach, U.; Prokosch, V. Does General Anesthesia Have a Clinical Impact on Intraocular Pressure in Children? *Paediatr. Anaesth.* **2016**, *26*, 936–941. [CrossRef]
17. Darlong, V.; Kalaiyarasan, R.; Baidya, D.K.; Pandey, R.; Sinha, R.; Punj, J.; Dada, T. Effect of Airway Device and Depth of Anesthesia on Intra-Ocular Pressure Measurement during General Anesthesia in Children: A Randomized Controlled Trial. *J. Anaesthesiol. Clin. Pharmacol.* **2021**, *37*, 226–230.
18. García-Resúa, C.; González-Meijome, J.M.; Gilino, J.; Yebra-Pimentel, E. Accuracy of the New ICare Rebound Tonometer vs. Other Portable Tonometers in Healthy Eyes. *Optom. Vis. Sci.* **2006**, *83*, 102. [CrossRef]
19. Nakakura, S.; Mori, E.; Yamamoto, M.; Tsushima, Y.; Tabuchi, H.; Kiuchi, Y. Intraocular Pressure of Supine Patients Using Four Portable Tonometers. *Optom. Vis. Sci.* **2013**, *90*, 700–706. [CrossRef]

20. Martinez-de-la-Casa, J.M.; Garcia-Feijoo, J.; Saenz-Frances, F.; Vizzeri, G.; Fernandez-Vidal, A.; Mendez-Hernandez, C.; Garcia-Sanchez, J. Comparison of Rebound Tonometer and Goldmann Handheld Applanation Tonometer in Congenital Glaucoma. *J. Glaucoma* **2009**, *18*, 49–52. [CrossRef]
21. Sakamoto, M.; Kanamori, A.; Fujihara, M.; Yamada, Y.; Nakamura, M.; Negi, A. Assessment of IcareONE Rebound Tonometer for Self-Measuring Intraocular Pressure. *Acta Ophthalmol.* **2014**, *92*, 243–248. [CrossRef] [PubMed]
22. Daxer, A.; Misof, K.; Grabner, B.; Ettl, A.; Fratzl, P. Collagen Fibrils in the Human Corneal Stroma: Structure and Aging. *Investig. Ophthalmol. Vis. Sci.* **1998**, *39*, 644–648. [PubMed]
23. Vaughan, D.; Asbury, T. General Ophthalmology. In *General Ophthalmology*; Lange Medical Publications: Los Altos, CA, USA, 1977; p. 379.
24. Schäfer, R.; Klett, J.; Auffarth, G.; Polarz, H.; Völcker, H.E.; Martin, E.; Böttiger, B.W. Intraocular Pressure More Reduced during Anesthesia with Propofol than with Sevoflurane: Both Combined with Remifentanil. *Acta Anaesthesiol. Scand.* **2002**, *46*, 703–706. [CrossRef] [PubMed]
25. Pirlich, N.; Grehn, F.; Mohnke, K.; Maucher, K.; Schuster, A.; Wittenmeier, E.; Schmidtmann, I.; Hoffmann, E.M. Anaesthetic Protocol for Paediatric Glaucoma Examinations: The Prospective EyeBIS Study Protocol. *BMJ Open* **2021**, *11*, e045906. [CrossRef]
26. Kontiola, A.I.; Goldblum, D.; Mittag, T.; Danias, J. The Induction/impact Tonometer: A New Instrument to Measure Intraocular Pressure in the Rat. *Exp. Eye Res.* **2001**, *73*, 781–785. [CrossRef]
27. Gloster, J.; Perkins, E.S. The Validity of the Imbert-Fick Law as Applied to Applanation Tonometry. *Exp. Eye Res.* **1963**, *2*, 274–283. [CrossRef]
28. Dobson, V.; Brown, A.M.; Harvey, E.M.; Narter, D.B. Visual Field Extent in Children 3.5–30 Months of Age Tested with a Double-Arc LED Perimeter. *Vision Res.* **1998**, *38*, 2743–2760. [CrossRef]
29. Mayer, D.L.; Dobson, V. Visual Acuity Development in Infants and Young Children, as Assessed by Operant Preferential Looking. *Vision Res.* **1982**, *22*, 1141–1151. [CrossRef]
30. Getz, L.; Dobson, V.; Muna, B. Grating Acuity Development in 2-Week-Old to 3-Year-Old Children Born prior to Term. *Clin. Version Sci.* **1992**, *7*, 251–256.
31. Salomao, S.R.; Ventura, D.F. Large Sample Population Age Norms for Visual Acuities Obtained with Vistech-Teller Acuity Cards. *Investig. Ophthalmol. Vis. Sci.* **1995**, *36*, 657–670.
32. Borrego Sanz, L.; Morales-Fernandez, L.; Martínez de-la-Casa, J.M.; Sáenz-Francés, F.; Fuentes, M.; García-Feijóo, J. The Icare-Pro Rebound Tonometer Versus the Hand-Held Applanation Tonometer in Congenital Glaucoma. *J. Glaucoma* **2016**, *25*, 149–154. [CrossRef] [PubMed]
33. Dahlmann-Noor, A.H.; Puertas, R.; Tabasa-Lim, S.; El-Karmouty, A.; Kadhim, M.; Wride, N.K.; Lewis, A.; Grosvenor, D.; Rai, P.; Papadopoulos, M.; et al. Comparison of Handheld Rebound Tonometry with Goldmann Applanation Tonometry in Children with Glaucoma: A Cohort Study. *BMJ Open* **2013**, *3*, e001788. [CrossRef] [PubMed]
34. Kageyama, M.; Hirooka, K.; Baba, T.; Shiraga, F. Comparison of ICare Rebound Tonometer with Noncontact Tonometer in Healthy Children. *J. Glaucoma* **2011**, *20*, 63–66. [CrossRef] [PubMed]
35. Flemmons, M.S.; Hsiao, Y.-C.; Dzau, J.; Asrani, S.; Jones, S.; Freedman, S.F. Icare Rebound Tonometry in Children with Known and Suspected Glaucoma. *J. AAPOS* **2011**, *15*, 153–157. [CrossRef]
36. Gandhi, N.G.; Prakalapakorn, S.G.; El-Dairi, M.A.; Jones, S.K.; Freedman, S.F. Icare ONE Rebound versus Goldmann Applanation Tonometry in Children with Known or Suspected Glaucoma. *Am. J. Ophthalmol.* **2012**, *154*, 843–849.e1. [CrossRef] [PubMed]
37. Molero-Senosiaín, M.; Morales-Fernández, L.; Saenz-Francés, F.; García-Feijoo, J.; Martínez-de-la-Casa, J.M. Analysis of Reproducibility, Evaluation, and Preference of the New iC100 Rebound Tonometer versus iCare PRO and Perkins Portable Applanation Tonometry. *Eur. J. Ophthalmol.* **2020**, *30*, 1349–1355. [CrossRef]
38. Takagi, D.; Sawada, A.; Yamamoto, T. Evaluation of a New Rebound Self-Tonometer, Icare HOME: Comparison with Goldmann Applanation Tonometer. *J. Glaucoma* **2017**, *26*, 613–618. [CrossRef]
39. Messenio, D.; Ferroni, M.; Boschetti, F. Goldmann Tonometry and Corneal Biomechanics. *Appl. Sci.* **2021**, *11*, 4025. [CrossRef]
40. Ehlers, N.; Bramsen, T.; Sperling, S. Applanation Tonometry and Central Corneal Thickness. *Acta Ophthalmol.* **1975**, *53*, 34–43. [CrossRef]
41. Barclay, K.; Wall, T.; Wareham, K.; Asai, T. Intra-Ocular Pressure Changes in Patients with Glaucoma. Comparison between the Laryngeal Mask Airway and Tracheal Tube. *Anaesthesia* **1994**, *49*, 159–162. [CrossRef]
42. Muir, K.W.; Jin, J.; Freedman, S.F. Central Corneal Thickness and Its Relationship to Intraocular Pressure in Children. *Ophthalmology* **2004**, *111*, 2220–2223. [CrossRef] [PubMed]
43. Deol, M.; Taylor, D.A.; Radcliffe, N.M. Corneal Hysteresis and Its Relevance to Glaucoma. *Curr. Opin. Ophthalmol.* **2015**, *26*, 96–102. [CrossRef] [PubMed]
44. Gatzioufas, Z.; Labiris, G.; Stachs, O.; Hovakimyan, M.; Schnaidt, A.; Viestenz, A.; Käsmann-Kellner, B.; Seitz, B. Biomechanical Profile of the Cornea in Primary Congenital Glaucoma. *Acta Ophthalmol.* **2013**, *91*, e29–e34. [CrossRef]
45. Touboul, D.; Roberts, C.; Kérautret, J.; Garra, C.; Maurice-Tison, S.; Saubusse, E.; Colin, J. Correlations between Corneal Hysteresis, Intraocular Pressure, and Corneal Central Pachymetry. *J. Cataract Refract. Surg.* **2008**, *34*, 616–622. [CrossRef] [PubMed]

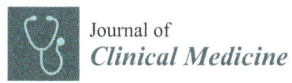

Journal of
Clinical Medicine

Article

Pulsatile Trabecular Meshwork Motion: An Indicator of Intraocular Pressure Control in Primary Open-Angle Glaucoma

Rong Du [1,†], Chen Xin [1,*,†], Jingjiang Xu [2], Jianping Hu [1], Huaizhou Wang [1], Ningli Wang [1] and Murray Johnstone [3]

1   Beijing Tongren Eye Center, Beijing Institute of Ophthalmology, Beijing Tongren Hospital, Capital Medical University, Beijing 100730, China; drdurong@ccmu.edu.cn (R.D.); hjp@mail.ccmu.edu.cn (J.H.); whz@ccmu.edu.cn (H.W.); wningli@ccmu.edu.cn (N.W.)
2   School of Physics and Optoelectronic Engineering, Foshan University, Foshan 528000, China; jjxu@uw.edu
3   Department of Ophthalmology, University of Washington, Seattle, WA 98195, USA; murrayj2@uw.edu
*   Correspondence: xinchen0322@ccmu.edu.cn
†   These authors contributed equally to this work.

Abstract: (1) Background: To investigate the value of pulsatile trabecular meshwork (TM) motion in predicting the diurnal intraocular pressure (IOP) fluctuation of primary open-angle glaucoma (POAG). (2) Methods: This cross-sectional study recruited 20 normal patients and 30 patients with POAG. Of the POAG group, 20 had stable diurnal IOP and 10 had high IOP fluctuation. A clinical prototype phase-sensitive optical coherence tomography (PhS-OCT) model was used to measure TM pulsatile motion with maximum velocity (MV) and cumulative displacement (CDisp). (3) Results: MV and CDisp were higher in the external region in both normal and POAG patients. All MV and CDisp reduced significantly in the POAG group ($p < 0.001$). In the POAG group, except MV in the external region ($p = 0.085$), MV and CDisp in the nasal area were significantly higher than those in the temporal area ($p < 0.05$). The MV and CDisp in the external region in the nasal area of POAG patients with high IOP fluctuation were much lower than those with stable IOP ($p_{EMV3} = 0.031$, $p_{ECDisp3} < 0.001$); (4) Conclusions: Pulsatile TM motion reduced in POAG patients relevant to the level of diurnal IOP fluctuation. This study presents the segmental variance of TM stiffness in human living eyes and suggests the clinical potential of the measurement of pulsatile TM motion with PhS-OCT for the evaluation of diurnal IOP fluctuation.

Keywords: trabecular meshwork; phase-sensitive optical coherent tomography; pulsatile motion; IOP fluctuation; primary open-angle glaucoma

Citation: Du, R.; Xin, C.; Xu, J.; Hu, J.; Wang, H.; Wang, N.; Johnstone, M. Pulsatile Trabecular Meshwork Motion: An Indicator of Intraocular Pressure Control in Primary Open-Angle Glaucoma. *J. Clin. Med.* **2022**, *11*, 2696. https://doi.org/10.3390/jcm11102696

Academic Editors: Maria Letizia Salvetat, Marco Zeppieri, Paolo Brusini and Emmanuel Andrès

Received: 18 December 2021
Accepted: 13 April 2022
Published: 10 May 2022

Publisher's Note: MDPI stays neutral with regard to jurisdictional claims in published maps and institutional affiliations.

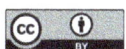
1. Introduction

Glaucoma is a leading cause of irreversible blindness around the world [1]. Primary open-angle glaucoma (POAG) is the most common type, with characteristics of optic neuropathy and visual field defects. Intraocular pressure (IOP) elevation is widely accepted as a major cause of POAG, and IOP control is the most reliable treatment [2,3]. Although IOP has become widely accepted as a major cause of POAG, how IOP is regulated and why it increases remain an enigma.

IOP measurement is the approach most frequently used to evaluate POAG treatment adequacy. Large and irregular IOP fluctuations may the cause loading and unloading of stress; the tissue is unable to compensate, and then damage occurs. Studies have proven that IOP is highly variable, and large IOP fluctuations are an independent risk factor for POAG development and progression [4,5]. Thus, 24 h IOP monitoring is recommended [6].

Because the measurement of IOP for 24 h is inconvenient and time-consuming [7], it would be valuable if we could estimate the fluctuation of IOP by less complex means. IOP homeostasis depends on the normal function of the aqueous outflow system, especially the trabecular meshwork (TM) outflow pathway [8]. Many experimental and clinical studies provide evidence that bulk aqueous humor outflow is characteristically pulse-dependent [9]. The pressure-sensitive bulk motion of the TM changes the dimensions of Schlemm's canal (SC), which functions as a compressible chamber and is a prerequisite for the pulsatile flow pattern [10].

Multiple lines of evidence document the progressive decrease and eventual loss of pulsatile flow in glaucoma patients as the disease progresses [11]. The elastic property of TM provides a grounding in the pumping of aqueoushumor. The TM pulsatile motion represents TM deformability to the cardiac-induced ocular pulse amplitude. As an important regulatory site, TM dysfunction plays a critical role in the pathogenesis of POAG [12,13]. TM stiffness, defined as the tissue's resistance to deform, is one of the essential factors that affects the ability to induce the pulsatile motion [14].

Phase-sensitive optical coherence tomography (PhS-OCT) has been found to quantify the pulsatile TM motion in vivo with high repeatability and reliability [15]. The quantified pulsatile motion is thought to be representative of TM stiffness. Recently, one study identified a reduced pulsatile TM motion in patients with PAOG by using PhS-OCT [16]. However, how effectively the pulsatile movement of TM measured by PhS-OCT reflects IOP fluctuation has not yet been evaluated. Here, we report a cross-sectional study designed to investigate the relationship between the pulsatile movement of TM and IOP fluctuation in normal and POAG subjects.

2. Materials and Methods

2.1. Subjects

This cross-sectional study was conducted at the Beijing Tongren Hospital, Capital Medical University, between August and December 2020. The study was approved by the Ethical Review Committee of Beijing Tongren Hospital (TRECKY2018-066). The study adhered to the tenets of the Declaration of Helsinki, and each subject signed an informed consent document.

All the recruited subjects received a comprehensive ocular examination of the right eye, including a review of their medical history, best-corrected visual acuity, refraction, a slit lamp, and a stereoscopic optic disc examination. Blood pressure (BP) was measured using an automatic BP device (OMRON Heem-907 blood pressure monitor, OMRON, Kyoto, Japan). IOP was measured by using Goldmann applanation tonometry (GAT). We used an IOL-Master 700 (Carl Zeiss Meditec AG, Jena, Germany) to measure the axial length (AL), central corneal thickness (CCT), and anterior chamber depth (ACD). We admitted POAG subjects to the hospital to provide 24 h IOP monitoring. We measured IOP in the seated position at the following seven times of day using GAT: 2:00 AM, 6:00 AM, 8:00 AM, 10:00 AM, 2:00 PM, 6:00 PM, and 10:00 PM. IOP fluctuation was defined as the difference between the maximum IOP and the minimum IOP in a day.

Normal subjects had no other ocular disease except dry eye or myopia (0~−3.0 Diopters). POAG was defined as the presence of a normal and open-angle gonioscopy, untreated IOP without medication > 21 mmHg, glaucomatous visual field loss confirmed on the subsequent visual field test, and corresponding glaucomatous optic nerve damage evidenced by stereoscopic fundus examination and the images of an optical coherence tomograph. All POAG patients were treated with topical medication for at least three months (18.6 ± 3.4 weeks). For these POAG patients, IOP was measured twice a week after medications were administered. The prescription for POAG was as follows: 1. Prostaglandins; 2. β-blocker; 3. Brinzolamide. All the recorded IOP values measured in the clinic during office hours were less than 21 mmHg while on medication. The exclusion criteria were as follows: (1) previous ocular trauma or surgery; (2) ocular diseases other than POAG; (3) high myopia with aspherical equivalent worse than −3.0 Diopters; (4) known diabetes or cardiac disease.

2.2. PhS-OCT Examination and Data Processing

The clinical PhS-OCT prototype (Figure 1) is composed of three parts: (1) a spectral-domain OCT system with the light source of a wavelength of 1310 nm with a spectral bandwidth of 100 nm; (2) a digital pulsimeter (Powerlab, ML 866, Colorado Springs, CO, USA) for cardiac signal recording; (3) an external controlling unit for synchronizing the OCT and cardiac signals. The theoretical axial resolution was ~5.5 μm, and the lateral resolution was ~16 μm in tissue. The subject was seated facing straight ahead in a slit-lamp style chin rest with a headrest support, and a digital pulsimeter was placed on the tip of the index finger. The subjects followed an external fixation target with their eyes without moving their head during PhS-OCT imaging. We scanned the temporal and nasal 3.5 mm limbal region of the TM. Each scan lasted for 5 s, creating a dataset containing 2000 OCT B-scans (400 B-scans/s).

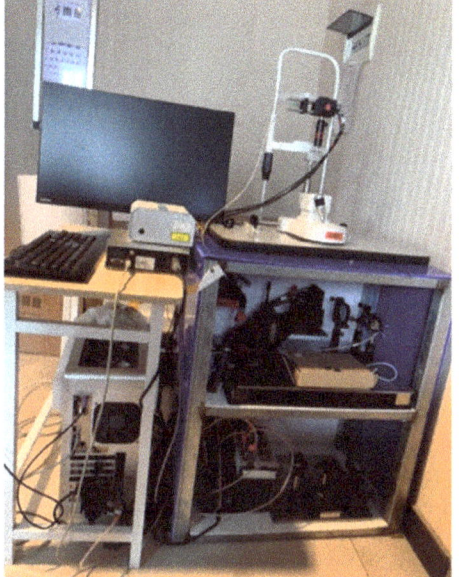
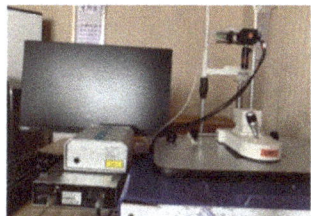
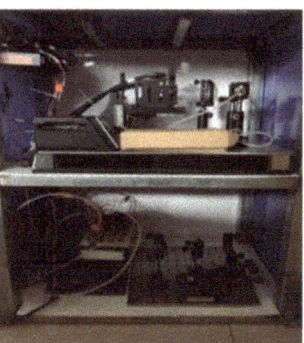

Figure 1. Photos of the clinic's phenotype of phase-sensitive optical coherence tomography.

For each dataset, the velocity waveform of each pixel was used to generate a velocity waveform tracing. A proprietary technique was used to compensate for the bulk involuntary motion occurring during the measurement. Between adjacent B-scans, we analyzed the phase shift of each pixel in the OCT signals, then calculated instantaneous velocity based on the difference between the two B-scan images. A mask derived from the cardiac pulse and harmonic frequency filtered the motion waveforms. We selected two regions of interest for each scan. The internal region of TM was defined as one-third of the distance anterior to the sclera spur along the line between Schwalbe's line and the sclera spur. The external region of the TM was selected as the area next to the SC lumen. The maximum velocity (MV) and cumulative displacement (CDisp) were then calculated (Figure 2), providing first an internal TM maximum velocity (IMV) and displacement (ICDisp), then an external TM Velocity (EMV) and displacement (ECDisp). For details on how to characterize the Phs-OCT system for dynamic displacement measurement, please refer to our previous studies [15,17].

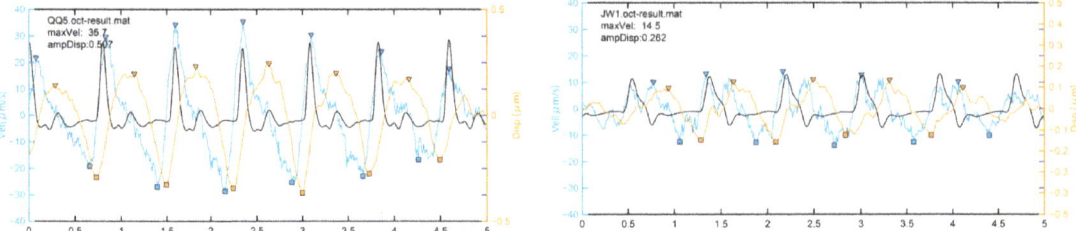

Figure 2. Representative of trabecular motion (TM) synchronized with heartbeat. The TM motion is synchronized with the heartbeat. The black curves represent the heartbeat. The blue curves indicate the instantaneous velocity of the TM in each cycle, while the orange lines demonstrate the cumulative displacement of the TM, which moves away from the original location at each check point. The inverted triangle indicates the peak value of the traced curve, while the square presents the valley value. The positive of the velocity or the displacement represents the TM moving outwards to the sclera in the systole; the negative velocities represent the TM moving inwards towards the anterior chamber during the diastole. The maximum velocity means the maximum instantaneous velocity during a cycle. The figures show two representatives of the TM motion in normal (**left**) and POAG patients (**right**).

All the examinations were performed by Dr. XC, who was masked to the diagnosis of the subjects. PhS-OCT imaging was performed at 10:00 AM, with the temporal and nasal limbal region scanned in each subject. Three successive datasets were collected in an examination on one day to assess the repeatability of the imaging. The scans were repeated two weeks later to determine the reliability of the PhS-OCT technique on separate exam days.

2.3. Statistical Analysis

Descriptive statistics are presented as the mean ± standard deviation (SD). The significant differences of the parameters of the pulsatile TM motion between normal patients and patients with POAG were determined using an unpaired t-test based on the analysis of normality (Shapiro–Wilk test). The intraclass correlation coefficient (ICC) was used to assess the repeatability and reproducibility of the pulsatile TM motion measurements in the PhS-OCT images. Each comparison was labeled as significant when $p < 0.05$.

3. Results

3.1. Demographic and Baseline Characteristics of the Subjects

Twenty normal and 30 POAG subjects were recruited in this study. The mean ages of the normal and POAG groups were 41.3 ± 9.3 years and 44.6 ± 9.5 years ($p = 0.992$), respectively. The IOP at 10:00 AM was not significantly different between groups ($p = 0.111$): 15.4 ± 1.6 mm Hg in the normal group and 15.3 ± 2.0 mmHg in the POAG group. The baseline characteristics of all participants are shown in Tables 1 and 2.

Table 1. Demographic of subjects.

	Normal	POAG	p-Value
Age (years)	41.3 ± 9.3	44.6 ± 9.5	0.992
Sex (F:M)	11/9	10/20	0.154
Axial length (mm)	24.04 ± 0.43	24.03 ± 0.28	0.069
Central corneal thickness (μm)	527 ± 28	540 ± 33	0.342
Heart rate	70.3 ± 8.8	72.9 ± 9.4	0.406
Mean arterial pressure (mmHg)	87.9 ± 7.5	90.4 ± 6.2	0.445
IOP (mmHg)	15.4 ± 1.6	15.3 ± 2.0	0.111
Mean deviation (dB)		−9.32 ± 1.58	

POAG—primary open-angle glaucoma; F:M—Female: Male; IOP—intraocular pressure.

Table 2. Demographic of POAG subjects.

	IOP Stable	IOP Fluctuant	*p*-Value
Age (years)	44.6 ± 14.5	46.4 ± 15.2	0.630
Sex (F:M)	8/12	4/6	0.833
Follow-up (weeks)	20.8 ± 4.2	19.7 ± 2.9	0.115
Axial length (mm)	24.34 ± 0.50	24.42 ± 0.50	0.982
Central corneal thickness (μm)	544 ± 37	537 ± 28	0.287
Heart rate	72.1 ± 4.6	73.5 ± 5.1	0.842
Mean arterial pressure (mmHg)	90.8 ± 9.5	89.4 ± 11.5	0.333
IOP (mmHg)	16.1 ± 3.1	16.2 ± 2.5	0.471
Mean deviation (dB)	−11.03 ± 3.09	−13.15 ± 4.01	0.127

3.2. Repeatability and Reliability

The ICCs of IMV, EMV, ICDisp, and ECDisp for the three continuous scans in the same region were 0.953, 0.937, 0.917, and 0.914, respectively. The ICCs of IMV, EMV, ICDisp, and ECDisp for the two images captured on separate days were 0.973, 0.884, 0.913, and 0.782, respectively.

3.3. Difference in MV and CDisp between Healthy and POAG Eyes

The results for pulsatile TM motion in all the recruited eyes are presented in Figure 3. In both the nasal and temporal areas, MV and CDisp in the internal and external regions were significantly lower in POAG eyes than in normal eyes ($p < 0.001$).

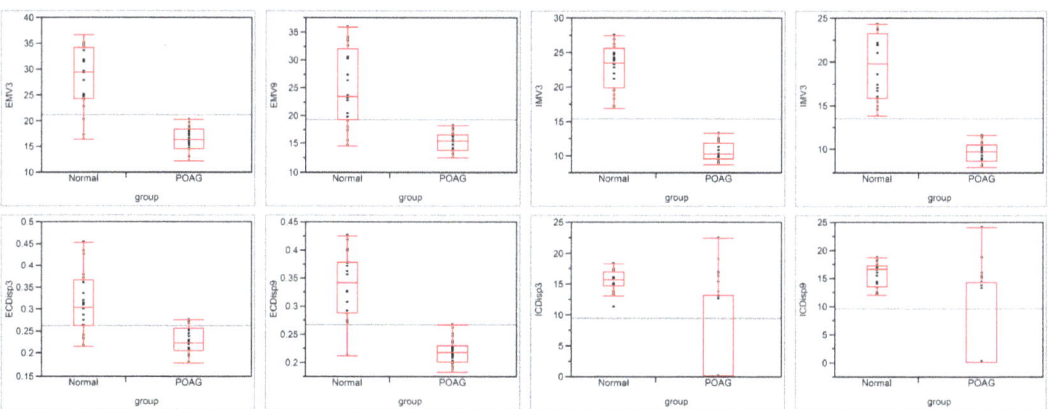

Figure 3. The pulsatile trabecular meshwork (TM) motion in normal and POAG eyes. MV—maximum velocity; CDisp—cumulative displacement; EMV3—MV in the external region of TM in the nasal area; EMV9—MV in the external region of TM in the temporal area; IMV3—MV in the internal region of TM in the nasal area; IMV9—MV in the internal region of TM in the nasal area; ECDisp3—CDisp in the external region of TM in the nasal area; ECDisp9—CDisp in the external region of TM in the temporal area; ICDisp3—CDisp in the external region of TM in the nasal area; ICDisp9—CDisp in the external region of TM in the temporal area. POAG—primary open-angle glaucoma.

In normal eyes, in both the internal and external regions, the MV in the nasal area was significantly higher than that in the temporal area. The CDisp in the external region of the TM in the nasal area was much higher than that in the temporal area. However, the CDisp in the internal region of the TM in the nasal area was similar to the temporal area (Table 2). Similar to normal subjects, the MVs in the nasal area were significantly higher than those in the temporal area of the eyes with glaucoma. However, in glaucoma eyes, the CDisp in both the external and internal regions of the TM in the nasal area was much higher than that in the temporal area (Table 3).

Table 3. The pulsatile TM motion in normal and POAG eyes.

	Nasal	Temporal	*p*-Value
Normal			
EMV, μm/s	28.5 ± 6.3	25.2 ± 6.8	0.002
IMV, μm/s	22.8 ± 3.2	19.5 ± 3.7	<0.001
ECDisp, μm	0.341 ± 0.063	0.305 ± 0.064	0.036
ICDisp, μm	0.271 ± 0.063	0.248 ± 0.064	0.253
POAG			
EMV, μm/s	16.3 ± 2.2	15.3 ± 1.6	0.085
IMV, μm/s	11.2 ± 1.9	9.7 ± 1.2	0.01
ECDisp, μm	0.231 ± 0.031	0.218 ± 0.021	0.037
ICDisp, μm	0.207 ± 0.038	0.156 ± 0.034	<0.001

TM—trabecular meshwork; POAG—primary open-angle glaucoma; MV—maximum velocity; CDisp—cumulative displacement; EMV—MV in the external region of TM; IMV—MV in the internal region of TM; ECDisp—CDisp in the external region of TM; ICDisp—CDisp in the internal region of TM.

Using the diurnal IOP amplitude ($IOP_{highest}$–IOP_{lowest}) as a categorical factor, the glaucoma eyes could be divided into two groups. Twenty eyes had stable IOP, defined as a diurnal IOP amplitude of ≤8 mm Hg, and ten eyes had fluctuating IOP (>8 mmHg). The mean IOP amplitudes were 4.0 ± 1.5 mmHg and 9.9 ± 2.2 mm Hg in the stable and fluctuating groups, respectively. The results showed that, compared with normal subjects, all the parameters of TM pulsatile motion decreased dramatically in both the stable and fluctuating groups ($p < 0.01$) in those with glaucoma. Moreover, the EMV3 (15.1 ± 2.3 μm/s) and ECDisp3 (0.205 ± 0.021 μm) in the fluctuating group were significantly lower than those in the stable group (19.9 ± 2.0 μm/s, pEMV3 = 0.031; 0.237 ± 0.030 μm, pECDisp3 < 0.001).

4. Discussion

In this study, we firstly demonstrated the good reliability and repeatability of TM motion quantification, as previously reported [15]. PhS-OCT was used to characterize the TM motion change with accommodation [15]. Our results showed that pulsatile TM motion was reduced in glaucoma compared with normal subjects. The pulsatile motion of TM originates from the ocular pulse caused by the oscillatory change in choroidal volume during the cardiac cycle [9]. Pulsatile TM motion reflects TM stiffness, which becomes abnormal in glaucoma [14,16]. Previously, the PhS-OCT system has been shown to be able to differentiate POAG from healthy subjects [17]. The study found that parameters of pulse-dependent TM motion were better able to predict the presence of glaucoma than measurements of outflow facility, or IOP measurements during clinic hours [17].

In this study, we matched the normal and POAG patients in terms of age, heart rate, and mean arterial pressure, which potentially correlate with TM motion. Although the IOP was well controlled with topical medication in the POAG patients, the TM motion was dramatically reduced nasally and temporally in both the internal and external TM regions. Recently, Li G et al. reported that, in corticosteroid-treated mice, SC was more resistant to collapse in elevated IOPs. The study, performed by estimates using inverse finite element modeling, was consistent with increased TM stiffness [18]. Additionally, Wang K et al. estimated human TM stiffness by numerical modeling and found that normal TM stiffness was lower than in glaucoma patients [16].

We also found that the pulsatile TM motion presented differently in different segments. Motion the in nasal region was much stronger than that in temporal area in both normal and glaucomatous eyes. However, we did not identify a regional progression difference of TM regions in glaucoma. Studies have documented that aqueous outflow is not homogeneous, but segmental [19,20]. Previous studies have reported that aqueous fluid is predominantly drained in the nasal and inferior quadrants [19]. The segmental labeling of the TM in multiple studies has provided evidence of regions of preferential aqueous outflow in both normal and glaucomatous eyes [21]. The circumference of the TM can be divided into regions of high, medium, and low flow, based on angiographic imaging or the distribution of fluorescent microspheres [22]. Moreover, a study showed that TM stiffness in high-flow wedges was softer than that in low-flow wedges for both normal and glaucomatous eyes [22].

Many studies have highlighted the importance of stable IOP fluctuations for preventing the progression of POAG. We found that the TM motion in the external region, next to SC, decreased dramatically in POAG eyes with high IOP variation during 24 h monitoring, compared to those with stable diurnal IOP. This high variance of 24 h IOP fluctuation reflects a loss of normal IOP homeostasis, and suggests the malfunctioning of the aqueous outflow system. The IOP peak typically occurs at night, reportedly related to the supine position and changes in ocular pulsations during sleep. The diurnal IOP fluctuation present in glaucoma, especially the IOP peak, correlates with the progression of visual field defects.

The TM plays a vital role in maintaining IOP homeostasis, reflecting the tissue's importance in preserving biomaterial properties, such as stiffness. It has been reported that pulsatile fluid in the aqueous vein was induced by an IOP increase after a water drinking test [11], which suggests that TM pumping functions in reaction to IOP variation. Recent studies report that SC shear stress and TM strain may act together as mechanosensory factors providing the homeostatic regulation of aqueous outflow and IOP [23]. A feed-forward loop involving alterations in TM stiffness may exacerbate malfunction of TM cells with further aberrations of the extracellular matrix of TM beams, the spaces between beams, and the juxtacanalicular tissue. Our study indicates that reduced TM motion, reflecting increased stiffness, may be relevant to the abnormal IOP homeostasis of glaucoma. Moreover, the results showed that the movement of the TM in the external region in glaucoma eyes with high IOP fluctuation decreased significantly. The external region of TM measured in this study mainly covered the juxtacanalicular TM region. Decreased movement indicates the TM becoming stiffer. This leads to the inability of TM to react to IOP transience, disturbing IOP homeostasis. The relationship between worse pulsatile TM motion and higher diurnal IOP fluctuation implicates the clinical potential of PhS-OCT for the differentiation of POAG and the efficient evaluation of POAG treatment.

There are several limitations to this study. (1) We have presented the segmental difference of TM pulsatile motion in normal and glaucoma subjects. Whether TM pulsatile motion represents regions that are especially vulnerable to damage requires further study. (2) The glaucoma subjects recruited in this study were relatively young, and they were treated with topical medications which might have altered the biomechanical properties of TM and affected aqueous outflow and IOP in currently unknown ways. Further studies are needed to compare normal tension glaucoma and healthy controls treated with the same medication.

5. Conclusions

Our study found segmental TM differences, with the nasal and inferior areas experiencing the greatest motion in both normal and glaucomatous eyes. The pulsatile motion was greater in the external than the internal portion of the TM. Pulsatile TM motion was decreased in glaucoma eyes compared with normal eyes, and imaging was able to detect glaucoma patients with large diurnal fluctuations. Imaging pulsatile TM motion may provide valuable insight into the pathophysiology of the aqueous outflow system in glaucoma. Imaging TM motion abnormalities may also help identify those at risk for fluctuations in IOP that are missed by measurements during clinic hours.

Author Contributions: Conceptualization, C.X. and H.W.; methodology, C.X., J.X. and M.J.; software, J.X.; formal analysis, R.D., C.X. and M.J.; data curation, R.D., C.X. and J.H., writing—original draft preparation, R.D. and C.X.; review and editing H.W., N.W. and M.J.; funding acquisition, C.X., R.D. and C.X. contributed equally to this paper. All authors have read and agreed to the published version of the manuscript.

J. Clin. Med. **2022**, *11*, 2696

Funding: Supported by the Open Research Fund from Beijing Advanced Innovation Center for Big Data-Based Precision Medicine, Beijing Tongren Hospital, Beihang University & Capital Medical University, Grant No. 202012 (BHTR-KFJJ-202012).

Institutional Review Board Statement: The study was conducted in accordance with the Declaration of Helsinki, and approved by the Ethical Review Committee of Beijing Tongren Hospital (TRECKY2018-066).

Informed Consent Statement: Informed consent was obtained from all subjects involved in the study.

Data Availability Statement: The data presented in this study are available from the corresponding author upon reasonable request.

Conflicts of Interest: The authors declare no conflict of interest.

References

1. Quigley, H.A.; Broman, A.T. The number of people with glaucoma worldwide in 2010 and 2020. *Br. J. Ophthalmol.* **2006**, *90*, 262–267. [CrossRef] [PubMed]
2. Tham, Y.-C.; Li, X.; Wong, T.Y.; Quigley, H.A.; Aung, T.; Cheng, C.-Y. Global Prevalence of Glaucoma and Projections of Glaucoma Burden through 2040: A systematic review and meta-analysis. *Ophthalmology* **2014**, *121*, 2081–2090. [CrossRef] [PubMed]
3. Bahrami, H. Causal Inference in Primary Open Angle Glaucoma: Specific Discussion on Intraocular Pressure. *Ophthalm. Epidemiol.* **2006**, *13*, 283–289. [CrossRef] [PubMed]
4. Matlach, J.; Bender, S.; König, J.; Binder, H.; Pfeiffer, N.; Hoffmann, E.M. Investigation of intraocular pressure fluctuation as a risk factor of glaucoma progression. *Clin. Ophthalmol.* **2018**, *13*, 9–16. [CrossRef] [PubMed]
5. Coleman, A.L.; Miglior, S. Risk Factors for Glaucoma Onset and Progression. *Surv. Ophthalmol.* **2008**, *53* (Suppl. 1), S3–S10. [CrossRef]
6. Leidl, M.C.; Choi, C.J.; Syed, Z.A.; Melki, S.A. Intraocular pressure fluctuation and glaucoma progression: What do we know? *Br. J. Ophthalmol.* **2014**, *98*, 1315–1319. [CrossRef]
7. Bhartiya, S.; Gangwani, M.; Kalra, R.B.; Aggarwal, A.; Gagrani, M.; Sirish, K.N. 24-hour Intraocular pressure monitoring: The way ahead. *Romanian J. Ophthalmol.* **2019**, *63*, 315–320. [CrossRef]
8. Acott, T.S.; Kelley, M.J.; Keller, K.E.; Vranka, J.A.; Abu-Hassan, D.W.; Li, X.; Aga, M.; Bradley, J.M. Intraocular pressure homeostasis: Maintaining balance in a high-pressure environment. *J. Ocul. Pharmacol. Ther.* **2014**, *30*, 94–101. [CrossRef]
9. Johnstone, M.; Xin, C.; Tan, J.; Martin, E.; Wen, J.; Wang, R.K. Aqueous outflow regulation – 21st century concepts. *Prog. Retin. Eye Res.* **2020**, *83*, 100917. [CrossRef]
10. Xin, C.; Wang, R.K.; Song, S.; Shen, T.; Wen, J.; Martin, E.; Jiang, Y.; Padilla, S.; Johnstone, M. Aqueous outflow regulation: Optical co-herence tomography implicates pressure-dependent tissue motion. *Exp. Eye Res.* **2017**, *158*, 171–186. [CrossRef]
11. Johnstone, M.; Martin, E.; Jamil, A. Pulsatile flow into the aqueous veins: Manifestations in normal and glaucomatous eyes. *Exp. Eye Res.* **2011**, *92*, 318–327. [CrossRef] [PubMed]
12. Buffault, J.; Labbé, A.; Hamard, P.; Brignole-Baudouin, F.; Baudouin, C. The trabecular meshwork: Structure, function and clinical implications. A review of the literature. *J. Fr. Ophtalmol.* **2020**, *43*, e217–e230. [CrossRef] [PubMed]
13. Kaufman, P.L. Deconstructing aqueous humor outflow—The last 50 years. *Exp. Eye Res.* **2020**, *197*, 108105. [CrossRef] [PubMed]
14. Wang, K.; Read, A.T.; Sulchek, T.; Ethier, C.R. Trabecular meshwork stiffness in glaucoma. *Exp. Eye Res.* **2016**, *158*, 3–12. [CrossRef]
15. Xin, C.; Song, S.; Johnstone, M.; Wang, N.; Wang, R. Quantification of Pulse-Dependent Trabecular Meshwork Motion in Normal Humans Using Phase-Sensitive OCT. *Investig. Opthalmol. Vis. Sci.* **2018**, *59*, 3675–3681. [CrossRef]
16. Wang, K.; Johnstone, M.A.; Xin, C.; Song, S.; Padilla, S.; Vranka, J.A.; Acott, T.S.; Zhou, K.; Schwaner, S.A.; Wang, R.; et al. Estimating Human Trabecular Meshwork Stiffness by Numerical Modeling and Advanced OCT Imaging. *Investig. Opthalmol. Vis. Sci.* **2017**, *58*, 4809–4817. [CrossRef]
17. Gao, K.; Song, S.; Johnstone, M.A.; Zhang, Q.; Xu, J.; Zhang, X.; Wang, R.K.; Wen, J.C. Reduced Pulsatile Trabecular Meshwork Motion in Eyes with Primary Open Angle Glaucoma Using Phase-Sensitive Optical Coherence Tomography. *Investig. Opthalmol. Vis. Sci.* **2020**, *61*, 21. [CrossRef]
18. Li, G.; Lee, C.; Agrahari, V.; Wang, K.; Navarro, I.; Sherwood, J.M.; Crews, K.; Farsiu, S.; Gonzalez, P.; Lin, C.-W.; et al. In vivo measurement of trabecular meshwork stiffness in a corticosteroid-induced ocular hypertensive mouse model. *Proc. Natl. Acad. Sci. USA* **2019**, *116*, 1714–1722. [CrossRef]
19. Saraswathy, S.; Bogarin, T.; Barron, E.; Francis, B.A.; Tan, J.C.; Weinreb, R.N.; Huang, A.S. Segmental differences found in aqueous angiographic-determined high–And low-flow regions of human trabecular meshwork. *Exp. Eye Res.* **2020**, *196*, 108064. [CrossRef]
20. Swaminathan, S.S.; Oh, D.-J.; Kang, M.H.; Rhee, D.J. Aqueous outflow: Segmental and distal flow. *J. Cataract Refract. Surg.* **2014**, *40*, 1263–1272. [CrossRef]
21. Vranka, J.A.; Bradley, J.M.; Yang, Y.-F.; Keller, K.E.; Acott, T.S. Mapping Molecular Differences and Extracellular Matrix Gene Expression in Segmental Outflow Pathways of the Human Ocular Trabecular Meshwork. *PLoS ONE* **2015**, *10*, e0122483. [CrossRef] [PubMed]

22. Vranka, J.A.; Staverosky, J.A.; Reddy, A.P.; Wilmarth, P.A.; David, L.L.; Acott, T.S.; Russell, P.; Raghunathan, V.K. Biomechanical Rigidity and Quantitative Proteomics Analysis of Segmental Regions of the Trabecular Meshwork at Physiologic and Elevated Pressures. *Investig. Opthalmol. Vis. Sci.* **2018**, *59*, 246–259. [CrossRef] [PubMed]
23. Sherwood, J.M.; Stamer, W.D.; Overby, D.R. A model of the oscillatory mechanical forces in the conventional outflow pathway. *J. R. Soc. Interface* **2019**, *16*, 20180652. [CrossRef] [PubMed]

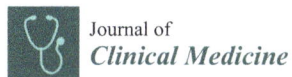

Journal of
Clinical Medicine

Article

Canaloplasty in Pseudoexfoliation Glaucoma. Can It Still Be Considered a Good Choice?

Paolo Brusini [1,*], Veronica Papa [1] and Marco Zeppieri [2]

[1] Department of Ophthalmology, Policlinico Città di Udine, Viale Venezia 410, 33100 Udine, Italy; papa.veronica87@gmail.com
[2] Department of Ophthalmology, University Hospital of Udine, 33100 Udine, Italy; markzeppieri@hotmail.com
* Correspondence: brusini@libero.it; Tel.: +39-432-239371; Fax: +39-432-545400

Abstract: Purpose: The aim of this study was to assess the long-term outcomes of canaloplasty surgery in pseudoexfoliation glaucoma (PEXG) patients. Material and Methods: A total of 116 PEXG patients with an intraocular pressure (IOP) > 21 mm/Hg and maximum tolerated local medical therapy who underwent canaloplasty from February 2008 to January 2022 were considered. Every six months, all subjects underwent a complete ophthalmic examination. The period of follow-up ranged from 2 to 167 months. Inclusion criteria included only patients for whom the entire procedure could be completed with a follow-up of at least 2 years. Results: Amongst the 116 PEXG patients, the entire procedure could not be performed in 10 eyes (8.6%), and thus they were not considered in the analysis. Twenty-three patients did not reach the two-year follow-up and another 16 patients during this time period were lost. A total of 67 patients with a mean follow-up of 49 ± 32.3 months were considered in the analysis. The pre-operative mean IOP was 31.2 ± 8.7 mm/Hg (range 20–60). The mean IOP at the two-year follow-up was 17.2 ± 6.7 mmHg, with a mean reduction from baseline of 44.9%. After two years, the qualified success rates according to three different criteria (IOP ≤ 21, ≤18 and ≤16 mmHg) were 80.6%, 73.1% and 61.0%, respectively. The total number of medications used pre- and at the follow-up at 2 years was 3.5 ± 0.8 and 1.2 ± 1.4, respectively. Early complications included: hyphema, in about 30% of cases; Descemet membrane detachment (4.9%); and IOP spikes > 10 mmHg (9.7%). A late failure with an acute IOP rise of up to 50 mmHg was observed in 41 cases (61.2%) after 3 to 72 months. Conclusions: Long-term post-operative outcomes of canaloplasty in PEXG patients appear to be quite good on average; however, an acute rise in IOP can be observed in more than 60% of the cases after a long period of satisfactory IOP control. For this reason, canaloplasty may not be suitable in eyes with PEXG, especially in patients with severe functional damage.

Keywords: canaloplasty; non-perforating surgical procedures; pseudoexfoliation glaucoma (PEXG); Schlemm's canal; intraocular pressure (IOP)

Citation: Brusini, P.; Papa, V.; Zeppieri, M. Canaloplasty in Pseudoexfoliation Glaucoma. Can It Still Be Considered a Good Choice? *J. Clin. Med.* **2022**, *11*, 2532. https://doi.org/10.3390/jcm11092532

Academic Editor: Andrzej Grzybowski

Received: 28 March 2022
Accepted: 28 April 2022
Published: 30 April 2022

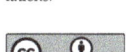
1. Introduction

Pseudoexfoliation glaucoma (PEXG) is a frequent form of secondary glaucoma due to deposits of fibrillary material in the juxtacanalicular portion of the trabecular meshwork [1]. It is known that PEXG is more aggressive than primary open-angle glaucoma (POAG) and scarcely responsive to medical treatment. Intraocular pressure (IOP) is usually higher and can show elevated spikes in eyes with PEXG compared to POAG, which may lead to a quicker progression of glaucomatous damage. Trabeculectomy using intra-operative antimetabolites remains the gold standard procedure in PEXG [2,3], even if the success rate seems to be lower in comparison with POAG [4,5]. Trabeculectomy is quite easy to perform and effective in reducing IOP; however, several late and early potentially serious complications can arise, such as hypotonus, atalamia, bleb infection, choroidal detachment, etc. Moreover, the scarring of conjunctival tissues, despite the use of antimetabolite drugs, often leads to a complete failure of this filtering operation over time.

Canaloplasty is a blebless, non-perforating technique, which became popular several years ago and involves the positioning and tensioning of a 10-0 prolene suture within Schlemm's canal, which is previously dilated using a viscoelastic agent. This surgical technique can facilitate aqueous outflow through the natural pathways [6–13]. The main indications for canaloplasty include POAG, juvenile glaucoma and pigmentary glaucoma. Even if PEXG is generally considered a good indication for canaloplasty, very few studies have specifically addressed this issue [14–16].

The aim of this paper is to evaluate the long-term outcomes and complications of canaloplasty in a group of PEXG patients.

2. Materials and Methods

The investigation was based on a retrospective, single-surgeon, observational, non-randomized study of patients with PEXG. One-hundred-and-sixteen eyes from 116 patients with uncontrolled pseudoexfoliation glaucoma under maximum tolerated medical therapy with significant visual field damage progression underwent canaloplasty under local anesthesia. Surgery was performed by the same surgeon (P.B.) in multi-subspecialty ophthalmic departments, either at the Department of Ophthalmology in the Azienda Ospedaliero-Universitaria "Santa Maria della Misericordia" Hospital or the Department of Ophthalmology in Policlinico "Città di Udine", in Udine, Italy, from February 2008 to January 2022.

The investigation was performed in accordance with the tenets of the Declaration of Helsinki and informed consent was obtained from all participants before surgery. The study was in compliance with institutional review boards (IRBs) and the HIPAA requirements of both clinics.

2.1. Inclusion Criteria

Inclusion criteria for this cohort included: patients diagnosed with PEXG having an IOP $\geq$ 20 mmHg with maximum tolerated medical therapy, typical optic nerve alterations and functional loss (based on the Glaucoma Staging System 2 (GSS2), ranging from early to moderate GSS2 stages 1–3) [17]. Visual fields had to show significant progression of defects in 2 consecutive tests assessed with the Guided Progression Analysis 2 (Carl Zeiss Meditec Inc., Dublin, CA, USA) program. Patients who underwent previous ocular surgeries (with the exception of cataract surgery) were excluded. Patients with narrow-angled eyes, other serious eye diseases and unwillingness to undergo surgery were also excluded. All patients in the analysis were older than 18 years.

2.2. Surgical Technique

All surgeries were performed under local anesthesia. Canaloplasty is widely used and well-reported in the current literature [6,12]. Briefly, this surgery commences with a conjunctival fornix-based flap and a 3×4 mm superficial scleral flap that is dissected forward by 1.5 mm into the clear cornea. Surgery continues with the creation of a deep scleral flap used to open Schlemm's canal. This flap is then removed. The exposed 2 ostia of the canal are dilated using hyaluronic acid of high molecular weight (Healon GV, Johnson & Johnson Surgical Vision, Inc., Santa Ana, CA, USA). A special 200-micron microcatheter is used which is connected to a flickering red light laser source, useful for easy identification through the sclera of the distal tip (Nova Eye Medical Limited, Fremont, CA, USA). The tip is inserted within Schlemm's canal and pushed forward for the whole 360° until it comes out of the other end. A 10-0 double prolene suture is then tied to the distal tip and the microcatheter is pulled back and withdrawn in the opposite direction from the canal. A small amount of viscoelastic agent is delivered during this step in Schlemm's canal every two hours of circumference using a special screw-driven syringe. Surgery then involves knotting the suture under tension to inwardly distend the trabecular meshwork. Using 5 to 7 10-0 vicryl sutures, the superficial scleral flap is then sutured to provide a closure that is watertight to avoid any bleb formation. Then, 8-0 vicryl sutures are used to close the conjunctival flap to complete the surgery.

2.3. Main Outcome Measures

Every 6 months, all patients underwent a complete ophthalmic examination that included slit lamp examination, Goldmann applanation tonometry IOP measurement, fundus examination using a 78 D Volk lens, best corrected visual acuity (BCVA) with visual field testing (Humphrey Field Analyzer 24-2 SITA standard test) and gonioscopy.

The definition of success was based on three different criteria: post-operative IOP $\leq$ 21 mmHg, $\leq$18 mmHg and $\leq$16 mmHg, without any medical treatment ("complete success") or with or without medical treatment ("qualified success"). The number of local medications taken before and after canaloplasty and the early and late complications were also taken into consideration.

In order to assess the long-term outcomes of canaloplasty, only patients with a minimum follow-up of 2 years for whom the full technique was successfully completed were taken into consideration.

3. Results

The whole standard surgical technique of canaloplasty could not be performed in 10 eyes (8.6%) due to the impossibility of cannulating the entire 360° of Schlemm's canal. In these cases, surgery was converted either in viscocanalostomy, which was carried out by injecting viscoelastic agent up to the intracanalicular obstacle, or in deep sclerectomy, whereby two nylon 10-0 stiches were used to suture the superficial scleral flap. These eyes were not included in the analysis. Twenty-three patients did not reach the two-year follow-up and another 16 patients were lost during follow-ups. A total of 67 patients (33 woman and 34 men) met the inclusion criteria and were considered in the analysis (mean age: 67.8 $\pm$ 12.5 years; range: 49 to 82 years). Six patients were treated with a combination of prostaglandin and timolol. Fifty-seven were using three to four topical medications (prostaglandin + timolol + dorzolamide + brimonidine) and four also used oral carbonic anhydrase inhibitors. Thirty-seven (55.2%) were pseudophakic. The best corrected visual acuity in decimal points ranged between 0.6 to 1.0 (mean 0.8). The optic disc showed glaucomatous cupping, ranging between 0.6 and 0.9 (mean cup/disc ratio 0.7). Visual field damage ranged between stage 1 and stage 3 of the Glaucoma Staging System, with a mean deviation ranging between -1.2 dB and -13.6 dB. The follow-up time ranged from 24 to 167 (mean 58.9 $\pm$ 28.8) months. The mean pre-operative IOP was 31.2 $\pm$ 8.7, ranging from 20 to 60 mmHg. After 24 months, the mean IOP was 17.2 $\pm$ 6.7 mmHg, with a reduction from baseline in mean IOP of 44.9%. The mean IOP values over a period of 7 years at various follow-up sessions are reported in the box plot diagram (Figure 1).

The scatter plot in Figure 2 shows the pre-operative IOP and post-operative IOP values after 2 years.

The qualified and complete success rates based on the three different IOP cut-offs after 2, 3 and 4 years are reported in Tables 1 and 2.

The number of medications used pre- and at the 2, 3, and 4-year follow-ups were 3.5 $\pm$ 0.9, 1.2 $\pm$ 1.4, and 1.3 $\pm$ 1.3, and 1.9 $\pm$ 1.3 respectively. A Wilcoxon matched-pairs signed-rank test revealed statistically significant reductions at all time points ($p < 0.001$).

Gonioscopy at each follow-up confirmed that the prolene suture was still in the right position within Schlemm's canal for the whole follow-up period, with the exception of one eye in which the tensioned prolene caused suture cheese-wiring through trabecular meshwork after surgery without any further complications.

Post-operative complications occurring early (within 4 weeks after surgery) included: hyphema in 14 eyes (34.1%), which completely reabsorbed within one week; hypotonus (IOP < 5 mm/Hg) in one eye (2.4%), in which the IOP returned to normal values (16 mmHg) in a couple of weeks; detachment of Descemet membrane in 2 eyes (4.9%), which spontaneously reattached without the need to be drained in one month; and IOP spikes > 10 mmHg in 4 eyes (9.7%). In the latter cases, no medical treatment was added in order to reduce IOP, a part one case, where acetazolamide tablets to be taken three times/day were prescribed for a few days. In all these four eyes, the IOP spontaneously dropped under 18 mmHg after about a month. A transient visual acuity decrease was reported in several patients within a few weeks after surgery which was brought on by induced according to-the-rule astigmatism that tended to disappear within one month. A late failure with an abrupt IOP rise, with values ranging between 26 and 50 mmHg, was observed after 3 to 72 months in 41 cases (61.2%). The number of these elevated IOP cases observed during the follow-up is reported in Figure 3. In 17 cases, it was possible to control IOP either with medical treatment or with selective laser trabeculoplasty, while in 22 eyes a trabeculectomy using the previous scleral flap was performed with good results in 18 cases (81.8%). In one case, we performed an ab interno trabeculotomy, stripping the prolene suture under gonioscopic control. In another case, a diode laser cyclophotocoagulation was performed. These last two patients were well controlled with medical therapy.

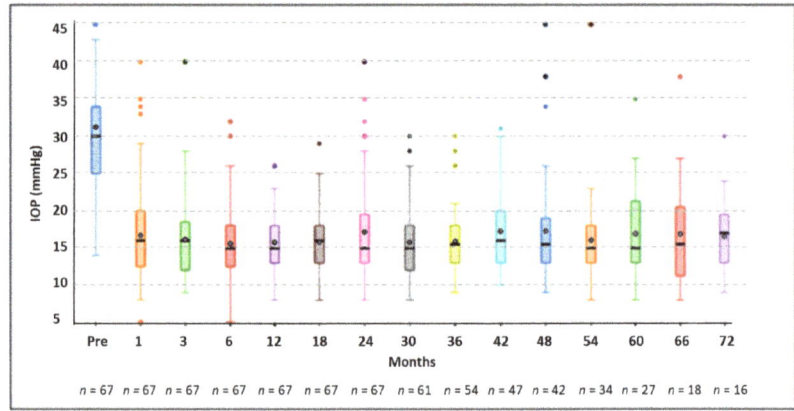

Figure 1. Box plot representation of IOP values over time in 7 years of follow-up in the cohort of 67 PEXG eyes that underwent canaloplasty.

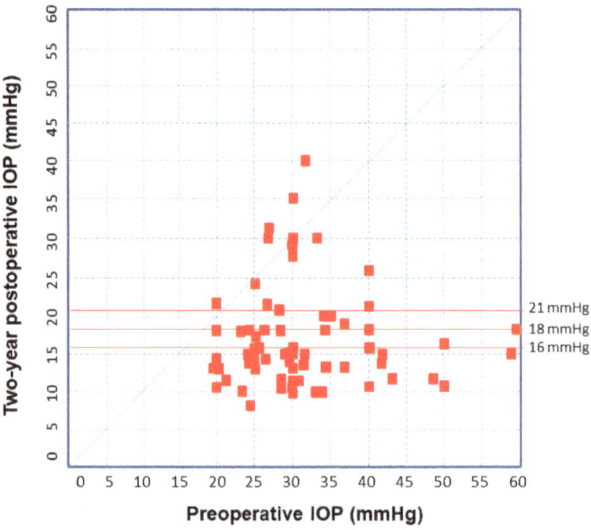

Figure 2. Scatter plot of IOP values before surgery and after canaloplasty in 67 PEXG eyes after 2 years.

Table 1. Qualified success rates after 2, 3 and 4 years.

	Post-operative IOP		
	≤ 21 mmHg	≤ 18 mmHg	≤ 16 mmHg
After 2 years (67 eyes)	54 (80.6%)	49 (73.1%)	41 (61.2%)
After 3 years (54 eyes)	50 (92.6%)	43 (79.6%)	31 (57.4%)
After 4 years (42 eyes)	35 (83.3%)	29 (69.0%)	23 (54.8%)

IOP: Intraocular pressure.

Table 2. Complete success rates after 2, 3 and 4 years.

	Post-operative IOP		
	≤ 21 mmHg	≤ 18 mmHg	≤ 16 mmHg
After 2 years (67 eyes)	28 (41.8%)	26 (38.8%)	24 (35.8%)
After 3 years (54 eyes)	22 (40.7%)	20 (37.0%)	14 (25.9%)
After 4 years (42 eyes)	9 (21.4%)	9 (21.4%)	9 (21.4%)

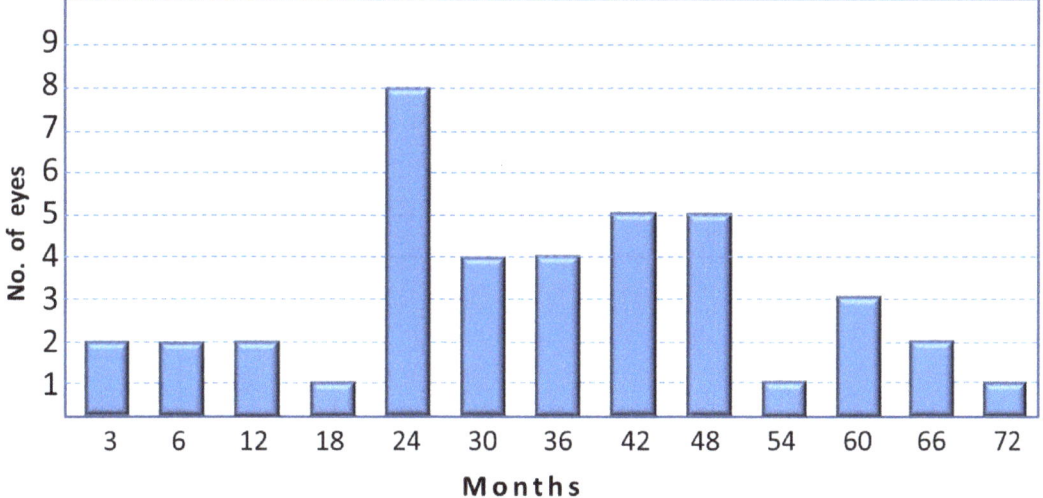

Figure 3. Number of eyes with an IOP increase >25 mmHg after canaloplasty.

4. Discussion

Surgery is often required to reduce ocular hypertension and limit damage progression in PEXG patients, especially considering that functional damage can be rapid and severe in PEXG patients [18–20]. In eyes with advanced visual field loss, very low post-operative IOP values are needed to preserve the remnants of vision. Only filtering procedures, such as trabeculectomy or ExPress implant using antimetabolites, can offer these low IOP values and should be the preferred choice in these patients [21].

In selected patients who show mild to moderate functional damage, however, minimally invasive glaucoma surgery (MIGS) techniques, such as i-Stent implant [22], gonioscopy-assisted transluminal trabeculotomy [23,24] and XEN gel implant [25,26], can be taken into consideration. Non-perforating techniques, such as deep sclerectomy [27–30] or canaloplasty, may be an interesting alternative, considering the higher hypotensive efficacy when compared to MIGS and the lower rate of complications compared to trabeculectomy.

One of the main advantages of canaloplasty is that this type of surgery reduces IOP without requiring the formation of a filtering bleb [31]. For this reason, canaloplasty could be a viable option in selected patients having a high risk of conjunctival bleb failure with filtrating surgery, which is typically seen in eyes that have been treated with multiple local drop therapy for numerous years. This issue, however, needs further investigation considering the lack of studies in the current literature in this field. Another important advantage of this surgical option is the simplified follow-up and lower post-operative complication rates compared to the relatively high number of manipulations for blebs required after trabeculectomy (up to 78.2% of cases) [32].

The drawbacks of canaloplasty include the need for specific and expensive instrumentation and a steep learning curve. Another disadvantage, especially for beginners, is the proper cannulation of Schlemm's canal, which can be difficult or not fully achieved in some cases. Canaloplasty, however, can be easily converted into a viscocanalostomy or a deep sclerectomy in these cases. In eyes that show mid-term failure after a successfully performed canaloplasty, a goniopuncture with YAG laser can be considered. In cases that do not show a sufficient reduction in IOP after canaloplasty and/or where medical therapy is not well tolerated or insufficient for lowering IOP, either a trabeculectomy or an implant of a drainage tube should be considered [33].

It is important to point out that in our cohort more than 60% of the PEXG eyes had an abrupt rise in IOP after years of satisfactory IOP stabilization. This long-term post-surgical complication, which is of utmost importance in these eyes at risk of functional progression, is poorly documented in the current literature [34]. According to our experience, this complication is more frequently observed two to four years after surgery.

The pathogenetic mechanisms behind such a late complication are not well known and need to be addressed in future studies. One possible reason could be related to the continuous production and accumulation of pseudoexfoliative material in the angle structures which can occlude the existing compromised aqueous humor outflow pathways after a short period of time, which may be due to the physiopathological mechanisms of the disease and by the effects of numerous years of medical drugs. This hypothesis is supported by the observation that a similar late IOP rise can be found only in 13.7% of POAG eyes (personal unpublished data obtained from a cohort of 117 POAG patients with a similar follow-up period who underwent canaloplasty performed by the same surgeon). The prolene suture inside Schlemm's canal could also be involved in the scarring process leading to the increase in outflow resistance.

Future studies based on ultrasound biomicroscopy, preferably with 80 MHz transducers, or high-resolution anterior segment OCT [35,36], could help clarify, at least in part, the anatomical changes in Schlemm's canal and in the trabecular meshwork in eyes showing long-term surgical failures. Histological studies conducted on human trabecular meshwork specimens could definitely provide a better comprehension behind the pathological post-operative induced structural changes in these eyes.

The onset of important IOP spikes can give rise to acute signs and symptoms in these patients, especially if IOP reaches high values. Urgent trabeculectomy can usually be effective in normalizing IOP in these situations, especially considering that the conjunctiva tends to in good condition after a long period without local medical treatment. Unfortunately, in some cases, this rise in IOP can be slower and less pronounced and can go totally unnoticed, leading to a worsening of the damage already present, which can cause a potentially devastating visual impairment. Based on these clinically important considerations and the post-surgical risks involved, all patients with PEXG who have undergone canaloplasty should be carefully managed and thoroughly monitored for life

Our study has several limitations, the most important being that it is based on retrospective results for a cohort of eyes and that a control group was not considered. The aim of our study, however, was not comparative in nature but to assess the long-term effectiveness of canaloplasty in pseudoexfoliation glaucoma, especially with regard to possible late complications of this procedure. The IOP cut-off values for the definition of success based on IOP values reported in the Methods section are not standardized and widely applicable in clinics; however, they have been used in several studies and are based on criteria reported in the World Glaucoma Association Guidelines published in 2009 [37].

The study adds to the very limited current literature in this field and could be of clinical importance to clinicians when managing post-surgical canaloplasty patients with PEXG. Our results may help pave the way to future studies regarding physiopathological mechanisms behind acute IOP spikes in these patients, which could be due to decreased outflow related to the effects of the prolene suture in Schlemm's canal. This could be of importance in those eyes with existing compromised angular tissue structures because of the long-term effects of PEX deposits, in addition to the cumulative side effects of numerous years of local medication. Comparative prospective studies based on traditional canaloplasty and surgery involving viscodilation of Schlemm's canal without the positioning of a prolene suture (i.e., ab interno canaloplasty) could be useful in clarifying the potential effects on outflow mechanisms.

5. Conclusions

Canaloplasty is a very interesting and fascinating surgical technique, which can offer good results, especially in POAG, juvenile and pigmentary glaucoma with very high IOP. The long-term outcomes in patients with PEXG may seem satisfactory at first glance, considering that canaloplasty can maintain post-operative IOP values at physiological values for numerous years in most cases. Unfortunately, our study showed that more than 60% of cases can develop an abrupt rise in IOP occurring several years after surgery. In some cases, these spikes can go unnoticed upon onset or be detected considerably late, leading to a potentially dramatic progression of the functional damage.

In order to limit the serious risks related to potential undetected IOP elevations after surgery, canaloplasty should either be avoided in PEXG eyes or only considered as a possible option in selected patients having a high risk of failure with filtrating surgery. These patients need to be carefully assessed after canaloplasty, even if it is apparently successful, and should be clearly informed about the advantages and potential risks of this surgical procedure. Moreover, patients need to be educated about the acute signs and symptoms of IOP spikes and be informed of the possible need for future filtrating surgery.

Author Contributions: Conceptualization and methodology, original draft preparation: P.B.; software, validation, formal analysis and investigation: P.B., V.P. and M.Z.; data collection: V.P.; critical revision and completion of final draft of the paper: P.B. and M.Z.; supervision: P.B. All authors have read and agreed to the published version of the manuscript.

Funding: This research received no external funding.

Institutional Review Board Statement: The study was conducted in accordance with the Declaration of Helsinki. Standardized surgical practices already in routine use were employed.

Informed Consent Statement: Informed consent was obtained from all subjects involved in the study.

Data Availability Statement: Not applicable.

Conflicts of Interest: The authors declare no conflict of interest.

References

1. Johnson, M.C.; Kamm, R.D. The role of Schlemm's canal in aqueous outflow from the human eye. *Invest. Ophthalmol. Vis. Sci.* **1983**, *24*, 320–325. [PubMed]
2. Edmunds, B.; Thompson, J.R.; Salmon, J.F.; Wormald, R.P. The National Survey of Trabeculectomy. I. Sample and methods. *Eye* **1999**, *13*, 524–530. [CrossRef] [PubMed]
3. Cairns, J.E. Trabeculectomy preliminary report of a new method. *Am. J. Ophthalmol.* **1968**, *66*, 673–679. [CrossRef]
4. Ayala, M. Lower Success in Trabeculectomies in Exfoliation Compared with Primary Open-angle Glaucoma Patients in Sweden. *J. Glaucoma.* **2021**, *30*, e237–e245. [CrossRef] [PubMed]
5. Li, F.; Tang, G.; Zhan, H.; Yan, X.; Ma, L.; Geng, Y. The Effects of Trabeculectomy on Pseudoexfoliation Glaucoma and Primary Open-Angle Glaucoma. *J. Ophthalmol.* **2020**, *2020*, 1723691. [CrossRef] [PubMed]
6. Lewis, R.A.; von Wolff, K.; Tetz, M.; Koerber, N.; Kearney, J.R.; Shingleton, B.; Samuelson, T.W. Canaloplasty: circumferential viscodilation and tensioning of Schlemm's canal using a flexible microcatheter for the treatment of open-angle glaucoma in adults. Interim clinical study analysis. *J. Cataract. Refract. Surg.* **2007**, *33*, 1217–1226. [CrossRef] [PubMed]

7. Lewis, R.A.; von Wolff, K.; Tetz, M.; Koerber, N.; Kearney, J.R.; Shingleton, B.; Samuelson, T.W. Canaloplasty: Circumferential viscodilation and tensioning of Schlemm's canal using a flexible microcatheter for the treatment of open-angle glaucoma in adults. Two-year interim clinical study analysis. *J. Cataract. Refract. Surg.* **2009**, *35*, 814–824. [CrossRef]
8. Grieshaber, M.C.; Pienaar, A.; Olivier, J.; Stegmann, R. Canaloplasty for primary open-angle glaucoma: Long term outcome. *Br. J. Ophthalmol.* **2010**, *94*, 1478–1482. [CrossRef]
9. Grieshaber, M.C.; Fraenkl, S.; Schoetzau, A.; Flammer, J.; Orgül, S. Circumferential viscocanalostomy and suture canal distension (canaloplasty) for whites with open-angle glaucoma. *J. Glaucoma* **2011**, *20*, 298–302. [CrossRef]
10. Lewis, R.A.; von Wolff, K.; Tetz, M.; Koerber, N.; Kearney, J.R.; Shingleton, B.; Samuelson, T.W. Canaloplasty. Three-year results of circumferential viscodilation and tensioning of Schlemm canal using a microcatheter to treat open-angle glaucoma. *J. Cataract. Refrac. Surg.* **2011**, *37*, 682–690. [CrossRef]
11. Bull, H.; von Wolff, K.; Körber, N.; Tetz, M. Three-year canaloplasty outcomes for the treatment of open-angle glaucoma: European study results. *Graefes. Arch. Clin. Exp. Ophthalmol.* **2011**, *249*, 1537–1545. [CrossRef] [PubMed]
12. Brusini, P.; Caramello, G.; Benedetti, S.; Tosoni, C. Canaloplasty in Open-angle Glaucoma: Mid-term Results from a Multicenter Study. *J. Glaucoma* **2016**, *25*, 403–407. [CrossRef] [PubMed]
13. Brusini, P. Canaloplasty in Open-Angle Glaucoma Surgery: A Four-Year Follow-Up. *Sci. World J.* **2014**, *2014*, 469609. [CrossRef] [PubMed]
14. Seuthe, A.M.; Szurman, P.; Januschowski, K. Canaloplasty with Suprachoroidal Drainage in Patients with Pseudoexfoliation Glaucoma—Four Years Results. *Curr. Eye Res.* **2021**, *46*, 217–223. [CrossRef] [PubMed]
15. Hasanov, J.V.; Kasimov, E.M. Late results of phaco-canaloplasty in patients with concomitant advanced pseudoexfoliation glaucoma and cataract. *Vestn. Oftalmol.* **2018**, *134*, 28–34. [CrossRef]
16. Łazicka-Gałecka, M.; Kamińska, A.; Gałecki, T.; Guszkowska, M.; Dziedziak, J.; Szaflik, J.; Szaflik, J.P. Canaloplasty—Efficacy and Safety in an 18-Month Follow Up Period, and Analysis of Outcomes in Primary Open Angle Glaucoma Pigmentary Glaucoma and Pseudoexfoliative Glaucoma. *Semin. Ophthalmol.* **2022**, 1–9. [CrossRef]
17. Brusini, P.; Filacorda, S. Enhanced Glaucoma Staging System (GSS 2) for Classifying Functional Damage in Glaucoma. *J. Glaucoma* **2006**, *15*, 40–46. [CrossRef]
18. Gillmann, K.; Meduri, E.; Niegowski, L.J.; Mermoud, A. Surgical Management of Pseudoexfoliative Glaucoma: A Review of Current Clinical Considerations and Surgical Outcomes. *J. Glaucoma* **2021**, *30*, e32–e39. [CrossRef]
19. Sayed, M.S.; Lee, R.K. Recent Advances in the Surgical Management of Glaucoma in Exfoliation Syndrome. *J. Glaucoma* **2018**, *27* (Suppl. 1), S95–S101. [CrossRef]
20. Desai, M.A.; Lee, R.K. The Medical and Surgical Management of Pseudoexfoliation Glaucoma. *Int. Ophthalmol. Clin.* **2008**, *48*, 95–113. [CrossRef]
21. Kornmann, H.L.; Gedde, S.J. Surgical Management of Pseudoexfoliation Glaucoma. *Int. Ophthalmol. Clin.* **2014**, *54*, 71–83. [CrossRef] [PubMed]
22. Ferguson, T.J.; Swan, R.; Ibach, M.; Schweitzer, J.; Sudhagoni, R.; Berdahl, J.P. Trabecular microbypass stent implantation with cataract extraction in pseudoexfoliation glaucoma. *J. Cataract Refract. Surg.* **2017**, *43*, 622–626. [CrossRef]
23. Hepşen, İ.F.; Güler, E.; Yalçin, N.G.; Kumova, D.; Aktaş, Z.P. Modified 360-degree Suture Trabeculotomy for Pseudoexfoliation Glaucoma: 12-Month Results. *J. Glaucoma* **2016**, *25*, e408–e412. [CrossRef] [PubMed]
24. Sharkawi, E.; Lindegger, D.J.; Artes, P.H.; Lehmann-Clarke, L.; El Wardani, M.; Misteli, M.; Pasquier, J.; Guarnieri, A. Outcomes of gonioscopy-assisted transluminal trabeculotomy in pseudoexfoliative glaucoma: 24-month follow-up. *Br. J. Ophthalmol.* **2021**, *105*, 977–982. [CrossRef]
25. Mansouri, K.; Gillmann, K.; Rao, H.L.; Guidotti, J.; Mermoud, A. Prospective Evaluation of XEN Gel Implant in Eyes With Pseudoexfoliative Glaucoma. *J. Glaucoma* **2018**, *27*, 869–873. [CrossRef] [PubMed]
26. Ibáñez-Muñoz, A.; Soto-Biforcos, V.S.; Chacón-González, M.; Rúa-Galisteo, O.; Arrieta-Los Santos, A.; Lizuain-Abadía, M.E.; Del Río Mayor, J.L. One-year follow-up of the XEN implant with mitomycin-C in pseudoexfoliative glaucoma patients. *Eur. J. Ophthalmol.* **2019**, *29*, 309–314. [CrossRef]
27. Drolsum, L. Deep sclerectomy in patients with capsular glaucoma. *Acta Ophthalmol. Scand.* **2003**, *81*, 567–572. [CrossRef]
28. Rekonen, P.; Kannisto, T.; Puustjärvi, T.; Teräsvirta, M.; Uusitalo, H. Deep sclerectomy for the treatment of exfoliation and primary open-angle glaucoma. *Acta Ophthalmol. Scand.* **2006**, *84*, 507–511. [CrossRef]
29. Suominen, S.M.; Harju, M.P.; Vesti, E.T. Deep sclerectomy in primary open-angle glaucoma and exfoliative glaucoma. *Eur. J. Ophthalmol.* **2016**, *26*, 568–574. [CrossRef]
30. Studeny, P.; Baxant, A.D.; Vranova, J.; Kuchynka, P.; Pokorna, J. Deep sclerectomy with nonabsorbable implant (T-Flux) in patients with pseudoexfoliation glaucoma. *J. Ophthalmol.* **2017**, *2017*, 6923208. [CrossRef]
31. Klink, T.; Panidou, E.; Kanzow-Terai, B.; Klink, J.; Schlunck, G.; Grehn, F.J. Are There Filtering Blebs After Canaloplasty? *J. Glaucoma* **2012**, *21*, 89–94. [CrossRef] [PubMed]
32. King, A.J.; Rotchford, A.P.; Alwitry, A.; Moodie, J. Frequency of bleb manipulations after trabeculectomy surgery. *Br. J. Ophthalmol.* **2007**, *91*, 873–877. [CrossRef] [PubMed]
33. Voykov, B.; Rohrbach, J.M. Revisionsmöglichkeiten nach Kanalplastik. *Ophthalmologe* **2016**, *113*, 910–913. [CrossRef] [PubMed]
34. Samuelson, T.W. Extreme intraocular pressure, mild glaucoma, and previous canaloplasty with indwelling suture: August consultation. *J. Cataract Refract. Surg.* **2018**, *44*, 1047. [CrossRef]

35. Kagemann, L.; Wollstein, G.; Ishikawa, H.; Bilonick, R.A.; Brennen, P.M.; Folio, L.S.; Gabriele, M.L.; Schuman, J.S. Identification and Assessment of Schlemm's Canal by Spectral-Domain Optical Coherence Tomography. *Investig. Opthalmology Vis. Sci.* **2010**, *51*, 4054–4059. [CrossRef]

36. Kagemann, L.; Wollstein, G.; Ishikawa, H.; Nadler, Z.; Sigal, I.A.; Folio, L.S.; Schuman, J.S. Visualization of the conventional outflow pathway in the living human eye. *Ophthalmology* **2012**, *119*, 1563–1568. [CrossRef]

37. *Guidelines on Design and Reporting of Glaucoma Surgical Trials*; Shaarawy, T.M.; Sherwood, M.B.; Grehn, F. (Eds.) Kugler Publication: Amsterdam, The Netherlands, 2009; p. 19.

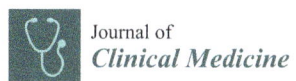

Journal of
Clinical Medicine

MDPI

Review

The Effects of Intranasal, Inhaled and Systemic Glucocorticoids on Intraocular Pressure: A Literature Review

Dries Wijnants [1,*], Ingeborg Stalmans [1,2] and Evelien Vandewalle [1,2]

[1] Department of Ophthalmology, University Hospitals UZ Leuven, Herestraat 49, 3000 Leuven, Belgium; ingeborg.stalmans@uzleuven.be (I.S.); evelien.vandewalle@uzleuven.be (E.V.)

[2] Biomedical Sciences Group, Department of Neurosciences, Research Group Ophthalmology, KU Leuven, Herestraat 49, 3000 Leuven, Belgium

* Correspondence: dries.wijnants@uzleuven.be

Abstract: Topical glucocorticoids are a well-known risk factor of intraocular pressure (IOP) elevation in one third of the general population and in up to 90% of glaucomatous patients. Whether this steroid response is caused by intranasal, inhaled or systemic glucocorticoids, is less known. This study presents an overview of the current literature on the topic, thereby providing guidance on when ophthalmological follow-up is indicated. A literature study was performed in Medline, and 31 studies were included for analysis. Twelve out of fourteen studies discussing intranasal glucocorticoids show no significant association with an elevated IOP. Regarding inhaled glucocorticoids, only three out of twelve studies show a significant association. The observed increase was either small or was only observed in patients treated with high inhaled doses or in patients with a family history of glaucoma. An elevated IOP caused by systemic glucocorticoids is reported by four out of the five included studies, with one study reporting a clear dose–response relationship. This review concludes that a steroid response can be triggered in patients treated with systemic glucocorticoids. Inhaled glucocorticoids may cause a significant IOP elevation when administered in high doses or in patients with a family history of glaucoma. At present, there is no evidence for a clinically significant steroid response caused by intranasally administered glucocorticoids.

Keywords: glucocorticoids; safety profile; intranasal administration; inhaled administration; systemic administration; intraocular pressure; steroid response

Citation: Wijnants, D.; Stalmans, I.; Vandewalle, E. The Effects of Intranasal, Inhaled and Systemic Glucocorticoids on Intraocular Pressure: A Literature Review. *J. Clin. Med.* **2022**, *11*, 2007. https://doi.org/10.3390/jcm11072007

Academic Editors: Maria Letizia Salvetat, Marco Zeppieri and Paolo Brusini

Received: 2 March 2022
Accepted: 31 March 2022
Published: 3 April 2022

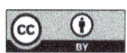
1. Introduction

Glaucoma is defined as a chronic progressive optic neuropathy with corresponding visual field defects and structural changes at the optic nerve head [1]. The most important risk factor for glaucoma development and progression is an elevated intraocular pressure (IOP), and depending on the cause of IOP elevation, different disease entities are described. Most glaucoma cases present as primary open angle glaucoma, in which the eye shows an elevated IOP with an open anterior chamber angle, without any underlying condition. Nevertheless, a smaller portion of patients present with secondary glaucoma, where an underlying cause for the IOP elevation can be identified. Treating the cause in such patients can prevent further glaucomatous damage to the optic nerve. Multiple causes of secondary IOP elevation have been identified, most importantly ocular inflammation and trauma, pigment dispersion and exfoliation, neovascularization, dense cataract formation, corneal pathologies and the use of glucocorticoids [2].

Since 1951, a steroid response is known as the ability of glucocorticoids to increase IOP [3]. However, the mechanisms by which this phenomenon is established still remain unclear to date. Three contributing factors have been identified. First, glucocorticoids have been demonstrated to alter the trabecular meshwork microstructure by causing cross-links in the actin fiber network [4]. Second, they stimulate the deposition of extracellular matrix components such as collagen and fibronectin in the juxtacanalicular region, contributing to an increased outflow resistance [5]. Finally, steroids reduce the breakdown of substances in the trabecular meshwork by inhibiting cellular phagocytotic activity, reducing arachidonic acid metabolism and reducing the activity of degradation enzymes such as metalloproteinases, stromelysin and tissue plasminogen activator [6]. All of these mechanisms cause an increase in aqueous humor outflow resistance in the trabecular meshwork, which is the key factor in the pathophysiology of glucocorticoid-induced IOP elevation.

Whether or not an individual patient is susceptible to develop a steroid response depends on both drug-related and patient-related factors. The administered dose and duration of glucocorticoid intake play an important role, and due to different pharmacokinetic and pharmacodynamic properties, different glucocorticoid classes have different risks of developing a steroid response [7]. Dexamethasone is a potent glucocorticoid and therefore a more frequent cause of a steroid response [8]. Prednisolone is considered safer, although associations with a higher IOP were also described [8]. Glucocorticoids with the lowest effect on IOP are Fluorometholone, Medrysone, Rimexolone and Loteprednol [8].

Only one third of the general population is a steroid responder, showing an increased IOP after using topical glucocorticoids for two weeks or more [9–11], which reflects the interindividual differences in susceptibility. In contrast to the general population, the percentage of steroid responders rises to more than 90% for patients with pre-existing primary open-angle glaucoma [10,11]. In the pediatric population, the incidence of a steroid response is comparable to the general adult population, with some studies even describing a more frequent occurrence of the phenomenon in children [8,12]. Steroid response in children has an earlier onset and a more rapid progression than in adults, with some individuals developing an increased IOP after only one day of glucocorticoid intake [8]. Moreover, glaucomatous damage to the optic nerve can be more severe than in the adult population [13]. Considering that a steroid response can develop rapidly without obvious symptoms, it is crucial that clinicians have a proper knowledge of the possible harming effects of glucocorticoids in order to detect an elevated IOP or glaucomatous damage to the optic nerve in an early stage.

In contrast to this well-established steroid response caused by topical ocular glucocorticoids, it is much less clear whether glucocorticoids administered by other routes also cause a steroid response. Since intranasal glucocorticoids are the main treatment of various inflammatory otolaryngeal and nasopharyngeal conditions, such as different phenotypes of rhinitis, sinusitis, and associated headaches, the question arises of whether the ocular side-effects are also caused by glucocorticoids administered by this route [14,15]. The aim of this study is to present a clear overview of the existing literature on the effects of intranasal, inhaled and systemic glucocorticoids on IOP up until 2022 and to provide guidance on when additional monitoring of IOP is indicated.

2. Methods

We conducted a systematic literature search in Medline, using PubMed as the search engine. The search was performed for the last time on 14 February 2022. All papers identified through database screening were assessed for eligibility for inclusion independently by two review authors. The PRISMA 2020 flow diagram was used for the identification, screening and inclusion of articles, which is graphically depicted for each glucocorticoid administration route separately in Figures 1–3. A detailed overview of MeSH-terms (medical subject headings) and search algorithms used is described in Table 1.

Before applying inclusion and exclusion criteria, this strategy yielded 38 results for intranasal glucocorticoids, 33 results for inhaled glucocorticoids and 57 results for systemic glucocorticoids. After the identification of these studies, they were screened for relevance, based on the PICO(TS) framework (patients, intervention, comparison, outcome, timing, setting) (Table 2). First, this was carried out by title and abstract, and for all articles considered relevant by title and abstract, a full-text assessment was carried out to determine eligibility for inclusion in this review. All original study types were included. Reviews, meta-analyses, case reports, case series and animal studies were excluded. Studies not published in English were also excluded.

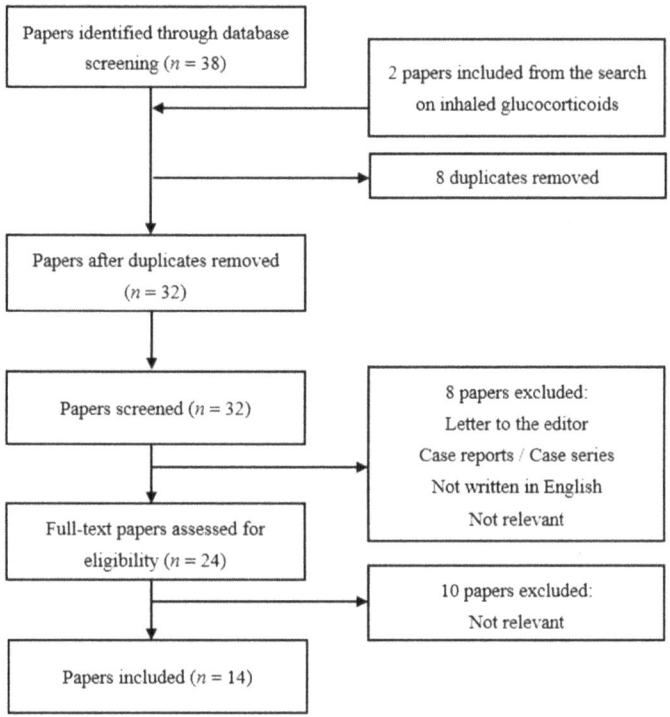

Figure 1. Study selection chart for intranasal glucocorticoids.

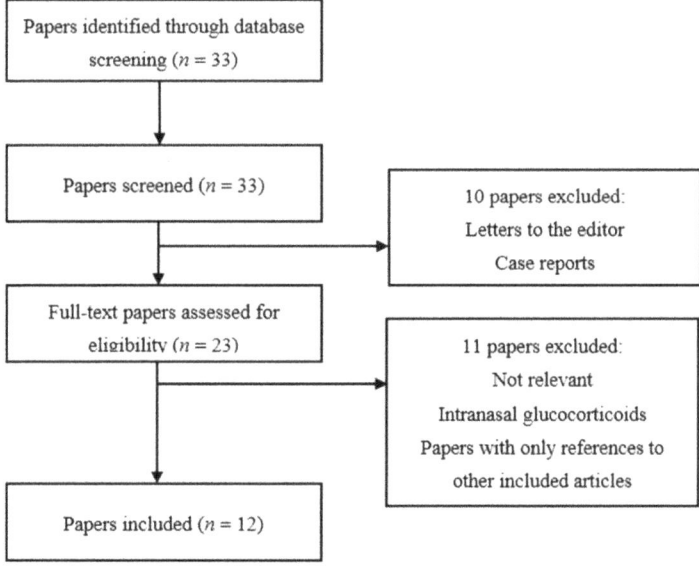

Figure 2. Study selection chart for inhaled glucocorticoids.

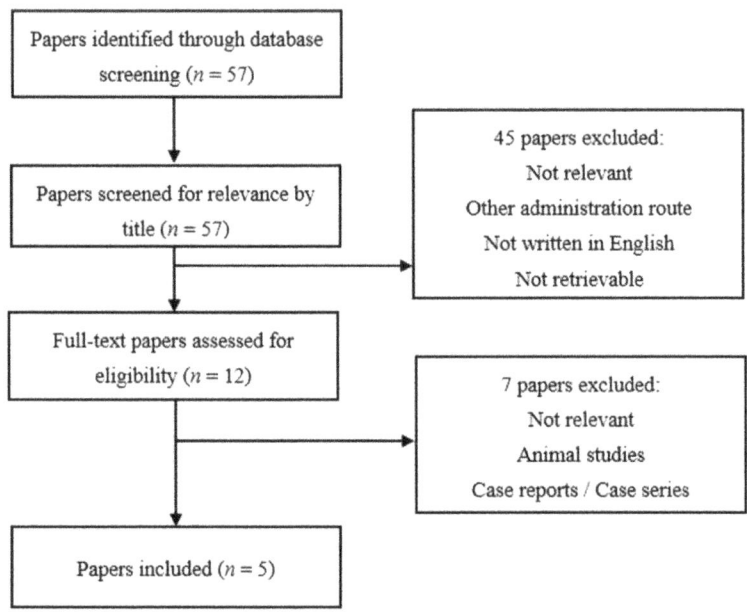

Figure 3. Study selection chart for systemic glucocorticoids.

Table 1. Search algorithms for each category of glucocorticoid administration.

Administration Form	Search Algorithm
Intranasal glucocorticoids	
Search 1	("Administration, Intranasal"(Mesh) OR "Nasal Sprays"(Mesh) OR "Nasal Lavage"(Mesh)) AND ("Glucocorticoids"(Mesh) OR "Steroids"(Mesh)) AND "Intraocular Pressure"(Mesh)
Search 2	("Rhinitis/drug therapy"(Mesh) OR "Sinusitis/drug therapy"(Mesh)) AND ("Glucocorticoids"(Mesh) OR "Anti-Inflammatory Agents"(Mesh) OR "Steroids"(Mesh)) AND ("Intraocular pressure"(Mesh) OR "eye/drug effects"(Mesh) OR "glaucoma"(Mesh) OR "ocular hypertension"(Mesh))
Inhaled glucocorticoids	
Search 1	("Administration, Inhalation"(Mesh) OR "Nebulizers and Vaporizers"(Mesh) OR "Respiratory Therapy"(Mesh) OR "Respiratory Tract Absorption"(Mesh)) AND ("Glucocorticoids"(Mesh) OR "Steroids"(Mesh)) AND ("Intraocular Pressure"(Mesh) OR "glaucoma"(Mesh) OR "ocular hypertension"(Mesh))
Systemic glucocorticoids	
Search 1	("Administration, Oral"(Mesh) OR "Capsules"(Mesh) OR "Tablets"(Mesh)) AND ("Glucocorticoids"(Mesh) OR "Steroids"(Mesh)) AND ("Intraocular Pressure"(Mesh) OR "glaucoma"(Mesh) OR "ocular hypertension"(Mesh))

J. Clin. Med. **2022**, *11*, 2007

Table 2. PICO(TS) framework for the literature search.

Patients	People with any medical condition requiring intranasal, inhaled or systemic glucocorticoid therapy.
Intervention	A treatment with intranasal, inhaled or systemic glucocorticoids.
Comparison	No treatment with intranasal, inhaled or systemic glucocorticoids.
Outcome	Intraocular pressure elevation.

Using the search terms mentioned above for the effect of intranasal glucocorticoids on IOP, the search yielded 38 results (Figure 1). Two other articles discussing the effect of intranasal glucocorticoids on IOP resulted from the search on inhaled glucocorticoids and were therefore also included here [16,17]. For intranasal glucocorticoids, we used two different combinations of search terms (Table 1) that yielded 8 overlapping studies, for which the duplicates were removed. The process of inclusion and exclusion of studies discussing intranasal glucocorticoids is demonstrated in Figure 1.

Using the search terms listed above for the effect of inhaled glucocorticoids on IOP, the search in Medline resulted in 33 studies (Figure 2). Two relevant papers were not retrievable online, and therefore a paper copy was retrieved from the library of the Faculty of Medicine, KU Leuven, Leuven, Belgium [17,18]. The further process of study selection is demonstrated in Figure 2.

Using the search terms for systemic glucocorticoids listed in Table 1, we retrieved 57 papers. The further process of study selection is demonstrated in Figure 3.

3. Results

After applying the inclusion and exclusion criteria for the study selection, we included 14 studies that discuss the effects of intranasal glucocorticoids on IOP, 12 discussing inhaled glucocorticoids, and five discussing systemically administered glucocorticoids.

3.1. Intranasal Glucocorticoids

An overview of the articles that discuss intranasally administered glucocorticoids is depicted in Table 3. Among the 14 included studies, 11 did not show any correlation between the use of intranasal glucocorticoids and an increased IOP [16,17,19–27]. In contrast to this finding, Bui et al. (2005) retrospectively reviewed twelve glaucoma patients taking intranasal glucocorticoids and found that the average IOP increased by 2.6 mmHg during steroid treatment compared with the pre-steroid examination ($p = 0.007$) [28]. In addition, after stopping the treatment with intranasal glucocorticoids, they observed a significant decrease in IOP ($p = 0.011$) [28]. The cross-sectional study conducted by Manji et al. in 2017 also suggests there is an increased risk of IOP elevation in long-term users of intranasal budesonide (administered daily for at least six months) [29]. Six percent of patients showed an increased IOP, although no significance level was mentioned [29]. More recently, the cross-sectional study by Mohd Zain et al. (2019) showed a significantly higher IOP in prolonged users of intranasal glucocorticoids for allergic rhinitis [30]. The rise of IOP was small (1.3 mmHg with a 95% confidence interval (CI) (0.72–1.9)), and no differences were shown in the cup–disc ratio. Exact treatment doses were not mentioned, but all patients received one or two puffs of intranasal momethasone, fluticasone or beclomethasone for an average of 5.42 years.

Table 3. Overview of the articles discussing intranasal glucocorticoid administration.

Study	Study Type (Evidence Level)	Patients Included	Age (Years)	Steroid + Daily Dose	IOP Increase?
Mohd Zain et al., 2019	Cross-sectional case control (3B)	95	10–40	Momethasone Fluticasone Beclomethasone	Yes

Table 3. *Cont.*

Study	Study Type (Evidence Level)	Patients Included	Age (Years)	Steroid + Daily Dose	IOP Increase?
Bui et al., 2005 *	Retrospective Chart Review (4)	12	35–83	variable	Yes
Manji et al., 2017	Cross-sectional observational (4)	100	>19	Budesonide 500 μg	Possible
Martino et al., 2015	Retrospective descriptive (4)	10	15–85	Dexamethasone 800 μg	No
Yuen et al., 2013 *	Randomized Controlled Trial (1B)	19	18–85	Beclomethasone 400 μg	No
Man et al., 2013	Prospective observational (4)	23	>18	Fluticasone 3000 μg [a]	No
LaForce et al., 2013	Randomized Controlled Trial (1B)	548	>12	Fluticasone 110 μg	No
Seiberling et al., 2013	Prospective observational (4)	18	>18	Budesonide 500 μg [a]	No
Ozkaya et al., 2011	Cross-sectional case control (3B)	240	7–15	Budesonide 100 μg	No
Spiliotopoulos et al., 2007	Prospective observational (4)	54	22–55	Dexamethasone 20 μg	No
Chervinsky et al., 2007	Randomized Controlled Trial (1B)	663	≥12	Ciclesonide 200 μg	No
Bross-Soriano et al., 2004	Prospective comparative (4)	360	18–60	Fluticasone 200 μg Mometasone 200 μg Beclomethasone 400 μg	No
Öztürk et al., 1998	Prospective observational (4)	26	18–66	Budesonide 400 μg Beclomethasone 400 μg	No
Garbe et al., 1997	Retrospective case control (3B)	48,118	>66	Fluticasone < or ≥200 μg Flunisolide < or ≥200 μg Beclomethasone < or ≥400 μg Budesonide < or ≥400 μg Triamcinolone < or ≥400 μg	No

* Studies including patients with pre-existing glaucoma. [a] Glucocorticoid doses were added to a 240 mL saline solution for administration by intranasal irrigation.

3.2. Inhaled Glucocorticoids

In Table 4, all included articles that discuss inhaled glucocorticoids are shown, among which three show an association with increased IOP. Mitchell et al. (1999) demonstrated an association between the use of inhaled glucocorticoids and an increased IOP in patients with a family history of glaucoma (odds ratio (OR) 3.1 with 95% CI (1.3–7.6)), although this association was not confirmed for people without such a family history [31]. Garbe et al. conducted a large case control study in 1997, showing a significantly increased risk of ocular hypertension or glaucoma in patients receiving high doses of inhaled glucocorticoids for at least three months continuously (OR 1.44 with 95% CI (1.01–2.06)). More recently, the cross-sectional case control study by Shroff et al. (2018) showed a higher IOP in chronic users of inhaled glucocorticoids (800 μg Budesonide or equivalents) compared to controls [32]. The difference in IOP was statistically significant ($p < 0.001$), although it was small: the observed pressure was 15.31 ± 3.27 mmHg for the inhaled glucocorticoid group versus 13.39 ± 1.95 mmHg for the control group. The study conducted by Nath et al. in 2017 showed 57 out of 405 subjects to have had an IOP higher than 22 mmHg after the intake of inhaled glucocorticoids, although no mention of statistical significance was made [33]. The eight remaining articles did not show any significant effect of inhaled glucocorticoids on IOP [11,18,34–39].

Table 4. Overview of the articles discussing inhaled glucocorticoid administration.

Study	Study Type (Evidence Level)	Patients Included	Age (Years)	Steroid + Daily Dose	IOP Increase?
Shroff et al., 2018	Cross-sectional case control (3B)	400	18–89	Budesonide 800 µg or equivalents	Yes
Mitchell et al., 1999	Cross-sectional observational (4)	3654	49–97	Beclomethasone ≤2 puffs >2 to ≤4 puffs >4 puffs	Yes [a]
Garbe et al., 1997	Retrospective case control (3B)	48,118	>66	Low versus high dose exposure: Beclomethasone < or ≥1600 µg Budesonide < or ≥1600 µg Triamcinolone < or ≥600 µg Flunisolide < or ≥1500 µg	Yes [b]
Nath et al., 2017	Prospective observational (4)	405	>50	Fluticasone equivalents [c]	Possible
Kerwin et al., 2019	Randomized Controlled Trial extension (1B)	456	40–80	Budesonide 320 µg	No
Moss et al., 2017 *	Randomized Controlled Trial (1B)	22	18–85	Fluticasone 500 µg	No
Alsaadi et al., 2012	Prospective observational (4)	93	5–15	Fluticasone 250 µg	No
Johnson et al., 2012 *	Retrospective case control (3B)	170	Not specified	Not specified	No
Gonzalez et al., 2010	Retrospective case control (3B)	15,736	≥66	Fluticasone equivalents [d]	No
Behbehani et al., 2005	Prospective observational (4)	95	<12	Budesonide 100–1050 µg Beclomethasone 100–1050 µg	No
Duh et al., 2000	Randomized Controlled Trials (1B)	1255	6–70	Budesonide 200–1600 µg	No
Samiy et al., 1996	Prospective observational (4)	187	20–79	Not specified	No

[a] IOP elevation only in patients with a family history of glaucoma. [b] IOP elevation only in patients receiving high doses continuously for at least 3 months. [c] Doses of different glucocorticoids were expressed as fluticasone equivalents: Low: 1–250 µg; Intermediate: 251–500 µg; High: 501–1000 µg. [d] Doses of different glucocorticoids expressed as fluticasone equivalents: Low: <500 µg; Intermediate: 500–999 µg; High: ≥1000 µg. * Studies including patients with pre-existing glaucoma.

3.3. Systemic Glucocorticoids

An overview of the included articles that discuss systemically administered glucocorticoids is depicted in Table 5. Four studies described a correlation between systemic glucocorticoids and an increased IOP. Prasad et al. (2019) prospectively observed 33 children with auto-immune hepatitis, for whom a treatment with systemic prednisone was started at the time of diagnosis [40]. An elevated IOP, defined as a value of ≥20 mmHg or an elevation of ≥6 mmHg compared to baseline IOP, was observed in 20 children (61%) after one month of treatment ($p < 0.001$). There was no difference in initial prednisone dose or total cumulative dose for patients who did or did not present with an elevated IOP [40]. Second, Kaur et al. (2016) retrospectively reviewed 150 patients of a pediatric glaucoma clinic and found that 36 (24%) cases were steroid-induced [41]. However, they included patients receiving topical or oral glucocorticoids, and only 12 received oral glucocorticoids alone. No significantly different effect on IOP was shown between orally and topically administered glucocorticoids [41]. Garbe et al. (1997) performed a retrospective case control study that proved IOP to be elevated compared to baseline in current users of oral glucocorticoids older than 65 (OR 1,41 with 95% CI (1.22–1.63)) [42]. They also discovered a dose–response relationship, in which the increase in IOP was narrowly significant for daily doses under 80 mg of hydrocortisone (OR 1.26 with 95% CI (1.01–1.56) for doses under 40 mg and OR 1.37 with 95% CI (1.06–1.76) for doses from 40 to 80 mg), but the response became clearer at daily doses higher than 80 mg (OR 1.88 with 95% CI (1.40–2.53)) [42]. Finally, in the cross-sectional study performed by Gaur et al. in 2014, 11% of the examined children with nephrotic syndrome developed an increased IOP after receiving oral glucocorticoids for at least six months [43]. There was no significant association between the administered dose or the duration of glucocorticoid intake and raised IOP [43]. Only cumulative glucocorticoid doses are mentioned in this study, which means that the exact dose delivered on a daily basis remains unclear.

Table 5. Overview of the articles discussing systemic glucocorticoid administration.

Study	Study Type (Evidence Level)	Patients Included	Age (Years)	Steroid + Daily Dose	IOP Increase?
Prasad et al., 2019	Prospective cohort (2B)	33	1–18	Prednisone 1–2 mg/kg/day, tapered after 2–4 weeks	Yes
Kaur et al., 2016	Retrospective observational (4)	150	<12	Not specified	Yes
Gaur et al., 2014	Cross-sectional observational (4)	82	4–18	Not specified	Yes
Garbe et al., 1997	Cross-sectional case control (3B)	48,118	>65	Hydrocortisone equivalents [a]	Yes
Gomes et al., 2014	Cross-sectional case control (3B)	106	>18	Variable, expressed as prednisone equivalents <10 mg	No

[a] Doses of different glucocorticoids were expressed as hydrocortisone equivalents: Low: <40 mg; Intermediate: 40–79 mg; High: ≥80 mg.

Only one study did not show a correlation between the intake of systemic glucocorticoids and an increased IOP. Gomes et al. (2014) found no correlation in patients with mixed connective tissue disease (MCTD) treated with low doses of prednisone (<10 mg daily for at least 6 months) [44].

4. Discussion

Since 1951, glucocorticoids are known to have the side effect of causing an increased IOP [3]. In contrast to topical ocular glucocorticoids, which are well known to cause a steroid response in a significant part of the general population [9,10], it is much less clear whether the same effect is to be expected for patients using intranasal, inhaled, or systemic glucocorticoids. A number of disquieting case reports on this topic have been published in the past, raising concerns about the possible ocular side effects following the administration of steroids by these routes. Opatowsky et al. (1995) described three patients, aged 60, 61 and 71, that developed ocular hypertension after starting therapy with beclomethasone diproprionate, administered by inhalation or nasal spray [45]. Second, Desnoeck et al. (2001) reported the case of an eight-year-old girl with bronchial asthma, treated with budesonide nasal spray 100 μg/day and budesonide inhalator 200 mg/day, in which ocular hypertension was discovered after two years of therapy [46]. Tham et al. (2004) described the case of a nine year old girl with leukemia that developed ocular hypertension after taking oral dexamethasone for only eight days [47]. Almost all patients described returned to an IOP within normal range after discontinuation of the glucocorticoid alone; only one patient needed IOP-lowering eyedrops. In addition to these examples, multiple other case reports and case series on the subject have been published [48–51]. These reports suggest the need for clear clinical guidance regarding the ophthalmological follow-up of glucocorticoid users. This review provides a relevant overview of the existing literature on the subject up until 2022 and serves as a first step toward a guideline for clinical practice.

4.1. Intranasal Glucocorticoids

Intranasal glucocorticoid administration specifically targets the nasal mucosa, which is the site where maximal drug effects are intended. As for all other topical administration forms, high local concentrations can be obtained without administering high systemic doses, and the amount of systemic adverse effects correlates with the drug fraction eventually reaching the systemic circulation. For intranasal glucocorticoids, this depends mostly on the absorption from the gastro-intestinal tract mucosa after swallowing [7]. The extent to which absorption from the upper airway mucosa contributes to the fraction reaching systemic circulation is almost negligible: Daley-Yates et al. (2001) measured a bioavailability of 44% for beclomethasone monopropionate, which fell to less than 1% after the administration of oral charcoal to exclude gastro-intestinal absorption [52]. This low absorption fraction from the upper airway mucosa can be explained by both the mucociliary transport toward the nasopharynx and the relatively small absorption surface [7]. The bioavailability of intranasally administered glucocorticoids depends on both the intestinal absorption and the liver's first pass effect, and it varies from under 1% (for fluticasone propionate) to 41% (for beclomethasone propionate) [7].

Different administration modalities are available for the use if intranasal glucocorticoids, among which intranasal sprays, intranasal drops, and high-volume intranasal irrigation solutions are most widely used. Although the efficacy of these different administration forms can be similar for certain diseases, one should always consider every patient individually to determine the most appropriate regimen, based on factors such as the inflammation phenotype, bioavailability, dosage, cost, tolerability and side effects [53].

Among the fourteen articles included in our review that discuss the use of intranasal glucocorticoids, twelve describe an administration by nasal sprays, of which nine show no correlation with increased IOP. Manji et al. (2017) noticed a possible correlation in their cross-sectional study, however they did not mention statistical significance [29]. Only two studies report a significant effect of intranasal glucocorticoids on IOP. Bui et al. (2005) was the first study to report this, although some study characteristics need to be taken into account. Their study sample consisted of only twelve patients, making it the second smallest sample of all fourteen included studies. Patients were also taking a wide variety of nasal glucocorticoid sprays with different potencies and in different doses, making it impossible to draw straightforward conclusions from this study alone. The more recent cross-sectional study of Mohd Zain et al. (2019) reports a significantly higher IOP in patients with allergic rhinitis, treated chronically with intranasal glucocorticoids (mean 5.42 years, standard deviation 3.22 years). The observed difference in IOP was—however significant—very small (1.30 mmHg, 95% CI (0.72–1.90)). Moreover, no significant differences in vertical cup–disc ratio were noticed; thus, the clinical relevance of this small IOP elevation can be debated.

The remaining two studies concerning intranasal glucocorticoids describe patients receiving high-volume intranasal irrigations, in which glucocorticoids were added to a 240 mL saline solution [22,24]. None of the studies discussing these irrigations showed an association with raised IOP.

As twelve out of the fourteen included studies do not show any significant association between the administration of intranasal glucocorticoids and elevated IOP, and considering the pharmacokinetic properties of intranasal glucocorticoids, we conclude that they can be used safely in clinical practice. Generally, no supplementary ophthalmological controls are needed, although clinicians should always consider each patient individually at the commencement of therapy, and risk factors for steroid response (such as pre-existing glaucoma) should be taken into consideration.

4.2. Inhaled Glucocorticoids

Inhaled glucocorticoids are administered topically to the lower airway mucosa, and the fraction reaching systemic circulation depends both on the absorption from the gastro-intestinal tract mucosa and from the lower airway mucosa [7]. When using inhaling devices, a substantial part of the medication dose is not inhaled but deposited into the oropharynx and swallowed afterward, to be absorbed by the gastro-intestinal tract mucosa. The extent to which both mechanisms play a role depends on the extent of pulmonary deposition, and on whether or not a correct inhalation technique is used [7]. This implies large interindividual differences of glucocorticoids reaching systemic circulation after inhaled administration.

Eight out of the twelve included studies discussing inhaled glucocorticoids do not show an association with an increased IOP. In contrast, Nath et al. (2017) noticed the possibility for an increased IOP in COPD (chronic obstructive pulmonary disease) patients receiving inhaled glucocorticoids, although their results were not marked as statistically significant [33]. Among all included patients, 16.0% developed an IOP higher than 22 mmHg, and 3.92% developed damage to the optic nerve head [33]. They described a dose–response relationship, with the highest prevalence of glaucoma among the patients in the high-dose group (501–1000 μg of fluticasone propionate equivalents daily) [33]. Mitchell et al. (1999) reported an elevated IOP in users of inhaled glucocorticoids with a family history of glaucoma, an association that was not confirmed in individuals without such family history [31]. Furthermore, Garbe et al. (1997) showed a significantly increased risk for IOP elevation in patients who had been continuously taking high doses of inhaled glucocorticoids for at least three months [17]. In contrast, no increased risk was observed for patients receiving low to medium doses of inhaled glucocorticoids [17]. Despite these results, previous oral glucocorticoid intake was not taken into account. Second, the glucocorticoid doses that posed an increased risk of ocular hypertension were much higher than those generally prescribed in daily practice, wherefore the results may not be clinically relevant for the majority of individual patients [54]. Finally, the study by Shroff et al., in 2019, shows a small but significant increase in chronic users of lower doses of intranasal glucocorticoids [32]. The question arises whether this small increase in IOP is clinically relevant and will trigger glaucomatous progression, but the results of this study certainly justify additional ophthalmological control visits in certain patients with glaucoma or glaucoma suspects, when they are long-term users of (moderately) high doses of inhaled glucocorticoids.

Combining all these results and considering the pharmacokinetic properties of inhaled glucocorticoids, we can conclude that they can be used safely for most patients in most circumstances. Extra precautions should be taken when prescribing high doses of inhaled glucocorticoids or for patients with a family history of glaucoma. The extent to which a family history of glaucoma contributes to a patient's predisposition to develop a steroid response following glucocorticoid inhalation still requires further investigation. Ophthalmological follow-up for IOP monitoring is recommended for these patients.

4.3. Systemic Glucocorticoids

Systemically administered glucocorticoids are expected to cause an increased IOP more often than intranasal or inhaled glucocorticoids because of higher doses reaching systemic circulation. In this case, not only the degree of side effects, but also the beneficial therapeutic effects depend on the systemic concentration that is reached [7].

Surprisingly, only a few studies on the subject have been published, varying greatly regarding patient age and glucocorticoid dosage. Five articles were retrieved, of which only the study by Gomes et al. (2014) did not demonstrate a correlation between the intake of systemic glucocorticoids and raised IOP [44]. The glucocorticoid doses administered in this study were low: all included patients were treated with less than 10 mg of prednisone equivalents daily. Among the included studies showing an association between systemic glucocorticoid intake and raised IOP, Kaur et al. (2016) [41] and Gaur et al. (2014) [43] did not mention daily doses. Prasad et al. (2019) mentioned a high incidence of IOP elevation in children treated with prednisone for auto-immune hepatitis [40]. Finally, Garbe et al. conducted a large case control study in 1997, in which a clear dose–response relationship was reported: the increase in IOP for daily doses under 80 mg of hydrocortisone equivalents was narrowly significant, but response became clearer at higher doses [42].

Since there are only a few articles discussing the IOP-related side effects of systemic glucocorticoids, caution is required when interpreting these results. Clinicians should be aware that patients receiving systemic glucocorticoids are at risk of developing an increased IOP. The highest risk is reported in users of high doses of glucocorticoids (>80 mg of hydrocortisone equivalents daily), whereas for low loses (<40 mg daily), the literature is contradictory. For every patient starting treatment with systemic glucocorticoids, especially children, regular ophthalmologic follow-up is warranted to detect steroid responders. Long-term systemic glucocorticoid users should also regularly be monitored for IOP elevation.

4.4. Glucocorticoids and Pre-Existing Glaucoma

Given that patients with pre-existing primary open-angle glaucoma (POAG) have a higher chance of being steroid-responders for topical intraocular glucocorticoids [10,11], the question arises of whether they are also more susceptible to an increased IOP caused by intranasal, inhaled, or systemic glucocorticoids. Among the articles discussed in this review, only four studied patients with pre-existing glaucoma. Regarding the effect of intranasal steroids, Bui et al. (2005) found a significant IOP elevation in intranasal steroid users with pre-existing glaucoma [28], although this association was denied by Yuen et al., in 2013 [21]. Both studies had small patient sample sizes, where definite conclusions cannot be drawn. The only two studies to discuss the effect of inhaled glucocorticoids on IOP in glaucoma patients both state that the risk of being a steroid responder does not increase [11,35]. Although no included articles discuss the use of systemic glucocorticoids in patients with pre-existing glaucoma, the phenomenon of a steroid response is especially important to diagnose in this patient group. If left unrecognized, even a small IOP elevation above the individual target pressure can induce progressive visual field defects and irreversible optic nerve head damage in glaucoma patients. Since patients with pre-existing glaucoma have a higher (up to 90%) risk of being a steroid responder, it is important to follow these patients on a regular basis at the start of their therapy. To determine whether patients with pre-existing POAG are at a higher risk of developing an increased IOP caused by intranasal or inhaled glucocorticoid administration forms, more research is needed.

5. Conclusions

The current literature indicates that patients receiving systemic glucocorticoids are at risk of developing an increased IOP, especially patients taking high daily doses. Regular ophthalmologic controls are therefore recommended for chronic steroid users and for patients starting with a new steroid treatment, especially for those with pre-existing glaucoma. Inhaled glucocorticoids may be associated with an increased IOP when delivered in high doses or in patients with a family history of glaucoma. Intranasal glucocorticoids have no clear IOP-elevating effect and can therefore be used safely without ophthalmologic follow-up in most circumstances. Clinicians should always consider each patient individually at the commencement of corticosteroid therapy in any form, and potential risk factors for a steroid response should be evaluated.

Author Contributions: Conceptualization: D.W., I.S. and E.V.; methodology: D.W. and E.V.; validation: D.W., I.S. and E.V.; data curation: D.W., I.S. and E.V.; investigation: D.W.; writing—original draft preparation: D.W.; writing—review and editing: I.S. and E.V.; visualization: D.W., I.S. and E.V.; supervision: I.S. and E.V.; project administration: I.S. and E.V. All authors have read and agreed to the published version of the manuscript.

Funding: This research received no external funding.

Institutional Review Board Statement: Not applicable.

Informed Consent Statement: Not applicable.

Data Availability Statement: Not applicable.

Conflicts of Interest: The authors declare no conflict of interest.

References

1. Schlote, T.; Mielke, J.; Grüb, M.; Rohrbach, J.M.; Gelisken, F. (Eds.) *Pocket Atlas of Ophthalmology*; Thieme: New York, NY, USA, 2006; pp. 2–8.
2. Agarwal, H.C.; Sood, N.N.; Kalra, B.R.; Ghosh, B. Secondary glaucoma. *Indian J. Ophthalmol.* **1982**, *30*, 121. [PubMed]
3. Gordon, D.M.; McLean, J.M.; Koteen, H.; Bousquet, F.P.; McCusker, W.D.; Baras, I.; Wetzig, P.; Norton, E. The Use of Acth and Cortisone in Ophthalmology. *Am. J. Ophthalmol.* **1951**, *34*, 1675–1686. [CrossRef]
4. Clark, A.F.; Wilson, K.; McCartney, M.D.; Miggans, S.T.; Kunkle, M.; Howe, W. Glucocorticoid-induced formation of cross-linked actin networks in cultured human trabecular meshwork cells. *Investig. Ophthalmol. Vis. Sci.* **1994**, *35*, 281–294.
5. Weinreb, R.; Cotlier, E.; Yue, B.Y. The extracellular matrix and its modulation in the trabecular meshwork. *Surv. Ophthalmol.* **1996**, *40*, 379–390. [CrossRef]
6. Jones, R.; Rhee, D.J. Corticosteroid-induced ocular hypertension and glaucoma: A brief review and update of the litera-ture. *Curr. Opin. Ophthalmol.* **2006**, *17*, 163–167. [PubMed]
7. Mortimer, K.J.; Tattersfield, A.E. Benefit Versus Risk for Oral, Inhaled, and Nasal Glucocorticosteroids. *Immunol. Allergy Clin. N. Am.* **2005**, *25*, 523–539. [CrossRef]
8. Nuyen, B.; Weinreb, R.N.; Robbins, S.L. Steroid-induced glaucoma in the pediatric population. *J. Am. Assoc. Pediatr. Ophthalmol. Strabismus* **2017**, *21*, 1–6. [CrossRef]
9. Armaly, M.F.; Becker, B. Intraocular pressure response to topical corticosteroids. *Fed. Proc.* **1965**, *24*, 1274–1278.
10. Tripathi, R.C.; Parapuram, S.K.; Tripathi, B.J.; Zhong, Y.; Chalam, K. Corticosteroids and Glaucoma Risk. *Drugs Aging* **1999**, *15*, 439–450. [CrossRef]
11. Moss, E.B.; Buys, Y.M.; Low, S.A.; Yuen, D.; Jin, Y.-P.; Chapman, K.R.; Trope, G.E. A Randomized Controlled Trial to Determine the Effect of Inhaled Corticosteroid on Intraocular Pressure in Open-Angle Glaucoma and Ocular Hypertension: The ICOUGH Study. *J. Glaucoma* **2017**, *26*, 182–186. [CrossRef]
12. Kwok, A.K.; Lam, D.S.; Ng, J.S.; Fan, D.S.; Chew, S.-J.; Tso, M.O. Ocular-hypertensive Response to Topical Steroids in Children. *Ophthalmology* **1997**, *104*, 2112–2116. [CrossRef]
13. Razeghinejad, M.R.; Katz, L.J. Steroid-Induced Iatrogenic Glaucoma. *Ophthalmic Res.* **2012**, *47*, 66–80. [CrossRef] [PubMed]
14. Gevorgyan, A.; Segboer, C.; Chusakul, S.; Kanjanaumporn, J.; Aeumjaturapat, S.; Reeskamp, R.; Fokkens, W.; Snidvongs, K. Intranasal corticosteroids for non-allergic rhinitis. *Cochrane Database Syst. Rev.* **2013**, *11*, 1465–1858. [CrossRef]
15. Maniaci, A.; Merlino, F.; Cocuzza, S.; Iannella, G.; Vicini, C.; Cammaroto, G.; Lechien, J.R.; Calvo-Henriquez, C.; La Mantia, I. Endoscopic surgical treatment for rhinogenic contact point headache: Systematic review and meta-analysis. *Eur. Arch. Oto-Rhino-Laryngol.* **2021**, *278*, 1743–1753. [CrossRef]
16. Öztürk, F.; Yücetürk, A.V.; Kurt, E.; Ünlü, H.H.; Ilker, S.S. Evaluation of Intraocular Pressure and Cataract Formation following the Long-Term Use of Nasal Corticosteroids. *Ear, Nose Throat J.* **1998**, *77*, 846–851. [CrossRef]
17. Garbe, E.; LeLorier, J.; Boivin, J.F.; Suissa, S. Inhaled and nasal glucocorticoids and the risks of ocular hypertension or open-angle glaucoma. *JAMA* **1997**, *277*, 722–727. [CrossRef]
18. Samiy, N.; Walton, D.S.; Dreyer, E.B. Inhaled steroids: Effect on intraocular pressure in patients without glaucoma. *Can. J. Ophthalmol.* **1996**, *31*, 120–123.
19. Bross-Soriano, D.; Hanenberg-Milver, C.; Schimelmitz-Idi, J.; Arrieta-Gomez, J.R.; Del Toro, R.A.; Bravo-Escobar, G. Effects of Three Nasal Topical Steroids in the Intraocular Pressure Compartment. *Otolaryngol. Neck Surg.* **2004**, *130*, 187–191. [CrossRef]
20. Martino, B.J.; Church, C.A.; Seiberling, K.A. Effect of intranasal dexamethasone on endogenous cortisol level and intraocular pressure. *Int. Forum Allergy Rhinol.* **2015**, *5*, 605–609. [CrossRef]
21. Yuen, D.; Buys, Y.M.; Jin, Y.-P.; Alasbali, T.; Trope, G.E. Effect of Beclomethasone Nasal Spray on Intraocular Pressure in Ocular Hypertension or Controlled Glaucoma. *J. Glaucoma* **2013**, *22*, 84–87. [CrossRef]
22. Man, L.-X.; Farhood, Z.; Luong, A.; Fakhri, S.; Feldman, R.M.; Orlander, P.R.; Citardi, M.J. The effect of intranasal fluticasone propionate irrigations on salivary cortisol, intraocular pressure, and posterior subcapsular cataracts in postsurgical chronic rhinosinusitis patients. *Int. Forum Allergy Rhinol.* **2013**, *3*, 953–957. [CrossRef] [PubMed]
23. LaForce, C.; Journeay, G.E.; Miller, S.D.; Silvey, M.J.; Wu, W.; Lee, L.A.; Chylack, L.T. Ocular safety of fluticasone furoate nasal spray in patients with perennial allergic rhinitis: A 2-year study. *Ann. Allergy, Asthma Immunol.* **2013**, *111*, 45–50. [CrossRef] [PubMed]
24. Seiberling, K.A.; Chang, D.F.; Np, J.N.; Park, F.; Church, C.A. Effect of intranasal budesonide irrigations on intraocular pressure. *Int. Forum Allergy Rhinol.* **2013**, *3*, 704–707. [CrossRef] [PubMed]
25. Ozkaya, E.; Ozsutcu, M.; Mete, F. Lack of Ocular Side Effects After 2 Years of Topical Steroids for Allergic Rhinitis. *J. Pediatr. Ophthalmol. Strabismus* **2011**, *48*, 311–317. [CrossRef] [PubMed]

26. Spiliotopoulos, C.; Mastronikolis, N.S.; Petropoulos, I.K.; Mela, E.K.; Goumas, P.D.; Gartaganis, S.P. The Effect of Nasal Steroid Administration on Intraocular Pressure. *Ear, Nose Throat J.* **2007**, *86*, 394–395. [CrossRef]

27. Chervinsky, P.; Kunjibettu, S.; Miller, D.L.; Prenner, B.M.; Raphael, G.; Hall, N.; Shah, T. Long-term safety and efficacy of intranasal ciclesonide in adult and adolescent patients with perennial allergic rhinitis. *Ann. Allergy Asthma Immunol.* **2007**, *99*, 69–76. [CrossRef]

28. Bui, C.M.; Chen, H.; Shyr, Y.; Joos, K.M. Discontinuing nasal steroids might lower intraocular pressure in glaucoma. *J. Allergy Clin. Immunol.* **2005**, *116*, 1042–1047. [CrossRef]

29. Manji, J.; Singh, G.; Okpaleke, C.; Dadgostar, A.; Al-Asousi, F.; Amanian, A.; Macias-Valle, L.; Finkelstein, A.; Tacey, M.; Thamboo, A.; et al. Safety of long-term intranasal budesonide delivered via the mucosal atomization device for chronic rhinosi-nusitis. *Int. Forum Allergy Rhinol.* **2017**, *7*, 488–493. [CrossRef]

30. Zain, A.M.; Noh, U.K.M.; Hussein, S.; Hamzah, J.C.; Khialdin, S.M.; Din, N.M. The Relationship Between Long-term Use of Intranasal Corticosteroid and Intraocular Pressure. *J. Glaucoma* **2019**, *28*, 321–324. [CrossRef]

31. Mitchell, P.; Cumming, R.G.; Mackey, D.A. Inhaled corticosteroids, family history, and risk of glaucoma. *Ophthalmology* **1999**, *106*, 2301–2306. [CrossRef]

32. Shroff, S.; Thomas, R.K.; D'Souza, G.; Nithyanandan, S. The effect of inhaled steroids on the intraocular pressure. *Digit. J. Ophthalmol.* **2018**, *24*, 6–9. [CrossRef] [PubMed]

33. Nath, T.; Roy, S.S.; Kumar, H.; Agrawal, R.; Kumar, S.; Satsangi, S.K. Prevalence of steroid-induced cataract and glaucoma in chronic obstructive pulmonary disease patients attending a tertiary care center in India. *Asia-Pac. J. Ophthalmol.* **2017**, *6*, 28–32. [CrossRef]

34. Osuagwu, U.L.; AlMubrad, T.M.; Alsaadi, M.M. Effects of inhaled fluticasone on intraocular pressure and central corneal thickness in asthmatic children without a family history of glaucoma. *Middle East Afr. J. Ophthalmol.* **2012**, *19*, 314–319. [CrossRef] [PubMed]

35. Johnson, L.N.; Soni, C.R.; Johnson, M.A.; Madsen, R.W. Short-term use of inhaled and intranasal corticosteroids is not associated with glaucoma progression on optical coherence tomography. *Eur. J. Ophthalmol.* **2012**, *22*, 695–700. [CrossRef] [PubMed]

36. Gonzalez, A.V.; Li, G.; Suissa, S.; Ernst, P. Risk of glaucoma in elderly patients treated with inhaled corticosteroids for chronic airflow obstruction. *Pulm. Pharmacol. Ther.* **2010**, *23*, 65–70. [CrossRef] [PubMed]

37. Behbehani, A.H.; Owayed, A.F.; Hijazi, Z.M.; A Eslah, E.; Al-Jazzaf, A.M. Cataract and ocular hypertension in children on inhaled corticosteroid therapy. *J. Pediatr. Ophthalmol. Strabismus* **2005**, *42*, 23–27. [CrossRef]

38. Duh, M.-S.; Walker, A.M.; Lindmark, B.; Laties, A.M. Association between intraocular pressure and budesonide inhalation therapy in asthmatic patients. *Ann. Allergy Asthma Immunol.* **2000**, *85*, 356–361. [CrossRef]

39. Kerwin, E.M.; Ferguson, G.T.; Mo, M.; DeAngelis, K.; Dorinsky, P. Bone and ocular safety of budesonide/glycopyrrolate/formoterol fumarate metered dose inhaler in COPD: A 52-week randomized study. *Respir. Res.* **2019**, *20*, 167. [CrossRef]

40. Prasad, D.; Poddar, U.; Kanaujia, V.; Yachha, S.K.; Srivastava, A. Effect of long-term oral steroids on intraocular pressure in children with autoimmune hepatitis: A prospective cohort study. *J. Glaucoma* **2019**, *28*, 929–933. [CrossRef]

41. Kaur, S.; Dhiman, I.; Kaushik, S.; Raj, S.; Pandav, S.S. Outcome of Ocular Steroid Hypertensive Response in Children. *J. Glaucoma* **2016**, *25*, 343–347. [CrossRef]

42. Garbe, E.; LeLorier, J.; Boivin, J.-F.; Suissa, S. Risk of ocular hypertension or open-angle glaucoma in elderly patients on oral glucocorticoids. *Lancet* **1997**, *350*, 979–982. [CrossRef]

43. Gaur, S.; Joseph, M.; Nityanandam, S.; Subramanian, S.; Koshy, A.S.; Vasudevan, A.; Phadke, K.D.; Iyengar, A. Ocular Com-plications in Children with Nephrotic Syndrome on Long Term Oral Steroids. *Indian J. Pediatr.* **2014**, *81*, 680–683. [CrossRef] [PubMed]

44. Gomes, B.F.; Moraes, H.V.; Kara-Junior, N.; de Azevedo, M.N.L.; de Lima, F.B.F.; Santhiago, M.R. Intraocular pressure in chronic users of low-dose oral corticosteroids for connective tissue disease. *Can. J. Ophthalmol.* **2014**, *49*, 363–366. [CrossRef] [PubMed]

45. Opatowsky, I.; Feldman, R.M.; Gross, R.; Feldman, S.T. Intraocular Pressure Elevation Associated with Inhalation and Nasal Corticosteroids. *Ophthalmology* **1995**, *102*, 177–179. [CrossRef]

46. Desnoeck, M.; Casteels, I.; Casteels, K. Intraocular pressure elevation in a child due to the use of inhalation steroids—A case report. *Bull. Soc. Belge Ophtalmol.* **2001**, *280*, 97–100.

47. Tham, C.C.; Ng, J.S.; Li, R.T.; Chik, K.W.; Lam, D.S. Intraocular pressure profile of a child on a systemic corticosteroid. *Am. J. Ophthalmol.* **2004**, *137*, 198–201. [CrossRef]

48. Yamashita, T.; Kodama, Y.; Tanaka, M.; Yamakiri, K.; Kawano, Y.; Sakamoto, T. Steroid-induced Glaucoma in Children with Acute Lymphoblastic Leukemia. *J. Glaucoma* **2010**, *19*, 188–190. [CrossRef]

49. Friling, R.; Weinberger, D.; Zeharia, A.; Lusky, M.; Mimouni, M.; Gaaton, D.; Snir, M. Elevated intraocular pressure associated with steroid treatment for infantile spasms. *Ophthalmology* **2003**, *110*, 831–834. [CrossRef]

50. Mogrovejo, S.; Moragón, E.M.; Climent, M. Ocular Hypertension Requiring Suspension of Inhaled Corticosteroids. *Arch. Bronconeumol.* **2017**, *1*, 34, (English Edition). [CrossRef]

51. Brito, P.; Silva, S.E.; Cotta, J.S.; Falcao-Reis, F. Severe ocular hypertension secondary to systemic corticosteroid treatment in a child with nephrotic syndrome. *Clin. Ophthalmol.* **2012**, *6*, 1675–1679. [CrossRef]

52. Daley-Yates, P.T.; Price, A.C.; Sisson, J.R.; Pereira, A.; Dallow, N. Beclomethasone dipropionate: Absolute bioavailability, pharmacokinetics and metabolism following intravenous, oral, intranasal and inhaled administration in man. *Br. J. Clin. Pharmacol.* **2001**, *51*, 400–409. [CrossRef] [PubMed]

53. Fowler, J.; Rotenberg, B.W.; Sowerby, L.J. The subtle nuances of intranasal corticosteroids. *J. Otolaryngol. Head Neck Surg.* **2021**, *50*, 18. [CrossRef] [PubMed]

54. Macris, N. Glucocorticoid Use and Risks of Ocular Hypertension and Glaucoma. *JAMA J. Am. Med. Assoc.* **1997**, *277*, 1929. [CrossRef]

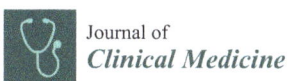

Journal of
Clinical Medicine

Article

Modification of Corneal Biomechanics and Intraocular Pressure Following Non-Penetrating Deep Sclerectomy

María Dolores Díaz-Barreda [1,2,3,*], Ignacio Sánchez-Marín [1], Ana Boned-Murillo [1,2,3], Itziar Pérez-Navarro [1], Juana Martínez [1], Elena Pardina-Claver [1], Diana Pérez [1,2,3], Francisco Javier Ascaso [1,2,3,*] and Juan Ibáñez [1,2,3]

[1] Department of Ophthalmology, Hospital Clínico Universitario Lozano Blesa, 50009 Zaragoza, Spain; nachosm89@gmail.com (I.S.-M.); anabomu@hotmail.com (A.B.-M.); ichuperez_87@hotmail.com (I.P.-N.); juanimarmor@hotmail.com (J.M.); elenapardina11@hotmail.com (E.P.-C.); dianapgpe@hotmail.com (D.P.); juanibanezalperte@msn.com (J.I.)
[2] Department of Surgery, School of Medicine, University of Zaragoza, 50009 Zaragoza, Spain
[3] Aragon Health Research Institute (IIS Aragón), 50009 Zaragoza, Spain
* Correspondence: lodiba92@gmail.com (M.D.D.-B.); jascaso@gmail.com (F.J.A.);
  Tel.: +34-629-863-827 (M.D.D.-B.); +34-686-574-389 (F.J.A.)

Citation: Díaz-Barreda, M.D.; Sánchez-Marín, I.; Boned-Murillo, A.; Pérez-Navarro, I.; Martínez, J.; Pardina-Claver, E.; Pérez, D.; Ascaso, F.J.; Ibáñez, J. Modification of Corneal Biomechanics and Intraocular Pressure Following Non-Penetrating Deep Sclerectomy. *J. Clin. Med.* **2022**, *11*, 1216. https://doi.org/10.3390/jcm11051216

Academic Editors: Maria Letizia Salvetat, Marco Zeppieri and Paolo Brusini

Received: 23 December 2021
Accepted: 21 February 2022
Published: 24 February 2022

Publisher's Note: MDPI stays neutral with regard to jurisdictional claims in published maps and institutional affiliations.

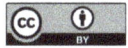
Abstract: Changes in the cornea can influence outcomes in patients with primary open-angle glaucoma (POAG). We aimed to evaluate the relevance of changes in corneal biomechanics and intraocular pressure (IOP) in patients undergoing non-penetrating deep sclerectomy (NPDS) with the Esnoper V2000 implant® (AJL Ophthalmic S.A., Gasteiz, Spain). We included 42 eyes of 42 patients with POAG scheduled for NPDS with the Esnoper V2000 implant. Biomechanical properties were measured by Ocular Response Analyzer® G3 (ORA; Reichert Inc., Depew, NY, USA). Corneal hysteresis (CH), corneal resistance factor (CRF), corneal compensated IOP (IOPcc), and Goldmann-correlated IOP (IOPg) were measured the day before surgery and on day 1, 7, and 30 and 2 and 3 months after surgery. CH initially increased, fell below the presurgical value at 30 days after the surgery, and increased again at 2 and 3 months. CRF, IOPcc, and IOPg decreased on the first day after surgery, then followed a trend of increasing but stayed below pre-surgery levels. All values reached statistical significance. While observed changes in corneal biomechanics after NPDS and Esnoper V2000 implant were significant, more studies are needed if we are to understand their influence on corneal biomechanics and their clinical relevance in POAG.

Keywords: corneal biomechanics; ocular response analyzer; ORA; corneal hysteresis; glaucoma; tonometry; non-penetrating deep sclerectomy; Esnoper V-2000 implant

1. Introduction

Glaucoma represents one of the main underlying causes of irreversible blindness worldwide, with the most frequent type being primary open-angle glaucoma (POAG) [1,2]. The main risk factor for disease progression, and the only one we can influence, is intraocular pressure (IOP); for this reason, its detailed study, along with the corneal properties (both structural and biomechanical) that can affect its measurement, is essential [3–6].

Goldmann applanation tonometry (GAT) is the gold standard in the measurement of the IOP, but the technique presents many inter-observer variations and is influenced by the curvature or central thickness of the cornea, biomechanical parameters of the cornea, and the age of the patient [7] (pp. 870–887) [8]. It has been shown, using a biomechanical model, that GAT does not always reflect true IOP values and that corneal compensated IOP (IOPcc) can become a fundamental parameter in the diagnosis and monitoring of this pathology [9]. Likewise, the resistance of the cornea to flattening by contact tonometry was the most determining factor to influence the differences in IOP between tonometers [6,10].

In an attempt to overcome the limitations of contact tonometers, other devices have been developed; the emergence of these new devices has resulted in new parameters, indices, and diagnostic algorithms that can help us to more quickly and reliably detect different pathological conditions [11]. One of the most recent is the Corvis® ST (OCULUS Optikgeräte GmbH, Wetzlar, Germany). It is a classical non-contact tonometer combined with an ultra-fast Scheimpflug camera capable not only of giving more reliable IOP measurements but also of analyzing biomechanical properties of the cornea and its dynamic deformation [12].

In this paper we focus on the Ocular Response Analyzer® G3 (ORA). Designed by Reichert Technologies (Reichert Inc., Depew, NY, USA), ORA is a non-contact device that measures, in vivo, the differential response of the cornea to applanation produced by a rapid air pulse over a period of approximately 20 milliseconds. By means of different parameters that we describe below, ORA provides information on the biomechanical and viscoelastic properties of the cornea [6,9]. Corneal hysteresis (CH) is a property that represents the dynamic resistance of the cornea to deformation (i.e., its ability to absorb and dissipate energy). The corneal resistance factor (CRF) represents static resistance and is proportional to the force applied to the cornea; CRF is related to the central corneal thickness (CCT), calculated by an ultrasonic pachymeter that forms part of the ORA, and the Goldmann-correlated IOP (IOPg). CRF is determined using the average of two IOP measurements made at the moment of maximum inward and outward applanation. A calculation is also made according to the air pressure required to flatten the central area of the cornea, using information provided by CH; this is known as the IOPcc. IOPcc offers several advantages over the IOP measured by GAT [7].

In recent years, the study of corneal biomechanics has been applied to the various branches of ophthalmology, including glaucoma [13]. Studies show that CH in subjects with glaucoma is significantly lower than in the general population [14–16]; this parameter has been associated with a greater defect in the optic disc. Further to this, a thinner layer of nerve fibers has been postulated as a risk factor for glaucoma progression, even in patients with well-controlled IOP measured by GAT [4,14,17–20]. In addition, the Ocular Hypertension Treatment Study (OHTS) concluded that CCT is a factor that can predict the evolution of ocular hypertension to POAG [21].

Studies also indicate that the continued use of certain prostaglandins (PGAs) can alter corneal biomechanics independent of the lowering of the IOP; this has also been observed in patients who had partial recovery of CH following therapy [22,23].

If we turn our attention to surgical treatments, there are a few isolated studies in the available literature that refer to biomechanical changes in the cornea following the different surgical techniques available to glaucoma patients. However, their limited number and heterogeneity make it very difficult to arrive at a conclusion; in fact, there is a general lack of studies on non-penetrating deep sclerectomy (NPDS), particularly in cases of implant-associated surgery, which is the technique of choice in our environment.

The purpose of this study was to evaluate changes in the parameters of corneal biomechanics (CH and CRF) and IOP (PIOg and PIOcc) in patients with POAG undergoing NPDS surgery associated with Esnoper V-2000 implant® (AJL Ophthalmic S.A., Gasteiz, Spain).

2. Materials and Methods

This was a consecutive non-randomized prospective study of 42 eyes corresponding to 42 patients diagnosed with POAG, selected for NPDS. It was carried out in the Department of Ophthalmology at the Lozano Blesa University Clinical Hospital, in Zaragoza, Spain, between September 2019 and July 2020. The study protocol was approved by the Review Committee of the Lozano Blesa University Clinical Hospital in Zaragoza and complied with Spanish legislation in the field of biomedical research; in the protection of personal data, Organic Law 3/2018 on the Protection of Personal Data; Basic Law 41/2002, regulating patient autonomy and rights; obligations regarding information and clinical documentation; and Law 14/2007 on biomedical research. All the research was carried out following the principles of the Declaration of Helsinki, and all patients signed an informed consent (IC) and were given a copy of it.

The inclusion criteria were as follows: The patient must be over 18 years old and present a diagnosis of POAG (requirement was for reproducible defects in the visual field (VF) detected by automated perimetry with Humphrey® 3 Field Analyzer (Carl Zeiss Meditec, Inc., Dublin, CA, USA) strategy 24-2 and corresponding defect in the retinal nerve fiber layer (RNFL) in the swept-source-optical coherence tomography (DRI OCT Triton™, Topcon, Tokyo, Japan); POAG had to have been treated for a minimum of the previous six months with at least two topical anti-glaucomatous drugs, one of which was supposed to be a PGA eye drop; despite topical treatment, the patient should not achieve adequate IOP control and the progression of POAG should continue, with the patient therefore a candidate for NPDS without associating phacoemulsification; no previous history of pathologies that could affect the cornea and no signs of retinopathy or optic neuropathy other than glaucoma; images obtained had to have a quality score higher than 20.

The exclusion criteria were as follows: The patient could not have a personal history of any ophthalmological condition other than glaucomatous damage caused by POAG (except senile cataract without surgery criteria); extreme axial lengths (below 22 mm and above 26 mm); surgery on any eye or have had an ocular trauma that required consultation with an ophthalmologist; any type of intraoperative complication, such as perforation of Descemet's membrane and conversion to trabeculectomy, or any postoperative complication; presentation of an IOP lower than 5 mmHg by GAT after surgery was also an exclusion criterion. Patients whose tests were not of sufficient quality to be analyzed were also excluded, as were patients who had required non-topical IOP lowering medication in the 6 months prior to surgery and those requiring topical medication (including hypotensive drops) three months after surgery (not counting the drops included in the post-surgical protocol).

Although 53 eyes of 53 patients with POAG were initially included, 1 was ruled out because of myopia magna with an axial length of 27.02 mm (not detected in the initial interview), 8 were ruled out for not meeting the time requirement for treatment with topical eye drops (also not recorded in the first interview), and 2 were ruled out for needing hypotensive eye drops after surgery. Finally, the data of 42 eyes of 42 patients were analyzed.

All surgeries were performed by the same surgeon (J.I.), as explained below. A fornix-based conjunctival flap was performed, followed by a superficial scleral flap of approximately one-third of the total thickness. A portion of 0.02% mitomycin C (MMC), prepared in the hospital pharmacy, was used for 2 min at both the scleral and subconjunctival levels. Finally, a small, deep flap was created, leaving a thin sheet of sclera to plane of the Schlemm's canal which was dissected. Esnoper V-2000 (AJL®) was used as a suprachoroidal implant without sutures. Finally, the surface flap was sutured with 10/0 Nylon (Dafilon®, B. Braun Surgical S.A., Barcelona, Spain) and the conjunctival flap with 8/0 Silk (Silkam®, B. Braun Surgical S.A., Barcelona, Spain). Postoperatively, patients followed a downward regimen of TobraDex® eye drops (Novartis, Basel, Switzerland) (1 mg of dexamethasone and 3 mg of tobramycin) according to postsurgical protocol.

The biomechanical properties of the cornea were measured with ORA: three measurements were made, and the mean all of them was expressed in millimeters of mercury (mmHg), calculated for the analysis. Values measured were CH, CRF, IOPcc, and IOPg; all were taken by the same ophthalmologist in the morning and in a time range of 3 h. All measurements were made the day before the surgery and on day 1, 7, and 30 and at 2 and 3 months after surgery.

Statistical Analysis

The statistical analysis was carried out using IBM SPSS v.23 (IBM, Armonk, NY, USA), calculating the means and standard deviations (SD), medians, and ranges for each variable and each time moment. To check the normality of the data to assess whether to apply the parametric or non-parametric tests corresponding to each analysis, the Kolmogorov–Smirnov test was used for a sample, obtaining significant deviations from the normal curve in most variables.

A value of $p < 0.05$ was used to consider the result statistically significant. The statistics were calculated using MedCalc ver.15.2 (MedCalc Software Bvba, Ostend, Belgium).

A global analysis was carried out for each variable using the Friedman test for non-parametric dependent or related samples to evaluate the differences in biomechanical parameters over time (day before surgery, and at day 1, 7, and 30 and at 2 and 3 months after surgery).

3. Results

The study sample consisted of 42 eyes from 42 different patients. The median age of the sample was 68.19 +/− 11.88 years. The demographic characteristics are set out in Table 1.

Table 1. Demographic characteristics of the 42 patients analyzed.

CHARACTERISTICS		VALUES
SEX, *N* (%)	Women	12 (28.57)
	Men	30 (71.43)
AGE, YEARS	Mean +/−SD	68.19 +/− 11.88 years
	Median (range)	70 (45–70)
LATERALITY OF THE TESTED EYE, *N* (%)	Right	21 (50)
	Left	21 (50)
NUMBER OF TOPICAL ANTIHYPERTENSIVE EYE DROPS PRIOR TO SURGERY, *N* (%)	1	0 (0)
	2	4 (9.53)
	3	21 (50)
	4	17 (40.47)

SD: standard deviation.

Table 2 shows the data on the changes in the ORA variables (CH, CRF, IOPcc, and IOPg) at the different study visits. These data are supported by Figure 1, where the four variables are shown across time. Regarding the presurgical values, CH increased on days 1 and 7, descending below the presurgical value at day 30, after which it increased again at 2 and 3 months after the intervention to above the values prior to surgery. The rest of the variables (CRF, IOPcc, IOPg) decreased the first day after surgery, then followed an increasing trend but stayed below pre-surgical levels. All values reached statistical significance.

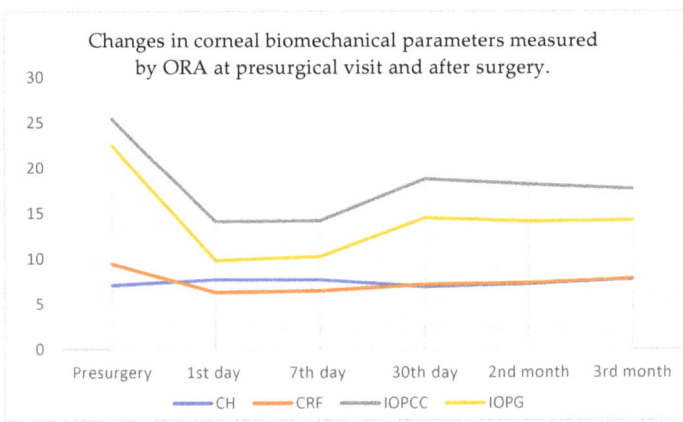

Figure 1. Data on biomechanical characteristics obtained by ORA before surgery and at days 1, 7, and 30 after surgery and at 2 and 3 months after surgery. The vertical axis on the left corresponds to mmHg, while the horizontal axis refers to time. The color legend for each variable studied is placed below. CH: corneal hysteresis; CRF: corneal resistance factor; IOPcc: compensated intraocular pressure; IOPg: Goldmann-correlated intraocular pressure.

Table 2. Data on biomechanical characteristics obtained by ORA day before surgery and at day 1, 7, and 30 and at 2 and 3 months after surgery. All data are measured in mmHg, with the mean and standard deviation (SD) in brackets on the first line. The second line shows the median and the range in brackets.

	N	Presurgery	1st Day	7th Day	30th Day	2nd Month	3rd Month	p
CH	42	7.10 (2.02) 7.3 (3.1–12.5)	7.74 (1.96) 7.9 (1.3–13.9)	7.72 (1.75) 7.35 (4.4–11)	6.95 (1.84) 6.9 (2.1–10.7)	7.25 (1.46) 7.55 (4.4–10.3)	7.81 (1.55) 8.15 (4.8–11.8)	0.031
CRF	42	9.44 (1.97) 9.25 (5.6–14.49)	6.34 (1.94) 6.45 (2.7–9.4)	6.5 (2.12) 6.5 (2.7–12.2)	7.19 (2.06) 6.65 (4.1–14)	7.35 (1.94) 7.35 (3.8–13.9)	7.85 (1.93) 7.2 (4.7–15.1)	<0.001
IOPcc	42	25.38 (7.48) 23.5 (11.2–43)	14.14 (9.03) 12.25 (0.2–42.7)	14.21 (6.75) 12.85 (4.7–32.2)	18.81 (7.69) 17.75 (6.2–43.5)	18.2 (5.82) 16.65 (6.2–36.9)	17.68 (6.09) 16.75 (6.3–31.9)	<0.001
IOPg	42	22.49 (7.47) 20.55 (11.9–39.1)	9.85 (7.63) 8.5 (5.1–30.7)	10.25 (6.78) 8.85 (5.0–26.8)	14.51 (7.54) 12.8 (5.4–31.3)	14.14 (6.1) 12.35 (5.2–25.9)	14.24 (6.24) 12.55 (5.9–26.1)	<0.001

CH: corneal hysteresis; CRF: corneal resistance factor; IOPcc: compensated intraocular pressure; IOPg: Goldmann-correlated intraocular pressure.

4. Discussion

IOP is the only risk factor in the development and progression of glaucomatous optic neuropathy that can be treated at the present time. It is essential to obtain a reliable measurement that allows us to reach a correct diagnosis and classification for the proper management and follow-up of the glaucoma patient. Nowadays, GAT is the gold standard. However, it is based on Imbert–Fick's law, which assumes conditions that are not real, such as that the cornea has a radius of constant curvature, which is always spherical, with minimal thickness, and that presents the same rigidity in all cases [24,25]. Further to this, a low degree of reproducibility of this measure has been demonstrated due to its interobserver variability [26]. In order to overcome these drawbacks, other devices have been developed, among which the ORA stands out. ORA is a non-contact instrument that provides a reproducible measurement of IOP that is not influenced by the person performing the test and that, perhaps most importantly, is based on biomechanical properties and parameters of the cornea [6,25]. Therefore, the ORA not only helps us to study and understand the properties of the cornea but also allows us to quantify the properties numerically. This allows us to compare the results obtained in order to standardize and look for ranges of normality, with which we can detect patients who deviate from them, and whose disease may be progressing due to the limitations of other devices.

Because ORA is a relatively new technology, available literature is limited. It is important to emphasize that in many studies, including ours, it is impossible to determine what proportion of the observed changes in corneal biomechanics and IOP are exclusively due to each of the interventions performed. New research would need to be designed in such a way as to isolate each factor that may affect these parameters.

In an attempt to address this issue, Touboul et al. [15] published a prospective study in 2008 in which they looked for correlations between the data provided by ORA across four different ophthalmological pathologies that they grouped into four groups: glaucoma ($n = 159$), keratoconus ($n = 88$), laser-assisted laser in situ keratomileusis (LASIK) ($n = 78$), and photorefractive keratectomy (PRK) ($n = 39$) (all vs. a control group without ophthalmic pathologies ($n = 122$)). The authors found statistically significant differences between GAT and IOPcc and IOPg in all pathological groups. It was also found that, in the general population, the higher the CH, the closer the values of GAT and IOPcc. CRF maintained similar values in the glaucoma group vs. the control group, while CH was lower and seemed independent of age.

Focusing on glaucomatous pathology, we know is that eyes with POAG show certain corneal characteristics that could also affect other structures of the eyeball. This could translate into a special susceptibility to increases in IOP at the level of structures such as lamina cribosa [27]. A significant decrease in CH is observed in patients with glaucoma (especially in cases of congenital glaucoma). With regard to CRF, elevated values were found in all glaucoma suspicion groups in different studies [25,28]. Of special interest is the research of Del Buey et al. [14], which analyzed 1065 eyes; the group describe a lower CH with a statistically significant difference in patients with glaucoma compared with healthy eyes. Additionally statistically significant was the difference with respect to IOPg and IOPcc in the group of patients with glaucoma and controls. Unexpectedly, the CRF was superior in all pathological groups with respect to control, but it was only significant in groups suspected of glaucoma, not in glaucoma patients. The data collected in our study were consistent with those discussed above, presenting a CH even lower with the IOPcc and the IOPg slightly higher. Perhaps the degree of severity of glaucoma can influence the parameters measured by ORA, our representative sample being of patients with moderate–severe glaucomatous damage with indication of surgery after the failure of other treatments and, therefore, being able to present more extreme averages than the group of glaucoma presented by Del Buey et al. [14].

Regarding eye surgery, the study of corneal biomechanical properties has centered mostly on phacoemulsification, and results have been obtained in different studies that indicate a decrease in CH values and an increase in CRF [24,29,30]. However, the evidence after glaucoma surgery is not very broad, despite being fundamental to understanding the intrinsic changes that may occur, and offers little evidence in terms of what real benefit surgical intervention will bring to the patient.

Our findings reflect those described for other glaucoma ophthalmological surgeries, such as those presented by Pakravan et al. [31]. Pakravan et al. found a significant increase in both CRF and CH in all groups of glaucomatous patients who were studied at 3 months following different surgeries (trabeculectomy with MMC (n = 23 eyes); trabeculectomy with MMC with phacoemulsification (n = 17 eyes)); Ahmed valve implantation (n = 17); cataract only in non-glaucomatous patients (n = 26 eyes)). This calls into question a possible relationship between the decrease in IOP (measured by GAT) and the increase in CH after treatment, which could be the first hypothesis to be considered for understanding the results of our study. The only ones who have described a weak correlation between both parameters, and only preoperatively, are Iordanidou et al. [32] and Sun et al. [22], who argue that ORA could make a mistake with the measurement of high pressures. It has even been shown that the change that occurs over 24 h in IOP does not affect biomechanical properties [33]. Sun et al. [22] analyzed a group of 40 patients with unilateral POAG who underwent trabeculectomy, achieving a statistically significant increase in CH only 2 weeks after the intervention. It would be comparable with what we obtained on day 1 and 7 after surgery. Unlike ours, one month after surgery its results do not reach statistical significance, although they remain above preoperative values, at which time we observed a marked decrease in CH. We should consider whether the changes produced by trabeculectomy (penetrating filter surgery) on corneal biomechanics are really more stable one month after the intervention than those caused by NPDS, therefore maintaining the upward trend despite not reaching statistically significant values.

If we search the literature for studies describing changes in corneal biomechanics through ORA produced by implant-associated surgery, there are very few results. Konstantinidis et al. [34] published a prospective study to compare corneal biomechanical changes in two groups: group 1 of patients with glaucoma who had an EX-PRESS® (Novartis, Basel, Switzerland) device implanted (n = 19) and group 2 who underwent a trabeculectomy (n = 11). Measurements were made of the eyes operated with ORA preoperatively and after surgery in months 1, 6, and 12. CH increased significantly for months 6 and 12 in group 1 and for all postoperative measures in group 2, compared with those obtained pre-surgery. Regarding the CRF parameter, it decreased significantly for both groups in all measures. Konstantinidis et al. found no correlation between CH and CRF. These results support our hypothesis that CH and CRF will follow the respective increasing and decreasing trend that we have found in our study. Similar changes between the two groups lead us to think that the introduction of an implant could have an influence similar to a piercing technique, although the sample size of each group was too small to validate this hypothesis by itself. On the other hand, it could be supported by the data provided by Casado et al. [35], which did not show statistically significant differences between two groups: the first formed by 20 eyes of 20 patients who underwent NPDS with implantation (Aquaflow; Staar Surgical AG, Nidau, Switzerland) and the second group by 20 eyes of the same 20 patients (the contralateral), with an intervention of sclerectomy converted to trabeculectomy. Group 1 had lower values (still reaching statistical significance) for both CH and CRF, which could be associated with a better prognosis due to worse results, which have been demonstrated in the visual field associated with lower CH values [17,20].

Special attention should be given to the work published by Iordanidou et al. [32], who were the first to use ORA technology to analyze 30 eyes of 30 patients with POAG to evaluate the biomechanical changes produced after an NPDS with a collagen implant (Staar Surgical AG, Nidau, Switzerland). They carried out a measurement on day 1 and 8, and at 1 month after surgery. Of the parameters studied, the only one whose variation remained statistically significant was CH, which increased the day after the surgery from 7.51 +/− 1.56 mmHg (in our study it was 7.10 +/− 2.02 mmHg) to 9.38 +/− 1.77 mmHg (7.74 +/− 1.96 mmHg), where it remained on day 8 with a value of 9.2 +/− 1.57 mmHg (in our case, on day 7 it was 7.72 +/− 1.75 mmHg) and then decreased to the figure of 8.41 +/− 1.72 mmHg per month after the NPDS (6.95 +/− 1.84 mmHg). The curve that CH draws was repeated in our study, presenting minor changes, although it also reached statistical significance, reaching the month of surgery, to descend below the preoperative level. Unlike Iordanidou et al. [32], who only follow up until the 30th postoperative day, we continued follow up for three months, analyzing the cases on days 1, 7, and 30 and at 2 and 3 months. We observed an increase in CH values at 2 and 3 months. In this study, IOPg had a preoperative mean value of 19.57 +/− 6.32 mmHg, which was drastically reduced the next day to a value of 5.2 +/− 3.49 mmHg, reaching statistical significance. Subsequently, IOPg began to increase without reaching statistical significance, reaching 8.32 +/− 5.37 mmHg on day 8 of the intervention and 12.71 +/− 7.43 mmHg one month after surgery. IOPcc and CRF initially decrease, to gradually increase without reaching the preoperative value, which makes us think that with a larger sample size or a longer monitoring time, these results could have reached statistical significance and support ours.

Following this same line, Díez-Álvarez et al. [19] published a prospective study of 49 patients with a mean age of 73.5 +/− 8.2 years who had been on anti-glaucomatous eye drops (77.6% with PGAs) and who were intervened with NPDS in combination with phacoemulsification (NPDS + P) in 26 cases or with and NPDS alone in the other 23 cases. The study analyses corneal biomechanics with ORA 3 months after surgery. Unlike the study presented above and ours, in no case did they accompany the surgery of an implant, which makes it difficult for us to compare results. Despite this, it presents a sample of size, age, and biomechanical data prior to surgery similar to ours. They performed a single postoperative measure, observing in both groups an increase in CH and a decrease in CRF, IOPcc, and IOPg. All measurements reached statistical significance and were consistent with our results. Based on their results, and despite preoperative values, the postoperative reduction in IOP was the independent factor that most influenced optic nerve changes after surgery.

We would like to point out that the first-month CH in our results followed a curve equal to that defined by Iordanidou et al. [32]; first ascends, and then descends, but after 3 months we find values greater than presurgical ones, as Díez-Álvarez et al. [19] also describe. This change in trend could be justified, or could at least be altered, by taking into account that an increase in CH associated with the use of PGAs has been demonstrated without being related to a decrease in IOP by GAT, by influencing extracellular matrix remodeling and modification of corneal properties [23,36,37]. In our study, all the participants had taken PGAs as a treatment prior to surgery, and PGAs are able to maintain their effect on corneal biomechanics after suspension for a few days and then gradually disappear [37]. On the other hand, the changes during the month after surgery could be altered by the use, according to the protocol, of eye drops with dexamethasone (TobraDex®) since it has been shown that it can increase IOP, although we have not found data in the literature on its effects on corneal biomechanics [38].

Our study has certain limitations, starting with the sample size, which might be limited due to the strict inclusion criteria of the study, which were put in place to ensure as homogeneous and reproducible a sample as possible, while avoiding as many confounding factors as possible. Another major limitation to highlight is the difficulty of comparing our results with other published studies. There are important works that establish biomechanical values in the healthy population, but not in a standardized way by age and sex groups. While we are able to find research in the literature on corneal biomechanics and glaucoma, the studies were quite heterogeneous in their methods and results. Regarding surgeries, the diversity was even greater since there are many techniques and devices to which the intrinsic variability is added with each surgeon who performs the procedure. In this sense, performing two different surgeries on the eyes of the same patient would be ideal to be able to compare them and thus establish differences, as Casado et al. [35] have reported. In the case of filtering surgery, it is necessary to consider the criteria of choice of each technique, which is usually determined by glaucomatous damage and its ability to decrease tension. Sclera deserves special consideration since it provides the anatomical support of the eye for many measurements we make, such as in the measurement of IOP by GAT and measurements by ORA. Therefore, surgeries such as trabeculectomy, in which the sclerectomy that is performed produces a thinning of the cornea–sclera interface, could clearly affect corneal biomechanics and its measurements. It has already been seen that structural changes of the eyeball affect its biomechanical properties, as described by Grost-Otero et al. [39] in a study in which they analyzed 20 patients who underwent surgery for pterygium in one eye and compared with the contralateral eye, finding a statistically significant decrease in CH in the first group with respect to the second. In addition, we must consider that there may be anatomical changes that are not completely restored, or that restore very slowly, after glaucoma surgery. That could be in favor of obtaining similar results, regardless of the technique or device used. Another limitation would be the failure to collect and analyze the data on CCT, axial length, and refraction, as these would be of interest. Regarding topical anti-glaucomatous hypotensive eye drops, there is evidence that affirms how PGAs influence corneal biomechanics, but evidence does not differ between the type of PGAs used, and the duration of treatment, or IOP prior to PGAs use [22,36]. The use of MMC (including duration and dose), as well as the use of an implant and in which location it is located, should also be considered. As we have already highlighted at the beginning of the discussion, other limitations would be that we were unable to determine what percentage of the biomechanical changes were due exclusively to the surgery, the implant, the use of MMC during surgery, the use of topical PGAs prior to surgery and its subsequent discontinuation, and the use of TobraDex® afterwards.

We believe our findings represent the first published study of which we are aware on variations in corneal biomechanics after an NPDS intervention, the surgery of choice in our environment, with Esnoper V-2000 implant, and the first whose evolution has been collected and analyzed throughout the first three post-surgical months. This would imply a greater sample size and a longer follow-up period than comparable studies presented in the existing literature, establishing how corneal biomechanics varies between the values before and after surgery.

5. Conclusions

According to our analysis, we conclude that at 3 months of follow-up, CRF remain below preoperative values, and CH above, after having decreased in the first month, reaching statistical significance in all measures. After the NPDS, as expected, the IOP was successfully maintained below preoperative values, being assessed by the IOPcc and IOPg values provided by the ORA.

More research is needed following this line with a larger sample size and longer follow-up periods and with more homogeneous groups in terms of age, glaucomatous damage, pre-surgery treatment, and surgical technique to evaluate the changes caused in corneal biomechanics and their relevance in clinical practice.

Author Contributions: Conceptualization, M.D.D.-B., I.S.-M., J.M. and J.I.; methodology, M.D.D.-B., I.S.-M. and J.I.; software, M.D.D.-B., I.P.-N. and J.I.; validation, M.D.D.-B., D.P. and J.I.; formal analysis, M.D.D.-B., I.S.-M. and J.I.; investigation, M.D.D.-B., I.S.-M., J.M. and J.I.; resources, M.D.D.-B., E.P.-C. and F.J.A.; data curation, M.D.D.-B., I.S.-M. and J.I.; writing—original draft preparation, M.D.D.-B., I.S.-M., J.M. and J.I.; writing—review and editing, M.D.D.-B., I.S.-M., A.B.-M. and J.I.; visualization, M.D.D.-B., A.B.-M. and J.I.; supervision, M.D.D.-B., I.S.-M., F.J.A. and J.I.; project administration, F.J.A. and J.I.; funding acquisition, F.J.A. and J.I. All authors have read and agreed to the published version of the manuscript.

Funding: This research received no external funding.

Institutional Review Board Statement: The study was conducted according to the guidelines of the Declaration of Helsinki, and the study was approved by the Review Committee of the Lozano Blesa University Clinical Hospital in Zaragoza C.P.—C.I. PI21/467.

Informed Consent Statement: Informed consent was obtained from all subjects involved in the study.

Conflicts of Interest: The authors declare no conflict of interest.

References

1. Bourne, R.R.A. Vision 2020: Where are we? *Curr. Opin. Ophthalmol.* **2020**, *31*, 81–84. [CrossRef]
2. Schuster, A.K.; Erb, C.; Hoffmann, E.M.; Dietlein, T.; Pfeiffer, N. The Diagnosis and Treatment of Glaucoma. *Dtsch Arztebl Int.* **2020**, *117*, 225–234. [CrossRef]
3. McMonnies, C.W. Glaucoma history and risk factors. *J. Optom.* **2017**, *10*, 71–78. [CrossRef]
4. Potop, V.; Corbu, C.; Coviltir, V.; Schmitzer, S.; Constantin, M.; Burcel, M.; Ionescu, C.; Dăscălescu, D. The importance of corneal assessment in a glaucoma suspect-A review. *Rom. J. Ophthalmol.* **2019**, *63*, 321–326. [CrossRef]
5. de Padua Soares Bezerra, B.; Chan, E.; Chakrabarti, R.; Vajpayee, R.B. Intraocular pressure measurement after corneal transplantation. *Surv. Ophthalmol.* **2019**, *64*, 639–646. [CrossRef]
6. Kaushik, S.; Pandav, S.S. Ocular Response Analyzer. *J. Curr. Glaucoma Pract.* **2012**, *6*, 17–19. [CrossRef]
7. del Buey Sayas, M.Á.; Peris Martínez, C. *Biomecánica y Arquitectura Corneal*; Elsevier Monografia Secoir: Amsterdam, The Netherlands, 2014.
8. Piñero, D.P.; Alcón, N. In vivo characterization of corneal biomechanics. *J. Cataract Refract. Surg.* **2014**, *40*, 870–887. [CrossRef]
9. Liu, J.; Roberts, C.J. Influence of corneal biomechanical properties on intraocular pressure measurement: Quantitative analysis. *J. Cataract Refract. Surg.* **2005**, *3*, 146–155. [CrossRef]
10. Tranchina, L.; Lombardo, M.; Oddone, F.; Serrao, S.; Schiano Lomoriello, D.; Ducoli, P. Influence of corneal biomechanical properties on intraocular pressure differences between an air-puff tonometer and the Goldmann applanation tonometer. *J. Glaucoma* **2013**, *22*, 416–421. [CrossRef]
11. Vinciguerra, R.; Ambrósio, R., Jr.; Elsheikh, A.; Roberts, C.J.; Lopes, B.; Morenghi, E.; Azzolini, C.; Vinciguerra, P. Detection of Keratoconus With a New Biomechanical Index. *J. Refract. Surg.* **2016**, *32*, 803–810. [CrossRef]
12. Jędzierowska, M.; Koprowski, R.; Wilczyński, S.; Krysik, K. A new method for detecting the outer corneal contour in images from an ultra-fast Scheimpflug camera. *Biomed. Eng. Online* **2019**, *18*, 115. [CrossRef]
13. Deol, M.; Taylor, D.A.; Radcliffe, N.M. Corneal hysteresis and its relevance to glaucoma. *Curr. Opin. Ophthalmol.* **2015**, *26*, 96–102. [CrossRef]
14. Del Buey-Sayas, M.; Lanchares-Sancho, E.; Campins-Falcó, P.; Pinazo-Durán, M.D.; Peris-Martínez, C. Corneal Biomechanical Parameters and Central Corneal Thickness in Glaucoma Patients, Glaucoma Suspects, and a Healthy Population. *J. Clin. Med.* **2021**, *10*, 2637. [CrossRef]
15. Touboul, D.; Roberts, C.; Kérautret, J.; Garra, C.; Maurice-Tison, S.; Saubusse, E.; Colin, J. Correlations between corneal hysteresis, intraocular pressure, and corneal central pachymetry. *J. Cataract Refract. Surg.* **2008**, *34*, 616–622. [CrossRef]
16. Shah, S.; Laiquzzaman, M.; Cunliffe, I.; Mantry, S. The use of the Reichert ocular response analyser to establish the relationship between ocular hysteresis, corneal resistance factor and central corneal thickness in normal eyes. *Contact Lens Anterior Eye* **2006**, *29*, 257–262. [CrossRef]
17. Liang, L.; Zhang, R.; He, L.Y. Corneal hysteresis and glaucoma. *Int. Ophthalmol.* **2019**, *39*, 1909–1916. [CrossRef]
18. Susanna, C.N.; Diniz-Filho, A.; Daga, F.B.; Susanna, B.N.; Zhu, F.; Ogata, N.G.; Medeiros, F.A. A Prospective Longitudinal Study to Investigate Corneal Hysteresis as a Risk Factor for Predicting Development of Glaucoma. *Am. J. Ophthalmol.* **2018**, *187*, 148–152. [CrossRef]
19. Díez-Álvarez, L.; Muñoz-Negrete, F.J.; Casas-Llera, P.; Oblanca, N.; de Juan, V.; Rebolleda, G. Relationship between corneal biomechanical properties and optic nerve head changes after deep sclerectomy. *Eur. J. Ophthalmol.* **2017**, *27*, 535–541. [CrossRef]

20. Susanna, B.N.; Ogata, N.G.; Jammal, A.A.; Susanna, C.N.; Berchuck, S.I.; Medeiros, F.A. Corneal Biomechanics and Visual Field Progression in Eyes with Seemingly Well-Controlled Intraocular Pressure. *Ophthalmology* **2019**, *126*, 1640–1646. [CrossRef]
21. Gordon, M.O.; Beiser, J.A.; Brandt, J.D.; Heuer, D.K.; Higginbotham, E.J.; Johnson, C.A.; Keltner, J.L.; Miller, J.P.; Parrish, R.K., 2nd; Wilson, M.R.; et al. The Ocular Hypertension Treatment Study: Baseline factors that predict the onset of primary open-angle glaucoma. *Arch Ophthalmol.* **2002**, *120*, 714–720; discussion 829–830. [CrossRef]
22. Sun, L.; Shen, M.; Wang, J.; Fang, A.; Xu, A.; Fang, H.; Lu, F. Recovery of corneal hysteresis after reduction of intraocular pressure in chronic primary angle-closure glaucoma. *Am. J. Ophthalmol.* **2009**, *147*, 1061–1066. [CrossRef]
23. Bolívar, G.; Sánchez-Barahona, C.; Teus, M.; Castejón, M.A.; Paz-Moreno-Arrones, J.; Gutiérrez-Ortiz, C.; Mikropoulos, D.G. Effect of topical prostaglandin analogues on corneal hysteresis. *Acta Ophthalmol.* **2015**, *93*, e495–e498. [CrossRef]
24. de Freitas Valbon, B.; Ventura, M.P.; da Silva, R.S.; Canedo, A.L.; Velarde, G.C.; Ambrósio, R., Jr. Central corneal thickness and biomechanical changes after clear corneal phacoemulsification. *J. Refract. Surg.* **2012**, *28*, 215–219. [CrossRef]
25. Doughty, M.J.; Zaman, M.L. Human corneal thickness and its impact on intraocular pressure measures: A review and meta-analysis approach. *Surv. Ophthalmol.* **2000**, *44*, 367–408. [CrossRef]
26. Pearce, J.G.; Maddess, T. The Clinical Interpretation of Changes in Intraocular Pressure Measurements Using Goldmann Applanation Tonometry: A Review. *J. Glaucoma* **2019**, *28*, 302–306. [CrossRef]
27. Grise-Dulac, A.; Saad, A.; Abitbol, O.; Febbraro, J.L.; Azan, E.; Moulin-Tyrode, C.; Gatinel, D. Assessment of corneal biomechanical properties in normal tension glaucoma and comparison with open-angle glaucoma, ocular hypertension, and normal eyes. *J. Glaucoma* **2012**, *21*, 486–489. [CrossRef]
28. Medeiros, F.A.; Weinreb, R.N. Evaluation of the influence of corneal biomechanical properties on intraocular pressure measurements using the ocular response analyzer. *J. Glaucoma* **2006**, *15*, 364–370. [CrossRef]
29. Kucumen, R.B.; Yenerel, N.M.; Gorgun, E.; Kulacoglu, D.N.; Oncel, B.; Kohen, M.C.; Alimgil, M.L. Corneal biomechanical properties and intraocular pressure changes after phacoemulsification and intraocular lens implantation. *J. Cataract Refract. Surg.* **2008**, *34*, 2096–2098. [CrossRef]
30. Hager, A.; Loge, K.; Füllhas, M.O.; Schroeder, B.; Grossherr, M.; Wiegand, W. Changes in corneal hysteresis after clear corneal cataract surgery. *Am. J. Ophthalmol.* **2007**, *144*, 341–346. [CrossRef]
31. Pakravan, M.; Afroozifar, M.; Yazdani, S. Corneal Biomechanical Changes Following Trabeculectomy, Phaco-trabeculectomy, Ahmed Glaucoma Valve Implantation and Phacoemulsification. *J. Ophthalmic Vis. Res.* **2014**, *9*, 7–13.
32. Iordanidou, V.; Hamard, P.; Gendron, G.; Labbé, A.; Raphael, M.; Baudouin, C. Modifications in corneal biomechanics and intraocular pressure after deep sclerectomy. *J. Glaucoma* **2010**, *19*, 252–256. [CrossRef] [PubMed]
33. Kida, T.; Liu, J.H.; Weinreb, R.N. Effect of 24-hour corneal biomechanical changes on intraocular pressure measurement. *Investig. Ophthalmol. Vis. Sci.* **2006**, *47*, 4422–4426. [CrossRef] [PubMed]
34. Konstantinidis, A.; Panagiotopoulou, E.K.; Panos, G.D.; Sideroudi, H.; Mehmet, A.; Labiris, G. The Effect of Antiglaucoma Procedures (Trabeculectomy vs. Ex-PRESS Glaucoma Drainage Implant) on the Corneal Biomechanical Properties. *J. Clin. Med.* **2021**, *10*, 802. [CrossRef]
35. Casado, A.; Cabarga, C.; Pérez-Sarriegui, A.; Fuentemilla, E. Differences in Corneal Biomechanics in Nonpenetrating Deep Sclerectomy and Deep Sclerectomy Reconverted into Trabeculectomy. *J. Glaucoma* **2017**, *26*, 15–19. [CrossRef]
36. Poostchi, A.; Nicholas, S.; Wells, A.P. Recovery of corneal hysteresis after reduction of intraocular pressure in chronic primary angle-closure glaucoma. *Am. J. Ophthalmol.* **2009**, *149*, 525. [CrossRef]
37. Meda, R.; Wang, Q.; Paoloni, D.; Harasymowycz, P.; Brunette, I. The impact of chronic use of prostaglandin analogues on the biomechanical properties of the cornea in patients with primary open-angle glaucoma. *Br. J. Ophthalmol.* **2017**, *101*, 120–125. [CrossRef]
38. Pleyer, U.; Ursell, P.G.; Rama, P. Intraocular pressure effects of common topical steroids for post-cataract inflammation: Are they all the same? *Ophthalmol. Ther.* **2013**, *2*, 55–72. [CrossRef] [PubMed]
39. Gros-Otero, J.; Pérez-Rico, C.; Montes-Mollón, M.A.; Gutiérrez-Ortiz, C.; Benítez-Herreros, J.; Teus, M.A. Effects of pterygium on the biomechanical properties of the cornea: A pilot study. *Arch Soc. Esp. Oftalmol.* **2013**, *88*, 134–138. [CrossRef]

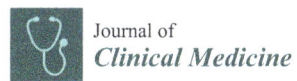

Journal of
Clinical Medicine

Review

Management of Childhood Glaucoma Following Cataract Surgery

Anne-Sophie Simons [1,2,*], Ingele Casteels [1,2], John Grigg [3], Ingeborg Stalmans [1,2], Evelien Vandewalle [1,2] and Sophie Lemmens [1,2]

1   Department of Ophthalmology, University Hospitals UZ Leuven, Herestraat 49, 3000 Leuven, Belgium; ingele.casteels@uzleuven.be (I.C.); ingeborg.stalmans@uzleuven.be (I.S.); evelien.vandewalle@uzleuven.be (E.V.); sophie.1.lemmens@uzleuven.be (S.L.)
2   Biomedical Sciences Group, Department of Neurosciences, Research Group Ophthalmology, KU Leuven, Herestraat 49, 3000 Leuven, Belgium
3   Faculty of Medicine and Health, Save Sight Institute, The University of Sydney, 8 Macquarie St., Sydney, NSW 2000, Australia; john.grigg@sydney.edu.au
*   Correspondence: anne-sophie.simons@uzleuven.be; Tel.: +32-16-34-62-28

Citation: Simons, A.-S.; Casteels, I.; Grigg, J.; Stalmans, I.; Vandewalle, E.; Lemmens, S. Management of Childhood Glaucoma Following Cataract Surgery. *J. Clin. Med.* **2022**, *11*, 1041. https://doi.org/10.3390/jcm11041041

Academic Editors: Maria Letizia Salvetat, Marco Zeppieri and Paolo Brusini

Received: 13 January 2022
Accepted: 14 February 2022
Published: 17 February 2022

Publisher's Note: MDPI stays neutral with regard to jurisdictional claims in published maps and institutional affiliations.

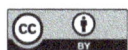
Abstract: Glaucoma remains a frequent serious complication following cataract surgery in children. The optimal approach to management for 'glaucoma following cataract surgery' (GFCS), one of the paediatric glaucoma subtypes, is an ongoing debate. This review evaluates the various management options available and aims to propose a clinical management strategy for GFCS cases. A literature search was conducted in four large databases (Cochrane, PubMed, Embase, and Web of Science), from 1995 up to December 2021. Thirty-nine studies—presenting (1) eyes with GFCS; a disease entity as defined by the Childhood Glaucoma Research Network Classification, (2) data on treatment outcomes, and (3) follow-up data of at least 6 months—were included. Included papers report on GFCS treated with angle surgery, trabeculectomy, glaucoma drainage device implantation (GDD), and cyclodestructive procedures. Medical therapy is the first-line treatment in GFCS, possibly to bridge time to surgery. Multiple surgical procedures are often required to adequately control GFCS. Angle surgery (360 degree) may be considered before proceeding to GDD implantation, since this technique offers good results and is less invasive. Literature suggests that GDD implantation gives the best chance for long-term IOP control in childhood GFCS and some studies put this technique forward as a good choice for primary surgery. Cyclodestruction seems to be effective in some cases with uncontrolled IOP. Trabeculectomy should be avoided, especially in children under the age of one year and children that are left aphakic. The authors provide a flowchart to guide the management of individual GFCS cases.

Keywords: childhood glaucoma; aphakia; pseudophakia; cataract surgery; lensectomy; management (or therapy); trabeculotomy; trabeculectomy; glaucoma drainage device; cyclodestruction

1. Introduction

Former terms used to describe childhood glaucoma, including 'developmental', 'congenital', or 'infantile', were often not clearly defined [1–3]. Therefore, the Childhood Glaucoma Research Network Classification recently developed a system for the classification of paediatric glaucoma to unify nomenclature (Figure 1) [3]. This review focuses on the subtype known as glaucoma following cataract surgery (GFCS), which accounts for 18% of childhood glaucoma [4].

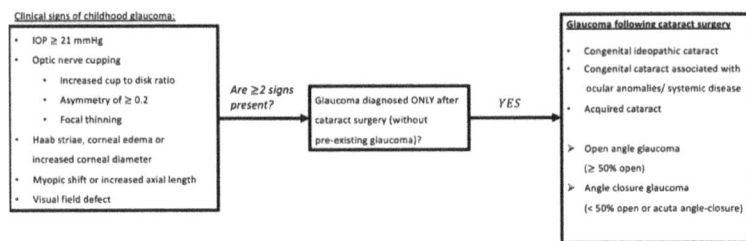

Figure 1. Glaucoma Following Cataract Surgery based on Childhood Glaucoma Research Network classification algorithm. Childhood: based on national criteria, <18 years old (USA); <16 years old (UK, Europe, UNICEF) (reproduced with permission from Grajewski, World Glaucoma Association Consensus Series 9: Childhood glaucoma, Kugler publications 2013 [5]). Abbreviations: IOP = Intra-Ocular Pressure.

After cataract extraction in early life, both aphakic and pseudophakic eyes are at high and lifelong risk for the development of glaucoma (GFCS, formerly known as aphakic or pseudophakic glaucoma). The incidence depends on duration of follow-up, age at time of surgery, corneal diameter, surgical techniques, and the definition of glaucoma among studies [6–8]. In the Infant Aphakia Treatment Study (IATS), a randomized clinical trial of 114 infants with unilateral congenital cataract who were aged 1 to 6 months at surgery, the incidence of GFCS was 22% after 10 years of follow-up [9]. Improved surgical techniques for childhood cataract extraction have reduced the incidence of angle-closure GFCS. The predominant type, accounting for 75 to 94% of GFCS, now has an open angle configuration [10]. Unlike angle-closure glaucoma, which is diagnosed in the early postoperative period, the incidence of open-angle glaucoma is known to rise with increasing postsurgical follow-up, and its presentation may occur any time after initially uneventful surgery [11]. Consequently, it is imperative that these patients receive lifelong follow-up in order to protect their vision.

The pathophysiological mechanism by which secondary glaucoma develops in these patients, who have a history of paediatric cataract, is still unclear and thought to be of multifactorial origin. A mechanical and a chemical theory have been hypothesized: (1) the mechanical support to the trabecular meshwork is lost after lensectomy and contributes to decreased trabecular spaces, potentially reducing outflow facility, or (2) the influence of chemical substances from the vitreous cavity and retained lens material may alter trabecular meshwork morphology and gene expression [12–14]. Further, early lensectomy and early use of high-dose steroids may also lead to structural alteration of the trabecular meshwork and associated impairment of normal angle maturation [11,15].

Age at time of lensectomy and microcornea are the two risk factors most commonly associated with a higher prevalence of GFCS [16]. The optimal timing of lensectomy is still under debate because the increased risk of developing GFCS must be balanced against the risk of irreversible deprivation amblyopia [10]. Until a few years ago, it was thought that pseudophakia was a protective factor for the development of GFCS [17]. However, selection bias in the possibility that children selected for intraocular lens placement have largely been those at lower risk for glaucoma may explain the observed lower incidence of glaucoma in pseudophakia in some initial small or non-randomised studies [16]. The IoLunder 2 Study and the Infant Aphakia Treatment Study (IATS) showed that the risk of glaucoma development at 5 and 10 years post lensectomy, respectively, is similar for aphakic and pseudophakic patients [9,18,19].

GFCS is often difficult to manage, and it is generally associated with a poor prognosis. The first-line treatment for most GFCS cases is medical [11,20]. When surgical intervention is indicated, the optimal surgical approach is subject to debate. Many studies reporting treatment outcomes of childhood glaucoma in general are available, but studies that focus on this particular glaucoma subtype are limited, resulting in a lack of consensus. This review summarizes the literature on the various medical and surgical options available for the management of GFCS, with the aim to suggest an appropriate management strategy for specific clinical GFCS cases. This paper provides a flowchart which may assist ophthalmologists treating GFCS patients in clinical decision-making.

2. Materials and Methods

This literature review was registered and approved by KU Leuven. In performing this review, the PRISMA statement (Preferred Reporting Items for Systematic Review and Meta-Analysis) was followed [21].

The databases Cochrane, PubMed, Embase, and Web of Science were systematically searched (from 1 January 1995 to 31 December 2021). A detailed search strategy for each database is presented in Appendix A. The individual references of each study were considered in order to identify additional relevant articles. Non-pertinent articles were rejected based on title and abstract screening. Thereafter, the full texts of the remaining articles were independently judged for eligibility by two independent reviewers (A.S., S.L.) according to the following inclusion criteria: the studies should (1) include eyes with GFCS; a disease entity as defined by the Childhood Glaucoma Research Network Classification (Figure 1), (2) report data on treatment outcomes, and (3) present follow-up data of at least six months after glaucoma therapy. Reviews that do not report original research results, non-English-language articles, and abstract-only articles were excluded. Inconsistencies were solved by consensus. The PRISMA flow diagram (Figure 2) gives details on the screening process. The authors performed a narrative synthesis because methodological heterogeneity precluded a meta-analysis. The Oxford Centre for Evidence-based Medicine classification was used to determine the Level Of Evidence (LOE) of the included papers [22].

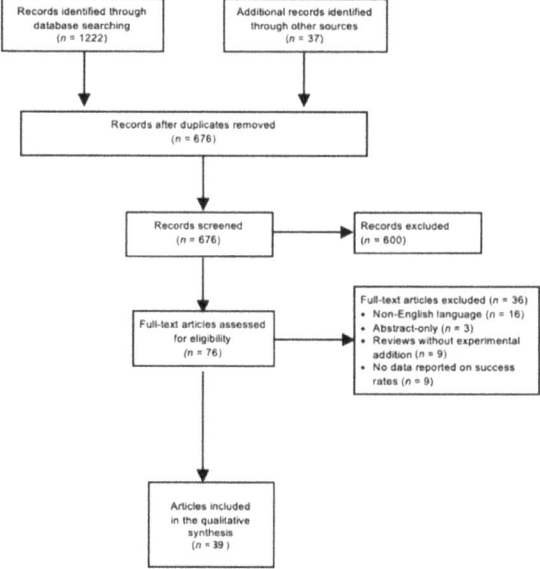

Figure 2. Literature search: PRISMA Consort flow diagram. According to THE PRISMA Statement 2009 [19]. Abbreviations: PRISMA = Preferred Reporting Items for Systematic Reviews and Meta-Analyses; *n* = amount of articles.

3. Results

A total of 676 studies were screened using the described search strategy. At the end of the selection process, 39 articles were judged eligible for qualitative synthesis: 1 randomized controlled trial, 21 cohort studies, and 17 case series were included in the systematic review. In the following sections, summary tables of findings of included papers are provided. Medical therapy, angle surgery, trabeculectomy, glaucoma drainage device (GDD) implantation, and cyclodestructive procedures are mainly discussed. Five out of 39 studies described success rate with medication alone, 7 studies examined success rates of angle surgery, 8 studies examined success rates of trabeculectomy, 14 studies examined success rates of drainage implants, and 9 out of 39 studies examined success rates of cyclodestructive procedures.

3.1. Medical Treatment

Only five studies in which initial treatment was medical in all of the included eyes with GFCS clearly described their success rates with medication alone (Table 1) [23–27].

Success rates between the five available studies range from 17 to 73%, with those three reporting success rates of 40% and more having the largest study cohorts. Unlike PCG, which responds inadequately to medical therapy, these studies showed that long-term intra-ocular pressure (IOP) control can be reached with medication alone in some patients with GFCS. Medical therapy consists of topical medications and systemic medications, alone or in combination, in order to achieve the best possible result. Beta-blockers, carbonic anhydrase inhibitors, miotics and prostaglandin analogues are the classes commonly used for treatment of GFCS [23,24]. In a retrospective series of 32 eyes with GFCS, the addition of echothiophate iodide (EI) 0.125%, a miotic, in combination with other medications reduced IOP about 33% over long-term follow-up. The side-effects of EI were limited to transient redness that did not necessitate cessation of treatment [27].

3.2. Surgical Treatment

According to the literature, surgery is required in 27–83% of GFCS cases (Table 1) [23–26]. Repeat surgery and multiple modalities are often indicated to avoid or at least slow down further glaucoma progression. Similar ratios regarding the number of required repeat surgeries are reported, with 30–40% of eyes needing only one surgery and more than half of included study eyes needing two or more sequential surgical interventions [23,24]. One study documented the need of four or more procedures in 7% of eyes after a follow-up period of 18.7 years [24].

Included papers report on GFCS treated with angle surgery, trabeculectomy, GDD implantation, and cyclodestructive procedures.

3.2.1. Angle Surgery

Data documenting this treatment modality in GFCS are limited and mostly presented by small retrospective cohorts with variably reported success rates (16–93%) (Table 2) [10,28–33]. Prior work found a success rate of only 16% after conventional angle surgery, including a 180-degee trabeculotomy or goniotomy [10]. This is in stark contrast with more recent studies in which success following angle surgery was achieved in the majority of eyes following a 360-degree trabeculotomy [28–30,32,33], with the most recent case series showing a success rate of 93% after a mean follow-up of 3.3 years [33]. The 360-degree trabeculotomy showed higher surgical success rates compared to conventional 180-degree goniotomy and trabeculotomy [29,32]. No visually devastating complications have been reported in the included studies.

Less favourable outcomes were reported in GFCS eyes with peripheral anterior synechiae [28,30].

3.2.2. Trabeculectomy (+Antimetabolites)

Results of trabeculectomy + Mitomycin C in eyes with GFCS are variable but generally poor (Table 3) [10,23,34–39] with the largest cohort on this subject reporting a 25% success rate after a mean follow-up of 8.6 years [10].

Table 1. Relevant studies involving success rates with medications alone and the need for surgical treatment in GFCS eyes.

Author, Year, Study Design (LOE) Reference	Inclusion and Exclusion Criteria	Mean Pre-Treatment IOP ± SD (mmHg)	Mean Age at GDx ± SD (Years)	n Eyes (a-p)	Success Criteria	Success Rate with Medications Alone (%) Number of Drugs (% of Cases)	Need for Surgery (%) Number of Operations (% of Cases)	Mean (*) Follow-Up ± SD (Years)
Bhola et al. (2006), retrospective cohort study (2b) [24]	Inclusion: • IOP > 25 mmHg following congenital cataract surgery. Exclusion: • Lensectomy > 10 y; • Ocular conditions; • Systemic syndromes; • Traumatic cataracts; • PCG; Follow-up < 1 y.	32 ± 6	7	55 (55-0)	IOP ≤ 25 mmHg	73 / 1–2 (36) / 3 (33) / ≥4 (31) / B-blockers, Cholinergic agents, Adrenergic agonists, Carbonic anhydrase inhibitors, Prostaglandin analogues.	27 / 1 (40) / 2–3 (53) / 4–6 (7) / Goniotomy, trabeculotomy, trabeculectomy ± MMC, GDD implantation, cyclodestruction.	18.7 ± 8
Comer et al. (2011), retrospective cohort study (2b) [25]	Inclusion: • Persistently elevated IOP, and/or evidence of corneal enlargement, and/or optic disc cupping. Exclusion: • Primary intraocular lens implantation; • Lensectomy > 1 y; • Pre-existing glaucoma; Ocular conditions	28.6 ± 5.9	2.6	18 (18-0)	IOP ≤ 20 mmHg	17 / *Not further specified*	83 ≥ 2 (61) GDD implantation, trabeculectomy + MMC, goniotomy, cyclodestruction.	6.5
Kraus et al. (2015), retrospective case series (4) [27]	Inclusion: • Aphakic and pseudophakic children < 18 y from 1992 to 2013 • EI Exposure • Glaucoma following cataract surgery was defined according to the consensus established by The Childhood Glaucoma Research Network Classification Exclusion: -	32.1	3.2	32 (27-5)	IOP-lowering effect of: • 5–10 mmHg • < 5 mmHg	41 / 37 / EI	12.5 / trabeculotomy, GDD implantation	7.88

Table 1. *Cont.*

Author, Year, Study Design (LOE) Reference	Inclusion and Exclusion Criteria	Mean Pre-Treatment IOP ± SD (mmHg)	Mean Age at GDx ± SD (Years)	n Eyes (a-p)	Success Criteria	Success Rate with Medications Alone (%) Number of Drugs (% of Cases)	Need for Surgery (%) Number of Operations (% of Cases)	Mean (*) Follow-Up ± SD (Years)
Baris et al. (2019), retrospective cohort study (2b) [23]	Inclusion: • IOP > 25 mmHg following congenital cataract surgery. Exclusion: • Pre-existing glaucoma; • Anterior segment dysgenesis; • Severe microphthalmia; • Previous laser.	29.8 ± 14.8	1 ± 2.1	40 (40-0)	IOP < 21 mmHg	50 1 (75) 2 (20) 3 (5) First choice: dorzolamide-timolol combination; Second choice: prostaglandin analogues.	50 1 (30) 2 (20) ≥3 (50) First choice: trabeculectomy +MMC (0.2 mg/mL for 4 min); Second choice: GDD implantation; Third choice: cyclodestruction	6.6 ± 2.6
Spiess et al (2020), retrospective cohort study (2b) [26]	Inclusion: • Paediatric patients with GFCS from 1996 to 2016; • Glaucoma following cataract surgery was defined according to the consensus established by The Childhood Glaucoma Research Network Classification • Glaucoma Association in 2018) as intraocular pressure (IOP) greater than 21 mmHg with associated anatomical optic disc changes or other signs of progressive myopia. Exclusion: • Acquired cataracts, trauma, aniridia, Lowe syndrome, an age of 2 years and older with congenital cataract surgery, and previous/concomitant ocular hypertension or primary intraocular lens (IOL) implantation	29.1 ± 5.6	-	58 (47-9)	IOP < 21 mmHg with or without medication	41 40% monotherapy 60% combination therapy The most frequently prescribed drugs were beta-blockers (82%), followed by carbonic anhydrase inhibitors, prostaglandins, and alpha-2 adrenergic agonists.	59 70% tube implantation 24% trabeculectomy 6% peripheral iridotomy	4.6 *

Abbreviations: GDx = Glaucoma diagnosis; LOE = level of evidence; SD = Standard Deviation; GFCS = Glaucoma Following Cataract Surgery; a = aphakic; p = pseudophakic; mg = milligram; mL = millilitre; min = minutes; GDD = Glaucoma Drainage Device; IOP = Intra-Ocular Pressure; PCG = Primary Congenital Glaucoma; MMC = Mitomycin C; IOL = Intra-Ocular Lens, n = amount; (*) = or median; EI = Echothiophate iodide.

Table 2. Relevant studies involving angle surgery in GFCS eyes.

Author, Year, Study Design (LOE) Reference	Inclusion and Exclusion Criteria	Mean Pre-Treatment IOP ± SD (mmHg)	Mean Age at GDx ± SD (y)	Mean (* Median) Age at Glaucoma Surgery ± SD (y)	n Eyes (a-p)	Procedure	Success Criteria	Success Rate (%)	Mean (*) Follow-Up ± SD (y)	Factors Affecting Treatment Outcomes % of Eyes That Had Prior Glaucoma Surgery
Chen et al. (2004), retrospective cohort study (2b) [10]	Inclusion: • IOP > 25 mmHg following congenital cataract surgery; • Lensectomy < 20 y. Exclusion: • Pre-existing glaucoma; • History of trauma; • Intraocular neoplasm; • Radiation therapy; • Anterior uveitis; • anterior segment dysgenesis; • Ocular syndromes; • PCG; • Corticosteroid use before lensectomy.	-	-	-	24 (24-0)	Goniotomy and rigid-probe Trabeculectomy Ab externo	IOP ≤ 21 mmHg with and without medications and with no need for further surgery.	16	8.6 ± 7.6	*Not specified*
Bothun et al. (2010), retrospective cohort study (2b) [28]	Inclusion: • Medically refractory glaucoma; • IOP > 25 mmHg following congenital cataract surgery; • Changes in corneal diameter or clarity; • Increased axial length; • Increased optic-nerve cupping; • A combination of the above. Exclusion: • Anterior segment dysgenesis; • Microcornea (corneal diameter < 9.5 mm); • Pre-existing glaucoma; • Follow-up < 1 y.	35 ± 10	-	3.1	14 (14-0)	Goniotomy and/or rigid-probe trabeculotomy (lateral 180° initially, repeat nasal 180°) Ab externo	IOP ≤ 24 mmHg with or without topical medication; a lack of sight-threatening complication; and avoidance of trabeculectomy or GDD.	57 (after a mean of 1.4 angle surgeries per eye) 43 (after a single procedure)	4.7	Eyes with initial trabeculotomy required fewer procedures than those with an initial goniotomy. 0%

Table 2. *Cont.*

Author, Year, Study Design (LOE) Reference	Inclusion and Exclusion Criteria	Mean Pre-Treatment IOP ± SD (mmHg)	Mean Age at GDx ± SD (y)	Mean (* Median) Age at Glaucoma Surgery ± SD (y)	n Eyes (a-p)	Procedure	Success Criteria	Success Rate (%)	Mean (*) Follow-Up ± SD (y)	Factors Affecting Treatment Outcomes % of Eyes That Had Prior Glaucoma Surgery
Beck et al. (2011), retrospective case series (4) [29]	Inclusion: • Glaucoma following congenital cataract surgery, diagnosed < 3 y. Exclusion: • Three or more clock hours of peripheral anterior synechiae; • Iridocorneal adhesions; • Pre-existing glaucoma.	33.0 ± 7.2	-	* 5.0	4 (4-0)	360-degree suture trabeculotomy Ab externo	IOP < 22 mmHg with and without medication.	75	* 1.6	- 0%
Dao et al. (2014), retrospective case series (4) [30]	Inclusion: • Medically refractory glaucoma following lensectomy. Exclusion: • Pre-existing glaucoma; • Anterior segment anomalies; • Extensive synechiae; • PCG; • Surgical interventions other than planned	35.4 ± 4.7	-	3.1	13 (10-3) All open angle	360° microcatheter trabeculotomy Ab externo	IOP ≤ 22 mmHg with 30% reduction, without disease progression, oral glaucoma medications or additional glaucoma surgery.	62	1.4	- 0%
Lim et al. (2017), retrospective case series (2b) [32]	Inclusion: • Medically refractory glaucoma following cataract surgery; • Micro-assisted trabeculotomy as initial surgical procedure. Exclusion: • Prior glaucoma surgery (laser or incisional); • Suture trabeculotomy; • Second eyes receiving subsequent 360-degree trabeculotomy; Coexisting ocular or systemic syndrome.	31.5 ± 7.5	3.3 ± 3.9	5.6 ± 5.6	25 (19-6)	360° microcatheter trabeculotomy Ab externo	IOP ≤ 22 mmHg and 20% reduction without additional glaucoma surgery or devastating complication.	72	2.7 ± 2.2	Lens status (p = 0.88) 0%

Table 2. *Cont.*

Author, Year, Study Design (LOE) Reference	Inclusion and Exclusion Criteria	Mean Pre-Treatment IOP ± SD (mmHg)	Mean Age at GDx ± SD (y)	Mean (* Median) Age at Glaucoma Surgery ± SD (y)	n Eyes (a-p)	Procedure	Success Criteria	Success Rate (%)	Mean (*) Follow-Up ± SD (y)	Factors Affecting Treatment Outcomes % of Eyes That Had Prior Glaucoma Surgery
El Sayed et al. (2020), prospective cohort study (2b) [31]	**Inclusion:** • Children ≤ 14 years who required surgery for GFCS. **Exclusion:** • Synechial angle closure over >90°; • Requirement of combined procedures; • Previous procedures other than lensectomy or IOL implantation; • Eyes in which the trabeculotomy involved < 180° of Schlemm's canal	26.8 ± 8.2	-	5.73 ± 1.79	29 (16-13)	Two-site rigid probe trabeculotomy 180–360° Ab externo	IOP <23 mmHg or 30% IOP reduction, on the same or fewer number of medications at 1 year, without the need for another glaucoma procedure	89.6 (51.7% without medications)	1.4	No significant difference in the final IOP of aphakic and pseudophakic eyes. 0%
Rojas et al. (2020), retrospective case series [33]	**Inclusion:** • Children ≤ 18 years who underwent trabeculotomy January 2013 and July 2019 **Exclusion:-**	27.1 ± 7	-	7.8 ± 5.8	15 (12-3)	360° microcatheter trabeculotomy Ab externo	5 < IOP < 20 without additional surgery	93	3.3 ± 2.4	- 0%

Abbreviations: GDx = Glaucoma diagnosis; LOE = level of evidence; SD = Standard Deviation; GFCS = Glaucoma Following Cataract Surgery; a = aphakic; p = pseudophakic; min = minute; GDD = Glaucoma Drainage Device; IOP = Intra-Ocular Pressure; PCG = Primary Congenital Glaucoma; mm = millimetres; y = years; (*) = or median; ° = degree.

Table 3. Relevant studies involving trabeculectomy in GFCS eyes.

Author, Year, Study Design (LOE) Reference	Inclusion and Exclusion Criteria	Mean Pre-Treatment IOP ± SD (mmHg)	Mean Age at GDx ± SD (y)	Mean (*) Age at Glaucoma Surgery ± SD (y)	n eyes (a-p)	Antimetabolites	Success Criteria	Success Rate (%)	Mean (*) Follow-Up ± sd (y)	Factors Affecting Treatment Outcomes % of Eyes That Had Prior Glaucoma Surgery
Beck et al. (1998), retrospective case series (4) [35]	Inclusion: • Glaucoma (not further defined) following congenital cataract surgery; • ≤17 y. Exclusion: -	35.8 ± 8.0	-	7.6	9 (7-2)	MMC 0.25 mg/mL for 5 min	IOP ≤ 22 mmHg with and without medication, no evidence of glaucoma progression, no further need of glaucoma surgery.	78	2.5 ± 1.3	Age < 1 y (p = 0.0005) Aphakia (p = 0.0364) Anterior segment dysgenesis/aniridia (p = 0.49) *Not specified*
Wallace et al. (1998), retrospective cohort study (2b) [39]	Inclusion: • Glaucoma (not further defined) after congenital cataract surgery; • Need of glaucoma surgery < 18 y. Exclusion: PCG.	35.9	6.1	8.7	13 (13-0)	MMC 0.2 to 0.4 mg/mL for 4 min	IOP ≤ 25 mmHg without medications and IOP ≤ 21 mmHg with medications.	62	4.2	– *Not specified*
Aztuara-Blanco et al. (1999), retrospective case series (4) [34]	Inclusion: • Glaucoma (not further defined) following congenital cataract surgery; • Aphakia; • <18 y. Exclusion: -	35.7 ± 10.5	-	5.7 ± 5.0	8 (8-0)	MMC 0.4 mg/mL for 1–5 min	Absolute success: IOP < 21 mmHg with no antiglaucoma medications, with apparently stable glaucoma and absence of severe complications. Relative success: No performance of or recommendation for further glaucoma surgery and absence of severe complications.	0 33	1.6 ± 1.2	Phakic cases (PCG) seemed to have a better outcome than aphakic cases. 12.5%
Freedman et al. (1999), retrospective case series (4) [36]	Inclusion: • Glaucoma refractory to maximum medical treatment, prior angle or filtration surgery (including goniotomy, trabeculotomy, or trabeculectomy) or both; • <17 y.; • Aphakia. (*Note: 2 aphakic glaucomatous eyes were uveitic, one aniridic and one case had PHPV*) Exclusion: -	35.6	-	7.2	7 (7-0)	MMC 0.4 mg/mL for 3–5 min and postoperative 5-fluorouracil, laser suture or both	4 mmHg < IOP < 16 mmHg without further glaucoma surgery or devastating complication.	29	1.9	Age < 1 y and aphakia (vs. phakic status in PCG and JOAG), taken together. (p = 0.013) The addition of postoperative 5-fluorouracil and suture lysis did not provide improvement and may have increased complication rate. 42.8%

Table 3. Cont.

Author, Year, Study Design (LOE) Reference	Inclusion and Exclusion Criteria	Mean Pre-Treatment IOP ± SD (mmHg)	Mean Age at GDx ± SD (y)	Mean (*) Age at Glaucoma Surgery ± SD (y)	n eyes (a-p)	Antimetabolites	Success Criteria	Success Rate (%)	Mean (*) Follow-Up ± sd (y)	Factors Affecting Treatment Outcomes % of Eyes That Had Prior Glaucoma Surgery
Mandal et al. (2003), retrospective case series (4) [37]	Inclusion: • Glaucoma with aphakia or pseudophakia after congenital cataract surgery. Exclusion: -	34.2 ± 8.9	9.6	9.9 ± 9.0	23 (21-2)	MMC 0.4 mg/mL for 3 min	Complete success: 6 mmHg < IOP < 21 mmHg without medication. Qualified success: 6 mmHg < IOP < 21 mmHg, with or without 1 topical medication, no further need of glaucoma surgery, and no visually devastating complication.	37 58	2.0 ± 1.5	- Not specified
Chen et al. (2004), retrospective cohort study (2b) [10]	Inclusion: • IOP > 25 mmHg following congenital cataract surgery; • Lensectomy < 20 y. Exclusion: • Pre-existing glaucoma; • History of trauma; • Intraocular neoplasm, radiation therapy, anterior uveitis, anterior segment dysgenesis, ocular syndromes; • PCG; • Corticosteroid use before lensectomy.	-	-	-	61 (61-0)	MMC (n = 43) 5-fluorouracil (n = 17) None (n = 1)	IOP ≤ 21 mmHg with and without medications and no need for further surgery.	25	8.6 ± 7.6	- Not specified
Pakravan et al. (2007), prospective randomized clinical trial (1) [37]	Inclusion: • Medically unresponsive glaucoma (not further defined) following congenital cataract surgery; • <16 y. Exclusion: • Any history of ocular surgery other than anterior lensectomy/vitrectomy; • Congenital cataract in the setting of PFV or intrauterine infections; Follow-up < 6 m.	31 ± 10.7	-	9.1 ± 4.1	15 (15-0)	MMC 0.02% for 2 min	Absolute success: 5 mmHg ≤ IOP < 21 without medications. Qualified success: 5 mmHg ≤ IOP < 21 with ≤2 medications. Overall success: absolute + qualified success. 5 mmHg ≤ IOP < 21	33 40 73	1.2 ± 0.9	- 0%

147

Table 3. *Cont.*

Author, Year, Study Design (LOE) Reference	Inclusion and Exclusion Criteria	Mean Pre-Treatment IOP ± SD (mmHg)	Mean Age at GDx ± SD (y)	Mean (*) Age at Glaucoma Surgery ± SD (y)	*n* eyes (a–p)	Antimetabolites	Success Criteria	Success Rate (%)	Mean (*) Follow-Up ± sd (y)	Factors Affecting Treatment Outcomes % of Eyes That Had Prior Glaucoma Surgery
Baris et al. (2019), retrospective cohort study (2b) [23]	Inclusion: • IOP > 25 mmHg following congenital cataract surgery. Exclusion: • Pre-existing glaucoma; • Independent risk factors for glaucoma development, such as anterior segment dysgenesis or severe microphthalmia; • Previous laser.	29.8 ± 14.8	1 ± 2.1	-	20	MMC 0.2 mg/mL for 4 min	Complete success: IOP < 21 mmHg without medication. Qualified success: IOP < 21 mmHg with and without medication.	5 30	6.6 ± 2.6	- 0%

Abbreviations: GDx = glaucoma diagnosis; LOE = level of evidence; SD = Standard Deviation, GFCS: Glaucoma Following Cataract Surger; a = aphakic; p = pseudophakic; (*): median; mg = milligram; mL = millilitre; min = minutes; GDD = Glaucoma Drainage Device; IOP = Intra-Ocular Pressure; PCG = Primary Congenital Glaucoma; JOAG = Juvenile open-angle glaucoma; MMC = Mitomycin C; *n* = amount; PHPV = persistent hyperplastic primary vitreous; y = years.

Certain patient-related factors have shown to be significant risk factors for trabeculectomy failure, including aphakia and age younger than one year, especially when combined [35].

The use of antimetabolites can improve success rates but at the cost of increased risk of complications, including blebitis and endophthalmitis [37].

3.2.3. Glaucoma Drainage Device Implantation

Most of the included studies report treatment outcomes of glaucoma drainage device implantation in eyes with GFCS with good success rates up to 95% (Table 4) [10,38–52]. Pakravan et al. demonstrated a 90% success rate after one year of follow-up following a glaucoma drainage device implantation as a primary procedure in eyes with GFCS. At five years, the success rate had fallen to 72% [49]. Other reports, analysing the effectiveness of GDDs in GFCS patients, noted similarly good success rates [40,41,48].

A prospective randomized clinical trial (RCT) found that GDD treatment outcome is superior to trabeculectomy. This RCT compared Ahmed glaucoma implant + MMC (AGI + MMC) with trabeculectomy + MMC (T + MMC) as the primary procedure for treatment of GFCS in children under 16 years of age. Each group consisted of 15 aphakic eyes, and although no statistically significant differences were found between both groups, the results were more favourable in the GDD + MMC group. The overall success rate was higher (87% vs. 73%), and the overall complication rate was lower (27% vs. 40%) in the AGI+MMC group versus T + MMC group, respectively [38]. Similarly, a retrospective study which revealed success rates of 44% after GDD implantation still shows more encouraging results when compared to a 24.6% success rate in patients who underwent trabeculectomy [10].

Similar to trabeculectomy, younger age at time of GDD surgery is associated with less favourable treatment outcomes. Nevertheless, in patients under two years of age, when compared to T + MMC, it was found that GDD implantation offered a significantly greater chance of successful IOP control. At the age of six, IOP was controlled in 19% in the trabeculectomy + MMC group versus in 53% in the GDD group [53]. A recent study demonstrated that the presence of persistent fetal vasculature (PFV) affects the outcome in a negative way; PFV-related cataracts showed a lower survival rate of the Ahmed glaucoma valve and a higher complication rate versus non-PFV-related cataracts [51]. Unlike for trabeculectomy, lens status is not consistently reported to be a significant risk factor for GDD failure. Patients with GFCS who have had multiple previous ocular surgeries may be at higher risk for tube failure, with better reported relative success rates in eyes with only one previous operation (83%) compared to those having had more than two previous operations (42%) [43].

Complications commonly described in the included studies after GDD implantation include suprachoroidal haemorrhage, choroidal detachment, hypotony, tube-corneal contact, and retinal detachment.

3.2.4. Cyclodestructive Procedures

Moderate success rates have been reported after cyclodestructive procedures in GFCS eyes with uncontrolled (Table 5) [10,39,54–60]. The highest success rate (54%) was presented in a cohort of 35 aphakic or pseudophakic GFCS eyes, after a follow-up of 7.2 years [55].

Table 4. Relevant studies involving glaucoma drainage device implantation in GFCS eyes.

Author, Year, Study Design (LOE) Reference	Inclusion and Exclusion Criteria	Mean Pre-Treatment IOP ± SD (mmHg)	Mean Age at GDx ± SD (y)	Mean (*) Age at Glaucoma Surgery ± SD (y)	Number of Eyes (a-p)	Device ± Antimetabolites	Success Criteria	Success Rate (%)	Mean (*) Follow-Up ± SD (y)	Factors Affecting Treatment Outcomes % of Eyes That Had Prior Glaucoma Surgery
Donahue et al. (1997), retrospective cohort study (2b) [43]	Inclusion: • <18 y; • Glaucoma (not further defined) after lensectomy. Indications for lensectomy were congenital cataract (*n* = 7), PHPV (*n* = 2) and Lowe syndrome (*n* = 1); Exclusion: -	33	-	-	10 (9-1)	Baerveldt 350 mm	Complete success: No further reoperation, no decrease in vision, and IOP at last follow-up <21 mmHg, without complication not associated with tube failure. Qualified success: With and without medication necessary to bring IOP < 21 mmHg, with or without complication not associated with tube failure.	40 / 70	1.6	It appeared that the aphakic patients who has had multiple previous procedures were at higher risk for shunt failure. 40%
Wallace et al. (1998), retrospective cohort study (2b) [39]	Inclusion: • Glaucoma (not further defined) after congenital cataract surgery; • Need of glaucoma surgery < 18 y. Exclusion: PCG.	35.9	6.1	8.7	9	Molteno	IOP ≤ 25 mmHg without medication and IOP ≤ 21 mmHg with medication.	67 at 6 m, 33 at 1 y	4.2	Not specified
Englert et al. (1999), retrospective case series (4) [45]	Inclusion: • <18 y; • Medically uncontrolled glaucoma or uncontrolled despite previous glaucoma surgery (goniotomy, trabeculotomy, trabeculectomy ± antimetabolites, and/or cycloablative procedures); Exclusion: -	32.8 ± 7.5	-	-	7 (7-0)	Ahmed S-2 model in the superotemporal quadrant	IOP ≤ 21 mmHg without medication without further surgery without visually devastating complication	86	1.0 ± 0.7	Previous cycloablation was not a significant risk factor for failure. 14.2%
Chen et al. (2004), retrospective cohort study (2b) [10]	Inclusion: • IOP > 25 mmHg following congenital cataract surgery; Exclusion: • Pre-existing glaucoma; • History of trauma; • Intraocular neoplasm, radiation therapy, anterior uveitis, anterior segment dysgenesis, ocular syndromes, PCG.	-	-	-	34	Ahmed (32 eyes) Molteno (2 eyes)	IOP ≤ 21 mmHg with and without medications and no need for further surgery.	44	8.6	Not specified
Chen et al. (2005), retrospective case series (4) [42]	Inclusion: • Aphakic glaucoma (not further defined) after congenital cataract surgery; • <18 y. Exclusion: -	38.1 ± 6.4	-	4.9 ± 6.5	19	Ahmed S-2 model	IOP ≤ 22 mmHg with or without medications, without further surgery, without visually devastating complications	68 (75 if GDD implantation was the initial surgery)	2.2 ± 1.8	57.9%

Table 4. Cont.

Author, Year, Study Design (LOE) Reference	Inclusion and Exclusion Criteria	Mean Pre-Treatment IOP ± SD (mmHg)	Mean Age at GDs ± SD (y)	Mean (*) Age at Glaucoma Surgery ± SD (y)	Number of Eyes (a-p)	Device ± Antimetabolites	Success Criteria	Success Rate (%)	Mean (*) Follow-Up ± SD (y)	Factors Affecting Treatment Outcomes % of Eyes That Had Prior Glaucoma Surgery
Kirwan et al. (2005), retrospective case series (4) [46]	Inclusion: • Paediatric aphakic glaucoma (diagnosis of glaucoma was mainly based on changes in optic disc and IOP, not further defined); • Uncontrolled glaucoma by medical therapy or other forms of surgery (cyclo ablation and/or trabeculectomy). Exclusion: -	31.1	-	8	19	Ahmed S-2 model in 10 eyes +MMC 0.5 mg/mL for 3 min	IOP < 15 with and without medical therapy.	95	2.7	- 47.4%
Pakravan et al. (2007), prospective randomized control trial (1) [38]	Inclusion: • Medically unresponsive glaucoma (not further defined) following congenital cataract surgery; • <16 y. Exclusion: • Any history of ocular surgery other than anterior lensectomy/vitrectomy; • Congenital cataract in the setting of PFV or intrauterine infections; • Follow-up < 6 m.	31 ± 7.5		10.9 ± 5.1	15 (15-0)	Ahmed + MMC 0.2 mg/mL for 2 min	Absolute success: 5 mmHg < IOP < 21 mmHg without medications. Qualified success: 5 mmHg < IOP < 21 mmHg, with < 2 medications. Overall success: absolute + qualified success.	20 67 87	1.1 ± 0.8	0%
O'Malley Schotthoefer et al. (2008), retrospective cohort study (2b) [48]	Inclusion: • Medically refractory glaucoma (not further defined) after cataract surgery; Exclusion: -	36		4.3 *	41 (38-3)	Ahmed S-2 or FP-7 (n = 16) Baerveldt (n = 22) Molteno (n = 3) All in superotemporal quadrant. PP + V in 5 eyes.	IOP < 21 mmHg without medication, without further surgery, without visually devastating complications.	90 at 1 y 82 at 2 y 55 at 10 y	0.5 *	Better reported outcomes with Ahmed valve implantation in aphakic glaucoma than refractory PCG, no statistically significant difference in Kaplan Meier. 0%
Banitt et al. (2009), retrospective cohort study (2b) [41]	Inclusion: • <18 y; • Uncontrolled glaucoma associated with aphakia or pseudophakia; • PCG (n = 1); • Secondary glaucoma (n = 29), Glaucoma following cataract surgery (n = 21), Glaucoma post ocular trauma (n = 5) Glaucoma associated with aniridia (n = 3). Exclusion: • Prior aqueous shunt surgery with anterior tube insertion.	32.9 ± 7.9		6.9 ± 5.0	30 (24-6)	Baerveldt PP + V in all eyes	5 mmHg < IOP < 21 mmHg, with and without medications, and without visually devastating complication or further surgery.	85 at 1 y 81 at 2 y 72 at 3 y	2.5 ± 2.2	Lens status (aphakia vs. pseudophakia) had comparable IOP results (p = 0.77). Not specified
Balekudaru et al. (2014), retrospective cohort study (2b) [40]	Inclusion: • Medically uncontrolled glaucoma (not further defined) in aphakia and pseudophakia; • <18 y; • Results of only the first implant were included in eyes that underwent surgery with more than one implant. Exclusion:	35.86 ± 9.57		-	47	Ahmed S-2 or FP-7 model in the superior-temporal quadrant	Complete success: 6 mmHg < IOP < 18 mmHg with and without medication. Qualified success: 6 mmHg < IOP < 18 mmHg, without visually devastating complication.	95 at 1 y 86 at 2 y	-	No significant differences in outcomes between the two Ahmed valve models. 76.6%

Table 4. *Cont.*

Author, Year, Study Design (LOE) Reference	Inclusion and Exclusion Criteria	Mean Pre-Treatment IOP ± SD (mmHg)	Mean Age at GDx ± SD (y)	Mean (*) Age at Glaucoma Surgery ± SD (y)	Number of Eyes (a-p)	Device ± Antimetabolites	Success Criteria	Success Rate (%)	Mean (*) Follow-Up ± SD (y)	Factors Affecting Treatment Outcomes % of Eyes That Had Prior Glaucoma Surgery
Elshatory et al. (2016), retrospective case series (4) [44]	Inclusion: • Aphakic glaucoma (not further defined) The causes of aphakia were congenital cataract extraction (n = 12), post-traumatic cataract extraction (n = 1) and Peter's anomaly (n = 1); • GDD implantation was the initial procedure; Exclusion: • Follow-up < 6 m.	33.9 ± 10.9	-	9.2 ± 5.7	14	Ahmed (36%), Baerveldt (64%) PP+V in all eyes	Improved postoperative IOP control without any intra- or postoperative complications.	Average decrease in IOP of 51%	1.0	- 0%
Pakravan et al. (2019), retrospective case series (4) [49]	Inclusion: • Aphakic glaucoma (not further defined) following cataract extraction; • Ahmed glaucoma valve implantation as primary procedure. Exclusion: • Follow-up < 6 m; • Prior cyclodestructive procedures.	28.9 ± 6.1	-	9.9 ± 5.6	33	Ahmed FP-7	5 mmHg < IOP < 21 mmHg with or without medication.	90 at 1 y; 72 at 5 y	4.1 ± 3.4	Better reported outcomes with Ahmed valve implantation in aphakic glaucoma than refractory PCG. 0%
Geyer et al. (2021) Retrospective case series (4) [52]	Inclusion: • Paediatric patients with GFCS; congenital cataract; • Ahmed glaucoma valve implantation between 2007 and 2018. Exclusion: -	35.8 ± 7.4	-	6.6 *	41	Ahmed	IOP ≤ 22 mmHg without glaucoma reoperations and without significant complications	95 at 1 y; 90 at 2 y; 83 at 5 y; 73 at 7 y	5 *	- 17%
Spiess et al. (2021), retrospective cohort study (2b) [51]	Inclusion: • Paediatric patients with GFCS from 1996 to 2016; • Glaucoma following cataract surgery was defined according to the consensus established by The Childhood Glaucoma Research Network (World Glaucoma Association in 2018) as intraocular pressure (IOP) greater than 21 mmHg with associated anatomical optic disc changes or other signs of progressive myopia. Exclusion: • Acquired cataracts, trauma, aniridia, Lowe syndrome, an age of 2 years and older with congenital cataract surgery, and previous/concomitant ocular hypertension or primary intraocular lens (IOL) implantation.	32.66 ± 6.73	Median 2.9 y after cataract surgery	2	29 (23 aphakic, 6 pseudophakic) 41% PHPV 59% non-PHPV	Ahmed: model FP7, model S2, and model FP8	IOP < 21 mmHg with or without medication. PHPV Non-PHPV	37.5 at 1 y, 28.1 at 5 y 88.2 at 1 y, 71.9 at 5 y	7.5	Eyes with PHPV and GFCS followed by AGV implantation had a higher number of complications and a decreased probability of success compared to the nonpersistent foetal vasculature group. Both groups achieved a significant decrease in intraocular pressure. Not specified

Abbreviations: GDx = glaucoma diagnosis; LOE = level of evidence; SD = Standard Deviation, GFCS: Glaucoma Following Cataract Surger; a = aphakic; p = pseudophakic; (*): median; mg = milligram; mL = millilitre; min = minutes; GDD = Glaucoma Drainage Device; IOP = Intra-Ocular Pressure; PCG = Primary Congenital Glaucoma; JOAG = Juvenile open-angle glaucoma; MMC = Mitomycin C; n = amount; PHPV = persistent hyperplastic primary vitreous; y = years; C/D = cup to disk ratio; PP+V: Posterior placement + vitrectomy.

Table 5. Relevant studies involving cyclodestruction in GFCS eyes.

Author, Year, Study Design (LOE) Reference	Inclusion and Exclusion Criteria	Mean Pre-Treatment IOP ± SD (mmHg)	Mean Age at GFCS Diagnosis ± SD (y)	Mean (* Median) Age at Glaucoma Surgery ± SD (y)	Number of Eyes (a-p)	Procedure	Success Criteria	Success Rate (%)	Mean (* Median) Follow-Up ± SD (y)	Factors Affecting Treatment Outcomes % of Eyes *That Had Prior Glaucoma Surgery*
Wallace et al. (1998), retrospective cohort study (2b) [39]	Inclusion: • Glaucoma (not further defined) following cataract surgery; • Need of surgery < 18 y. Exclusion: • PCG.	35.9	6.1	8.7	4	ECP	IOP ≤ 25 mmHg without medications and IOP ≤ 21 mmHg with medications.	50	4.2	Not specified
Neely and Plager (2001), retrospective cohort study (2b) [59]	Inclusion: • 5) ECP procedures performed on 36 eyes of 29 paediatric patients with glaucoma. Aphakic glaucoma (n = 19, 53%) PCG (n = 10), Sturge-Weber syndrome (n = 2), Anterior segment dysgenesis (n = 1) Microphthalmia (n = 1) Note: In addition to the 19 eyes with aphakic glaucoma after removal of congenital cataracts, 3 additional ones	35.06 ± 8.55	-	4.90 ± 4.17	22 aphakic eyes (19 GFCS, 3 PCG)	ECP	IOP < 21 mmHg, with and without antiglaucoma medications.	50	1.6 ± 1.6	Aphakic patients may have an increased risk of significant postoperative complications, such as retinal detachment. Not specified
Kirwan (2002), retrospective cohort study (2b) [58]	Inclusion: • <18 y. • Aphakic glaucoma (n = 34, 45%) and PCG (n = 26, 35%), other types of glaucoma (aniridia, anterior segment dysgenesis, uveitic glaucoma, Sturge-Weber, silicone-oil-associated glaucoma, naevus- or Ota-associated glaucoma, secondary angle-closure glaucoma) Note: Of 28 eyes that underwent primary cyclodiode, 23 were aphakic; • Advanced glaucoma with previous failed surgical procedures; • Markedly elevated IOP on acute presentation; • Blind, painful eyes; • Markedly elevated IOP, where the fellow eye had recently undergone surgery; • Moderately elevated IOP with maximum therapy, where risks of drainage surgery were considered high or where surgery was declined by the patient or parents. Exclusion: • Follow-up < 1 y.	32.0 ± 6.4	-	7.4	34	TDLC (300°)	IOP < 22 mmHg or reduction by 30%, with and without antiglaucoma medications.	42 at 1 y	1.8	Aphakic eyes had a more sustained IOP control than phakic eyes (PCG, aniridia, anterior segment dysgenesis, uveitic glaucoma, Sturge-Weber, silicone-oil-associated glaucoma, naevus- or Ota-associated glaucoma, secondary angle-closure glaucoma). Aphakic patients had a 42% IOP control at one year versus 14% in phakic eyes. (p < 0.001 log rank test). Success rate is lower than in adults, and younger eyes may recover from treatment more rapidly. Not specified

Table 5. *Cont.*

Author, Year, Study Design (LOE) Reference	Inclusion and Exclusion Criteria	Mean Pre-Treatment IOP ± SD (mmHg)	Mean Age at GFCS Diagnosis ± SD (y)	Mean (* Median) Age at Glaucoma Surgery ± SD (y)	Number of Eyes (a-p)	Procedure	Success Criteria	Success Rate (%)	Mean (* Median) Follow-Up ± SD (y)	Factors Affecting Treatment Outcomes % of Eyes That Had Prior Glaucoma Surgery
Autrata and Lokaj (2003), retrospective cohort study (2b) [54]	Inclusion: • Glaucomatous eyes that underwent TDLC. • aphakic glaucoma (n = 26), PCG (n = 21), Other glaucomas (uveitic glaucoma, secondary angle closure, Sturge-Weber, aniridia); • Advanced glaucoma with previous failed surgical procedures; • Markedly elevated IOP where an IOP control was required before undertaking definitive surgery; • Moderately elevated IOP with maximum medical therapy where the risks of drainage surgery were considered high; • Blind, painful eyes with an elevated IOP. Exclusion: • Follow-up < 1 y.	34.08 ± 7.13	-	6.1	26	TDLC (300°)	IOP ≤ 21 mmHg, with and without adjunctive antiglaucoma medications.	47 at 1 y	5.6 ± 2.8	Aphakic patients had a more sustained IOP-lowering response after their first treatment session. Of aphakic eyes, 47% had IOP control at one year versus 19% of the phakic eyes (PCG, uveitic glaucoma, secondary angle closure, Sturge-Weber, aniridia). The data suggest that multiple repeated cyclodiode treatments may still have an IOP-lowering effect. *Not specified.*
Chen et al. (2004), retrospective cohort study (2b) [10]	Inclusion: • IOP > 25 mmHg following congenital cataract surgery; • Lensectomy < 20 y. Exclusion: • Pre-existing glaucoma; • History of trauma; • Intraocular neoplasm, radiation therapy, anterior uveitis, anterior segment dysgenesis, ocular syndromes, PCG.	-	-	-	21 (21.0)	Cyclocryotherapy, TDLC, contact Nd:YAG laser cyclotherapy	IOP ≤ 21 mmHg with and without medications and no need for further surgery.	14	8.6 ± 7.6	*Not specified*
Carter et al. (2007), Retrospective case series (4) [56]	Inclusion: • Aphakic or pseudophakic glaucoma (unacceptable IOP combined with evidence of optic nerve damage) *Note: 3 eyes with unilateral cataract associated with PFV were included;* <16 y; • Medical, and in some cases surgical therapy was performed in most patients prior to ECP treatment. Exclusion: • PCG; • Anterior segment dysgenesis; • Follow-up < 1 y.	32.6	3.3	4.2	34 (32.2)	ECP (180°–270°)	IOP ≤ 24 mmHg and IOP decrease of more than 15% despite the addition of glaucoma medications, without sight-threatening complications.	53	3.7	Retreatment of eyes increased the overall success rate. *18%*

Table 5. Cont.

Author, Year, Study Design (LOE) Reference	Inclusion and Exclusion Criteria	Mean Pre-Treatment IOP ± SD (mmHg)	Mean Age at GFCS Diagnosis ± SD (y)	Mean (* Median) Age at Glaucoma Surgery ± SD (y)	Number of Eyes (a-p)	Procedure	Success Criteria	Success Rate (%)	Mean (* Median) Follow-Up ± SD (y)	Factors Affecting Treatment Outcomes % of Eyes That Had Prior Glaucoma Surgery
Schlote et al. (2008), retrospective cohort study (2b) [60]	Inclusion: • Glaucoma in aphakia Note: Of the 21 patients with glaucoma in aphakia, lensectomy was performed for congenital cataracts (n = 11) and acquired cataracts (n = 10); • IOP levels > 21 mmHg despite maximal medical therapy; • Progression of glaucoma damage despite maximal medical therapy. Exclusion: Follow-up < 1 y.	31.1 ± 8.8	-	53.1 ± 23.6	21	TDLC	5 <IOP ≤ 21 mmHg with and without medication.	19 after 1 TDLC; 48 after repeated TDLC	3.5 ± 2.4	Translimbal or pars-plana-modified GDD may be associated with a better long-term prognosis, and should be used prior to TDLC to avoid the increasing risk of hypotonia using a filtering procedure after cyclodestruction. 42.9%
Cantor et al. (2018), Retrospective cohort study (2b) [55]	Inclusion: • Glaucoma (not further defined) following cataract surgery; • <16 y. Exclusion: -	34.1 ± 8.3	4.0 ± 2.5	6.0 ± 3.8	35 (27.8)	ECP (average 230° for first ECP, average of 151° for repeat ECP)	IOP ≤ 24 mmHg, no alternative glaucoma procedure following ECP, or occurrence of devastating complications With and without medications.	54; 48 in a 75 in p; Successful eyes had 1.1 ± 0.2 ECP treatments (average).	7.2 ± 3.6	The failure rate was not increased in pseudophakic patients relative to aphakic patients. 0%
Glaser et al. (2019), retrospective cohort study (2b) [57]	Inclusion: • Childhood glaucoma (not further defined) • 80 eyes of 70 patients were included The most common glaucoma diagnoses were GFCS (60%), anterior segment dysgenesis (13%), and PCG (9%). The majority of eyes were aphakic (n = 45, 46%) or pseudophakic (n = 28, 35%). Exclusion: -	30.8 ± 7.9	-	9.5 ± 6.0 (for all eyes)	48 (60% of all eyes)	ECP	IOP ≤ 24 mmHg with and without medications, without any additional glaucoma surgery, without devastating complications, without progression to NLP visual acuity.	64 at 1 y; 36 at 3 y; 16 at 5 y (after single ECP) (for all eyes)	*2.2	In multivariable analysis, of many risk factors considered, only a preoperative IOP < 32 mmHg was significantly associated with treatment success. Not specified

Abbreviations: GDx = glaucoma diagnosis; LOE = level of evidence; SD = Standard Deviation, GFCS: Glaucoma Following Cataract Surger; a = aphakic; p = pseudophakic; (*): median; mg = milligram; mL = millilitre; min = minutes; GDD = Glaucoma Drainage Device; IOP = Intra-Ocular Pressure; PCG = Primary Congenital Glaucoma; n = amount; PHPV = persistent hyperplastic primary vitreous; y = years; ECP = endoscopic cyclophotocoagulation; TDLC = transscleral diode laser cyclodestruction.

In the study of Schlote et al., cyclodestruction showed better outcomes in older patients than in younger patients [60]. No effect of prior glaucoma interventions was found [53,55,56]. No significant differences in success rates between aphakic and pseudophakic eyes were found [55,57]. The only finding repeatedly associated with reduced outcomes was a higher pretreatment IOP; those eyes may need more sessions of cyclodestruction in order to control the IOP [55,57].

Postoperative hypotony, chronic uveitis, and rarely phthisis are complications reported after cyclodestruction [10,39,54–60]. Aphakic eyes with GFCS after endoscopic cyclophotocoagulation were at higher risk of postoperative complications, including retinal detachment, compared to eyes with other types of glaucoma [59].

4. Discussion

Medical therapy should be tried first in GFCS cases since long-term IOP control can be reached with medication alone in some cases. For example, Bhola et al. noted that 73% of patients achieved IOP with medication alone after a mean follow-up of 18.7 years [24]. The choice of medication varies between clinicians and depends on efficacy, potential adverse effects, cost, and availability across different health systems [5]. Kraus et al. found that EI had an impressive IOP-lowering effect in children with GFCS. Unfortunately, this medication was discontinued in 2021 and is currently no longer commercially available [27]. The decision to proceed to surgery should be a well-argued one, because younger age is frequently associated with reduced surgical outcomes; hence, medical therapy should be considered the initial strategy of choice in GFCS, possibly to bridge the time to surgery. On the other hand, topical IOP-lowering drugs have a higher potential for systemic adverse effects, and adherence to complex regimens is more difficult in young age groups [10]. When IOP control is inadequate, surgery should not be delayed because of fear of poor results.

Surgical treatment modalities for GFCS include angle surgery (trabeculotomy and goniotomy), GDD implantation, trabeculectomy with MMC, and cyclodestructive procedures. Given their normal life expectancy, children with GFCS may need multiple repeat interventions. Hence, the development of a long-term surgical strategy allowing a step-wise escalation of risk is strongly advisable. Selecting the most appropriate operation technique is crucial since the primary surgical intervention chosen for the child is often his or her best chance for long-term success.

Some patient-related factors are associated with reduced outcomes of particular surgical procedures, making particular procedures more suitable than others for individual clinical cases. Since glaucoma surgery suffers from poor success rates in GFCS, knowledge about these patient-related factors affecting the outcomes helps in choosing the optimal approach for each individual patient. Considering the identified risk factors after reviewing the current literature, the authors suggest a flowchart for the management of GFCS (Figure 3). The flowchart was adapted from a previously published flowchart (Childhood Glaucoma, 9th Consensus Report of the World Glaucoma Association) [16].

It should be stressed that this is not intended as a pre-set algorithm that must be followed unconditionally as clinical decision-making will always be influenced by several factors (including surgeon preference/experience and local facilities/equipment availability). The next paragraphs may clarify the flowchart by summarising and interpreting the main findings of each surgical option.

Although angle surgery is more often reserved for cases of PCG, some recent studies have shown promising results in GFCS (Table 2); these studies are associated with the recent resurgence of interest in this treatment modality. This is not surprising since angle dysgenesis plays a role in the pathogenesis of GFCS and angle surgery addresses the physiological outflow pathways. In particular, 360-degree trabeculotomy maximises the therapeutic effect by providing both a temporal and nasal trabeculotomy at initial surgery, whether by two-site rigid probe or via microcatheter assisted suture placement. This technique is less invasive when compared to trabeculectomy, GDD implantation, and cyclodestructive procedures. Additionally, 360-degree trabeculotomy is beneficial because it spares the conjunctiva for potential future surgeries. Angle surgery was not mentioned in the previous flowchart of suggested management approach in 2013 (Childhood Glaucoma, 9th Consensus Report of the World Glaucoma Association) [16]. However, studies after 2013 showed good success rates in GFCS cases and the authors of this review suggest that a 360-degree trabeculotomy could be attempted as the primary surgical procedure in cases of relatively early-onset GFCS when the angle is deep and in the absence of peripheral anterior synechiae [20]. Some studies in the literature, mainly in the form of case reports, describe the performance of goniotomy with a 23 or 25 gauge straight cystotome or a Sinskey hook. These devices are much less expensive than other devices on the market for goniotomy such as Kahook blade, Goniotome, and Trabectome. It is a good option in resource-poor areas that cannot afford more expensive goniotomy devices [61–66].

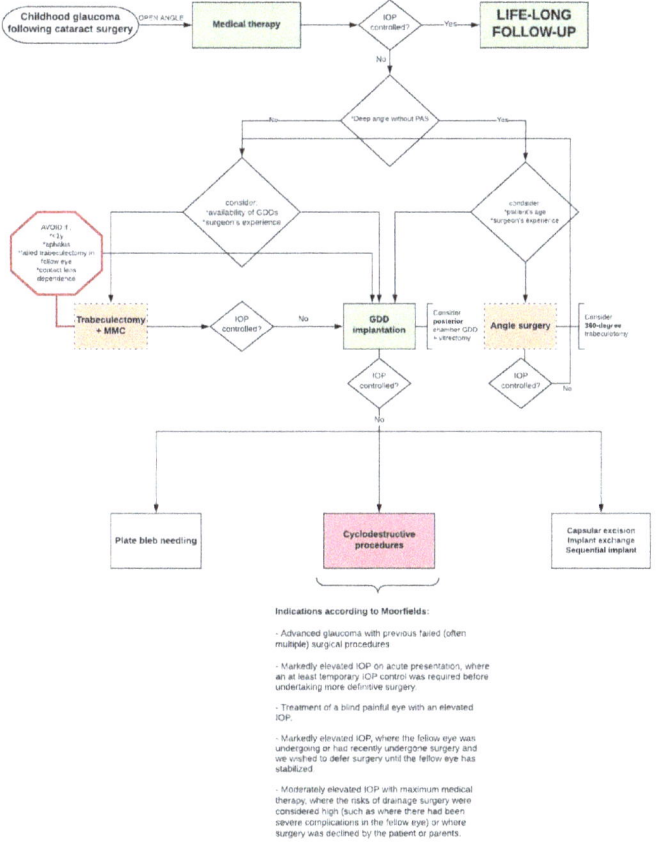

Figure 3. Suggested flowchart for the management of childhood GFCS with open-angle configuration (adapted with permission from Grigg, World Glaucoma Association Consensus Series 9: Childhood glaucoma, Kugler publications 2013 [16]). Abbreviations: IOP = Intra-Ocular Pressure; MMC = Mitomycin C; y = years; GDD = Glaucoma drainage device; PAS = peripheral anterior synechiae.

Trabeculectomy has traditionally been the first choice of the remaining surgical options in childhood glaucoma, but it has shown limited success in GFCS (Table 3). Due to this limited success rates, the concern about bleb-related complications post trabeculectomy + MMC and due to the high success rates of up to 95% following GDD implantation in GFCS eyes (Table 4), there is a growing interest in selecting a GDD at primary surgery. Although large RCTs are lacking in this domain, the current literature does suggest that GDD implantation gives the best chance for long-term IOP control. Some studies put this technique forward as a good choice for primary surgery [38,44,48,49]. Where trabeculectomy was still considered as the primary procedure of choice in the previous flowchart (Childhood Glaucoma, 9th Consensus Report of the World Glaucoma Association) [16], the authors of this review suggest that glaucoma drainage implantation is preferred over trabeculectomy in GFCS cases. The complication of tube-cornea contact and corneal decompensation can be minimised by placing the tube in the sulcus in pseudophakic patients or pars plana with concomitant (or prior) vitrectomy in aphakic/pseudophakic patients [41].

Cyclodestructive procedures (Table 5), plate bleb needling, and exchange or sequential implant have proven to be effective in patients with uncontrolled IOP after a GDD implantation [67–69]. Cyclodestruction is generally considered when other options have failed. Although initially reserved for end-stage glaucomatous eyes in which multiple procedures have failed, indications for this procedure have expanded, and it can be considered an initial surgical approach in selected cases (Figure 3, indications according to Moorfields).

The aetiology of GFCS is largely not understood and thought to be multifactorial in origin. A significant reduction in Schlemm's canal (SC) size and loss of SC dilation during physiologic accommodation in children with GFCS has recently been demonstrated, suggesting that targeting SC may potentially offer a new management approach [70] 3. Future research directed at better understanding the underlying aetiology is necessary since such an understanding may have implications for the clinical management of GFCS.

One of the major strengths of this review is that it specifically focuses on the management of the glaucoma subtype GFCS. Many reports in the literature offer a comparison of different procedures for childhood glaucoma in general; however, the mix of diagnoses of subjects differs between studies and different aetiologies of glaucoma do not respond in the same manner to a particular surgical intervention. For that reason, the authors chose to extract and analyse the outcomes separately for patients with GFCS. However, it must be noted that the differing study results are limited by their retrospective nature, varying study populations (including patient age and the severity of glaucoma), varying techniques and devices, and varying number of previous surgeries as well differences in the definitions of success and failure.

5. Conclusions

Although medical therapy is usually the first-line treatment for GFCS, multiple surgical procedures are often required to adequately control the condition. It might be worth trying a 360-degree trabeculotomy before proceeding to glaucoma drainage device implantation, since this technique offers good results and is less invasive. Glaucoma drainage device implantation seems to give the best chance for long-term IOP control in childhood GFCS and some studies put this technique forward as a good choice for primary surgery. Cyclodestruction seems to be effective in some GFCS cases with uncontrolled IOP after a glaucoma drainage device implantation. Trabeculectomy offers poor success rates in children with GFCS, especially in children under the age of one year and children that are left aphakic. The authors provide a flowchart to guide the management of individual GFCS cases.

Author Contributions: Conceptualization, S.L. and E.V.; methodology, A.-S.S. and S.L.; software, not applicable; validation, S.L., E.V., I.S., I.C. and J.G.; formal analysis, not applicable; investigation, A.-S.S. and S.L.; resources, not applicable; data curation, not applicable; writing—original draft preparation, A.-S.S.; writing—review and editing, S.L., E.V., I.S., I.C. and J.G.; visualization, E.V.; supervision, S.L., E.V., I.S., I.C. and J.G.; project administration, E.V.; funding acquisition, not applicable. All authors have read and agreed to the published version of the manuscript.

Funding: This research received no external funding.

Institutional Review Board Statement: Not applicable.

Informed Consent Statement: Not applicable.

Conflicts of Interest: The authors declare no conflict of interest.

Appendix A

Search conducted on 23 June 2019–last updated on 31 December 2021 in Pubmed (Medline): ("Glaucoma"[Mesh] OR Glaucoma[tiab]) AND (("Aphakia, Postcataract"[Mesh] OR "Aphakia"[Mesh] OR Aphak*[tiab]) OR ("Pseudophakia"[Mesh] OR "Pseudophak"[tiab])) AND ("therapy"[Mesh] OR therap*[tiab] OR treatment[tiab] OR management[tiab]).

Search conducted on 23 June 2019–last updated on 31 December 2021 in Embase: Concept 1: ('disease management'/exp OR 'management':ti,ab) AND Concept 2: ('aphakic glaucoma'/exp OR 'aphakic':ti,ab) OR Concept 3: ('pseudophakic glaucoma' OR 'pseudophak':ti,ab) Combine.

Search conducted on 23 June 2019–last updated on 31 December 2021 in Web of Science Concept 1: TS = (Glaucoma AND Aphak* OR Pseuphak*) Concept 2: TS = (therap*OR treatment OR management) Combine.

Search conducted on 23 June 2019–last updated on 31 December 2021 in Cochrane: Concept 1: disease management AND Concept 2: aphakic glaucoma OR Concept 3: pseudophakic glaucoma.

References

1. Roy, F.H. Comprehensive Developmental Glaucoma Classification. *Ann. Ophthalmol.* **2005**, *37*, 237–244. [CrossRef]
2. Yeung, H.H.; Walton, D.S. Clinical Classification of Childhood Glaucomas. *Arch. Ophthalmol.* **2010**, *128*, 680–684. [CrossRef] [PubMed]
3. Thau, A.; Lloyd, M.; Freedman, S.; Beck, A.; Grajewski, A.; Levin, A.V. New classification system for pediatric glaucoma. *Curr. Opin. Ophthalmol.* **2018**, *29*, 385–394. [CrossRef] [PubMed]
4. Hoguet, A.; Grajewski, A.; Hodapp, E.; Chang, T.C.P. A retrospective survey of childhood glaucoma prevalence according to Childhood Glaucoma Research Network classification. *Indian J. Ophthalmol.* **2016**, *64*, 118–123. [CrossRef]
5. Weinreb, R.N.; Grajewski, A.L.; Papadopoulos, M. Definition, classification, differential diagnosis. In *Childhood Glaucoma: The 9th Consensus Report of the World Glaucoma Association*; Kugler Publications: Amsterdam, The Netherlands, 2013.
6. Rabiah, P.K. Frequency and predictors of glaucoma after pediatric cataract surgery. *Am. J. Ophthalmol.* **2004**, *137*, 30–37. [CrossRef]
7. Chen, T.C.; Chen, P.P.; Francis, B.A.; Junk, A.K.; Smith, S.D.; Singh, K.; Lin, S.C. Pediatric Glaucoma Surgery. *Ophthalmology* **2014**, *121*, 2107–2115. [CrossRef]
8. Swamy, B.N.; Billson, F.; Martin, F.; Donaldson, C.; Hing, S.; Jamieson, R.; Grigg, J.; Smith, J.E.H. Secondary glaucoma after paediatric cataract surgery. *Br. J. Ophthalmol.* **2007**, *91*, 1627–1630. [CrossRef]
9. Freedman, S.F.; Beck, A.D.; Nizam, A.; Vanderveen, D.K.; Plager, D.A.; Morrison, D.G.; Drews-Botsch, C.D.; Lambert, S.R.; Infant Aphakia Treatment Study Group. Glaucoma-Related Adverse Events at 10 Years in the Infant Aphakia Treatment Study: A Secondary Analysis of a Randomized Clinical Trial. *JAMA Ophthalmol.* **2021**, *139*, 165–173. [CrossRef]
10. Walton, D.S.; Chen, T.C.; Bhatia, L.S. Aphakic Glaucoma After Congenital Cataract Surgery. *Int. Ophthalmol. Clin.* **2008**, *48*, 87–94. [CrossRef]
11. Mandal, A.K.; Netland, P.A. Glaucomas in aphakia and pseudophakia after congenital cataract surgery. *Indian J. Ophthalmol.* **2006**, *52*, 93–102. Available online: http://www.ncbi.nlm.nih.gov/pubmed/15510457 (accessed on 9 April 2019).
12. Asrani, S.; Freedman, S.; Hasselblad, V.; Buckley, E.G.; Egbert, J.; Dahan, E.; Parks, M.; Johnson, D.; Maselli, E.; Gimbel, H.; et al. Does primary intraocular lens implantation prevent 'aphakic' glaucoma in children? *J. Am. Assoc. Pediatr. Ophthalmol. Strabismus* **2000**, *4*, 33–39. [CrossRef]
13. Michael, I.; Shmoish, M.; Walton, D.S.; Levenberg, S. Interactions between Trabecular Meshwork Cells and Lens Epithelial Cells: A Possible Mechanism in Infantile Aphakic Glaucoma. *Investig. Opthalmol. Vis. Sci.* **2008**, *49*, 3981–3987. [CrossRef] [PubMed]
14. Kirwan, C.; O'Keefe, M. Paediatric aphakic glaucoma. *Acta Ophthalmol. Scand.* **2006**, *84*, 734–739. [CrossRef] [PubMed]
15. Lam, D.S.C.; Fan, D.S.P.; Ng, J.S.K.; Yu, C.B.O.; Wong, C.Y.; Cheung, A.Y.K. Ocular hypertensive and anti-inflammatory responses to different dosages of topical dexamethasone in children: A randomized trial. *Clin. Exp. Ophthalmol.* **2005**, *33*, 252–258. [CrossRef] [PubMed]
16. Fenerty, C.; Grigg, J.; Freedman, S. Glaucoma Following Cataract Surgery. In *Childhood Glaucoma: The 9th Consensus Report of the World Glaucoma Association*; Kugler Publications: Amsterdam, The Netherlands, 2013.
17. Mataftsi, A.; Haidich, A.-B.; Kokkali, S.; Rabiah, P.K.; Birch, E.; Stager, D.R.; Cheong-Leen, R.; Singh, V.; Egbert, J.E.; Astle, W.F.; et al. Postoperative Glaucoma Following Infantile Cataract Surgery: An individual patient data meta-analysis. *JAMA Ophthalmol.* **2014**, *132*, 1059–1067. [CrossRef]
18. Freedman, S.F.; Lynn, M.J.; Beck, A.D.; Bothun, E.D.; Örge, F.H.; Lambert, S.R. Glaucoma-Related Adverse Events in the First 5 Years After Unilateral Cataract Removal in the Infant Aphakia Treatment Study. *JAMA Ophthalmol.* **2015**, *133*, 907–914. [CrossRef] [PubMed]

19. Solebo, A.; Cumberland, P.; Rahi, J.S. 5-year outcomes after primary intraocular lens implantation in children aged 2 years or younger with congenital or infantile cataract: Findings from the IoLunder2 prospective inception cohort study. *Lancet Child Adolesc. Health* **2018**, *2*, 863–871. [CrossRef]
20. Dosunmu, E.; Freedman, S. Aphakic/pseudophakic glaucoma. In *Practical Management of Pediatric Ocular Disorders and Strabismus: A Case-Based Approach*; Springer: New York, NY, USA, 2016; pp. 459–470.
21. Moher, D.; Liberati, A.; Tetzlaff, J.; Altman, D.G.; Prisma Group. Preferred reporting items for systematic reviews and meta-analyses: The PRISMA statement. *BMJ* **2009**, *339*, b2535. [CrossRef]
22. Philips, B. *Oxford Centre for Evidence-Based Medicine–Levels of Evidence*; Centre for Evidence Based Medicine: Oxford, UK, 2014.
23. Baris, M.; Biler, E.D.; Yilmaz, S.G.; Ates, H.; Uretmen, O.; Kose, S. Treatment results in aphakic patients with glaucoma following congenital cataract surgery. *Int. Ophthalmol.* **2017**, *39*, 11–19. [CrossRef]
24. Bhola, R.; Keech, R.V.; Olson, R.; Petersen, D.B. Long-Term Outcome of Pediatric Aphakic Glaucoma. *J. Am. Assoc. Pediatr. Ophthalmol. Strabismus* **2006**, *10*, 243–248. [CrossRef]
25. Comer, R.M.; Kim, P.; Cline, R.; Lyons, C.J. Cataract surgery in the first year of life: Aphakic glaucoma and visual outcomes. *Can. J. Ophthalmol.* **2011**, *46*, 148–152. [CrossRef] [PubMed]
26. Spiess, K.; Calvo, J.P. Clinical Characteristics and Treatment of Secondary Glaucoma After Pediatric Congenital Cataract Surgery in a Tertiary Referral Hospital in Spain. *J. Am. Assoc. Pediatr. Ophthalmol. Strabismus* **2020**, *57*, 292–300. [CrossRef] [PubMed]
27. Kraus, C.L.; Trivedi, R.H.; Wilson, M.E. Intraocular pressure control with echothiophate iodide in children's eyes with glaucoma after cataract extraction. *J. Am. Assoc. Pediatr. Ophthalmol. Strabismus* **2015**, *19*, 116–118.e1. [CrossRef] [PubMed]
28. Bothun, E.D.; Guo, Y.; Christiansen, S.P.; Summers, C.G.; Anderson, J.S.; Wright, M.M.; Kramarevsky, N.Y.; Lawrence, M.G. Outcome of angle surgery in children with aphakic glaucoma. *J. Am. Assoc. Pediatr. Ophthalmol. Strabismus* **2010**, *14*, 235–239. [CrossRef] [PubMed]
29. Beck, A.D.; Lynn, M.J.; Crandall, J.; Mobin-Uddin, O. Surgical outcomes with 360-degree suture trabeculotomy in poor-prognosis primary congenital glaucoma and glaucoma associated with congenital anomalies or cataract surgery. *J. Am. Assoc. Pediatr. Ophthalmol. Strabismus* **2011**, *15*, 54–58. [CrossRef] [PubMed]
30. Dao, J.B.; Sarkisian, S.R.; Freedman, S.F. Illuminated Microcatheter–facilitated 360-Degree Trabeculotomy for Refractory Aphakic and Juvenile Open-angle Glaucoma. *J. Glaucoma* **2014**, *23*, 449–454. [CrossRef]
31. El Sayed, Y.M.; Elhusseiny, A.M.; Gawdat, G.I.; Elhilali, H.M. One-year results of two-site trabeculotomy in paediatric glaucoma following cataract surgery. *Eye* **2020**, *35*, 1637–1643. [CrossRef]
32. Lim, M.E.; Dao, J.B.; Freedman, S.F. 360-Degree Trabeculotomy for Medically Refractory Glaucoma Following Cataract Surgery and Juvenile Open-Angle Glaucoma. *Am. J. Ophthalmol.* **2017**, *175*, 1–7. [CrossRef]
33. Rojas, C.; Bohnsack, B.L. Rate of Complete Catheterization of Schlemm's Canal and Trabeculotomy Success in Primary and Secondary Childhood Glaucomas. *Am. J. Ophthalmol.* **2019**, *212*, 69–78. [CrossRef]
34. Azuara-Blanco, A.; Wilson, R.P.; Spaeth, G.L.; Schmidt, C.M.; Augsburger, J.J. Filtration procedures supplemented with mitomycin C in the management of childhood glaucoma. *Br. J. Ophthalmol.* **1999**, *83*, 151–156. [CrossRef]
35. Beck, A.D.; Wilson, W.R.; Lynch, M.G.; Lynn, M.J.; Noe, R. Trabeculectomy with adjunctive mitomycin C in pediatric glaucoma. *Am. J. Ophthalmol.* **1998**, *126*, 648–657. Available online: http://www.ncbi.nlm.nih.gov/pubmed/9822228 (accessed on 1 June 2019). [CrossRef]
36. Freedman, S.F.; Mccormick, K.; Cox, T.A. Mitomycin C-augmented trabeculectomy with Postoperative Wound Modulation in Pediatric Glaucoma. *J. Am. Assoc. Ped. Ophthalmol. Strabismus* **1999**, *3*, 117–124. [CrossRef]
37. Mandal, A.K.; Bagga, H.; Nutheti, R.; Gothwal, V.K.; Nanda, A.K. Trabeculectomy with or without mitomycin-C for paediatric glaucoma in aphakia and pseudophakia following congenital cataract surgery. *Eye* **2003**, *17*, 53–62. [CrossRef]
38. Pakravan, M.; Homayoon, N.; Shahin, Y.; Reza, B.R.A. Trabeculectomy With Mitomycin C Versus Ahmed Glaucoma Implant With Mitomycin C for Treatment of Pediatric Aphakic Glaucoma. *J. Glaucoma* **2007**, *16*, 631–636. [CrossRef] [PubMed]
39. Wallace, D.K.; Plager, D.A.; Snyder, S.K.; Raiesdana, A.; Helveston, E.M.; Ellis, F.D. Surgical results of secondary glaucomas in childhood. *Ophthalmology* **1998**, *105*, 101–111. [CrossRef]
40. Balekudaru, S.; Vadalkar, J.; George, R.; Vijaya, L. The use of Ahmed glaucoma valve in the management of pediatric glaucoma. *J. Am. Assoc. Pediatr. Ophthalmol. Strabismus* **2014**, *18*, 351–356. [CrossRef] [PubMed]
41. Banitt, M.R.; Sidoti, P.A.; Gentile, R.C.; Tello, C.; Liebmann, J.M.; Rodriguez, N.; Dhar, S. Pars Plana Baerveldt Implantation for Refractory Childhood Glaucomas. *J. Glaucoma* **2009**, *18*, 412–417. [CrossRef]
42. Chen, T.C.; Bhatia, L.S.; Walton, D.S. Ahmed valve surgery for refractory pediatric glaucoma: A report of 52 eyes. *J. Am. Assoc. Pediatr. Ophthalmol. Strabismus* **2005**, *42*, 274–283. [CrossRef]
43. Donahue, S.P.; Keech, R.V.; Munden, P.; Scott, W.E. Baerveldt implant surgery in the treatment of advanced childhood glaucoma. *J. Am. Assoc. Pediatr. Ophthalmol. Strabismus* **1997**, *1*, 41–45. [CrossRef]
44. Elshatory, Y.M.; Gauger, E.H.; Kwon, Y.; Alward, W.L.M.; Boldt, H.C.; Russell, S.; Mahajan, V. Management of Pediatric Aphakic Glaucoma With Vitrectomy and Tube Shunts. *J. Am. Assoc. Pediatr. Ophthalmol. Strabismus* **2016**, *53*, 339–343. [CrossRef]
45. Englert, J.A.; Freedman, S.; Cox, T.A. The Ahmed Valve in refractory pediatric glaucoma. *Am. J. Ophthalmol.* **1999**, *127*, 34–42. [CrossRef]
46. Kirwan, C.; O'Keefe, M.; Lanigan, B.; Mahmood, U. Ahmed valve drainage implant surgery in the management of paediatric aphakic glaucoma. *Br. J. Ophthalmol.* **2005**, *89*, 855–858. [CrossRef] [PubMed]

47. Mills, R.P.; Reynolds, A.; Emond, M.J.; Barlow, W.E.; Leen, M.M. Long-term Survival of Molteno Glaucoma Drainage Devices. *Ophthalmology* **1996**, *103*, 299–305. [CrossRef]

48. O'Malley Schotthoefer, E.; Yanovitch, T.L.; Freedman, S.F. Aqueous drainage device surgery in refractory pediatric glaucomas: I. Long-term outcomes. *J. Am. Assoc. Pediatr. Ophthalmol. Strabismus* **2008**, *12*, 33–39. [CrossRef]

49. Pakravan, M.; Esfandiari, H.; Yazdani, S.; Doozandeh, A.; Dastborhan, Z.; Gerami, E.; Kheiri, B.; Pakravan, P.; Yaseri, M.; Hassanpour, K. Clinical outcomes of Ahmed glaucoma valve implantation in pediatric glaucoma. *Eur. J. Ophthalmol.* **2018**, *29*, 44–51. [CrossRef]

50. Rotsos, T.; Tsioga, A.; Andreanos, K.; Diagourtas, A.; Petrou, P.; Georgalas, I.; Papaconstantinou, D. Managing high risk glaucoma with the Ahmed valve implant: 20 years of experience. *Int. J. Ophthalmol.* **2018**, *11*, 240–244. [CrossRef]

51. Spiess, K.; Calvo, J.P. Outcomes of Ahmed glaucoma valve in paediatric glaucoma following congenital cataract surgery in persistent foetal vasculature. *Eur. J. Ophthalmol.* **2020**, *31*, 1070–1078. [CrossRef]

52. Geyer, O.; Segal, A.; Melamud, A.; Wolf, A. Clinical Outcomes After Ahmed Glaucoma Valve Implantation for Pediatric Glaucoma After Congenital Cataract Surgery. *J. Glaucoma* **2020**, *30*, 78–82. [CrossRef]

53. Beck, A.D.; Freedman, S.; Kammer, J.; Jin, J. Aqueous shunt devices compared with trabeculectomy with Mitomycin-C for children in the first two years of life. *Am. J. Ophthalmol.* **2003**, *136*, 994–1000. [CrossRef]

54. Autrata, R.; Lokaj, M. Trans-scleral diode laser cyclophotocoagulation in children with refractory glaucoma. Long-term outcomes. *Scripta Med. Fac. Med. Univ. Brun. Masaryk.* **2003**, *76*, 67–78.

55. Cantor, A.J.; Wang, J.; Li, S.; Neely, D.E.; Plager, D.A. Long-term efficacy of endoscopic cyclophotocoagulation in the management of glaucoma following cataract surgery in children. *J. Am. Assoc. Pediatr. Ophthalmol. Strabismus* **2018**, *22*, 188–191. [CrossRef] [PubMed]

56. Carter, B.C.; Plager, D.A.; Neely, D.E.; Sprunger, D.T.; Sondhi, N.; Roberts, G.J. Endoscopic diode laser cyclophotocoagulation in the management of aphakic and pseudophakic glaucoma in children. *J. Am. Assoc. Pediatr. Ophthalmol. Strabismus* **2006**, *11*, 34–40. [CrossRef] [PubMed]

57. Glaser, T.S.; Mulvihill, M.S.; Freedman, S.F. Endoscopic cyclophotocoagulation (ECP) for childhood glaucoma: A large single-center cohort experience. *J. Am. Assoc. Pediatr. Ophthalmol. Strabismus* **2019**, *23*, 84.e1–84.e7. [CrossRef] [PubMed]

58. Kirwan, J.F.; Shah, P.; Khaw, P.T. Diode laser cyclophotocoagulation: Role in the management of refractory pediatric glaucomas. *Ophthalmology* **2002**, *109*, 316–323. [CrossRef]

59. Neely, D.E.; Plager, D.A. Endocyclophotocoagulation for management of difficult pediatric glaucomas. *J. Am. Assoc. Pediatr. Ophthalmol. Strabismus* **2001**, *5*, 221–229. [CrossRef]

60. Schlote, T.; Grüb, M.; Kynigopoulos, M. Long-term results after transscleral diode laser cyclophotocoagulation in refractory posttraumatic glaucoma and glaucoma in aphakia. *Glaucoma* **2007**, *246*, 405–410. [CrossRef]

61. Hirabayashi, M.T.; Lee, D.; King, J.T.; Thomsen, S.; An, J.A. Comparison of Surgical Outcomes of 360° Circumferential Trabeculotomy Versus Sectoral Excisional Goniotomy with the Kahook Dual Blade At 6 Months. *Clin. Ophthalmol.* **2019**, *13*, 2017–2024. [CrossRef]

62. Laroche, D.; Rickford, K.; Sakkari, S. Case report: Cataract extraction/lensectomy, excisional goniotomy and transscleral cyclophotocoagulation: Affordable combination MIGS for plateau iris glaucoma. *J. Natl. Med. Assoc.* **2022**. [CrossRef]

63. Laroche, D.; Nkrumah, G.; Ng, C. Combination microinvasive glaucoma surgery: 23-gauge cystotome goniotomy and intra-scleral ciliary sulcus suprachoroidal microtube surgery in refractory and severe glaucoma: A case series. *Indian J. Ophthalmol.* **2020**, *68*, 2557–2561. [CrossRef]

64. Laroche, D.; Okaka, Y.; Ng, C. A Novel Low Cost Effective Technique in Using a 23 Gauge Straight Cystotome to Perform Goniotomy: Making Micro-invasive Glaucoma Surgery (MIGS) Accessible to the Africans and the Diaspora. *J. Natl. Med. Assoc.* **2019**, *111*, 193–197. [CrossRef]

65. Tanito, M.; Sano, I.; Ikeda, Y.; Fujihara, E. Short-term results of microhook ab interno trabeculotomy, a novel minimally invasive glaucoma surgery in Japanese eyes: Initial case series. *Acta Ophthalmol.* **2017**, *95*, e354–e360. [CrossRef] [PubMed]

66. Tanito, M. Microhook ab interno trabeculotomy, a novel minimally invasive glaucoma surgery. *Clin. Ophthalmol.* **2018**, *12*, 43–48. [CrossRef] [PubMed]

67. Chen, P.P.; Palmberg, P.F. Needling Revision of Glaucoma Drainage Device Filtering Blebs. *Ophthalmology* **1997**, *104*, 1004–1010. [CrossRef]

68. Zuo, W.; Lesk, M.R. Surgical Outcome of Replacing a Failed Ahmed Glaucoma Valve by a Baerveldt Glaucoma Implant in the Same Quadrant in Refractory Glaucoma. *J. Glaucoma* **2018**, *27*, 421–428. [CrossRef] [PubMed]

69. Anand, A.; Tello, C.; Sidoti, P.A.; Ritch, R.; Liebmann, J.M. Sequential Glaucoma Implants in Refractory Glaucoma. *Am. J. Ophthalmol.* **2010**, *149*, 95–101. [CrossRef] [PubMed]

70. Daniel, M.C.; Adams, G.G.W.; Dahlmann-Noor, A. Medical Management of Children with Congenital/Infantile Cataract Associated with Microphthalmia, Microcornea, or Persistent Fetal Vasculature. *J. Am. Assoc. Pediatr. Ophthalmol. Strabismus* **2019**, *56*, 43–49. [CrossRef]

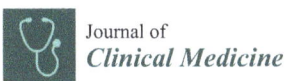

Journal of
Clinical Medicine

Article

The Dual Effect of Rho-Kinase Inhibition on Trabecular Meshwork Cells Cytoskeleton and Extracellular Matrix in an In Vitro Model of Glaucoma

Juliette Buffault [1,2,3,*], Françoise Brignole-Baudouin [2,4], Élodie Reboussin [2], Karima Kessal [2], Antoine Labbé [1,2,3], Stéphane Mélik Parsadaniantz [2] and Christophe Baudouin [1,2,3]

1   Department of Ophthalmology III, Quinze-Vingts National Ophthalmology Hospital, IHU Foresight, 75012 Paris, France; alabbe@15-20.fr (A.L.); cbaudouin@15-20.fr (C.B.)
2   Institut de la Vision, Sorbonne Université, INSERM, CNRS, IHU Foresight, 75012 Paris, France; fbaudouin@15-20.fr (F.B.-B.); elodie.reboussin@inserm.fr (É.R.); karima.kessal@inserm.fr (K.K.); stephane.melik-parsadaniantz@inserm.fr (S.M.P.)
3   Department of Ophthalmology, Ambroise Paré Hospital, APHP, Université de Paris Saclay, 92100 Boulogne-Billancourt, France
4   Department of Biology, CHNO des Quinze-Vingts, IHU Foresight, 75012 Paris, France
*   Correspondence: jbuffault@15-20.fr

Citation: Buffault, J.; Brignole-Baudouin, F.; Reboussin, É.; Kessal, K.; Labbé, A.; Mélik Parsadaniantz, S.; Baudouin, C. The Dual Effect of Rho-Kinase Inhibition on Trabecular Meshwork Cells Cytoskeleton and Extracellular Matrix in an In Vitro Model of Glaucoma. *J. Clin. Med.* **2022**, *11*, 1001. https://doi.org/10.3390/jcm11041001

Academic Editors: Maria Letizia Salvetat and Michele Lanza

Received: 29 December 2021
Accepted: 11 February 2022
Published: 15 February 2022

Publisher's Note: MDPI stays neutral with regard to jurisdictional claims in published maps and institutional affiliations.

Abstract: The trabecular meshwork (TM) is the main site of drainage of the aqueous humor, and its dysfunction leads to intraocular pressure elevation, which is one of the main risk factors of glaucoma. We aimed to compare the effects on cytoskeleton organization and extracellular matrix (ECM) of latanoprost (LT) and a Rho-kinase inhibitor (ROCKi) on a transforming growth factor beta2 (TGF-β2)-induced glaucoma-like model developed from primary culture of human TM cells (pHTMC). The TGF-β2 stimulated pHTMC were grown and incubated with LT or a ROCKi (Y-27632) for 24 h. The expression of alpha-smooth muscle actin (αSMA) and fibronectin (FN), and phosphorylation of the myosin light chain (MLC-P) and Cofilin (Cofilin-P) were evaluated using immunofluorescence and Western blot. The architectural modifications were studied in a Matrigel™ 3D culture. TGF-β2 increased the expression of αSMA and FN in pHTMC and modified the cytoskeleton with cross-linked actin network formation. LT did not alter the expression of αSMA but decreased FN deposition. The ROCKi decreased TGF-β2-induced αSMA and FN expression, as well as MLC-P and Cofilin-P, and stimulated the cells to recover a basal cytoskeletal arrangement. In the preliminary 3D study, pHTMC organized in a mesh conformation showed the widening of the TM under the effect of Y-27632. By simultaneously modifying the organization of the cytoskeleton and the ECM, with fibronectin deposition and overexpression, TGF-β2 reproduced the trabecular degeneration described in glaucoma. The ROCKi was able to reverse the TGF-β2-induced cytoskeletal and ECM rearrangements. LT loosened the extracellular matrix but had no action on the stress fibers.

Keywords: glaucoma; trabecular meshwork; Matrigel; 3D culture; intraocular pressure; outflow; cytoskeleton; rho-kinase inhibitor; prostaglandin analog

1. Introduction

Primary open-angle glaucoma (POAG) is a leading cause of irreversible blindness. This optic neuropathy affected more than 50 million people worldwide in 2020 [1]. Its main risk factor is elevated intraocular pressure (IOP) [2]. The trabecular meshwork (TM), in the iridocorneal angle, is the main site of drainage of the aqueous humor, and its dysfunction results in IOP elevation. The TM is a complex, three-dimensional structure composed of multiple layers of extracellular matrix (ECM) covered with trabecular meshwork cells (TMC) [3].

In POAG, abnormal resistance is generated in the outflow pathway including the juxtacanalicular TM, the inner wall of Schlemm's canal, and its basement membrane [4]. In the TM, increase in resistance is linked to a mixed mechanism, including loss of TMC and changes in their architecture and remodeling of the ECM [4–7]. Changes in the morphology and stiffness of juxtacanalicular TM cells have been described [6]. TGF-β2 is a profibrotic cytokine known to be involved in glaucoma pathophysiology. It is significantly elevated in the aqueous humor of patients with POAG [8]. TM exposure to TGFβ 2 has been used to induce ocular hypertension in animal models and cultured human anterior segment perfusion studies [9,10]. In vitro studies have shown that TGF-β induced the synthesis by TM cells of components of the ECM not degradable by metalloproteinases, which could lead to increased outflow resistance [11]. TGF-β2 also increases cell stiffness by the formation of cross-linked actin networks (CLANs) via the Rho-ROCK pathway [12].

However, this primum movens of the glaucomatous pathology is still rarely targeted by glaucoma treatments. The only demonstrated therapeutic strategy to stop the progression of the visual field deterioration in glaucoma is to reduce IOP [2,13]. Among the medical treatments, prostaglandin analogs (PGA) are the most effective. PGAs increase the aqueous humor outflow. The mechanism of the hypotonic action of PGA is still imperfectly understood. It is mainly due to a promotion of the aqueous humor outflow through the uveoscleral route. However, an action of PGA on the TM, acting by remodeling the ECM, was described [14,15]. In recent years, studies in the field aimed to develop medication that act directly on the trabecular cytoskeleton. Rho-kinase inhibitors (ROCKi) represent a new therapeutic strategy in glaucoma, which precisely target a major pathway involved in the modifications observed in the TM [16].

The Rho GTPase/Rho kinase (ROCK) signaling pathway plays an important role in the modulation of the cytoskeleton of cells and the synthesis of ECM [16,17]. Rho GTPase activates its effector molecules, Rho-kinase ROCK1 and ROCK2. ROCK1 and 2 inhibit the myosin light chain phosphatase complex of Type 1 (MYPT1), thereby modifying the actin cytoskeleton. ROCK1 and 2 also activate LIM kinases (LIMKs), leading to the inhibition of Cofilin. This results in actin polymerization [18,19] (Figure 1). Activation of this pathway increases resistance to outflow, while its inhibition reduces IOP [12,20]. Rho-kinase inhibitors were recently approved for clinical use [21–26].

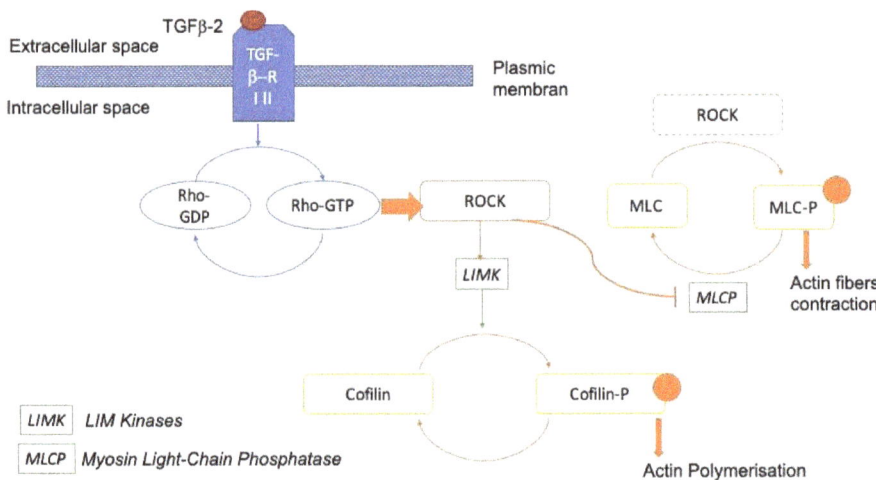

Figure 1. Rho-kinase signaling pathway. The TGF-β receptor (TRF-β RI-II) activates its effector molecules, ROCKs (Rho-kinases ROCK1 and 2). ROCKs inhibit myosin light chain phosphatase (MLCP). Phosphorylation of the myosin light chain induces actin fiber contraction. ROCKs activate LIM kinases, which phosphorylate cofilin, leading to actin stabilization [27].

We aimed to study the effect of a ROCK-inhibitor on two major targets in glaucoma pathophysiology: the organization of both the trabecular ECM and TM cytoskeleton. We used a pathological TM model induced by TGF-β2 on 2D and 3D primary cultures of human TMC (pHTMC). Indeed, 2D cell culture models may not fully reflect the actual architecture of the TM. Cell culture in 3D could allow us to better mimic the microenvironmental conditions encountered in vivo. We compared the effects of ROCKi Y-27632 on the cytoskeleton of pHTMC and the TM ECM, with LT, the lead compound of the PGA family.

2. Materials and Methods

2.1. Primary Human Trabecular Meshwork Cell Isolation and Culture

Primary human TMC (pHTMC) was isolated from non-glaucomatous donor tissue rings. All donor tissues were obtained and managed following the guidelines of the Declaration of Helsinki for research involving human tissue. The human tissues used in our study came from corneoscleral rings discarded after the corneal graft. Human tissues were provided by the French eye bank, which ensured complete anonymization. The TM was carefully dissected under a microscope from a corneoscleral ring and transported in an Optisol-GS conservation medium (Bausch and Lomb Surgical, Inc.; Irvine, CA, USA) at room temperature (RT). The TM samples were digested with collagenase (Gibco^{TM} Collagenase, Type IV, Fisher Scientific, Cat. # 17-104-019) diluted to 10 mg/mL in culture medium for TMC (Trabecular Meshwork Cell Medium (TMCM), ScienCell Cat. # 6591, composition: basic medium, 2% fetal calf serum (FBS), 1% trabecular cell growth supplement, and 1% penicillin and streptomycin solution (penicillin 10,000 U/mL, streptomycin 10,000 µg/mL)) for 30 min at 37 °C and then stirred at RT for 30 min. After digestion, the cells were centrifuged at $1500 \times g$ for 5 min before being suspended in 250 µL of TMCM and seeded into a 24-well plate. Cells were seeded at 100,000 cells/mL (25,000 cells per well). The cultured cells were incubated at 37 °C in a humid atmosphere with 5% carbon dioxide. At 48 h, we added 250 µL of TMCM. Fresh culture medium was supplied every 3 to 4 days. Cells were maintained at 37 °C in a humidified atmosphere until 80–90% confluence was achieved, at which point cells were trypsinized using 0.05% Trypsin/0.5 mM EDTA (Gibco^{TM}, Cat. #25300062, Grand Island, NY, USA) and subcultured at 1.8×10^5 cells/mL in 25 cm^2 or 75 cm^2 cell culture flasks with TMCM. At each passage (P), a part of the pHTMC was seeded in 48-well plates for immunofluorescence analysis. Before use in experiments, all pHTMC strains were characterized by immunohistochemistry. All studies were conducted using cells before the 7th passage, and at least three different donors' human primary cell cultures were used for each experiment. Information about pHTMC lines are available in supplementary data (Table S1).

2.2. Trabecular Meshwork Cell Characterization

Before use in experiments, all pHTMC strains were characterized by immunohistochemistry for expression of α-smooth muscle actin (alpha-SMA), aquaporin 1 (AQP1), chitinase-3-like 1 (CHI3L1), and CD44. Characterization was performed between the 1st and 4th passages. The induction of alpha-SMA in response to dexamethasone (DXM) at 100 nM for 7 days was also used. It represents a reliable marker for characterizing trabecular cells. The pHTMC were fixed with 4% paraformaldehyde for 15 min. Then, a saturation/permeation solution containing 0.1% Triton X-100 and 5% NGS in PBS was employed for 1 h at RT before incubation with specific primary antibodies overnight at 4 °C. Primary antibodies and dilutions used are listed in Table 1. After washing with PBS, the cells were incubated with the corresponding secondary antibodies (Thermo Fisher, donkey anti-mouse conjugated with Alexa fluor 594 (A21203), and donkey anti-rabbit conjugated to Alexa fluor 488 (A21206)), at a dilution of 1/1000 for 1 h at RT. The nuclei were stained with DAPI (1/1000 dilution).

Western immunoblot analysis of the myocilin induction in response to DXM was also used to characterize the pHTMC in accordance with the consensus recommendations [28]. The analysis of myocilin induction by DXM compared two conditions: 1/TMCM + 2.10^{-3}% ethanol (control) for 6 days, and 2/TMCM + 100 nM DXM (Sigma D8893, stock solution 20 µg/mL) dissolved in ethanol for 6 days. Mouse anti-myocilin (Santa Cruz sc-137233, dilution 1/100), anti-β-actin (Cell signaling 3700, 1/5000) primary antibodies, and HRP-linked anti-mouse secondary antibody (Invitrogen) were used. Protein expression was analyzed using Quantity One software and normalized with β-actin protein.

Table 1. Primary antibodies used in immunofluorescence for the characterization of cells.

Antibody	Dilution	Host	Supplier	Reference
Alpha-SMA	1/100	Rabbit polyclonal	Abcam	ab 5694
CD44	1/125	Rabbit monoclonal	Abcam	ab 189524
Aquaporin 1 (AQP1)	1/100	Mouse monoclonal	Santa Cruz	sc 25287
Chitinase-3like 1 (CHI3L1)	1/125	Rabbit polyclonal	Thermo Fisher	PAS-43746

2.3. Exposure to TGF-β2 and Therapeutic Molecules

pHTMC were seeded at 100,000 cells/mL in 48-well plates (100 μL/well; 10,000 cells/well); At subconfluence, TGF-β2 (5 ng/mL) was introduced in the TMCM and incubated for 24 h [29]. Then, the pHTMC were incubated for 24 h with TGF-β2 (5 ng/mL), combined either with the ROCKi Y-27632 (Santa Cruz Biotechnology) at 25 nM [30,31] or with Monoprost® (LT) at 1/100 (i.e., 1.15 μM) (latanoprost 50 μg/mL, Laboratoires Théa, France). We used Y-27632 (25 nM), a ROCKi, which acts upstream of the phosphorylation of MYPT1 and Cofilin. The controls were vehicle (TMCM only) or TGF-β2 (5 ng/mL) for 48 h.

2.4. Immunocytochemistry

The effects on the organization of the cytoskeleton and of the ECM were characterized in immunocytochemistry using the anti-alpha-SMA and the anti-fibronectin (FN) antibodies, respectively. Involvement of the Rho-kinase pathway was studied using the anti-Phospho-Myosin Light Chain 2 (Ser19) (MLC-P) and anti-Phospho-Cofilin (Ser3) (Cofilin-P). The pHTMC were fixed with 4% paraformaldehyde for 15 min. Primary antibodies and dilution used are listed in Table 2. After washing with PBS, the cells were incubated with the corresponding secondary antibodies (donkey anti-rabbit, conjugated to Alexa fluor 488 (Thermo Fisher, A21206)), at a dilution of 1/1000 for 1 h at RT. The nuclei were stained with DAPI (1/1000). Phalloidin (Alexa 546 (A22283) 1/200) was used to label actin filaments in the cytoplasm.

Table 2. Primary antibodies used in immunofluorescence staining.

Antibody	Dilution	Host	Supplier	Reference
Alpha-SMA	1/100	Rabbit	Abcam	ab5694
Fibronectin	1/100	Rabbit	Abcam	ab2413
Phospho-Myosin Light Chain 2 (Ser19)	1/100	Rabbit	Cell signaling	3671S
Phospho-Cofilin (Ser3)	1/100	Rabbit	Cell signaling	3313S

The immunofluorescence images were taken using a Nikon ECLIPSE Ti fluorescence inverted microscope; the images were acquired with $100\times$ and $200\times$ magnifications and then processed using ImageJ software (NIH, Bethesda, MD, USA).

The quantification was carried out using the Cellomics ArrayScanVTI (Thermo Fisher Scientific, MA, USA), an imaging system that detects, analyzes, and quantifies immunofluorescence staining on adherent cells. In each well, a central zone of 16 mm² was analyzed. Using the HCS Studio Cellomics Scan software (Thermo Scientific, version 6.6.0), we measured the total area of positive labeling, which we related to the number of nuclei. An annular analysis pattern around each nucleus was drawn. The positive labeling area was measured in each of these rings. This area was then related to the number of nuclei.

2.5. Protein Extraction and Western Blot Analysis

The protein levels of fibronectin (FN) were quantified by Western blotting. Cellular proteins were extracted with ice-cold radioimmunoprecipitation assay (RIPA) buffer (RIPA Buffer, Sigma-Aldrich R0278) containing protease inhibitors (Complete Protease Inhibitor, Roche, Manheim, Germany) on ice. Proteins were quantified using a bicinchoninic acid assay (Thermo Fischer Scientific). Proteins from each sample (1 μg) were separated by electrophoresis on a NuPAGE™ 3–8% Tris-Acetate Protein Gel (Invitrogen EA03752PK2) in SDS running buffer (Invitrogen). The proteins were then transferred onto a polyvinylidene fluoride (PVDF) membrane and probed with the following primary antibodies: rabbit anti-fibronectin (Abcam ab2413, 1/500) and anti-β-actin (Cell signaling 3700, 1/1000). HRP-linked anti-rabbit secondary antibodies (Invitrogen) were used. Bound antibody was detected using Pierce™ ECL Plus Western Blotting Substrate (Thermo Scientific). Protein expression was analyzed by densitometry using ImageJ and normalized to the housekeeping proteins β-actin.

2.6. Three-Dimensional (3D) Trabecular Meshwork Cell Culture

For the 3D pHTMC culture, we used Matrigel® (Corning Inc., Tewksbury, MA, USA), a basement membrane matrix secreted by Engelbreth–Holm–Swarm (EHS) mouse sarcoma cells [32]. Its composition is close to that of trabecular ECM, as it contains laminin-11, collagen IV, heparin sulfate proteoglycans, entactin/nidogen, and growth factors (FGF, EGF, TGF beta, IGF, and PDGF) [33]. The pHTMC stained with DiO (Vybrant™ DiO Cell-Labeling Solution, Invitrogen, V-22886) were gently mixed at a concentration of 10^5 cells/mL in Matrigel® diluted 1/2 in the TMCM culture medium and then sewn onto inserts in a 12-well plate (Greiner Bio-One ThinCert cell culture insert for 12 well plates, sterile, polyethylene terephthalate (PET) transparent membrane, pore diameter: 0.4 μm. Cat. N° 665641). The cells were incubated at 37 °C for 30 min, and then 800 μL of TMCM medium was added to the bottom of the well, and 200 μL in the inserts. The cells were then let incubate at 37 °C in a humid atmosphere with 5% CO_2. Fresh culture medium was supplied every 3 to 4 days. The cells were exposed to TGF-β2 (5 ng/mL) for 48 h and LT and Y-27632 for 24 h, according to the same protocol as for the two-dimensional model. At 7 days, the 3D cultures obtained were fixed with 4% paraformaldehyde for one hour. Actin was stained with phalloidin (1/100), and the nuclei were stained with DAPI (1/1000) before analysis using confocal microscopy. Confocal laser scanning microscopy was performed using an Olympus IX81 confocal microscope coupled to Fluoview software (Olympus, Ver 4.2), and the images were acquired at 200× magnification. Confocal 3D images were processed using Imaris3D® software (Bitplane AG, Zurich, Switzerland). All confocal images from the same experiment were captured using the same laser intensity and gain settings, so that the intensities of different samples could be compared.

2.7. Statistical Analysis

At least three different donors' human primary cell cultures were used for each experiment. Data are expressed as mean ± standard deviation. The differences between vehicle-treated (controls), TGF-β2-treated, and TGF-β2/LT- or TGF-β2/Y27632-treated pHTMC were analyzed using ANOVA followed by Tukey's multiple comparisons test (GraphPad Prism 9, LLC). p values < 0.05 were considered significant.

3. Results

3.1. Trabecular Meshwork Cell Characterization

Experiments conducted to validate our pHTMC culture are available in the supplementary data (Figure S1). There are no specific markers for trabecular cells, so we used a set of molecules known to be expressed by trabecular cells. pHTMC expressed alpha-SMA in relation to their important contractile property in the mechanotransduction process [3]. As expected, the AQP1 and CD44 antigens were located at the pHTMC plasma membrane. Nuclear localization of the protein CHI3L1 was found, compatible with the macrophagic activity of trabecular cells [34] (Figure S1b). Then, we used dexamethasone (DXM) exposure (100 nM) for 7 days to further characterize the pHTMC through alpha-SMA induction of and actin skeleton reorganization (Figure S1c).

Western immunoblot analysis of the myocilin induction in response to DXM confirmed the TMC characterization in accordance with the consensus recommendations [28] (Figure S1d).

3.2. Exposure to TGF-β2

Unlike the untreated primary trabecular cells, which displayed aligned actin fibers, after 48 h of exposure to TGF-β2 at 5 ng/mL, pHTMC exhibited rearrangements of the actin cytoskeleton, appearing disorganized and more extended. While labeling of alpha-SMA was more diffuse in the cytosol of untreated cells, there was a reorganization of fibers under the effect of TGF-β2. An increase in cell stress fibers was thus observed accompanied by the formation of CLANs (Figures 2 and 3). These CLANs were present in 38.7% (±12%) of cells exposed to TGF-β2 and were not present in the control. Quantification of the alpha-SMA expression was also greater after treatment with TGF-β2 compared with the control (1.8-fold, $p = 0.0116$) (Figure 3b, alpha-SMA).

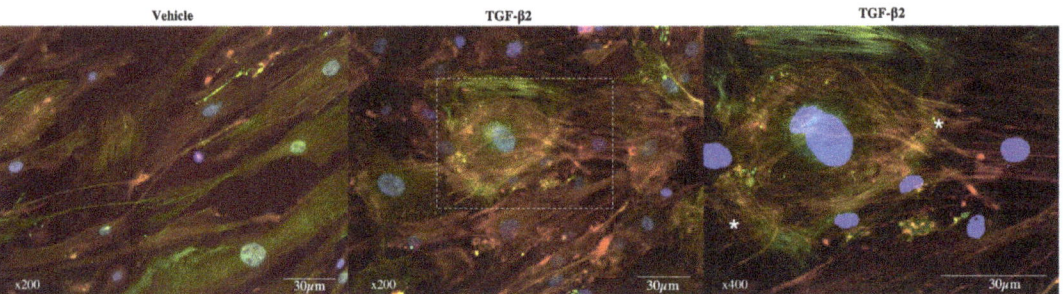

Figure 2. Cytoskeletal remodeling after TGF-β2 exposure. pHTMC were treated for 48 h with TMCM only (Vehicle) or with TGF-β2 (5 ng/mL). F-actin filaments were visualized by phalloidin staining (red) and alpha-SMA antibody (green), and nuclei were counterstained with DAPI (blue). Right: enlarged images from corresponding areas. Asterisks indicate CLANs.

The Rho-ROCK downstream signaling pathway for TGF-β2 induces phosphorylation of MYPT1, which inhibits the dephosphorylation of MLC and the phosphorylation of the intracellular protein Cofilin. After 48 h of exposure to TGF-β2 at 5 ng/mL, there was an activation of the ROCK pathway, with increased expressions of MLC-P and Cofilin-P compared to the vehicle-treated pHTMC (Figure 3b, MLC-P and Cofilin-P) (respectively 1.5 and 2.0-fold, $p < 0.05$). MLC-P immunofluorescence labeling presented the same distribution as actin: rather diffuse in the cytosol of untreated cells and organized into fibers after exposure to TGF-β2 (Figure 3a, MLC-P). Cofilin-P was located in the cytosol of pHTMC, and the staining was more intense after TGF-β2 exposure (Figure 3a, Cofilin-P).

Regarding the ECM, immunofluorescence analysis showed that following exposure to TGF-β2 at 5 ng/mL, fibronectin organized differently, with multiple joint fibrils forming a network that appeared thicker and denser than that found in the controls (Figure 3a, fibronectin). Quantification of the fibronectin expression was also greater after treatment with TGF-β2 vs. control (1.8-fold, $p = 0.0119$) (Figure 3b, fibronectin).

Western blot analysis confirmed the induction of fibronectin expression in pHTMC cultures after TGFβ2 treatment compared with the control (Figure 4a,b).

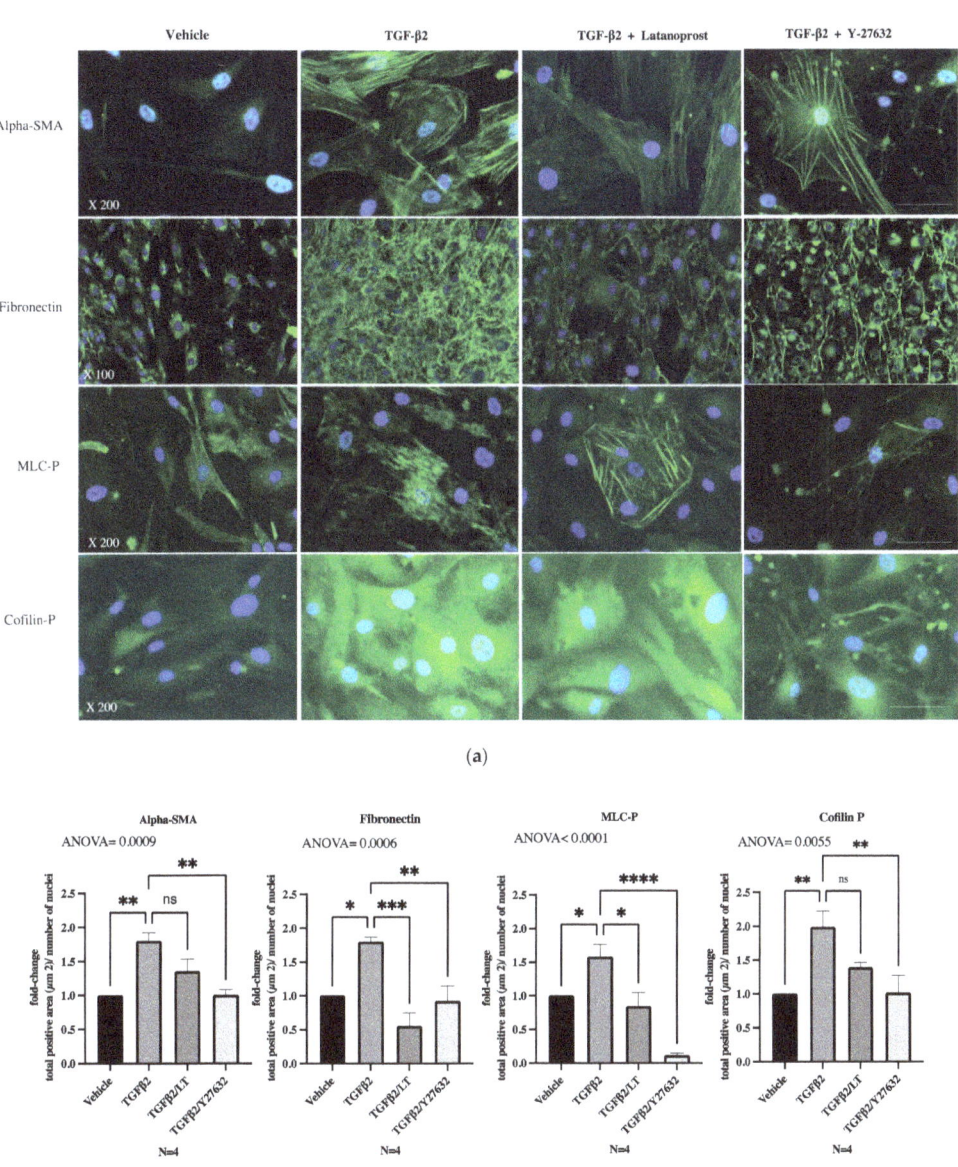

(a)

(b)

Figure 3. (**a**) Immunofluorescence analysis of the effect of LT 0.5 μg/mL or the ROCK-inhibitor Y-27632 25 nM for 24 h on pHTMC. pHTMC were treated for 48 h with TMCM only (Vehicle) or with TGF-β2 5 ng/mL or with 24 h of TGF-β2 5 ng/mL followed by 24 h of TGF-β2 5 ng/mL along with LT 0.5 μg/mL or Y-27632 25 nM. Nuclei are stained with DAPI (blue). The green staining corresponds to the antibodies indicated. Scale bar = 30 μm. This figure shows the major effect of LT on the density of ECM with no effect on the cytoskeleton itself. The ROCKi modified both the cytoskeleton and the ECM relaxation. (**b**) Quantification, with Arrayscan, of the total positive labeling area related to the number of cells (μm^2) in fold-change (mean ± SEM). * $p < 0.05$, ** $p < 0.01$, *** $p < 0.001$, **** $p < 0.0001$.

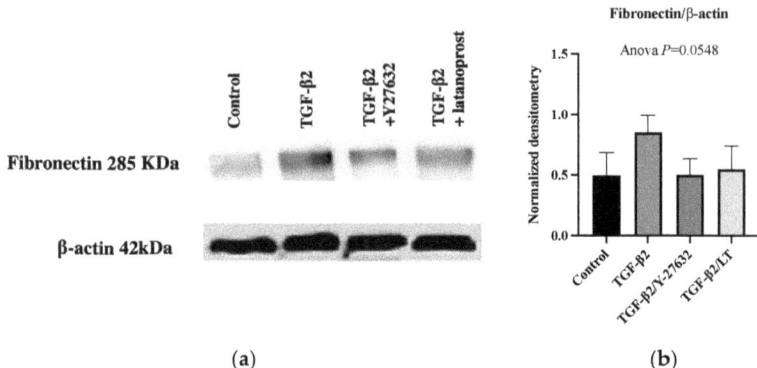

(a)   (b)

Figure 4. Protein expressions in pHTMC cultures after treatment with 5 ng/mL TGFβ2 for 48 h in the absence or presence of 25 nM Y27632 or 0.5 µg/mL LT for 24 h. (**a**) Representative Western blots of fibronectin and β-actin (mean ± SEM). (**b**) Densitometry of Western blot analysis of fibronectin normalized to β-actin.

3.3. Effects of Therapeutic Molecules on TGF-β2-Induced Pathological Trabecular Meshwork Model

Cytoskeletal rearrangements induced by TGF-β2 persisted under the effect of LT (Figure 3a, alpha-SMA). The expression of alpha-SMA remained more intense than in vehicle-treated pHTMC, which was confirmed after quantification using Arrayscan (Figure 3b, alpha-SMA) (ANOVA, $p < 0.0001$, TGFβ2 vs. TGFβ2/LT ns). CLANs were also present, and the expression profile of MLC-P and Cofilin-P did not differ qualitatively from TGFβ2-exposed cells in immunofluorescence images, even though the quantification showed a significant decrease in the total positive labeling area (Figure 3a,b).

Regarding the ECM, following exposure to TGF-β2 at 5 ng/mL, fibronectin increased in density compared to that of the controls. LT greatly reduced the expression of fibronectin, resulting in the formation of a much looser mesh compared with TGF-β2-exposed pHTMCs (Figure 3a, fibronectin). The total positive area related to the number of nuclei was reduced (0.55-fold) when treating the TGF-β2-exposed pHTMC with LT ($p = 0.0004$) compared with TGF-β2-exposed pHTMC (Figure 3b, fibronectin). While non-significant, Western blot analysis revealed that the TGF-β2-exposed pHTMC with LT (0.5 µg/mL) seemed to decrease the TGF-β2-stimulated expression of fibronectin (ANOVA, $p = 0.0548$) (Figure 4a,b).

The cytoskeletal rearrangements induced by TGF-β2 were modified by Y-27632. The intensity of α-SMA labeling was reduced compared to TGF-β2-exposed pHTMC ($p = 0.017$) (Figure 3b, alpha-SMA). Inhibition of ROCK was associated with relaxation of the cells and disassembly of stress fibers and CLANs. A new distribution of actin fibers in the periphery was observed in response to the alteration of the actin cytoskeleton (Figure 3a, alpha-SMA). TGF-β2-induced MLC-P and Cofilin-P overexpression were also inhibited by Y-27632 ($p < 0.01$) (Figure 3a,b, MLC-P and Cofilin-P).

Regarding the ECM, the ROCK inhibitor Y-27632 decreased fibronectin expression, with a looser mesh and enlarged intercellular spaces compared with TGF-β2-exposed pHTMC (Figure 3a, fibronectin). The labeling quantification revealed a reduction in fibronectin expression compared to TGF-β2-exposed pHTMC ($p = 0.0062$) (Figure 3b, fibronectin). Western blot analysis showed that treating the TGF-β2-exposed pHTMC with the ROCK inhibitor Y-27632 (25 nM) for 24 h decreased the TGF-β2-induced overexpression of fibronectin (Figure 4a,b).

3.4. Three-Dimensional Trabecular Meshwork Cell Cultures

Figure 5 shows the 3D organization of pHTMC in Matrigel^{TM}. The pHTMC organized in a mesh conformation with interconnections and the formation of intercellular spaces. Visual observations show that TGF-β2 induced rearrangements of the cytoskeleton with an organization of actin into more extensive fibers and decreased intercellular space. There was no modification of the actin disposition nor of the intercellular spaces after exposure to LT. However, the changes induced by TGF-β2 were modified under the effect of Y-27632. Actin fibers were less extensive, resulting in the widening of spaces between cells (Figure 5).

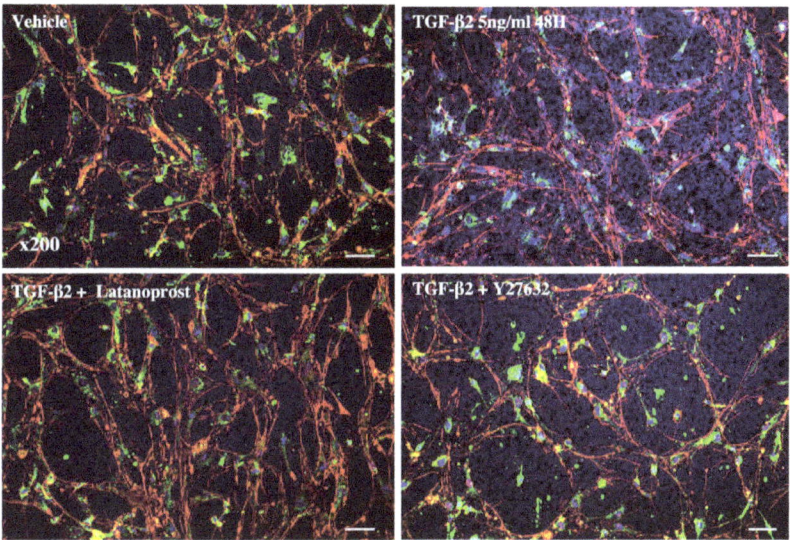

Figure 5. Confocal microscopy images of the 3D cultured pHTMC. Analysis of the effect of the ROCK inhibitor Y27632 at 25 nM for 24 h and the effect of LT at 0.5 µg/mL on primary human pHTMC treated with TGF-β2 at 5 ng/mL for 48 h. The cells were treated with TMCM alone (vehicle), 5 ng/mL of TGF-β2 for 48 h, or with TGF-β2 (5 ng/mL) for 24 h followed by a combination of TGF-β2 at 5 ng/mL and with Y-27632 (25 nM) or LT (0.5 µg/mL) for 24 h. Actin fibers are stained in red by phalloidin, membranes with DiO (green), and nuclei with DAPI (blue). Magnification 200×. Scale bar = 30 µm.

4. Discussion

In the present study, we used an in vitro TGF-β-induced pathological TM model from primary cultures of human trabecular cells. We first showed an effect of TGF-β2 on the organization of the cytoskeleton, with the formation of CLANs, and an increase in its contractibility, as well as an effect on the ECM, with an increase in fibronectin deposits. We also demonstrated activation of the ROCK pathway. We then showed that ROCKi has a dual effect on pHTMC with action on both the fibronectin deposition and the cytoskeleton, whereas latanoprost only acts on ECM degradation.

The family of TGF-β cytokines is known to be associated with impairment of several cellular functions, including differentiation, proliferation, and remodeling of the ECM [35]. The profibrotic role of TGF-β2 and its presence in the aqueous humor of patients with glaucoma implicates its potential role in the pathogenesis of ocular hypertension through TM degeneration/dysfunction [36]. In our study, we showed that TGF-β2 activated the Rho-ROCK pathway in TMC and induced actin fiber rearrangement and co-localization of alpha-SMA to stress fibers. TGF-β2 also induced fibronectin deposition. By simultaneously modifying the organization of the cytoskeleton and the ECM, with fibronectin deposition and overexpression, TGF-β2 allows the trabecular degeneration described in glaucoma to develop. TGF-β2 was also used in a TM model by Torrejon et al., who described the production of ECM and increased resistance to the aqueous humor outflow in vitro [37]. Ota et al. also showed that TGF-β2 enhances transendothelial electrical resistance in a culture of HTM [38]. Glucocorticoids such as dexamethasone are often used to model trabecular degeneration because they modify the cytoskeleton of TMC and the ECM. However, this corresponds more to the modifications obtained in corticosteroid-induced iatrogenic glaucoma, which constitutes a subtype of open-angle glaucoma [39]. This constitutes an advantage of the TGF-β2-induced model of TM alteration compared to the use of glucocorticoids. One of the limitations of our study is that we did not study the effect of therapeutic molecules in the absence of TGF-β2. Torrejon et al. studied the effect of Y-27632 alone on fibronectin expression of TMC and found no difference with the control. However, they demonstrated that Y-27632 in combination with TGF-β2 substantially decreased the expression of fibronectin compared to samples treated with TGF-β2 alone. Compared to vehicle control, TGF beta2/Y-27632 combined treatment increased fibronectin, demonstrating that the ROCKi counteracts the otherwise fibrotic effect of TGF-β2, effectively lowering ECM accumulation [37].

We highlighted an action of latanoprost on the fibronectin deposition without action on the cytoskeleton. This is consistent with the literature. Kalouche et al. showed that latanoprost decreased the accumulation of collagen onto cultured human trabecular cells [40]. Bahler et al. studied the effect of latanoprost on histologic sections of the anterior segment of the eye and observed focal losses of ECM in the juxtacanalicular region of the TM [15].

Moreover, in our study, we enriched our result on a three-dimensional (3D) TM cellular model. Our preliminary results presented an interesting tool to advance research on this pathology by taking into account biomechanics, which is a key element in the pathophysiology of glaucoma [41]. Nevertheless, for the moment, the results provided are only qualitative, which constitutes a limitation of the study. Quantification work is in progress. The 3D cell cultures in Matrigel^{TM} allowed us to obtain a meshed organization of trabecular cells with interconnections and the formation of intercellular spaces, which we did not find in 2D, and which better reflects the real anatomy of the TM. We were able to show with this model that the ROCKi Y-27632 widened the meshes between the cells by modifying the cytoskeleton of pHTMC. Cell culture in 3D recreates the conditions of the microenvironment encountered in vivo and provides cells with an environment allowing them to interact with each other and with the ECM. It would also help to better understand not only the physiological function of the TM but also its behavior under conditions of stress or toxicity, as well as the effect of medications [42]. This 3D TM model was first used by Bouchemi et al. to study the effect of benzalkonium chloride (BAK), a preservative commonly used in eye drops [29]. They showed that BAK induced inflammatory chemokines and inhibited the activity of MMPs, which play a crucial role in ECM degradation and increased outflow facility. Further research will be necessary to better exploit all the information provided by this model. Indeed, the main biomechanical cues experienced by TMC are not investigated in this article. For example, TMC in vivo are subjected to a significant pressure change, shear stress, and mechanical stretch. Rigidity and outflow measurement systems using this model might also be implemented to improve the relevance of the model. Analysis and understanding of the pathophysiology of the TM are essential for understanding and treating glaucoma.

We also showed the involvement of the ROCK signaling pathway in the stiffening of the TM and that the inhibitor Y-27632 modified the TGF-β2-induced cytoskeletal rearrangements. Previous studies have demonstrated the changes in pHTMC cytoskeleton organization with a modification of cell shape and actomyosin organization [43–45]. A new distribution of actin fibers in the periphery was observed in response to the alteration of the actin cytoskeleton. This redistribution was first described by Murphy et al. and qualified as cortical actin arrays (CAA) [46]. In our study, there was also reversibility of ECM deposition induced by TGF-β2 after treatment with ROCKi. Indeed, the ROCKi Y-27632 decreased TGF-β2-induced fibronectin deposition. A recent study by Li et al. also demonstrated the antifibrotic activity of a rho-kinase inhibitor on an in vivo glucocorticoid-induced ocular hypertension model [39]. Our work confirmed the anti-fibrotic action of

ROCK inhibitors to prevent cell contractility and accumulation of ECM, consistent with studies by Torrejon et al., Pattabiraman et al., and Ota et al. [12,37,38].

Although it is known that the mechanism of action of PGA relies on increased expression of MMP in the TM, few studies have investigated the remodeling of the ECM by MMPs under the effect of ROCKi [47]. Torrejon et al. showed that after 3 and 5 days, TMC exposed to MMP2 mRNA-level in TMC was enhanced after a 3-days co-treatment with Y27632 and TGF-β2 [37]. Watanabe et al. showed that the addition of a pan-ROCKi (ripasudil 10 nM) to TGF-β2 (5 ng/mL)-exposed TMC induced significant up-regulation of MMP2, MMP9, and MMP14 at Day 6 [48]. Further studies exploring MMP and TIMP expression in TMC after PGA and ROCKi exposure would be of interest.

A ROCK inhibitor, 0.02% netarsudil (Rhopressa® (US)/Rhokiinsa® (EU), Aerie Pharmaceuticals, Inc., NC) received Food and Drug Administration approval in December 2017 and marketing authorization to the European Medicines Agency in November 2019 for lowering IOP in patients with POAG [49]. Another molecule from the same family, ripasudil (Glanatec®, Kowa Pharmaceuticals, Japan) was approved by the Japanese health authorities in 2014 for the treatment of glaucoma, or ocular hypertension, as a second line after prostaglandin therapy [50]. In addition, the combination of netarsudil with latanoprost was clinically developed and led to a new formulation (Rocklatan® (US)/Roclanda® (EU), Aerie Pharmaceuticals, Inc., Bedminster, NC, USA), which had a greater effect on the reduction of IOP than either of its two components, by reducing IOP by an additional 1.8 mmHg on average compared to netarsudil, and 2.7 mmHg compared to latanoprost [51,52]. Although we have not tested the combination of the two molecules, our work suggests that the significant effect of latanoprost on fibronectin deposition associated with the remodeling of the ROCK inhibitor cytoskeleton could effectively lead to a significant decrease in resistance to the aqueous humor outflow.

5. Conclusions

We used an in vitro TGF-β2-induced TM remodeling mimicking glaucomatous trabeculopathy to confirm the effects of both a ROCKi and a PGA on the TM. We showed that ROCK inhibition had an action on the TM cells' cytoskeleton by reducing actin stress fibers, as well as on ECM release. In our model, we also demonstrated that latanoprost loosened the ECM.

Supplementary Materials: The following supporting information can be downloaded at https://www.mdpi.com/article/10.3390/jcm11041001/s1. Table S1: HTMC lines information, Figure S1: Characterization of the normal human trabecular meshwork cells.

Author Contributions: J.B. performed, analyzed, and interpreted the experiments and wrote the manuscript. É.R. performed and analyzed the experiments. F.B.-B., K.K., A.L., S.M.P. and C.B. made substantial contributions to the conception and design of the study. F.B.-B., C.B. and S.M.P. supervised the study. All authors read and approved the final manuscript.

Funding: This work was funded by IHU FOReSight.

Institutional Review Board Statement: Not applicable.

Informed Consent Statement: Not applicable.

Data Availability Statement: The datasets used and/or analyzed during the current study are included in this published article or available from the corresponding author upon reasonable request.

Acknowledgments: This work was completed with the support of the Programme Investissements d'Avenir IHU FOReSIGHT (ANR-18-IAHU-01) and an unrestricted grant from the Fondation des Aveugles de Guerre.

Conflicts of Interest: Christophe Baudouin: Financial support and consultant (Alcon; Allergan; Santen; Laboratoires Théa). The other authors declare no conflict of interest.

References

1. Zhang, N.; Wang, J.; Li, Y.; Jiang, B. Prevalence of Primary Open Angle Glaucoma in the Last 20 Years: A Meta-Analysis and Systematic Review. *Sci. Rep.* **2021**, *11*, 13762. [CrossRef]
2. Kass, M.A.; Heuer, D.K.; Higginbotham, E.J.; Johnson, C.A.; Keltner, J.L.; Miller, J.P.; Parrish, R.K.; Wilson, M.R.; Gordon, M.O. The Ocular Hypertension Treatment Study: A Randomized Trial Determines That Topical Ocular Hypotensive Medication Delays or Prevents the Onset of Primary Open-Angle Glaucoma. *Arch. Ophthalmol.* **2002**, *120*, 701–713; discussion 829–830. [CrossRef]
3. Stamer, W.D.; Clark, A.F. The Many Faces of the Trabecular Meshwork Cell. *Exp. Eye Res.* **2017**, *158*, 112–123. [CrossRef] [PubMed]
4. Tektas, O.-Y.; Lütjen-Drecoll, E. Structural Changes of the Trabecular Meshwork in Different Kinds of Glaucoma. *Exp. Eye Res.* **2009**, *88*, 769–775. [CrossRef] [PubMed]
5. Keller, K.E.; Aga, M.; Bradley, J.M.; Kelley, M.J.; Acott, T.S. Extracellular Matrix Turnover and Outflow Resistance. *Exp. Eye Res.* **2009**, *88*, 676–682. [CrossRef] [PubMed]
6. Tamm, E.R. The Trabecular Meshwork Outflow Pathways: Structural and Functional Aspects. *Exp. Eye Res.* **2009**, *88*, 648–655. [CrossRef]
7. Liton, P.B.; Challa, P.; Stinnett, S.; Luna, C.; Epstein, D.L.; Gonzalez, P. Cellular Senescence in the Glaucomatous Outflow Pathway. *Exp. Gerontol.* **2005**, *40*, 745–748. [CrossRef]
8. Tripathi, R.C.; Li, J.; Chan, W.F.; Tripathi, B.J. Aqueous Humor in Glaucomatous Eyes Contains an Increased Level of TGF-Beta 2. *Exp. Eye Res.* **1994**, *59*, 723–727. [CrossRef]
9. Gottanka, J.; Chan, D.; Eichhorn, M.; Lütjen-Drecoll, E.; Ethier, C.R. Effects of TGF-B2 in Perfused Human Eyes. *Investig. Ophthalmol. Vis. Sci.* **2004**, *45*, 153–158. [CrossRef]
10. Kasetti, R.B.; Maddineni, P.; Kodati, B.; Nagarajan, B.; Yacoub, S. Astragaloside IV Attenuates Ocular Hypertension in a Mouse Model of TGFβ2 Induced Primary Open Angle Glaucoma. *Int. J. Mol. Sci.* **2021**, *22*, 12508. [CrossRef]
11. Wang, J.; Harris, A.; Prendes, M.A.; Alshawa, L.; Gross, J.C.; Wentz, S.M.; Rao, A.B.; Kim, N.J.; Synder, A.; Siesky, B. Targeting Transforming Growth Factor-β Signaling in Primary Open-Angle Glaucoma. *J. Glaucoma* **2017**, *26*, 390–395. [CrossRef]
12. Pattabiraman, P.P.; Rao, P.V. Mechanistic Basis of Rho GTPase-Induced Extracellular Matrix Synthesis in Trabecular Meshwork Cells. *Am. J. Physiol. Cell Physiol.* **2010**, *298*, C749–C763. [CrossRef] [PubMed]
13. Heijl, A.; Leske, M.C.; Bengtsson, B.; Hyman, L.; Bengtsson, B.; Hussein, M.; Early Manifest Glaucoma Trial Group. Reduction of Intraocular Pressure and Glaucoma Progression: Results from the Early Manifest Glaucoma Trial. *Arch. Ophthalmol.* **2002**, *120*, 1268–1279. [CrossRef] [PubMed]
14. Winkler, N.S.; Fautsch, M.P. Effects of Prostaglandin Analogues on Aqueous Humor Outflow Pathways. *J. Ocul. Pharmacol. Ther.* **2014**, *30*, 102–109. [CrossRef]
15. Bahler, C.K.; Howell, K.G.; Hann, C.R.; Fautsch, M.P.; Johnson, D.H. Prostaglandins Increase Trabecular Meshwork Outflow Facility in Cultured Human Anterior Segments. *Am. J. Ophthalmol.* **2008**, *145*, 114–119. [CrossRef] [PubMed]
16. Rao, P.V.; Pattabiraman, P.P.; Kopczynski, C. Role of the Rho GTPase/Rho Kinase Signaling Pathway in Pathogenesis and Treatment of Glaucoma: Bench to Bedside Research. *Exp. Eye Res.* **2017**, *158*, 23–32. [CrossRef] [PubMed]
17. Amano, M.; Nakayama, M.; Kaibuchi, K. Rho-Kinase/ROCK: A Key Regulator of the Cytoskeleton and Cell Polarity. *Cytoskeleton* **2010**, *67*, 545–554. [CrossRef]
18. Prunier, C.; Prudent, R.; Kapur, R.; Sadoul, K.; Lafanechère, L. LIM Kinases: Cofilin and Beyond. *Oncotarget* **2017**, *8*, 41749. [CrossRef]
19. Liao, J.K.; Seto, M.; Noma, K. Rho Kinase (ROCK) Inhibitors. *J. Cardiovasc. Pharmacol.* **2007**, *50*, 17–24. [CrossRef]
20. Wang, J.; Liu, X.; Zhong, Y. Rho/Rho-Associated Kinase Pathway in Glaucoma (Review). *Int. J. Oncol.* **2013**, *43*, 1357–1367. [CrossRef]
21. Tanihara, H.; Inoue, T.; Yamamoto, T.; Kuwayama, Y.; Abe, H.; Araie, M.; K-115 Clinical Study Group. Phase 1 Clinical Trials of a Selective Rho Kinase Inhibitor, K-115. *JAMA Ophthalmol.* **2013**, *131*, 1288–1295. [CrossRef] [PubMed]
22. Serle, J.B.; Katz, L.J.; McLaurin, E.; Heah, T.; Ramirez-Davis, N.; Usner, D.W.; Novack, G.D.; Kopczynski, C.C.; ROCKET-1 and ROCKET-2 Study Groups. Two Phase 3 Clinical Trials Comparing the Safety and Efficacy of Netarsudil to Timolol in Patients With Elevated Intraocular Pressure: Rho Kinase Elevated IOP Treatment Trial 1 and 2 (ROCKET-1 and ROCKET-2). *Am. J. Ophthalmol.* **2018**, *186*, 116–127. [CrossRef] [PubMed]
23. Tanihara, H.; Inoue, T.; Yamamoto, T.; Kuwayama, Y.; Abe, H.; Suganami, H.; Araie, M.; K-115 Clinical Study Group. Intra-Ocular Pressure-Lowering Effects of a Rho Kinase Inhibitor, Ripasudil (K-115), over 24 Hours in Primary Open-Angle Glaucoma and Ocular Hypertension: A Randomized, Open-Label, Crossover Study. *Acta Ophthalmol.* **2015**, *93*, e254–e260. [CrossRef] [PubMed]
24. Tanihara, H.; Inoue, T.; Yamamoto, T.; Kuwayama, Y.; Abe, H.; Araie, M.; K-115 Clinical Study Group. Phase 2 Randomized Clinical Study of a Rho Kinase Inhibitor, K-115, in Primary Open-Angle Glaucoma and Ocular Hypertension. *Am. J. Ophthalmol.* **2013**, *156*, 731–736. [CrossRef]
25. Bacharach, J.; Dubiner, H.B.; Levy, B.; Kopczynski, C.C.; Novack, G.D.; AR-13324-CS202 Study Group. Double-Masked, Randomized, Dose-Response Study of AR-13324 versus Latanoprost in Patients with Elevated Intraocular Pressure. *Ophthalmology* **2015**, *122*, 302–307. [CrossRef] [PubMed]
26. Tanihara, H.; Inoue, T.; Yamamoto, T.; Kuwayama, Y.; Abe, H.; Fukushima, A.; Suganami, H.; Araie, M.; K-115 Clinical Study Group. One-Year Clinical Evaluation of 0.4% Ripasudil (K-115) in Patients with Open-Angle Glaucoma and Ocular Hypertension. *Acta Ophthalmol.* **2016**, *94*, e26–e34. [CrossRef] [PubMed]

27. Wang, S.K.; Chang, R.T. An Emerging Treatment Option for Glaucoma: Rho Kinase Inhibitors. *Clin. Ophthalmol.* **2014**, *8*, 883–890. [CrossRef]

28. Keller, K.E.; Bhattacharya, S.K.; Borrás, T.; Brunner, T.M.; Chansangpetch, S.; Clark, A.F.; Dismuke, W.M.; Du, Y.; Elliott, M.H.; Ethier, C.R.; et al. Consensus Recommendations for Trabecular Meshwork Cell Isolation, Characterization and Culture. *Exp. Eye Res.* **2018**, *171*, 164–173. [CrossRef]

29. Bouchemi, M.; Roubeix, C.; Kessal, K.; Riancho, L.; Raveu, A.-L.; Soualmia, H.; Baudouin, C.; Brignole-Baudouin, F. Effect of Benzalkonium Chloride on Trabecular Meshwork Cells in a New in Vitro 3D Trabecular Meshwork Model for Glaucoma. *Toxicol. Vitr.* **2017**, *41*, 21–29. [CrossRef]

30. Fujimoto, T.; Inoue, T.; Inoue-Mochita, M.; Tanihara, H. Live Cell Imaging of Actin Dynamics in Dexamethasone-Treated Porcine Trabecular Meshwork Cells. *Exp. Eye Res.* **2016**, *145*, 393–400. [CrossRef]

31. Hamard, P.; Blondin, C.; Debbasch, C.; Warnet, J.-M.; Baudouin, C.; Brignole, F. In Vitro Effects of Preserved and Unpreserved Antiglaucoma Drugs on Apoptotic Marker Expression by Human Trabecular Cells. *Graefes Arch. Clin. Exp. Ophthalmol.* **2003**, *241*, 1037–1043. [CrossRef] [PubMed]

32. Benton, G.; Arnaoutova, I.; George, J.; Kleinman, H.K.; Koblinski, J. Matrigel: From Discovery and ECM Mimicry to Assays and Models for Cancer Research. *Adv. Drug Deliv. Rev.* **2014**, *79–80*, 3–18. [CrossRef] [PubMed]

33. Hughes, C.S.; Postovit, L.M.; Lajoie, G.A. Matrigel: A Complex Protein Mixture Required for Optimal Growth of Cell Culture. *Proteomics* **2010**, *10*, 1886–1890. [CrossRef] [PubMed]

34. Di Rosa, M.; Tibullo, D.; Saccone, S.; Distefano, G.; Basile, M.S.; Di Raimondo, F.; Malaguarnera, L. CHI3L1 Nuclear Localization in Monocyte Derived Dendritic Cells. *Immunobiology* **2016**, *221*, 347–356. [CrossRef]

35. Kottler, U.B.; Jünemann, A.G.M.; Aigner, T.; Zenkel, M.; Rummelt, C.; Schlötzer-Schrehardt, U. Comparative Effects of TGF-Beta 1 and TGF-Beta 2 on Extracellular Matrix Production, Proliferation, Migration, and Collagen Contraction of Human Tenon's Capsule Fibroblasts in Pseudoexfoliation and Primary Open-Angle Glaucoma. *Exp. Eye Res.* **2005**, *80*, 121–134. [CrossRef]

36. Connor, T.B.; Roberts, A.B.; Sporn, M.B.; Danielpour, D.; Dart, L.L.; Michels, R.G.; de Bustros, S.; Enger, C.; Kato, H.; Lansing, M. Correlation of Fibrosis and Transforming Growth Factor-Beta Type 2 Levels in the Eye. *J. Clin. Investig.* **1989**, *83*, 1661–1666. [CrossRef]

37. Torrejon, K.Y.; Papke, E.L.; Halman, J.R.; Bergkvist, M.; Danias, J.; Sharfstein, S.T.; Xie, Y. TGFβ2-Induced Outflow Alterations in a Bioengineered Trabecular Meshwork Are Offset by a Rho-Associated Kinase Inhibitor. *Sci. Rep.* **2016**, *6*, 38319. [CrossRef] [PubMed]

38. Ota, C.; Ida, Y.; Ohguro, H.; Hikage, F. ROCK Inhibitors Beneficially Alter the Spatial Configuration of TGFβ2-Treated 3D Organoids from a Human Trabecular Meshwork (HTM). *Sci. Rep.* **2020**, *10*, 20292. [CrossRef]

39. Li, G.; Lee, C.; Read, A.T.; Wang, K.; Ha, J.; Kuhn, M.; Navarro, I.; Cui, J.; Young, K.; Gorijavolu, R.; et al. Anti-Fibrotic Activity of a Rho-Kinase Inhibitor Restores Outflow Function and Intraocular Pressure Homeostasis. *Elife* **2021**, *10*, e60831. [CrossRef]

40. Kalouche, G.; Beguier, F.; Bakria, M.; Melik-Parsadaniantz, S.; Leriche, C.; Debeir, T.; Rostène, W.; Baudouin, C.; Vigé, X. Activation of Prostaglandin FP and EP2 Receptors Differently Modulates Myofibroblast Transition in a Model of Adult Primary Human Trabecular Meshwork Cells. *Investig. Ophthalmol. Vis. Sci.* **2016**, *57*, 1816–1825. [CrossRef]

41. Wang, K.; Read, A.T.; Sulchek, T.; Ethier, C.R. Trabecular Meshwork Stiffness in Glaucoma. *Exp. Eye Res.* **2017**, *158*, 3–12. [CrossRef] [PubMed]

42. Hongisto, V.; Jernström, S.; Fey, V.; Mpindi, J.-P.; Kleivi Sahlberg, K.; Kallioniemi, O.; Perälä, M. High-Throughput 3D Screening Reveals Differences in Drug Sensitivities between Culture Models of JIMT1 Breast Cancer Cells. *PLoS ONE* **2013**, *8*, e77232. [CrossRef]

43. Ramachandran, C.; Patil, R.V.; Combrink, K.; Sharif, N.A.; Srinivas, S.P. Rho-Rho Kinase Pathway in the Actomyosin Contraction and Cell-Matrix Adhesion in Immortalized Human Trabecular Meshwork Cells. *Mol. Vis.* **2011**, *17*, 1877–1890.

44. Saha, B.C.; Kumari, R.; Kushumesh, R.; Ambasta, A.; Sinha, B.P. Status of Rho Kinase Inhibitors in Glaucoma Therapeutics— An Overview. *Int. Ophthalmol.* **2021**, *42*, 281–294. [CrossRef] [PubMed]

45. Rao, P.V.; Deng, P.F.; Kumar, J.; Epstein, D.L. Modulation of Aqueous Humor Outflow Facility by the Rho Kinase-Specific Inhibitor Y-27632. *Investig. Ophthalmol. Vis. Sci.* **2001**, *42*, 1029–1037.

46. Murphy, K.C.; Morgan, J.T.; Wood, J.A.; Sadeli, A.; Murphy, C.J.; Russell, P. The Formation of Cortical Actin Arrays in Human Trabecular Meshwork Cells in Response to Cytoskeletal Disruption. *Exp. Cell Res.* **2014**, *328*, 164–171. [CrossRef]

47. Heo, J.Y.; Ooi, Y.H.; Rhee, D.J. Effect of Prostaglandin Analogs: Latanoprost, Bimatoprost, and Unoprostone on Matrix Metalloproteinases and Their Inhibitors in Human Trabecular Meshwork Endothelial Cells. *Exp. Eye Res.* **2020**, *194*, 108019. [CrossRef]

48. Watanabe, M.; Ida, Y.; Ohguro, H.; Ota, C.; Hikage, F. Diverse Effects of Pan-ROCK and ROCK2 Inhibitors on 2 D and 3D Cultured Human Trabecular Meshwork (HTM) Cells Treated with TGFβ2. *Sci. Rep.* **2021**, *11*, 15286. [CrossRef]

49. US Department of Health and Human Services, Food and Drug Administration Rhopressa Approval Letter 208254. 2017. Available online: https://www.accessdata.fda.gov/drugsatfda_docs/nda/2017/208254Orig1s000TOC.cfm (accessed on 10 February 2022).

50. Tanna, A.P.; Johnson, M. Rho Kinase Inhibitors as a Novel Treatment for Glaucoma and Ocular Hypertension. *Ophthalmology* **2018**, *125*, 1741–1756. [CrossRef]

51. Lewis, R.A.; Levy, B.; Ramirez, N.; Kopczynski, C.C.; Usner, D.W.; Novack, G.D.; PG324-CS201 Study Group. Fixed-Dose Combination of AR-13324 and Latanoprost: A Double-Masked, 28-Day, Randomised, Controlled Study in Patients with Open-Angle Glaucoma or Ocular Hypertension. *Br. J. Ophthalmol.* **2016**, *100*, 339–344. [CrossRef]
52. Tanihara, H.; Inoue, T.; Yamamoto, T.; Kuwayama, Y.; Abe, H.; Suganami, H.; Araie, M.; K-115 Clinical Study Group. Additive Intraocular Pressure-Lowering Effects of the Rho Kinase Inhibitor Ripasudil (K-115) Combined With Timolol or Latanoprost: A Report of 2 Randomized Clinical Trials. *JAMA Ophthalmol.* **2015**, *133*, 755–761. [CrossRef] [PubMed]

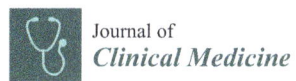

Journal of
Clinical Medicine

Article

Mid-Term Impact of Anti-Vascular Endothelial Growth Factor Agents on Intraocular Pressure

Marc-Antoine Hannappe [1,†], Florian Baudin [1,2,3,*,†], Anne-Sophie Mariet [3,4], Pierre-Henri Gabrielle [1,5], Louis Arnould [1,3,5], Alain M. Bron [1,5] and Catherine Creuzot-Garcher [1,5]

1   Ophthalmology Department, University Hospital of Dijon, 21000 Dijon, France; ma.hannappe@gmail.com (M.-A.H.); pierre-henri.gabrielle@chu-dijon.fr (P.-H.G.); louis.arnould@chu-dijon.fr (L.A.); alain.bron@chu-dijon.fr (A.M.B.); catherine.creuzot-garcher@chu-dijon.fr (C.C.-G.)
2   Physiopathologie et Epidémiologie Cérébro-Cardiovasculaires (PEC2, EA 7460), Burgundy University, 21000 Dijon, France
3   INSERM, CIC 1432, Clinical Investigation Center, Clinical Epidemiology/Clinical Trials Unit, Burgundy University, 21000 Dijon, France; anne-sophie.mariet@chu-dijon.fr
4   Service de Biostatistique et d'Informatique Médicale (DIM), University Hospital of Dijon, 21000 Dijon, France
5   Eye and Nutrition Research Group, CSGA, UMR 1324 INRA, 6265 CNRS, Burgundy University, 21000 Dijon, France
*   Correspondence: florian.baudin@chu-dijon.fr; Tel.: +33-380-293-536; Fax: +33-380-293-879
†   These authors contributed equally as co-first authors.

Citation: Hannappe, M.-A.; Baudin, F.; Mariet, A.-S.; Gabrielle, P.-H.; Arnould, L.; Bron, A.M.; Creuzot-Garcher, C. Mid-Term Impact of Anti-Vascular Endothelial Growth Factor Agents on Intraocular Pressure. *J. Clin. Med.* **2022**, *11*, 946. https://doi.org/10.3390/jcm11040946

Academic Editors: Maria Letizia Salvetat, Marco Zeppieri and Paolo Brusini

Received: 28 January 2022
Accepted: 7 February 2022
Published: 11 February 2022

Publisher's Note: MDPI stays neutral with regard to jurisdictional claims in published maps and institutional affiliations.

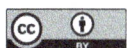
Abstract: The effect of intraocular injections of anti-vascular endothelial growth factor (VEGF) on intraocular pressure (IOP) has not been clearly stated. We extracted data from the electronic health records at Dijon University Hospital of 750 patients who were unilaterally injected with anti-VEGF agents between March 2012 and March 2020. These were treatment-naïve patients who had received at least three injections of the same treatment (aflibercept, bevacizumab, or ranibizumab) in one eye only, and had IOP measurements before and after the injections. Fellow untreated eyes were used as comparators. A clinically significant IOP rise was determined as an IOP above 21 mmHg and an increase of at least 6 mmHg compared to baseline, or the need for IOP-lowering agents. We found an overall slight increase in IOP between treated and untreated eyes at 6 months ($+0.67 \pm 3.33$ mmHg, 95% confidence interval 0.33–1.02, $p < 0.001$). Ranibizumab had a higher final IOP at 1 and 3 months. Age, sex, and the number of injections were not associated with IOP variation. Ranibizumab was associated with a higher rate of increase in clinically significant IOP at 6 months ($p = 0.03$). Our study confirms that anti-VEGF injections constitute a relatively safe treatment regarding their impact on IOP.

Keywords: intravitreal injection; anti-VEGF agents; intraocular pressure

1. Introduction

Various retinal diseases can lead to central vision impairment. In high-income countries, population aging has led to an increase in chronic diseases, such as choroidal neovascularization in age-related macular degeneration (AMD), which is one of the main causes of irreversible blindness [1]. Other retinal conditions, such as high myopia, retinal vein occlusion (RVO), and diabetic macular edema (DME), may also lead to severe central vision impairment if left untreated, and these conditions have also seen a significant increase in prevalence [2]. These diseases have a major impact on the quality of life of patients and represent a heavy burden on public health costs [3,4]. Their prognosis has critically improved with the availability of intravitreal injections (IVTs) of anti-vascular endothelial growth factor (anti-VEGF) agents. However, the maintenance of visual acuity requires regular injections over several months or years. Protocols have been established, such as treat and extend, to limit the number of injections and, thereby, the cumulative risk of complications; however, the average number of injections remains at 7–8 injections per year of treatment [5]. According to the French medical–administrative database, the use of IVTs doubled between 2012 and 2015 [6]. It is, therefore, important to study the occurrence of adverse events after IVTs, such as increased intraocular pressure (IOP) [7].

Indeed, it has been shown that IVTs are responsible for a transient elevation in IOP, with a return to normal levels within 1 h of IVT administration [8–10]. This increase in IOP is related to the mechanical consequences of injecting a volume of liquid into an inextensible globe [8,11]. However, the effect of anti-VEGF agents on long-term IOP elevation is still debated. A recent meta-analysis found mixed results regarding the effect of anti-VEGF agents on long-term IOP elevation [12]. Eight studies demonstrated that between 2.6% and 14.8% of patients exhibited IOP elevation 9–24 months after treatment, according to predetermined criteria. Six studies did not find a change in IOP during follow-up, which ranged from 1 to 36 months, or when compared with a control group that did not receive IVT. Moreover, the results were unclear as to whether the type of anti-VEGF agent, the number of injections, or pre-existing glaucoma were associated with sustained IOP elevation.

Here, we aimed to study the impact of intravitreal anti-VEGF injections on mid-term IOP variations.

2. Materials and Methods

2.1. Study Design and Population

This study included patient data from a tertiary-center electronic health record (EHR) registry in the Ophthalmology Department of Dijon University Hospital. From this registry, treatment-naïve patients receiving unilateral IVTs for any retinal disease from 5 March 2012 to 27 March 2020 were included in the study. Exclusion criteria were any patient who had previous anti-VEGF or steroid treatments, patients injected in both eyes, patients under the age of 18 years, patients treated with fewer than 3 injections, patients who had a change in anti-VEGF agent during their treatment without a period of wash-out and IOP measurements. Patients treated with at least three unilateral anti-VEGF injections of the same drug were included in the analysis and were defined as completers; the data of 750 patients were therefore analyzed (Figure 1). Our study complied with the Declaration of Helsinki, and the locally appointed ethics committee gave approval for the research protocol.

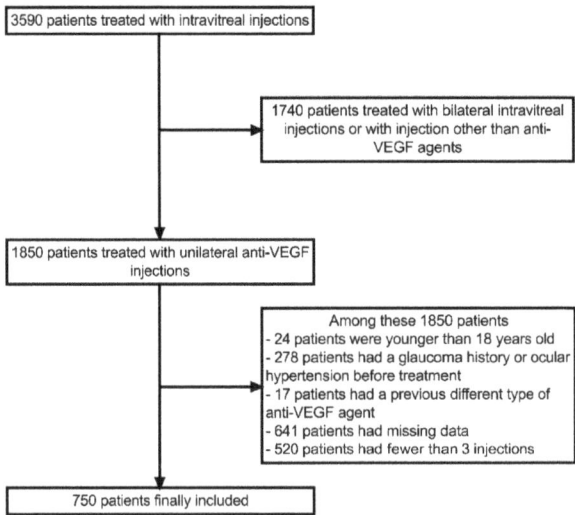

Figure 1. Flowchart of the study.

2.2. EHR Description

Data were extracted from specific software designed for ophthalmology practice (Softalmo Corilus SA, Gembloux, Belgium). This software is autonomous, with an administrative part for patient identification and a medical part for eye examination follow-up. Patients' files are updated at each consultation by practitioners to create a single and exhaustive individual medical record. The software is organized into different examination fields, such as "refraction," "retina," "angiography," "intravitreal injection," "surgery," "prescriptions," etc., which allow for precise and quick browsing. IOP was measured with the air puff tonometer Tonoref II (Nidek, Tokyo, Japan) by trained technicians. In the "intravitreal injection" field, specific items were systematically entered, such as "diagnosis" and "type of injection." An associated research software (Ophtalmo Query, Softalmo Corilus SA, Gembloux, Belgium) was used to extract specific data from the Softalmo Software database.

2.3. Algorithm Elaboration

To create the algorithm used in this study, we first extracted data using Ophtalmo Query. The variables retained were age, sex, consultation dates, IOP, diagnosis, type, and number of injections, surgeries, and prescriptions. The SAS statistical analysis software package (version 9.4; SAS Institute Inc., Cary, NC, USA) was then used to elaborate the different extraction programs. The analysis included any patient for whom a single eye was treated with a minimum of three injections of the same anti-VEGF agent. The anti-VEGF treatments under study were aflibercept, bevacizumab, or ranibizumab. Patients who met these criteria were defined as completers. The end of treatment occurred when exudation regressed, when a different type of anti-VEGF agent or steroid was used, or if the contralateral eye had to be injected. For each patient, we calculated the change in IOP from baseline to the end of treatment. Baseline IOP was calculated as the mean of the different IOP measurements available in the year preceding the anti-VEGF treatment. The final IOP was classified into the following three groups: IOP at 1, 3, or 6 months after the end of treatment. A clinically significant IOP elevation was determined as an IOP above 21 mmHg and a rise of at least 6 mmHg compared to baseline, or the need for an IOP-lowering treatment (medical treatment for at least 3 months or surgery) [13,14]. IOP data were collected for the treated eye and the contralateral, untreated eye. We also considered glaucoma (surgery and medical treatments) and any eye surgery impacting IOP, such as cataract surgery or vitrectomy, during the study.

2.4. Statistical Analysis

Continuous variables were tested with a Shapiro–Wilk test and are expressed as mean ± standard deviation (SD). Dichotomous variables are expressed as numbers (percentages). A Wilcoxon test was used for univariate analysis. A generalized linear model for continuous outcome (IOP variation) on repeated measures was used and controlled for potential confounders, such as sex, age, baseline IOP, type of anti-VEGF agent, number of anti-VEGF injections, history of glaucoma, history of vitrectomy, history of cataract surgery, and glaucoma surgery or medication during the treatment, including the random subject effect. Factors associated with the incidence of clinically significant IOP elevation were evaluated via binary logistic regression. Statistical significance was set at $p < 0.05$ (two-tailed tests). All data processing and statistical analyses were performed using the SAS statistical analysis software package (version 9.4; SAS Institute Inc., Cary, NC, USA).

3. Results

3.1. Population

From our registry of 3590 patients with IVTs, a total of 750 patients met the inclusion criteria (Figure 1). The completers were younger (71.9 ± 13.7 vs. 73.6 ± 13.0 years, $p = 0.002$), and presented with a higher rate of RVO (25.5% vs. 13.0%, $p < 0.001$) and a lower rate of DME (16.8% vs. 21.2%, $p = 0.005$) when compared with the non-included patients. The baseline characteristics of the patients included in the analysis are displayed in Table 1.

Table 1. Baseline characteristics of patients injected with anti-vascular endothelial growth factor agents.

Number of Eyes Enrolled (Patients)	1500 (750)
Mean ± SD Age, Years	71.9 ± 13.7
Sex, *n* (%)	
Female	435 (58.0%)
Baseline IOP, mmHg ± SD	
Treated eyes	14.6 ± 2.7
Untreated eyes	15.0 ± 2.8
Mean ± SD IOP measurement, days	
1 month after the last injection	323 ± 340
3 months after the last injection	374 ± 333
6 months after the last injection	458 ± 327
Retinal disease, *n* (%)	
AMD	347 (46.3%)
RVO	191 (25.5%)
DME	126 (16.8%)
Myopic CNV	27 (3.6%)
Others	59 (7.8%)
Mean ± SD number of injections	6.3 ± 4.7
Cataract surgery during the study, *n* (%)	54 (7.2%)
Vitrectomy during the study, *n* (%)	18 (2.4%)

n = number of eyes; IOP = intraocular pressure; AMD = age-related macular degeneration; RVO = retinal vein occlusion; DME = diabetic macular edema; CNV = choroidal neovascularization; SD = standard deviation.

3.2. IOP Variation

We found an IOP elevation in treated versus untreated eyes from baseline to IOP, measured at 1, 3, and 6 months after the end of the treatment, of +0.15 ± 2.96 mmHg (95% confidence interval (CI), −0.08–0.38, $p = 0.09$), +0.46 ± 2.94 mmHg (95% CI, 0.18–0.78, $p < 0.001$), and +0.67 ± 3.33 mmHg (95% CI, 0.33–1.02, $p < 0.001$), respectively. A significant difference between treated and untreated eyes was also found, depending on the injected drug (Table 2).

Table 2. Intraocular pressure variation in treated eyes compared with untreated fellow eyes.

Anti-VEGF Agent	*n*	Delta IOP at 1 Month, mmHg	*p* Value	Delta IOP at 3 Months, mmHg	*p* Value	Delta IOP at 6 Months, mmHg	*p* Value
Aflibercept	205	−0.68	<0.001	−0.19	0.40	0.71	0.01
Bevacizumab	17	−0.48	0.48	0.37	0.68	0.02	0.98
Ranibizumab	528	0.48	<0.001	0.73	<0.001	0.61	0.001

IOP = intraocular pressure; delta IOP = difference between baseline IOP and IOP at x month after the last injection; VEGF = vascular endothelial growth factor; *p* value of the paired difference test (Wilcoxon test).

When considering the anti-VEGF agent injected in treated eyes, the IOP at 1 month and 3 months was significantly higher with ranibizumab than with aflibercept or bevacizumab ($p < 0.001$ and $p = 0.004$, respectively), but there was no difference at 6 months (Figure 2). The change in IOP was not correlated with the number of injections at any time (Figure 3). Other factors, such as age at treatment initiation ($p = 0.11$), sex ($p = 0.27$), retinal disease treated ($p = 0.13$), and vitrectomy surgery ($p = 0.36$), were not found to impact the IOP in treated eyes. Cataract surgery was associated with a lower IOP in treated eyes at 1, 3, and 6 months after the last injection ($p < 0.001$, $p = 0.006$, $p < 0.001$, respectively), while a higher IOP at 1 month was found in patients treated for glaucoma ($p = 0.019$), but not at 3 and 6 months.

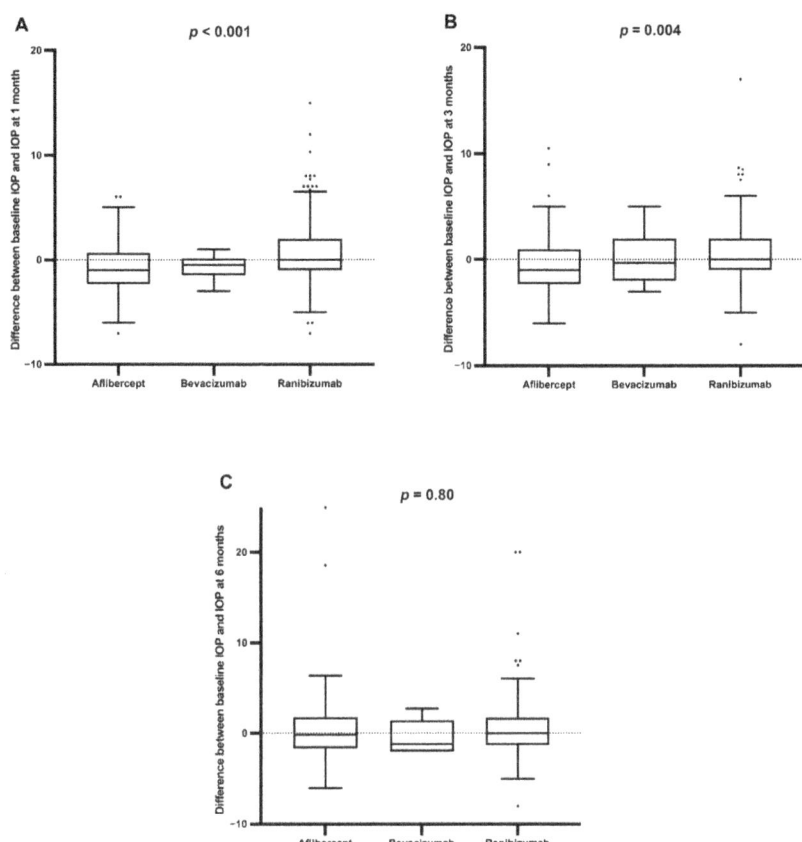

Figure 2. Variation between baseline intraocular pressure and intraocular pressure at 1, 3, or 6 months (**A–C**, respectively) depending on anti-VEGF agent used in treated eyes.

Multivariate analysis confirmed that after adjusting for cataract surgery and anti-glaucomatous treatment, the type of anti-VEGF agent was still associated with variation in IOP in treated eyes at 1 and 3 months ($p = 0.001$ and $p = 0.005$, respectively). However, this effect disappeared 6 months after the last injection.

3.3. Clinically Significant IOP Rise

No difference in IOP elevation was observed between treated and untreated eyes, as defined previously. Regarding anti-VEGF agents, ranibizumab was associated with a higher rate of IOP elevation at 6 months than aflibercept (3.60% vs. 3.41%, $p = 0.031$). The administration of six injections or more was associated with a higher rate of IOP increase at 1 month from the last injection (6.36% vs. 2.97%, $p = 0.040$), but this effect was no longer observed at 3 and 6 months. Other factors, such as age, sex, retinal disease treated, cataract surgery, or vitrectomy surgery, were not associated with a higher rate of clinically significant IOP elevation.

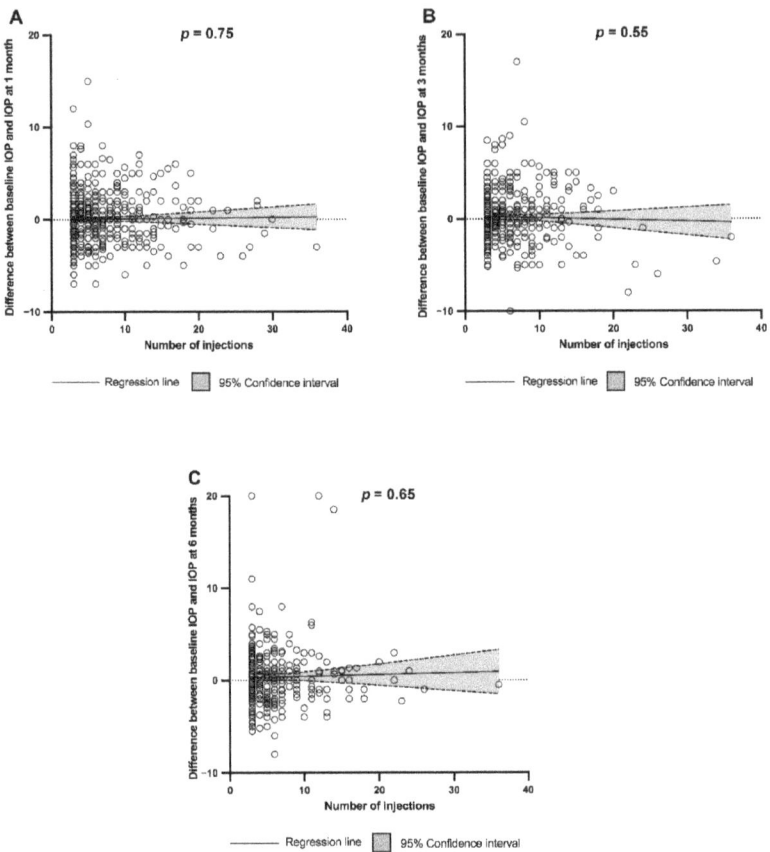

Figure 3. Variation between baseline intraocular pressure and intraocular pressure at 1, 3, or 6 months (**A–C**, respectively) according to the number of injections. IOP = intraocular pressure; *p* value testing the null hypothesis that the linear regression line slope is zero.

4. Discussion

In this study, we found a minimal IOP elevation after anti-VEGF injections, taking into account potential confounders. This change in IOP increased with time. A previous study did not find a difference in the mean change in IOP between treated and untreated fellow eyes during follow-up, but IOP was not measured after the end of anti-VEGF treatment [15]. Another study comparing IOP changes between treated and untreated eyes after the end of anti-VEGF treatment found a slight decrease in IOP in treated eyes, but the timing of the final IOP measurement was not reported [16]. However, these results are probably not clinically relevant in terms of the range in variations, as outlined in a recent review of the literature [17], and this study does not outweigh the positive effects of injections on visual acuity gain.

The anti-VEGF agent ranibizumab was associated with a significantly higher IOP change from baseline at all times, while aflibercept showed an IOP decrease at 1 month. In the Intelligent Research in Sight (IRIS) study, a decrease in IOP in treated versus untreated eyes was observed with bevacizumab and aflibercept, but not with ranibizumab [16]. In the present study, we observed that IOP variation was time dependent, which could explain the difference in results with the IRIS study. The size of the study population in the latter study was also significantly larger. Closer to our results, Freund et al. showed that the IOP in the aflibercept group decreased during follow-up compared with the baseline measurements, while the IOP was consistently higher in the ranibizumab group [15]. In a recent study, a lower mean IOP change and fewer cases of IOP elevation were found in eyes treated with aflibercept compared to those that received bevacizumab or ranibizumab [18]. In our study, 6 months after aflibercept treatment, the IOP had returned to baseline. We could presume that the IOP-lowering effect of aflibercept was transient. There is no clear explanation as to why IOP was lower with aflibercept; in contrast, arguments for a higher IOP with ranibizumab have already been proposed, such as larger protein aggregates, worse vitreal solubility, and endotoxin-induced trabeculitis, since ranibizumab is produced within *Escherichia coli* cells [15,19]. Interestingly, in the HAWK and HARRIER studies of the efficacy and safety of a new anti-VEGF agent, brolucizumab, the incidence of increased IOP was reported to be similar in the brolucizumab and aflibercept groups, 30 min after injection [20]. It would be interesting to know its effect on IOP in the long term, especially because this molecule would require fewer injections. As found in the IRIS study, our analysis showed that cataract surgery was a factor that modified the IOP in treated eyes, while the number of injections was not [16]. While cataract surgery, and, thus, pseudophakic status, was associated with lowered IOP, as in other studies [21,22], this was not the case for vitrectomy. One hypothesis is that intraocular lenses, because of their smaller size than native lenses, offer less resistance to the flow of fluids from the vitreous cavity to the anterior chamber [22]. The effect on the decrease in intraocular pressure after cataract surgery has been widely demonstrated. Conversely, vitrectomy would be responsible for a transient increase in IOP, possibly related to the oxidative stress of the trabecular meshwork [23], and then, in the long term, an unchanged IOP [24].

We did not find any difference in the occurrence of clinically significant IOP elevation when comparing treated eyes with untreated fellow eyes, which is in accordance with a previous study with a similar design to ours [25]. Our results differed from those of the IRIS study, where a clinically significant rise in IOP was more common in treated than in untreated eyes [16]. Our study found a higher rate of IOP elevation in both treated and untreated eyes than the rate reported in the IRIS study. This difference could be explained by our composite criteria for clinically significant IOP elevation, which included IOP-lowering treatment, contrary to the IRIS study. However, we share a similar finding regarding the higher rate of significant IOP elevation with ranibizumab compared with untreated eyes. In our study, 3.60% of the patients treated with ranibizumab experienced an IOP rise versus 2.55% in untreated eyes. In the IRIS study, the rate in treated eyes was 2.80% versus 1.30% for untreated eyes. The MARINA and ANCHOR trials also found a higher rate of clinically significant IOP elevation with ranibizumab compared with controls [26]. Similar findings were reported in the Diabetic Retinopathy Clinical Research Network (DRCRnet) study between eyes treated with ranibizumab and those treated with laser surgery, but only in a population of patients with diabetes [27]. As found in other studies, the clinically significant IOP rise was not related to the number of injections [13,26]. Some studies showed a possible link between higher rates of IOP elevation and repeated injections, but they also showed a higher mean number of injections, especially the study by Hoang et al., which included 20.8 injections compared to the 6.3 included in our study [16,28,29]. Older age, male gender, and retinal disease were not associated with IOP elevation in our study; however, a recent study that did not use controls and allowed switching in the analysis, but had a longer follow-up of 3 years, found an association [30].

Regarding the characteristics of the pathologies treated in our population, there was a significant prevalence of RVO, which can be explained by our inclusion criteria. This disease is more frequently unilateral, and, thus, patients with RVO were more likely to be included than patients with frequently bilateral diseases, such as AMD or DME. Although RVO is associated with IOP changes and glaucoma, our results were adjusted for retinal disease to address this potential confounding bias. However, a recent study by Ahmad et al. found that a significant proportion of patients treated with anti-VEGF for RVO had an increase in IOP of more than 10 mmHg at 5 years after the initiation of anti-VEGF therapy [31]. It would, therefore, be interesting to study the evolution of IOP in these patients treated for RVO in a few years.

We acknowledge several limitations in our study. Firstly, the retrospective design does not meet the quality of prospective clinical trials, especially regarding data collection. Secondly, a minority of patients were treated with bevacizumab compared to those treated with aflibercept and ranibizumab, limiting our conclusions on bevacizumab. Thirdly, IOP is subject to diurnal fluctuations, and the IOP of patients in our study was not measured at the same time at each visit [32]. However, we calculated a mean IOP for baseline and at 1, 3, and 6 months after the last injection, when more than one measurement was available. Fourthly, although the IOP was not measured with Goldmann applanation tonometry, a strength of our study was that the same non-contact tonometer (NCT) was used for every patient. Finally, although this study considered IOP-lowering treatments, it did not address other direct indications of glaucoma risk or progression, including optic nerve function and structure assessments. One of the strengths of our study that only unilateral injections were considered, taking the contralateral eye as a comparator, using mixed models stratified at the patient level.

In conclusion, this study confirms the relative safety of anti-VEGF injections regarding IOP changes. The slight IOP elevation found in treated versus untreated eyes was not clinically relevant. Injections were not associated with more cases of clinically significant IOP elevation compared with untreated fellow eyes, except for ranibizumab at 6 months after the last injection.

Author Contributions: Conceptualization, M.-A.H. and F.B.; Methodology, M.-A.H. and F.B.; Software, F.B.; Formal Analysis, F.B. and A.-S.M.; Validation, P.-H.G., L.A., C.C.-G. and A.M.B.; Writing—Original Draft Preparation, M.-A.H. and F.B.; Writing—Review and Editing, P.-H.G., L.A., C.C.-G. and A.M.B.; Supervision; C.C.-G. and A.M.B. All authors contributed to this manuscript and have approved the submitted version, and agree to be personally accountable for their contribution and for ensuring that questions related to the accuracy or integrity of any part of the work, even ones in which the author was not personally involved, are appropriately investigated, resolved, and documented in the literature. All authors have read and agreed to the published version of the manuscript.

Funding: This research received no external funding.

Institutional Review Board Statement: Our study complied with the Declaration of Helsinki, and the locally appointed ethics committee gave approval for the research protocol. Dijon University Hospital Ethic Committee, retrospective study on IOP after IVT-4 July 2020.

Informed Consent Statement: Because all patients received standard medical care and because the dataset contained no information that could enable patient identification, the study was exempt from informed consent requirements.

Conflicts of Interest: F.B. is a consultant for Novartis, Théa; P.-H.G. is a consultant for Allergan, Bayer, Novartis; L.A. is a consultant for Novartis; A.M.B. is a consultant for Aerie, Allergan, Bausch and Lomb, Santen Pharmaceutical, Théa; C.C.-G. is a consultant for Allergan, Bayer, Horus Pharma, Novartis, Roche, Théa. The following authors declare no conflict of interest: M.-A.H. and A.-S.M.

References

1. Bourne, R.R.; Jonas, J.B.; Flaxman, S.R.; Keeffe, J.; Leasher, J.; Naidoo, K.; Parodi, M.B.; Pesudovs, K.; Price, H.; White, R.A.; et al. Prevalence and causes of vision loss in high-income countries and in Eastern and Central Europe: 1990–2010. *Br. J. Ophthalmol.* **2014**, *98*, 629–638. [CrossRef] [PubMed]
2. Flaxman, S.R.; Bourne, R.R.A.; Resnikoff, S.; Ackland, P.; Braithwaite, T.; Cicinelli, M.V.; Das, A.; Jonas, J.B.; Keeffe, J.; Kempen, J.H.; et al. Global causes of blindness and distance vision impairment 1990-2020: A systematic review and meta-analysis. *Lancet Glob Health* **2017**, *5*, e1221–e1234. [CrossRef]
3. Taylor, D.J.; Hobby, A.E.; Binns, A.M.; Crabb, D.P. How does age-related macular degeneration affect real-world visual ability and quality of life? A systematic review. *BMJ Open* **2016**, *6*, e011504. [CrossRef] [PubMed]
4. Mulligan, K.; Seabury, S.A.; Dugel, P.U.; Blim, J.F.; Goldman, D.P.; Humayun, M.S. Economic Value of Anti-Vascular Endothelial Growth Factor Treatment for Patients With Wet Age-Related Macular Degeneration in the United States. *JAMA Ophthalmol.* **2019**, *138*, 40–47. [CrossRef]

5. Volkmann, I.; Knoll, K.; Wiezorrek, M.; Greb, O.; Framme, C. Individualized treat-and-extend regime for optimization of real-world vision outcome and improved patients' persistence. *BMC Ophthalmol.* **2020**, *20*, 122. [CrossRef]
6. Baudin, F.; Benzenine, E.; Mariet, A.S.; Bron, A.M.; Daien, V.; Korobelnik, J.F.; Quantin, C.; Creuzot-Garcher, C. Association of Acute Endophthalmitis with Intravitreal Injections of Corticosteroids or Anti-Vascular Growth Factor Agents in a Nationwide Study in France. *JAMA Ophthalmol* **2018**, *136*, 1352–1358. [CrossRef]
7. Solomon, S.D.; Lindsley, K.; Vedula, S.S.; Krzystolik, M.G.; Hawkins, B.S. Anti-vascular endothelial growth factor for neovascular age-related macular degeneration. *Cochrane Database Syst. Rev.* **2019**, *3*, CD005139. [CrossRef]
8. Kim, J.E.; Mantravadi, A.V.; Hur, E.Y.; Covert, D.J. Short-term intraocular pressure changes immediately after intravitreal injections of anti-vascular endothelial growth factor agents. *Am. J. Ophthalmol.* **2008**, *146*, 930–934.e1. [CrossRef]
9. Gismondi, M.; Salati, C.; Salvetat, M.L.; Zeppieri, M.; Brusini, P. Short-term effect of intravitreal injection of Ranibizumab (Lucentis) on intraocular pressure. *J Glaucoma* **2009**, *18*, 658–661. [CrossRef]
10. De Vries, V.A.; Bassil, F.L.; Ramdas, W.D. The effects of intravitreal injections on intraocular pressure and retinal nerve fiber layer: A systematic review and meta-analysis. *Sci. Rep.* **2020**, *10*, 13248. [CrossRef]
11. Bakri, S.J.; Pulido, J.S.; McCannel, C.A.; Hodge, D.O.; Diehl, N.; Hillemeier, J. Immediate intraocular pressure changes following intravitreal injections of triamcinolone, pegaptanib, and bevacizumab. *Eye* **2009**, *23*, 181–185. [CrossRef] [PubMed]
12. Hoguet, A.; Chen, P.P.; Junk, A.K.; Mruthyunjaya, P.; Nouri-Mahdavi, K.; Radhakrishnan, S.; Takusagawa, H.L.; Chen, T.C. The Effect of Anti-Vascular Endothelial Growth Factor Agents on Intraocular Pressure and Glaucoma: A Report by the American Academy of Ophthalmology. *Ophthalmology* **2019**, *126*, 611–622. [CrossRef] [PubMed]
13. Choi, D.Y.; Ortube, M.C.; McCannel, C.A.; Sarraf, D.; Hubschman, J.P.; McCannel, T.A.; Gorin, M.B. Sustained elevated intraocular pressures after intravitreal injection of bevacizumab, ranibizumab, and pegaptanib. *Retina* **2011**, *31*, 1028–1035. [CrossRef] [PubMed]
14. Tseng, J.J.; Vance, S.K.; Della Torre, K.E.; Mendonca, L.S.; Cooney, M.J.; Klancnik, J.M.; Sorenson, J.A.; Freund, K.B. Sustained increased intraocular pressure related to intravitreal antivascular endothelial growth factor therapy for neovascular age-related macular degeneration. *J. Glaucoma* **2012**, *21*, 241–247. [CrossRef]
15. Freund, K.B.; Hoang, Q.V.; Saroj, N.; Thompson, D. Intraocular Pressure in Patients with Neovascular Age-Related Macular Degeneration Receiving Intravitreal Aflibercept or Ranibizumab. *Ophthalmology* **2015**, *122*, 1802–1810. [CrossRef]
16. Atchison, E.A.; Wood, K.M.; Mattox, C.G.; Barry, C.N.; Lum, F.; MacCumber, M.W. The Real-World Effect of Intravitreous Anti-Vascular Endothelial Growth Factor Drugs on Intraocular Pressure: An Analysis Using the IRIS Registry. *Ophthalmology* **2018**, *125*, 676–682. [CrossRef]
17. Levin, A.M.; Chaya, C.J.; Kahook, M.Y.; Wirostko, B.M. Intraocular Pressure Elevation Following Intravitreal Anti-VEGF Injections: Short- and Long-term Considerations. *J. Glaucoma* **2021**, *30*, 1019–1026. [CrossRef]
18. Gabrielle, P.H.; Nguyen, V.; Wolff, B.; Essex, R.; Young, S.; Hunt, A.; Gemmy Cheung, C.M.; Arnold, J.J.; Barthelmes, D.; Fight Retinal Blindness! Study Group; et al. Intraocular Pressure Changes and Vascular Endothelial Growth Factor Inhibitor Use in Various Retinal Diseases: Long-Term Outcomes in Routine Clinical Practice: Data from the Fight Retinal Blindness! Registry. *Ophthalmol Retin.* **2020**, *4*, 861–870. [CrossRef]
19. Dedania, V.S.; Bakri, S.J. Sustained Elevation of Intraocular Pressure After Intravitreal Anti-Vegf Agents: What Is the Evidence? *Retina* **2015**, *35*, 841–858. [CrossRef]
20. Dugel, P.U.; Koh, A.; Ogura, Y.; Jaffe, G.J.; Schmidt-Erfurth, U.; Brown, D.M.; Gomes, A.V.; Warburton, J.; Weichselberger, A.; Holz, F.G. HAWK and HARRIER: Phase 3, Multicenter, Randomized, Double-Masked Trials of Brolucizumab for Neovascular Age-Related Macular Degeneration. *Ophthalmology* **2020**, *127*, 72–84. [CrossRef]
21. Cui, Q.N.; Gray, I.N.; Yu, Y.; VanderBeek, B.L. Repeated intravitreal injections of antivascular endothelial growth factors and risk of intraocular pressure medication use. *Graefes Arch. Clin. Exp. Ophthalmol.* **2019**, *257*, 1931–1939. [CrossRef] [PubMed]
22. Foss, A.J.; Scott, L.J.; Rogers, C.A.; Reeves, B.C.; Ghanchi, F.; Gibson, J.; Chakravarthy, U. Changes in intraocular pressure in study and fellow eyes in the IVAN trial. *Br. J. Ophthalmol.* **2016**, *100*, 1662–1667. [CrossRef]
23. Siegfried, C.J.; Shui, Y.-B. Intraocular Oxygen and Antioxidant Status: New Insights on the Effect of Vitrectomy and Glaucoma Pathogenesis. *Am. J. Ophthalmol.* **2019**, *203*, 12–25. [CrossRef] [PubMed]
24. Tognetto, D.; Pastore, M.R.; Cirigliano, G.; D'Aloisio, R.; Borelli, M.; De Giacinto, C. Long-term intraocular pressure after uncomplicated pars plana vitrectomy for idiopathic epiretinal membrane. *Retina* **2019**, *39*, 163–171. [CrossRef] [PubMed]
25. Wehrli, S.J.; Tawse, K.; Levin, M.H.; Zaidi, A.; Pistilli, M.; Brucker, A.J. A lack of delayed intraocular pressure elevation in patients treated with intravitreal injection of bevacizumab and ranibizumab. *Retina* **2012**, *32*, 1295–1301. [CrossRef] [PubMed]
26. Bakri, S.J.; Moshfeghi, D.M.; Francom, S.; Rundle, A.C.; Reshef, D.S.; Lee, P.P.; Schaeffer, C.; Rubio, R.G.; Lai, P. Intraocular pressure in eyes receiving monthly ranibizumab in 2 pivotal age-related macular degeneration clinical trials. *Ophthalmology* **2014**, *121*, 1102–1108. [CrossRef] [PubMed]
27. Bressler, S.B.; Almukhtar, T.; Bhorade, A.; Bressler, N.M.; Glassman, A.R.; Huang, S.S.; Jampol, L.M.; Kim, J.E.; Melia, M. Repeated intravitreous ranibizumab injections for diabetic macular edema and the risk of sustained elevation of intraocular pressure or the need for ocular hypotensive treatment. *JAMA Ophthalmol.* **2015**, *133*, 589–597. [CrossRef]
28. Hoang, Q.V.; Mendonca, L.S.; Della Torre, K.E.; Jung, J.J.; Tsuang, A.J.; Freund, K.B. Effect on intraocular pressure in patients receiving unilateral intravitreal anti-vascular endothelial growth factor injections. *Ophthalmology* **2012**, *119*, 321–326. [CrossRef]

29. Hoang, Q.V.; Tsuang, A.J.; Gelman, R.; Mendonca, L.S.; Della Torre, K.E.; Jung, J.J.; Freund, K.B. Clinical predictors of sustained intraocular pressure elevation due to intravitreal anti-vascular endothelial growth factor therapy. *Retina* **2013**, *33*, 179–187. [CrossRef]

30. Bilgic, A.; Kodjikian, L.; Chhablani, J.; Sudhalkar, A.; Trivedi, M.; Vasavada, V.; Vasavada, V.; Vasavada, S.; Srivastava, S.; Bhojwani, D.; et al. Sustained Intraocular Pressure Rise after the Treat and Extend Regimen at 3 Years: Aflibercept versus Ranibizumab. *J. Ophthalmol.* **2020**, *2020*, 7462098. [CrossRef]

31. Aref, A.A.; Scott, I.U.; VanVeldhuisen, P.C.; King, J.; Ip, M.S.; Blodi, B.A.; Oden, N.L. Intraocular Pressure-Related Events after Anti-Vascular Endothelial Growth Factor Therapy for Macular Edema Due to Central Retinal Vein Occlusion or Hemiretinal Vein Occlusion: SCORE2 Report 16 on a Secondary Analysis of a Randomized Clinical Trial. *JAMA Ophthalmol.* **2021**, *139*, 1285–1291. [CrossRef] [PubMed]

32. Chakraborty, R.; Read, S.A.; Collins, M.J. Diurnal variations in axial length, choroidal thickness, intraocular pressure, and ocular biometrics. *Investig. Ophthalmol. Vis. Sci.* **2011**, *52*, 5121–5129. [CrossRef] [PubMed]

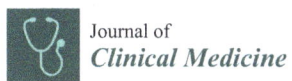

Journal of
Clinical Medicine

Article

Elevated Levels of Growth/Differentiation Factor-15 in the Aqueous Humor and Serum of Glaucoma Patients

Rupalatha Maddala [1,†], Leona T. Y. Ho [1,†], Shruthi Karnam [1,‡], Iris Navarro [1], Anja Osterwald [2], Sandra S. Stinnett [1], Christoph Ullmer [2], Robin R. Vann [1], Pratap Challa [1,3,*] and Ponugoti V. Rao [1,3,*]

[1] Department of Ophthalmology, Duke University School of Medicine, Durham, NC 27710, USA; rupa.maddala@duke.edu (R.M.); leona24ho@gmail.com (L.T.Y.H.); shruthi.karnam@berkeley.edu (S.K.); iris.navarro@duke.edu (I.N.); sandra.stinnett@duke.edu (S.S.S.); Robin.Vann@duke.edu (R.R.V.)

[2] Pharma Research and Early Development, Roche Innovation Center Basel, F. Hoffmann-La Roche Ltd., 4070 Basel, Switzerland; anja.osterwald@roche.com (A.O.); christoph.ullmer@roche.com (C.U.)

[3] Duke Eye Center, Duke University, Durham, NC 27710, USA

* Correspondence: pratap.challa@duke.edu (P.C.); p.rao@duke.edu (P.V.R.); Tel.: +919-684-3282 (P.C.); +919-681-5883 (P.V.R.); Fax: +919-681-8267 (P.C.); +919-684-8983 (P.V.R.)

† These authors contributed equally to this work.

‡ Current address: Department of Optometry and Vision Science, School of Optometry, University of California, Berkeley, CA 94720, USA.

Citation: Maddala, R.; Ho, L.T.Y.; Karnam, S.; Navarro, I.; Osterwald, A.; Stinnett, S.S.; Ullmer, C.; Vann, R.R.; Challa, P.; Rao, P.V. Elevated Levels of Growth/Differentiation Factor-15 in the Aqueous Humor and Serum of Glaucoma Patients. *J. Clin. Med.* 2022, 11, 744. https://doi.org/10.3390/jcm11030744

Academic Editors: Maria Letizia Salvetat, Marco Zeppieri and Paolo Brusini

Received: 9 January 2022
Accepted: 26 January 2022
Published: 29 January 2022

Publisher's Note: MDPI stays neutral with regard to jurisdictional claims in published maps and institutional affiliations.

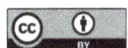

Abstract: Dysregulated levels of growth/differentiation factor-15 (GDF15), a divergent member of the transforming growth factor-beta super family, have been found to be associated with the pathology of various diseases. In this study, we evaluated the levels of GDF15 in aqueous humor (AH) and serum samples derived from primary open-angle glaucoma (POAG) and age- and gender-matched non-glaucoma (cataract) patients to assess the plausible association between GDF15 and POAG. GDF15 levels were determined using an enzyme-linked immunosorbent assay, and data analysis was performed using the Wilcoxon rank sum test, or the Kruskal–Wallis test and linear regression. GDF15 levels in the AH ($n = 105$) of POAG patients were significantly elevated (by 7.4-fold) compared to cataract patients ($n = 117$). Serum samples obtained from a subgroup of POAG patients ($n = 41$) also showed a significant increase in GDF15 levels (by 50%) compared to cataract patients. GDF15 levels were elevated in male, female, African American, and Caucasian POAG patients. This study reveals a significant and marked elevation of GDF15 levels in the AH of POAG patients compared to non-glaucoma cataract control patients. Although serum GDF15 levels were also elevated in POAG patients, the magnitude of difference was much smaller relative to that found in the AH.

Keywords: glaucoma; aqueous humor; GDF15; serum; intraocular pressure

1. Introduction

Glaucoma, a group of optic neuropathies, is the second leading cause of irreversible blindness worldwide. Among the various characterized types of glaucoma, primary-open angle glaucoma (POAG) accounts for more than 70% [1,2]. Although the etiology of POAG is poorly understood, elevated intraocular pressure (IOP) due to impaired aqueous humor (AH) drainage through the trabecular pathway has been identified as a major risk factor for POAG [3,4]. Lowering of IOP has been demonstrated to slow down retinal ganglion cell death and vision loss in glaucoma patients, and is a mainstay of treatment for glaucoma [3–5]. Though several IOP-lowering drugs are currently available, many of them do not possess adequate efficacy to control IOP in glaucoma patients, with several posing considerable adverse effects [3]. Therefore, a better understanding of the etiology of ocular hypertension and impaired AH outflow through the trabecular pathway, which accounts for more than 80% of AH outflow in glaucoma patients, is necessary to enable the development of targeted and efficacious IOP-lowering drugs [4,6].

Dysregulated levels of various secretory proteins in the AH, including transforming growth factor-beta (TGF-β), endothelin-1, connective tissue growth factor, and lysophospholipid-producing enzyme autotaxin, have been shown to be associated with POAG and elevated IOP [7,8]. We recently reported that human trabecular meshwork cells express and secrete growth/differentiation factor 15 (GDF15), suggesting its plausible role in the regulation of IOP [9]. GDF15 is a distant member of the TGF-β superfamily, and is widely expressed in multiple mammalian tissues albeit in low concentrations [10,11]. GDF15 is often induced under stress and with aging [12], and is involved in the homeostasis of cell and tissue function [11]. Elevated GDF15 levels are linked to various pathological conditions, including inflammation, cardiovascular disease, cancer, obesity, and kidney disease [13–15]. GDF15 has thus been widely explored as a prognostic biomarker in several diseases [11,14].

Previous studies have reported significant elevations in AH and serum levels of GDF15 protein in small cohorts of POAG and pseudoexfoliation glaucoma patients, where the increased levels of AH GDF15 exhibited a positive correlation with disease severity [16–18]. The findings from these studies were inconsistent, however [18], and did not include an evaluation of GDF-15 in AH and serum derived from the same cohort of patients [16,19]. Therefore, to undertake an independent evaluation of the status of GDF15 levels in the AH and serum from the same population of glaucoma patients, and to understand the plausible role of GDF15 in the pathobiology of ocular hypertension, we determined the levels of GDF15 in AH and serum samples derived from POAG and age- and gender-matched non-glaucoma (cataract) patients. The findings of this study reveal elevated levels of GDF15 in the AH, as well as the serum, of POAG patients, indicating the plausible role for GDF15 in the pathobiology of ocular hypertension.

2. Materials and Methods

Human Subjects: Research involving the collection of human AH and blood samples was approved by the Institutional Review Board (IRB; Protocol No. Pro00093311)/Ethics Committee of Duke University Medical Center, in compliance with Health Insurance Portability and Accountability Act guidelines, and the tenets of the Declaration of Helsinki. Written informed consent was obtained from patients prior to the collection of AH and blood samples. All samples analyzed in the study were obtained from patients who underwent cataract or glaucoma surgeries at the academic Duke University Eye Center. Only one eye per patient was enrolled for glaucoma and non-glaucoma subjects. Samples were collected starting from the beginning of 2017 to the end of 2020.

Clinical Assessment: Patients underwent a review of medical history, measurement of best-corrected visual acuity and refraction, slit lamp biomicroscopy, gonioscopy, and Goldmann applanation tonometry (Haag-Streit Diagnostics, Essex, UK). In glaucoma patients, disc and red-free fundus photography, gonioscopy, and optical coherence tomography (OCT; Heidelberg Engineering Inc., Franklin, MA, USA) were performed. POAG was defined as the presence of glaucomatous optic neuropathy associated with typical reproducible glaucomatous visual field defects without any other ocular disease or conditions that might elevate IOP, and an open angle on gonioscopy. A glaucomatous visual field change was defined either as: (1) an outside normal limit result on the glaucoma hemifield test; (2) three abnormal points with a <5% probability of being normal, including one with a probability <1% by pattern deviation; or (3) a pattern standard deviation of 5% if the visual field was otherwise full, as confirmed on two consecutive tests. Disease severity of glaucoma, including mild, moderate, and severe classification, was based on the ICD-10 coding of each patient. Pigment dispersion syndrome and psuedoexfoliation syndrome cases were excluded. In the cataract and POAG patients, the rate of comorbidities (systemic diseases), medications (including cholesterol-, glucose-, and hypertension-lowering drugs; atropine, multivitamin supplement, calcium supplement, Tylenol, gabapentin, and Flonase), and smoking were found to be very close. Use of sildenafil was identified in some of the cataract patients, but was not significant. As anticipated, most of the POAG patients were on one or more IOP-lowering medications prior to glaucoma surgery.

Collection of aqueous humor and blood samples: AH samples were collected at the initiation of cataract or glaucoma surgery. A tuberculin syringe with a 30-gauge needle was inserted into the anterior chamber through a limbal paracentesis tract at the start of the surgery, and approximately 40–100 µL of AH was slowly aspirated. The AH samples were transferred from the syringe to a 1.5 mL Eppendorf tube, and centrifuged at $1000 \times g$ for 10 min at 4 °C. The supernatant obtained from the AH samples was collected and stored at -80 °C until further use.

Blood samples from the patients were collected by venipuncture by the triage nurse using a BD Vacutainer push button blood collection set, and the blood was carefully dispensed into serum blood collection tubes from Becton, Dickinson, and Company, Franklin Lakes, NJ. Tubes containing blood samples were inverted gently five times, rested at room temperature for 30 min, and centrifuged for 15 min at $1000 \times g$ using a benchtop Eppendorf centrifuge at room temperature. Serum samples were collected into bio-safe tubes, and stored at -80 °C until further use.

Detection of GDF15: A human GDF15 enzyme-linked immunosorbent assay kit (Human GDF15 DuoSet ELISA, R&D Systems, Inc., Minneapolis, MN, USA) was used to determine the levels of GDF15 in both AH and serum samples. Analysis was performed in a masked manner, and per the manufacturer's protocol, which included appropriate standards and background controls, using a SpectraMax M3 plate reader (Molecular Devices, San Jose, CA, USA). Ten microliters of AH was used in duplicate for each sample analyzed. Serum samples were diluted 10-fold with diluent buffer provided in the kit, and 10 µL of the diluted sample was used in duplicate per sample. Results for both AH and serum samples were expressed as picograms of GDF15/milliliter (pg/mL).

Statistical Analysis: The significance of differences in continuous variables between categories of disease (POAG and cataract), diagnosis (cataract, mild POAG, moderate POAG, severe POAG), race (Asian, African American, Caucasian), and gender were assessed using the Wilcoxon rank sum test or the Kruskal–Wallis test. Relationships between continuous variables were assessed using linear regression. The data analysis was performed using SAS/STAT software, Version 9.4 of the SAS System for Windows (Copyright © 2022–2012 SAS Institute Inc.).

3. Results

3.1. Elevated Levels of GDF15 in Both AH and Serum Samples of POAG Patients

In this study, we aimed to investigate whether dysregulated AH and serum GDF15 levels relate to POAG. To address this goal, we initially compared the levels of GDF15 in AH and serum samples from the same cohort of POAG patients ($n = 40$ and 41, respectively) with age- and gender-matched controls (non-glaucomatous, cataract patients, $n = 32$). Although this cohort was matched for gender and age, race was not matched between the glaucoma and cataract patients in the study (Supplementary Table S1 describes the demography details of human patients included in the study). The GDF15 levels in AH and serum samples from POAG patients were significantly elevated ($p < 0.001$ and $p < 0.011$, respectively) by >9 fold and 1.5-fold, respectively, compared to the respective samples derived from non-glaucoma (cataract) patients based on the Wilcoxon rank sum test of difference between medians (Figure 1, Table S2). AH GDF15 levels were significantly ($p < 0.001$) elevated in both male (by 11.6-fold) and female (by 5.4-fold) POAG patients compared to cataract patients (Table S3). In the case of serum samples (Table S3), although there was an increase (median values: 2228.0 pg/mL, $n = 19$) in male POAG patients compared to male cataract patients (1850.0 pg/mL, $n = 19$), the difference did not achieve statistical significance ($p < 0.148$). Serum GDF15 levels in female POAG patients ($n = 22$), however, were significantly ($p < 0.015$) elevated (by 64%) compared to female cataract patients ($n = 13$).

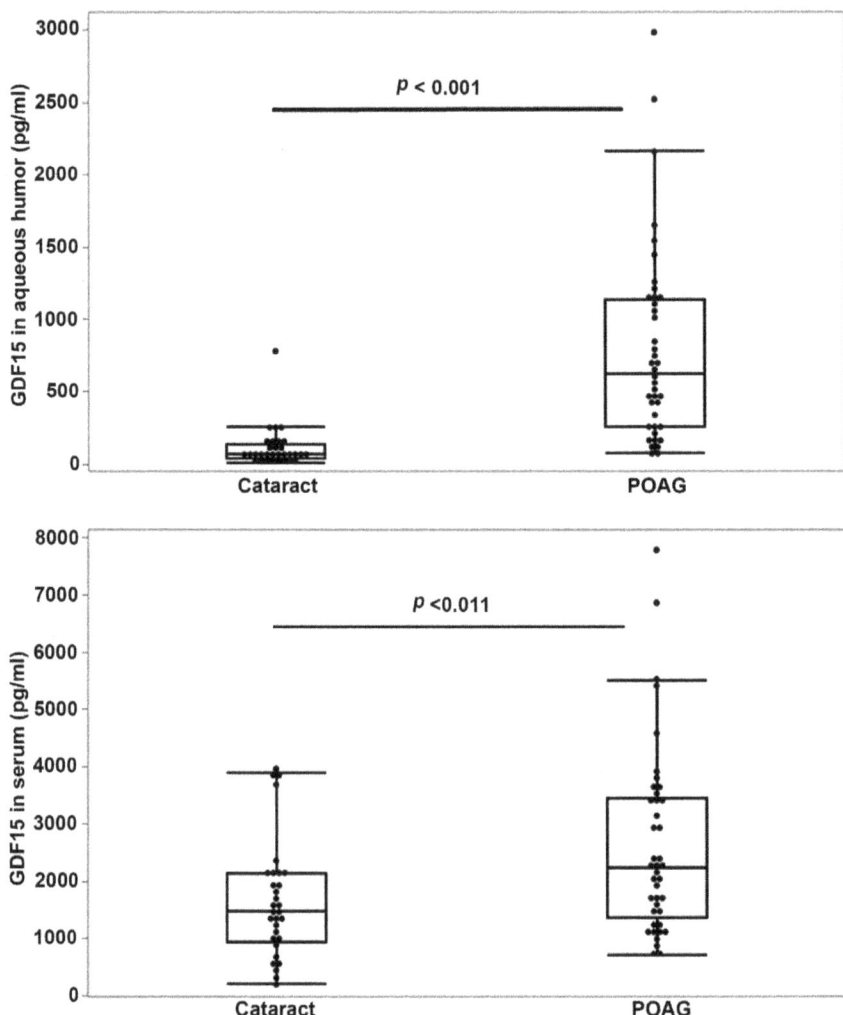

Figure 1. Elevated levels of GDF15 in aqueous humor and serum samples of POAG patients. Aqueous humor (*n* = 40) and serum (*n* = 41) samples derived from POAG patients revealed significantly elevated levels of growth/differentiation factor-15 (GDF15) (by >9-fold and 50%, respectively) compared to age- and gender-matched cataract patient samples (*n* = 32). The box and whisker plots represent median and the interquartile range in the distribution. *p*-values were based on the Wilcoxon rank sum test of difference between medians. Abbreviations: GDF15, growth/differentiation factor-15; POAG, primary open-angle glaucoma.

3.2. Robust Elevation of GDF15 Levels in the Aqueous Humor of a Large Cohort of POAG Patients

We then expanded the scope of our investigation to include analysis of GDF15 in AH samples from additional POAG and cataract patients. Analysis of GDF15 was performed as described above, with the data set comprised of a total of 105 POAG AH samples and 117 non-glaucoma cataract AH samples derived from gender- and age-matched, but not race-matched, patient populations (Table S4 describes the demography details for all of the POAG patients of this study). Median GDF15 levels in the AH from this large cohort of subjects were significantly ($p < 0.001$) and robustly (by 7.4-fold) elevated in the

POAG group relative to the cataract group (Figure 2, Table S5). The coefficient of variation for GDF15 in POAG is 104.9. In this large cohort of POAG patients, males ($n = 52$) and females ($n = 53$), and African Americans ($n = 53$) and Caucasians ($n = 50$), all showed significantly increased median levels of AH GDF15 ($p < 0.001$) compared to their respective non-glaucoma (cataract) controls (males, $n = 53$; females, $n = 64$; African Americans, $n = 16$; Caucasians, $n = 94$). These results are summarized in Tables 1 and 2. Within the POAG patient group, there was no gender or racial (African American versus Caucasians) difference in the AH GDF15 levels (data not shown). Interestingly, although there was no racial difference in the AH GDF15 levels within the cataract group, the male subjects ($n = 53$) have significantly ($p < 0.046$) higher median levels (by 33%) of AH GDF15 compared to female subjects ($n = 64$, Table S6). This gender difference in the levels of GDF15 was also consistent in the serum samples derived from the cataract subjects (Table S6). Serum samples derived from male cataract ($n = 19$) subjects have significantly ($p < 0.025$) higher (by 42%) median levels of GDF15 compared to the female cataract subjects ($n = 13$).

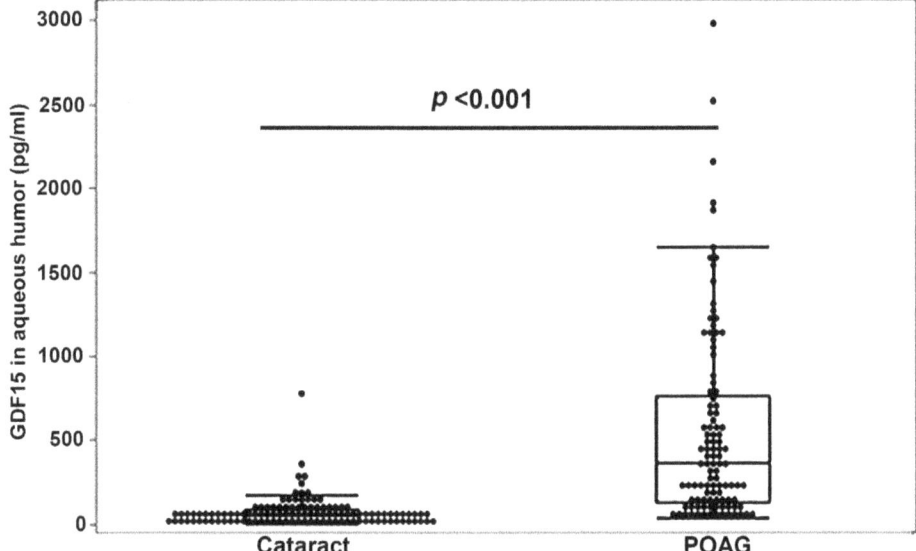

Figure 2. Elevated levels of GDF15 in aqueous humor samples from POAG patients. Aqueous humor samples derived from POAG patients ($n = 105$) showed significantly increased levels of GDF15 (by 7.4-fold) compared to age- and gender-matched non-glaucoma cataract patient samples ($n = 117$). The box and whisker plots represent median and the interquartile range in the distribution. *p*-values were based on Wilcoxon rank sum test of difference between medians. Abbreviations: GDF15, growth/differentiation factor-15; POAG, primary open-angle glaucoma.

Table 1. GDF15 levels in the aqueous humor of male and female POAG and cataract patients.

	Gender		Cataract	POAG	*p*-Value *
GDF-15 (AH)	Female	*n*	64	53	
		Mean (SD)	60.41 (65.33)	543.55 (664.30)	
		Min, Median, Max	0.3, 39.0, 357.1	36.1, 246.0, 2978.0	<0.001
GDF-15 (AH)	Male	*n*	53	52	
		Mean (SD)	80.07 (108.36)	556.95 (478.73)	
		Min, Median, Max	1.5, 52.0, 776.0	48.0, 438.6, 1868.2	<0.001

* *p*-value based on Wilcoxon rank sum test of difference between medians.

Table 2. GDF15 levels in the aqueous humor of Caucasian and African American POAG and cataract patients.

Variable	Race	Statistic	Cataract	POAG	*p*-Value *
GDF-15 (AH)	African American	*n*	16	53	
		Mean (SD)	54.90 (43.12)	515.41 (561.68)	
		Min, Median, Max	2.0, 49.0, 146.0	44.7, 225.0, 2156.0	<0.001
	Caucasian	*n*	94	50	
		Mean (SD)	74.26 (95.43)	571.55 (591.09)	
		Min, Median, Max	0.3, 51.0, 776.0	36.1, 419.5, 2978.0	<0.001

* *p*-value based on Wilcoxon rank sum of difference between medians.

3.3. Aqueous Humor GDF15 Levels, IOP, and Age Relationships in POAG Patients

Intraocular pressure was significantly higher ($p < 0.001$) in POAG patients ($n = 105$; 20.79 ± 6.974 (mean $\pm$ SD) compared to non-glaucoma cataract patients ($n = 43$; 14.97 ± 2.923; Figure S1). The coefficient of variation for IOP in POAG is 33.5. However, AH and serum GDF15 and IOP did not reveal a significant relationship in POAG patients (Figure S2A,B, respectively). Similarly, there was no significant relationship between the AH GDF15 levels and age, and between the serum GDF15 and age in POAG patients (Figure S3A,B, respectively).

3.4. Relationship between AH GDF15 and POAG Disease Severity

To explore a plausible relationship between the levels of AH GDF15 and disease severity of glaucoma, we sub-classified glaucoma patients from the smaller cohort described above (Table S1) into mild ($n = 10$), moderate ($n = 8$), and severe ($n = 20$) POAG subgroups, based on the ICD-10 coding of each patient. The mean deviation was taken from the last visual field prior to surgery. All visual fields were within 3 months of surgery. The median deviation was significantly different between the mild POAG and severe POAG patients, and between the moderate POAG and severe POAG subgroup, but not between mild POAG and moderate POAG subgroups (Figure 3A). As expected, cup-to-disk ratio was significantly higher in mild, moderate, and severe POAG compared to that of cataract patients ($n = 43$). The cup-to-disk ratio was significantly higher in moderate POAG compared to mild POAG, and in severe POAG compared to mild POAG patients (Figure 3B). AH GDF15 levels were significantly elevated in mild, moderate, and severe POAG patients compared to cataract patients. However, although there was an increase in GDF15 levels in the severe POAG patient subgroup relative to mild POAG patients, there was no statistical difference in AH GDF15 levels between the mild and moderate POAG, and between the mild and severe POAG patients (Figure 3C). Additionally, we examined for an association between the serum GDF15 levels and severity of POAG. Though there was a significant increase in the serum GDF15 levels in moderate ($n = 8$) and severe ($n = 21$) POAG patients compared to cataract patients ($n = 32$), there was no difference between the mild POAG ($n = 10$) and severe POAG patients (Figure 3D). Interestingly, serum GDF15 levels were found to be significantly higher in the moderate POAG patients compared to mild POAG patients (Figure 3D). Overall, although there is an increase in the levels of both AH and serum GDF15 levels in severe POAG patients compared to mild POAG patients, there was no statistical difference between these two groups in the small cohort of glaucoma patients examined.

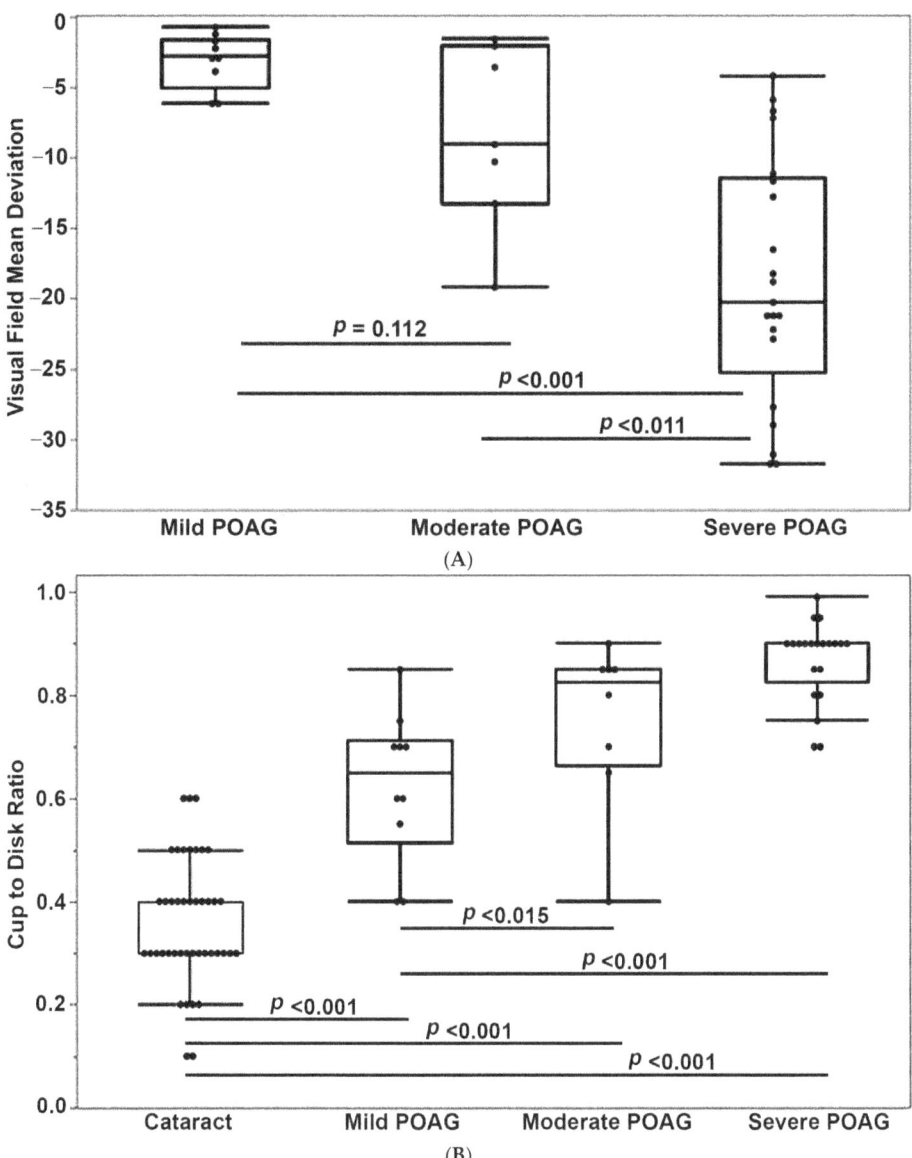

Figure 3. *Cont.*

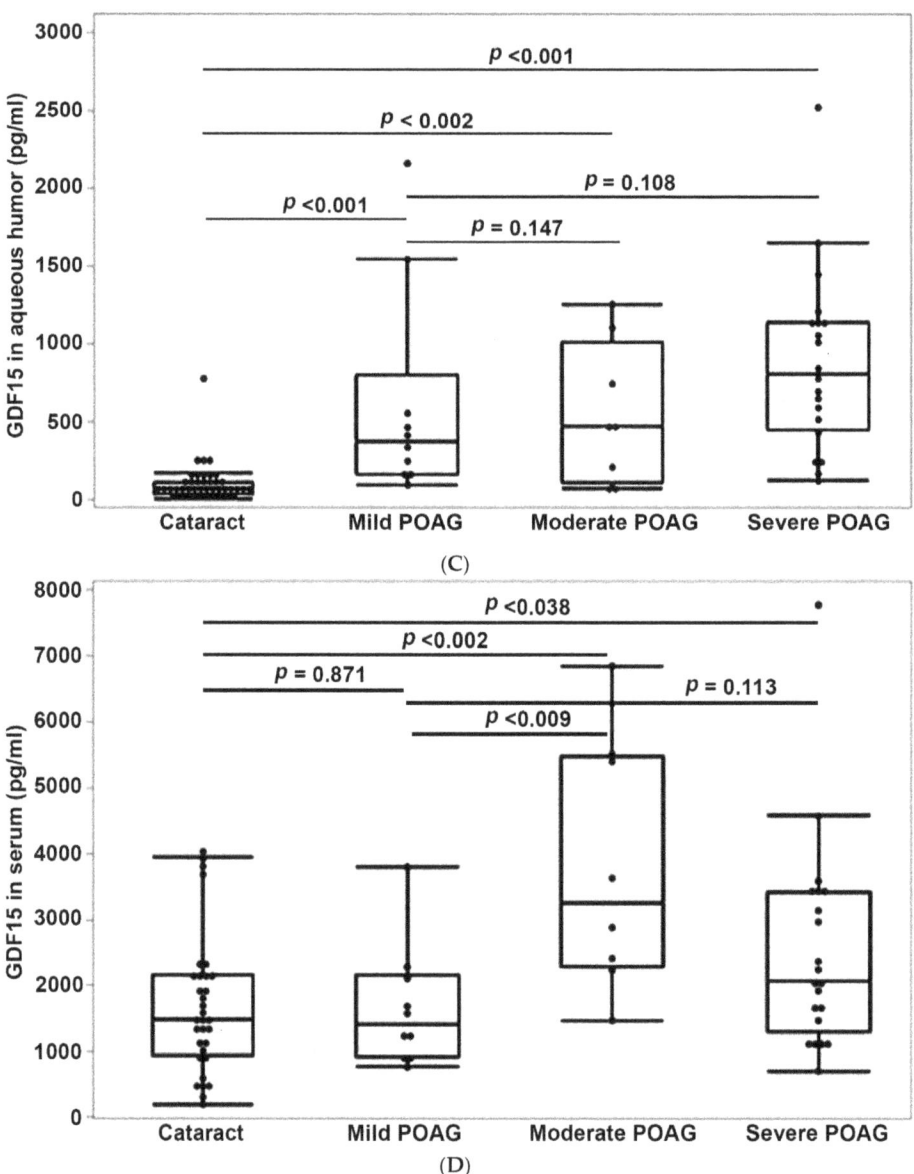

Figure 3. Relationship between aqueous humor and serum GDF15 levels and disease severity of POAG. To determine whether elevated levels of GDF15 either in the AH or serum reveal a positive association with disease severity of glaucoma, POAG patients from a small cohort study were divided into mild, moderate, and severe glaucoma based on median deviation of visual field loss and GDF15 levels from the categories analyzed. (**A**) Overall, there was a significant difference in median deviation of visual field loss among the three groups, based on the Kruskal–Wallis test ($p < 0.001$). Though the median deviation was not found to be significant between mild and moderate POAG, it was significant between mild to severe, and moderate to severe POAG based on the Wilcoxon rank sum test. (**B**) Cup-to-disk ratio showed a significant difference between cataract patients versus mild, moderate, and severe POAG, and between mild to moderate, and mild to severe POAG based on the

J. Clin. Med. **2022**, *11*, 744

Wilcoxon rank sum test. (**C**) AH GDF15 levels were significantly elevated between cataract and mild, moderate, and severe POAG, but not different between mild and moderate, and mild and severe POAG, based on the Wilcoxon rank sum test. (**D**) Serum GDF15 levels were also significantly elevated in moderate and severe POAG samples compared to cataract samples, but not different between mild and severe POAG, although there was a significant difference between mild and moderate POAG based on the Wilcoxon rank sum test. In all panels, the box and whisker plots represent median and the interquartile range in the distribution. Abbreviations: GDF15, growth/differentiation factor-15; POAG, primary open-angle glaucoma.

4. Discussion

GDF15 is a well-characterized secretory stress cytokine that possesses several physiological activities [11,13]. Our previous study identified GDF15, a divergent member of the TGF-β superfamily of growth factors, as a common constituent of the extracellular matrix secreted by trabecular meshwork cells [9]. The results of this study revealed a robust increase in AH GDF15 levels, with a moderate and significant increase in serum GDF15 levels of POAG patients relative to the corresponding samples from control (non-glaucomatous cataract) patients, suggesting a potential association between GDF15 and POAG.

GDF15, which was also identified as macrophage inhibitory cytokine-1 and nonsteroidal anti-inflammatory drug activated gene-1, has gained increased attention because of its role in several diseases [11,13]. Increased GDF15 levels have been reported under various disease conditions, including cancer, cardiovascular disease, liver and kidney diseases, and with inflammation, age, smoking, stress, and tissue injury [11,14,15,20]. Although it was initially thought to act through the TGF-β receptors and possess TGF-β-like biological activities, recent studies have revealed that GDF15 binds to the GDNF family receptor α–like (GFRAL) orphan receptor with high affinity, with GFRAL playing a crucial role in GDF15-induced weight loss and decreased food intake [21–23]. However, GFRAL is reported to be expressed only in a distinct region of the brain known as the postrema [10,23]. Therefore, it is presumed that the widely distributed GDF15 may also act through an alternative, but yet to be characterized, molecular pathway(s), and to be involved in different physiological activities [13].

Interestingly, in the eye, GDF15 has been shown to promote retinal ganglion cell (RGC) differentiation [24], and neuroprotection of RGC under optic nerve crush injury [25], with GDF15 expression and secretion by RGCs being increased under tissue injury [16]. Moreover, GDF15 was found to be elevated in the RGC and AH in different glaucoma experimental models [16], wherein a good correlation has been documented between RGC loss and increased expression and protein levels of GDF15 [16]. Importantly, elevated AH GDF15 has also been shown to correlate with disease severity (based on the median deviation of visual field loss) in POAG and pseudoexfoliation glaucoma patients [16,17]. Based on these findings, GDF15 has been suggested to serve as a molecular marker for glaucomatous neurodegeneration [16]. However, these latter conclusions were drawn mainly based on findings from one laboratory study [16,17]. Moreover, although serum derived from both POAG and pseudoexfoliation glaucoma patients has been reported to contain elevated levels of GDF15 [19], a recent study using plasma derived from both POAG and pseudoexfoliation glaucoma patients showed no difference in GDF15 levels compared to non-glaucoma (cataract) patients [18]. The reason for the noted discrepancy between levels of GDF15 in serum and plasma derived from glaucoma patients is not clear. However, in the above referenced studies, there was no evaluation of GDF15 levels in the AH and serum derived from the same cohort of patients.

In this study, using serum and AH from the same cohort of patients, we found significantly elevated levels of GDF15 in POAG patients relative to cataract patients, with a more robust difference in AH GDF15 levels compared to serum GDF15 levels. A total of 105 POAG and 117 cataract patient derived samples were utilized for the analysis of AH GDF15 levels. In this relatively large cohort of POAG patients, the AH GDF15 levels were robustly elevated (by 7.4-fold) relative to the respective age- and gender-matched non-glaucoma cataract patient subgroup. This increase in AH GDF15 levels was consistent in males, females, African American, and Caucasian POAG patients. However, when the subset of POAG patients was categorized into mild, moderate, and severe POAG subgroups based on the median deviation of visual field loss, we did not find a definitive correlation between the levels of AH or serum GDF15 and disease severity of glaucoma, although there was an increasing trend in GDF15 levels in AH and serum with an increasing disease severity of glaucoma. The sample size in our cohort of glaucoma patients was very close to that described by Lin et al. [17], and Ban et al. [16], in which they found a positive correlation between the levels of GDF15 of AH and the disease severity of glaucoma.

Interestingly, consistent with previous reports [18,26], AH and serum samples from male cataract patients contained significantly higher levels of GDF15 relative to female patients, suggesting a definitive gender difference in GDF15 levels. Coincidently, the gender prevalence of open angle glaucoma is mixed, but some studies have reported higher rates in males compared to females [1,27,28]. However, within POAG patients, there was no statistical difference in AH GDF15 levels between male and female patients.

5. Limitations

We want to recognize the limitations of this study in regards to a lack of a definitive correlation between the levels of AH GDF15 and the disease severity of glaucoma. The sample size in our study was one limitation for establishing this correlation. Additionally, though this study matched the gender and age of subgroups, race was not matched between the POAG and cataract (non-glaucoma) subgroups, and race and ethnicity have been found to influence the incidence of glaucoma [1]. Additionally, this study did not reveal a correlation between the levels of AH or serum GDF15 and IOP in POAG patients. Two reasons could likely account for this observation, with the first being that all POAG patients were already on IOP-lowering medications as part of their glaucoma therapy; as a result of which, their IOP readings would be lower. Since we did not have access to all of the patients' pre-treatment IOPs, this possibility could not be verified. The second reason is that we do not know the implications of prior eye surgeries for GDF15 levels, since some POAG patients had previously undergone cataract removal and glaucoma procedures, and corneal, or retinal intraocular surgery.

6. Conclusions

This study reveals increased levels of GDF15 in both the AH and serum of POAG patients compared to age- and gender-matched non-glaucoma cataract patients, suggesting a strong association between elevated levels of GDF15 and POAG.

Supplementary Materials: The following supporting information can be downloaded at https://www.mdpi.com/article/10.3390/jcm11030744/s1: Figure S1: Elevated IOP in POAG patients compared to non-glaucoma (cataract patients). The box and whisker plots represent median and the interquartile range in the distribution. *p*-values were based on Wilcoxon rank sum test of difference between medians; Figure S2. Relationship between aqueous humor and serum growth/differentiation factor-15 (GDF15) levels and IOP in POAG patients. AH GDF15 (A), serum GDF15 (B), and IOP of POAG patients did not reveal a significant relationship; Figure S3. Relationship between aqueous humor and serum GDF15 levels and age in POAG patients. AH GDF15 (A), serum GDF15 (B), and age of POAG patients did not reveal a significant relationship; Table S1: Demography details of the subgroup of POAG and cataract patient study; Table S2: GDF15 levels in the aqueous humor and serum of POAG and non-glaucoma (cataract) subjects; Table S3: GDF15 levels in the aqueous humor and serum of male and female POAG and cataract patients; Table S4: Demography details of the large cohort POAG and cataract patient study; Table S5: GDF15 levels in the aqueous humor of POAG and cataract patients; Table S6: GDF15 levels in aqueous humor and serum samples from male and female cataract patients.

J. Clin. Med. **2022**, *11*, 744

Author Contributions: Conceptualization, R.M., L.T.Y.H., C.U., P.C. and P.V.R.; Methodology, R.M., L.T.Y.H., S.K., A.O., I.N., R.R.V. and P.C.; Software, R.M., A.O., L.T.Y.H. and S.S.S.; Validation, R.M., P.C. and P.V.R.; Formal Analysis, R.M., L.T.Y.H., A.O. and S.S.S.; Investigation, R.M., L.T.Y.H., C.U., P.C. and P.V.R.; Resources, I.N., R.R.V., P.C., C.U. and P.V.R.; Data Curation, R.M., L.T.Y.H., S.S.S. and P.V.R.; Writing—Original Draft Preparation, R.M., L.T.Y.H., P.C. and P.V.R.; Writing—Review and Editing, R.M., L.T.Y.H., S.K., A.O., S.S.S., C.U., R.R.V., C.U., P.C. and P.V.R.; Visualization, R.M., S.S.S. and P.V.R.; Supervision, P.V.R. and C.U.; Project Administration, P.C. and P.V.R.; Funding Acquisition, P.V.R. All authors have read and agreed to the published version of the manuscript.

Funding: Supported by the National Eye Institute, National Institutes of Health, Bethesda, Maryland (investigator grant no. R01EY018590 and R01-EY028823 (PVR)). The funding organization had no role in the design or conduct of this research.

Institutional Review Board Statement: The study was conducted according to the guidelines of the Declaration of Helsinki, and was approved by the Institutional Review Board (IRB; Protocol No. Pro00093311; date approved, 20 July 2018)/Ethics Committee of Duke University Medical Center, in compliance with Health Insurance Portability and Accountability Act guidelines.

Informed Consent Statement: Written informed consent was obtained from all subjects involved in the study.

Data Availability Statement: Authors will make all data available upon request.

Conflicts of Interest: The authors have made the following disclosure(s): No conflicts: R.M., L.T.Y.H., K.S., I.N., R.R.V., P.C., S.S.S. and P.V.R.; Employed by the F. Hoffmann-La Roche Ltd.: A.O. and C.U.

References

1. Allison, K.; Patel, D.; Alabi, O. Epidemiology of Glaucoma: The Past, Present, and Predictions for the Future. *Cureus* **2020**, *12*, e11686. [CrossRef] [PubMed]
2. Tham, Y.C.; Li, X.; Wong, T.Y.; Quigley, H.A.; Aung, T.; Cheng, C.Y. Global prevalence of glaucoma and projections of glaucoma burden through 2040: A systematic review and meta-analysis. *Ophthalmology* **2014**, *121*, 2081–2090. [CrossRef] [PubMed]
3. Weinreb, R.N.; Leung, C.K.; Crowston, J.G.; Medeiros, F.A.; Friedman, D.S.; Wiggs, J.L.; Martin, K.R. Primary open-angle glaucoma. *Nat. Rev. Dis. Primers* **2016**, *2*, 16067. [CrossRef] [PubMed]
4. Weinreb, R.N.; Aung, T.; Medeiros, F.A. The pathophysiology and treatment of glaucoma: A review. *JAMA* **2014**, *311*, 1901–1911. [CrossRef] [PubMed]
5. Kwon, Y.H.; Fingert, J.H.; Kuehn, M.H.; Alward, W.L. Primary open-angle glaucoma. *N. Engl. J. Med.* **2009**, *360*, 1113–1124. [CrossRef] [PubMed]
6. Stamer, W.D.; Acott, T.S. Current understanding of conventional outflow dysfunction in glaucoma. *Curr. Opin. Ophthalmol.* **2012**, *23*, 135–143. [CrossRef] [PubMed]
7. Rao, P.V.; Pattabiraman, P.P.; Kopczynski, C. Role of the Rho GTPase/Rho kinase signaling pathway in pathogenesis and treatment of glaucoma: Bench to bedside research. *Exp. Eye Res.* **2017**, *158*, 23–32. [CrossRef] [PubMed]
8. Ho, L.T.Y.; Osterwald, A.; Ruf, I.; Hunziker, D.; Mattei, P.; Challa, P.; Vann, R.; Ullmer, C.; Rao, P.V. Role of the autotaxin-lysophosphatidic acid axis in glaucoma, aqueous humor drainage and fibrogenic activity. *Biochim. Biophys. Acta Mol. Basis Dis.* **2020**, *1866*, 165560. [CrossRef]
9. Muralidharan, A.R.; Maddala, R.; Skiba, N.P.; Rao, P.V. Growth Differentiation Factor-15-Induced Contractile Activity and Extracellular Matrix Production in Human Trabecular Meshwork Cells. *Invest. Ophthalmol. Vis. Sci.* **2016**, *57*, 6482–6495. [CrossRef]
10. Mullican, S.E.; Rangwala, S.M. Uniting GDF15 and GFRAL: Therapeutic Opportunities in Obesity and Beyond. *Trends Endocrinol. Metab.* **2018**, *29*, 560–570. [CrossRef]
11. Breit, S.N.; Brown, D.A.; Tsai, V.W. The GDF15-GFRAL Pathway in Health and Metabolic Disease: Friend or Foe? *Annu. Rev. Physiol.* **2021**, *83*, 127–151. [CrossRef] [PubMed]
12. Basisty, N.; Kale, A.; Jeon, O.H.; Kuehnemann, C.; Payne, T.; Rao, C.; Holtz, A.; Shah, S.; Sharma, V.; Ferrucci, L.; et al. A proteomic atlas of senescence-associated secretomes for aging biomarker development. *PLoS Biol.* **2020**, *18*, e3000599. [CrossRef] [PubMed]
13. Baek, S.J.; Eling, T. Growth differentiation factor 15 (GDF15): A survival protein with therapeutic potential in metabolic diseases. *Pharmacol. Ther.* **2019**, *198*, 46–58. [CrossRef] [PubMed]
14. Desmedt, S.; Desmedt, V.; De Vos, L.; Delanghe, J.R.; Speeckaert, R.; Speeckaert, M.M. Growth differentiation factor 15: A novel biomarker with high clinical potential. *Crit. Rev. Clin. Lab. Sci.* **2019**, *56*, 333–350. [CrossRef] [PubMed]
15. Breit, S.N.; Johnen, H.; Cook, A.D.; Tsai, V.W.; Mohammad, M.G.; Kuffner, T.; Zhang, H.P.; Marquis, C.P.; Jiang, L.; Lockwood, G.; et al. The TGF-beta superfamily cytokine, MIC-1/GDF15: A pleotrophic cytokine with roles in inflammation, cancer and metabolism. *Growth Factors* **2011**, *29*, 187–195. [CrossRef]

16. Ban, N.; Siegfried, C.J.; Lin, J.B.; Shui, Y.B.; Sein, J.; Pita-Thomas, W.; Sene, A.; Santeford, A.; Gordon, M.; Lamb, R.; et al. GDF15 is elevated in mice following retinal ganglion cell death and in glaucoma patients. *JCI Insight* **2017**, *2*, e91455. [CrossRef] [PubMed]
17. Lin, J.B.; Sheybani, A.; Santeford, A.; De Maria, A.; Apte, R.S. Increased Aqueous Humor GDF15 Is Associated with Worse Visual Field Loss in Pseudoexfoliative Glaucoma Patients. *Transl. Vis. Sci. Technol.* **2020**, *9*, 16. [CrossRef]
18. Hubens, W.H.G.; Kievit, M.T.; Berendschot, T.; de Coo, I.F.M.; Smeets, H.J.M.; Webers, C.A.B.; Gorgels, T. Plasma GDF-15 concentration is not elevated in open-angle glaucoma. *PLoS ONE* **2021**, *16*, e0252630.
19. Bourouki, E.; Oikonomou, E.; Moschos, M.; Siasos, G.; Siasou, G.; Gouliopoulos, N.; Deftereos, S.; Miliou, A.; Zacharia, E.; Tousoulis, D. Pseudoexfoliative Glaucoma, Endothelial Dysfunction, and Arterial Stiffness: The Role of Circulating Apoptotic Endothelial Microparticles. *J. Glaucoma* **2019**, *28*, 749–755. [CrossRef] [PubMed]
20. Luan, H.H.; Wang, A.; Hilliard, B.K.; Carvalho, F.; Rosen, C.E.; Ahasic, A.M.; Herzog, E.L.; Kang, I.; Pisani, M.A.; Yu, S.; et al. GDF15 Is an Inflammation-Induced Central Mediator of Tissue Tolerance. *Cell* **2019**, *178*, 1231–1244 e11. [CrossRef]
21. Yang, L.; Chang, C.C.; Sun, Z.; Madsen, D.; Zhu, H.; Padkjaer, S.B.; Wu, X.; Huang, T.; Hultman, K.; Paulsen, S.J.; et al. GFRAL is the receptor for GDF15 and is required for the anti-obesity effects of the ligand. *Nat. Med.* **2017**, *23*, 1158–1166. [CrossRef] [PubMed]
22. Mullican, S.E.; Lin-Schmidt, X.; Chin, C.N.; Chavez, J.A.; Furman, J.L.; Armstrong, A.A.; Beck, S.C.; South, V.J.; Dinh, T.Q.; Cash-Mason, T.D.; et al. GFRAL is the receptor for GDF15 and the ligand promotes weight loss in mice and nonhuman primates. *Nat. Med.* **2017**, *23*, 1150–1157. [CrossRef] [PubMed]
23. Hsu, J.Y.; Crawley, S.; Chen, M.; Ayupova, D.A.; Lindhout, D.A.; Higbee, J.; Kutach, A.; Joo, W.; Gao, Z.; Fu, D.; et al. Non-homeostatic body weight regulation through a brainstem-restricted receptor for GDF15. *Nature* **2017**, *550*, 255–259. [CrossRef] [PubMed]
24. Chang, K.C.; Sun, C.; Cameron, E.G.; Madaan, A.; Wu, S.; Xia, X.; Zhang, X.; Tenerelli, K.; Nahmou, M.; Knasel, C.M.; et al. Opposing Effects of Growth and Differentiation Factors in Cell-Fate Specification. *Curr. Biol.* **2019**, *29*, 1963–1975 e5. [CrossRef] [PubMed]
25. Iwata, Y.; Inagaki, S.; Morozumi, W.; Nakamura, S.; Hara, H.; Shimazawa, M. Treatment with GDF15, a TGFbeta superfamily protein, induces protective effect on retinal ganglion cells. *Exp. Eye Res.* **2021**, *202*, 108338. [CrossRef]
26. Lind, L.; Wallentin, L.; Kempf, T.; Tapken, H.; Quint, A.; Lindahl, B.; Olofsson, S.; Venge, P.; Larsson, A.; Hulthe, J.; et al. Growth-differentiation factor-15 is an independent marker of cardiovascular dysfunction and disease in the elderly: Results from the Prospective Investigation of the Vasculature in Uppsala Seniors (PIVUS) Study. *Eur. Heart J.* **2009**, *30*, 2346–2353. [CrossRef]
27. Kalayci, M.; Cetinkaya, E.; Erol, M.K. Prevalence of primary open-angle glaucoma in a Somalia population. *Int. Ophthalmol.* **2021**, *41*, 581–586. [CrossRef]
28. Rahman, M.M.; Rahman, N.; Foster, P.J.; Haque, Z.; Zaman, A.U.; Dineen, B.; Johnson, G.J. The prevalence of glaucoma in Bangladesh: A population based survey in Dhaka division. *Br. J. Ophthalmol.* **2004**, *88*, 1493–1497. [CrossRef]

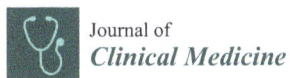

Journal of
Clinical Medicine

Article

360° Ab-Interno Schlemm's Canal Viscodilation with OMNI Viscosurgical Systems for Open-Angle Glaucoma—Midterm Results

Giacomo Toneatto [1], Marco Zeppieri [1,*], Veronica Papa [2], Laura Rizzi [3], Carlo Salati [1], Andrea Gabai [1] and Paolo Brusini [2]

[1] Department of Ophthalmology, University Hospital of Udine, 33100 Udine, Italy; giacomo.toneatto@gmail.com (G.T.); carlo.salati66@gmail.com (C.S.); andrea.gabai@gmail.com (A.G.)
[2] Department of Ophthalmology, Policlinico "Città di Udine", 33100 Udine, Italy; papa.veronica87@gmail.com (V.P.); brusini@libero.it (P.B.)
[3] Department of Economics and Statistics, University of Udine, 33100 Udine, Italy; laura.rizzi@uniud.it
* Correspondence: markzeppieri@hotmail.com; Tel.: +43-255-2743

Citation: Toneatto, G.; Zeppieri, M.; Papa, V.; Rizzi, L.; Salati, C.; Gabai, A.; Brusini, P. 360° Ab-Interno Schlemm's Canal Viscodilation with OMNI Viscosurgical Systems for Open-Angle Glaucoma—Midterm Results. *J. Clin. Med.* **2022**, *11*, 259. https://doi.org/10.3390/jcm11010259

Academic Editor: Stephen Andrew Vernon

Received: 9 November 2021
Accepted: 29 December 2021
Published: 4 January 2022

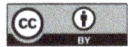
Abstract: Purpose: To evaluate the effectiveness of ab-interno microcatheterization and 360° viscodilation of Schlemm's canal (SC) performed with OMNI viscosurgical system in open angle glaucoma (OAG) together or not with phacoemulsification. Setting: Two surgical sites. Design: Retrospective, observational. Methods: Eighty eyes from 73 patients with mild to moderate OAG underwent ab-interno SC viscodilation performed with OMNI system. Fifty eyes (Group 1) underwent only SC viscodilation, while 30 eyes (Group 2) underwent glaucoma surgery + cataract extraction. Primary success endpoint at 12 months was an intraocular pressure (IOP) reduction higher than 25% from baseline with an absolute value of 18 mmHg or lower, either on the same number or fewer ocular hypotensive medications, without further interventions. Secondary effectiveness endpoints included mean IOP, number of medications and comparison of outcomes between groups. Safety endpoints consisted of best-corrected visual acuity (BCVA), adverse events (AEs), and subsequent surgical procedures. Results: Primary success was achieved in 40.0% and 67.9% in Groups 1 and 2, respectively. Mean IOP at 12-month follow-up showed a significant reduction in both groups (from 23.0 to 15.6 mmHg, $p < 0.001$, and from 21.5 to 14.1, $p < 0.001$, in Groups 1 and 2, respectively). Mean medication number decreased in both groups (from 3.0 to 2.0, $p < 0.001$ and from 3.4 to 1.9, $p < 0.001$, in Groups 1 and 2, respectively). AEs included hyphema (2 eyes), mild hypotony (4 eyes), IOP spikes one month after surgery (1 eye). Twelve eyes (15.0%) required subsequent surgical procedures. No BCVA reduction was observed. Conclusions: Viscodilation of SC using OMNI viscosurgical systems is safe and relatively effective in reducing IOP in adult patients with OAG.

Keywords: open angle glaucoma (OAG); Schlemm's canal viscodilation; OMNI viscosurgical system; minimally invasive glaucoma surgeries (MIGS); trabeculotomy; cataract extraction

1. Introduction

Glaucoma is one of the leading worldwide causes of blindness [1]. The most important risk factor for development and progression of glaucoma is elevated intraocular pressure (IOP) [2]. Important clinical trials such as the Ocular Hypertension Treatment Study (OHTS) and Advanced Glaucoma Intervention Study (AGIS) established the importance of IOP reduction in glaucoma management [3,4]. The first therapeutic option is the use of ocular hypotensive eye drops; however, medical treatment tends to be associated with poor compliance and tolerability [5,6]. When medical treatment proves to be insufficient to reach the target IOP or drops are not well tolerated, laser or surgical treatment need to be considered to avoid irreversible damage progression.

Trabeculectomy, usually with antimetabolites, is still considered the gold standard surgical procedure [7], however, it is not free of potentially serious complications [8,9]. In addition, strict postoperative care is mandatory to obtain clinically successful results. Minimally invasive glaucoma surgeries (MIGS) have been developed as safer and less invasive techniques. MIGS are characterized by an ab-interno approach, minimal trauma and disruption of eye anatomy with conjunctiva sparing, high safety profile, rapid recovery and the possibility of performing the procedure during routine cataract surgery [10].

Ab-interno Schlemm's canal (SC) viscodilation, performed with the OMNI device is a novel MIGS angle surgical procedure. The aim of this study was to evaluate the effectiveness of ab-interno microcatheterization and 360° viscodilation of SC performed with the OMNI viscosurgical system in adult patients with open angle glaucoma (OAG).

2. Materials and Methods

The investigation was based on a double-center, retrospective, observational, consecutive design. All patients underwent surgery with the OMNI viscosurgical system (Sight Sciences Inc., Menlo Park, CA, USA) by 3 ophthalmic surgeons (G.T., C.S., P.B.) from 2 multi-subspecialty ophthalmic departments (University Hospital of Udine and Policlinico "Città di Udine"). All surgeries were performed between March 2017 and January 2020. All adult patients (>18 years old) with mild to moderate (Glaucoma Staging System 2 Stages 1 to 3) [10]. OAG who had undergone ab-interno SC viscodilation were enrolled retrospectively. The types of OAGs considered included primary open angle glaucoma (POAG), pigmentary glaucoma (PG) and pseudoexfoliative glaucoma (XFG). Patients underwent surgery for uncontrolled IOP values on maximally tolerated therapy or to reduce medical therapy due compliance and/or tolerance issues. The ab-interno SC viscodilation surgical procedure was combined with cataract extraction when indicated.

2.1. Main Outcome Measures

Each patient underwent a complete baseline ophthalmologic examination, including ocular history, ophthalmic and systemic medication used, best corrected visual acuity (BCVA) using Snellen charts, IOP measured by Goldmann applanation tonometry, central corneal thickness, gonioscopy, undilated and dilated slit-lamp biomicroscopic examination. Cup disc ratio (CDR), measured by slit-lamp fundus biomicroscopy in relation with disc size, visual field examination using 24-2 SITA Standard test (Humphrey Field Analyzer II; Carl Zeiss Meditec Inc., Dublin, CA, USA), and measurement of macular ganglion cell and retinal nerve fiber layer thickness using optical coherence tomography (OCT RS-3000 Advance; Nidek CO. LTD., 34-14 Maehama, Hiroishi-cho, Gamagori, Aichi 443-0038, JAPAN and DRI-OCT Triton, Topcon, Inc, Tokyo, Japan) were used to evaluate the severity of glaucomatous damage and to determine target pressure before planning glaucoma surgery. Follow-up examinations were performed at Week 1, Week 2, Month 1, Month 3, Month 6, and Month 12. At each follow-up, information regarding IOP, number of antiglaucoma medications, BCVA, postoperative AEs and any other interventions was recorded and used in the analysis.

The study cohort was divided into two groups based on whether or not combined cataract surgery was performed. Group 1 included all eyes that underwent ab interno microcatheterization and viscodilation of SC as a standalone procedure, while Group 2 included all eyes with glaucoma surgery combined with cataract extraction. Our primary success endpoint at the 12-month follow-up visit was defined as a reduction of IOP equal to or greater than 25% from baseline with an absolute value of 18 mmHg or lower, either with the same number of ocular hypotensive medications or fewer, with no additional IOP-lowering surgery. The eyes who reached this endpoint without any medical treatment were considered as complete success, whereas those where this result was obtained using medical treatment were labelled as qualified success. The secondary endpoints included mean IOP and mean number of ocular hypotensive medications at each follow-up time up to 12 months. Outcomes were also compared between groups.

The investigation was performed in accordance with the tenets of the Declaration of Helsinki, and informed consent was obtained from all participants before surgery. The study was in compliance with institutional review boards (IRBs) and HIPAA requirements of the University Hospital of Udine, Italy.

2.2. Statistical Methods

The mean levels of IOP at different follow up times were compared to baseline by means of paired sample *t*-test, which was also used to compare IOP mean reduction at 12 months in Groups 1 and 2. The decrease of medications in each group was analyzed by means of non-parametric Wilcoxon matched-pairs signed rank test. The comparison between Group 1 and 2 on the ordinal variable of the difference between medications at 12 months and at pre-surgery time was performed using Mann–Whitney U test. Descriptive and survival analysis was used to describe proportions of success, which was defined in terms of specific levels of IOP target reached with or without antiglaucoma medications, and to compare failure probabilities in the two groups. BCVA changes at follow-up times were evaluated and compared at group level with parametric *t*-test for paired data.

2.3. Surgical Technique

The surgical technique for ab-interno SC viscodilation as a sole procedure includes the following steps.

After a 1.5 mm paracentesis, pupil miosis was obtained by injecting acetylcholine chloride 1% (Miovisin; Farmigea SPA, Pisa, Italy) into the anterior chamber. Space and stability were achieved by cohesive ophthalmic viscosurgical device (Healon GV; Johnson & Johnson Surgical Vision, Santa Ana, CA, USA). A moderate intraocular pressure was maintained in order to enhance visualization of SC during surgery. The head was tilted and positioned about 40° from the surgeon, while the microscope was tilted 40° towards the surgeon for gonioscopic visualization of the trabecular meshwork.

The OMNI Viscosurgical System (Figure 1a shows the detail of the cannula and the microcatheter) was prepared by removing the retainer pin on the back of the handle and by loading the reservoir with Healon GV (Figure 1b). The cannula was then introduced into the anterior chamber by a 1.5 mm, self-sealing, clear corneal incision performed in the temporal region. The cannula tip was brought near the nasal trabecular meshwork under gonioscopic view (ocular surgical gonioprism for direct viewing gonioscopy, Figure 1c) and used to gently but firmly open the SC. The microcatheter was then advanced into SC for 180° by rotating a finger wheel on the handle of the device (Figure 1d). As the microcatheter was retracted into the cannula, the infusion pump delivered a controlled volume of Healon GV to achieve viscodilation of SC and collectors. The same procedure was then repeated to expand the other 180° of SC.

The surgeon had to be careful to pinch the trabecular meshwork in the right location and to clearly see the blue microcannula into the SC to avoid undesirable suprachoroidal advancement of the tip. Blood reflux indicates a successful catheterization of SC. As the cannula was retracted out the eye, the anterior chamber was irrigated to entirely remove Healon GV.

With regards to ab-interno SC viscodilation combined with cataract surgery, the surgical steps are slightly modified. A 2.2 mm microincision cataract surgery (MICS) was performed with the Constellation Vision System (Alcon Laboratories, Fort Worth, TX, USA). All IOLs were implanted in the capsular bag, which were all hydrophobic, acrylic and monofocal. Acetylcholine chloride 1% (Miovisin; Farmigea SPA, Pisa, Italy) was then injected into the anterior chamber to obtain pupil miosis. Viscodilation of SC was achieved with the method previously described.

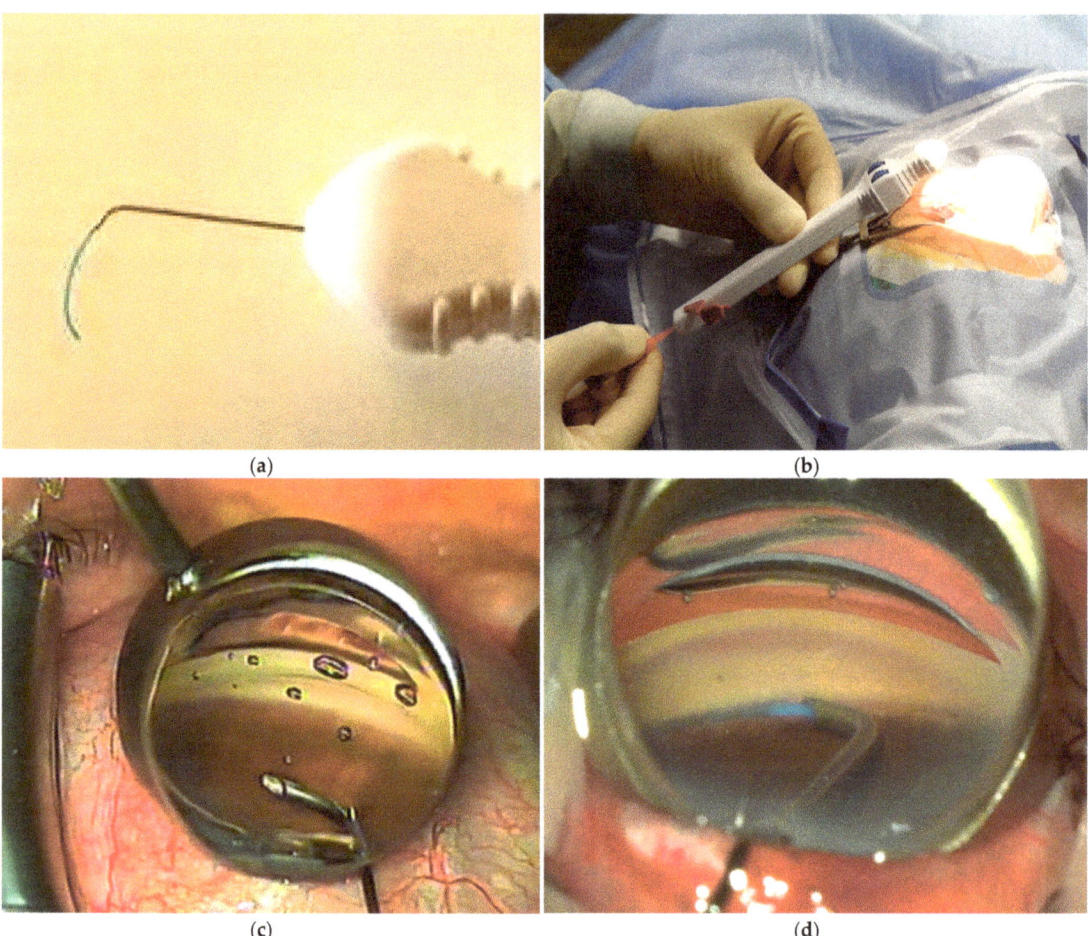

Figure 1. The OMNI device ends with a cannula and microcatheter at the tip (**a**). The preparation of the device includes loading the reservoir with high-molecular weight hyaluronic acid (**b**). The cannula is inserted into the anterior chamber under gonioscopic view to reach the nasal trabecular meshwork (**c**). The procedure involves the opening of trabecular meshwork and advancement of the microcatheter in Schlemm's canal (**d**).

3. Results

The study cohort consisted of 80 eyes of 73 patients that met the inclusion criteria and completed the baseline evaluation, with 66 eyes (82%) completing the 12-month visit. Of the remaining 14 eyes, 12 (15%) had additional glaucoma surgery and 2 (2.5%) were lost to follow-up. The patients were divided into two groups according to the type of surgery performed: Group 1 (SC viscodilation alone) consisted of 50 eyes (62.5%) while Group 2 (SC viscodilation combined with phaco) included 30 eyes (37.5%). Table 1 shows the baseline characteristics. The patients were predominantly female, with the majority diagnosed with POAG (63.8%). The most common previous anti-glaucoma procedure was laser trabeculoplasty (19%). Thirteen patients (16.2%) had previous glaucoma surgery (10 cases underwent deep sclerectomy, and three cases had trabeculectomy) that did not interfere with the complete catheterization of Schlemm's canal. Forty-four eyes (55%) were pseudophakic at baseline. Of the remaining 36 eyes, 30 of them (83%) had combined cataract extraction with IOL implantation. Successful circumferential catheterization of the canal was achieved in all eyes and no significant adverse events were recorded intraoperatively, other than small bleeding from the SC.

Table 1. Demographic and baseline characteristics.

	All Eyes	Group 1 (SC Viscodilation)	Group 2 (SC Vscd + Phaco)	Test on Differences (Statistical Significance)
Eyes, *n*	80	50	30	
Patients, *n*	73	47	26	
Age in years				
Mean Age ± SD (years)	74.5 ± 7.5	74.2 ± 8.0	75.0 ± 6.6	t test (*p* = 0.32)
Age Range (years)	56–93	56–93	62–89	
Gender, *n* (%)				
Female	43 (58.9)	26 (55.3)	17 (65.4)	Chi² test on gender
Male	30 (41.1)	21 (44.7)	9 (34.6)	distribution (*p* = 0.35)
Preoperative IOP, mean ± SD	22.5 ± 5.3	23.0 ± 5.7	21.5 ± 4.7	t test (*p* = 0.11)
Preoperative medications, mean n ± SD	3.2 ± 1.0	3.0 ± 1.1	3.4 ± 0.8	t test (*p* = 0.03)
Preoperative BCVA, mean ± SD	7.5 ± 2.5	7.9 ± 2.4	6.8 ± 2.1	t test (*p* = 0.02)
Glaucoma diagnosis, *n* (%)				
Primary open angle glaucoma	51 (63.8)	37 (74.0)	14 (46.7)	Chi² test (*p* = 0.01)
Pseudoexfoliative glaucoma	27 (33.7)	12 (24.0)	15 (50.0)	Chi² test (*p* = 0.01)
Pigmentary dispersion glaucoma	2 (2.5)	1 (2.0)	1 (3.3)	Chi² test (*p* = 0.71)
Baseline lens status, *n* (%)				
Pseudophakic	44 (55.0)	44 (88.0)	0 (0)	Chi² test (*p* = 0.00)
Phakic	36 (45.0)	6 (12.0)	30 (100)	Chi² test (*p* = 0.00)
Previous surgery, *n* (%)	-	-	-	
Cataract	44 (55.0)	44 (88.0)	0 (0.0)	Chi² test (*p* = 0.00)
Laser trabeculoplasty	15 (18.8)	10 (20.0)	5 (16.7)	Chi² test (*p* = 0.71)
Deep sclerectomy	10 (12.5)	10 (20.0)	0 (0.0)	Chi² test (*p* = 0.01)
Trabeculectomy	3 (3.8)	3 (6.0)	0 (0.0)	Chi² test (*p* = 0.01)

SC = Schlemm's canal; SD = standard deviation; IOP = intraocular pressure; BCVA = best corrected visual acuity.

3.1. Differences in Intraocular Pressure and Antiglaucoma Medication Used

Table 2 shows the differences in intraocular pressure and antiglaucoma medications used at the different time points overall and in the two groups. Mean IOP values at baseline were 22.5 ± 5.3 mmHg for all eyes, and 23.0 ± 5.7 mmHg and 21.5 ± 4.7 mmHg in Group 1 and 2, respectively. After 12 months, mean IOP reduced to 15.0 ± 3.6 mmHg, 15.6 ± 3.6 mmHg, and 14.1 ± 3.3 mmHg, respectively. IOP reduction was statistically significant in both groups at 1, 3, 6 and 12 months ($p < 0.001$). The difference between mean IOP reduction in Groups 1 and 2, however, was not statistically significant at 12 months ($p = 0.21$). Figure 2A reports the box plots of IOP distributions at different follow up times in all the patients and in the two groups.

The mean number of medications at baseline was 3.0 ± 1.1 and 3.4 ± 0.8 in Group 1 and 2, respectively, and decreased at 12 months to 2.0 ± 1.4 and 1.9 ± 1.4, respectively (Figure 2B). Wilcoxon matched pairs signed rank test showed statistically significant reductions in all the groups and at all time points ($p < 0.001$). The reduction of medications at 12 months between the two groups was not significantly different ($p = 0.26$).

Table 2. Differences in intraocular pressure and antiglaucoma medications.

		BL	7 Days	15 Days	1 Month	3 Months	6 Months	12 Months
All eyes	Eyes, *n*	80	80	79	77	70	68	66
	Mean IOP, mmHg ± SD	22.5 ± 5.3	17.8 ± 7.5	20.5 ± 8.4	17.8 ± 5.5	15.6 ± 4.0	15.3 ± 4.6	15.0 ± 3.6
	Mean IOP reduction from BL, mmHg (%)		4.7 (18%)	1.8 (5.3%)	4.5 (16.6%)	6.5 (26.9%)	6.8 (28.4%)	6.9 (29.0%)
	p-Value		(*p* < 0.001)	(*p* = 0.035)	*p* < 0.001	*p* < 0.001	*p* < 0.001	*p* < 0.001
	Mean MEDs, *n* ± SD	3.2 ± 1.0	0.7 ± 1.2	0.9 ± 1.3	1.3 ± 1.4	1.6 ± 1.4	1.7 ± 1.4	1.9 ± 1.4
	Mean MEDs reduction from BL, *n* (*p*-Value)		2.5 (*p* < 0.001)	2.2 (*p* < 0.001)	1.8 (*p* < 0.001)	1.6 (*p* < 0.001)	1.5 (*p* < 0.001)	1.2 (*p* < 0.001)
Group 1	Eyes, *n*	50	50	49	47	43	42	40
	Mean IOP, mmHg ± SD	23.0 ± 5.7	17.8 ± 7.9	21.1 ± 9.5	18.6 ± 6.0	16.4 ± 4.4	15.8 ± 5.1	15.6 ± 3.6
	Mean IOP reduction from BL, mmHg (%)		5.2 (20.3%)	1.6 (4.6%)	4.2 (15.1%)	5.9 (23.8%)	6.5 (27.0%)	6.5 (26.8%)
	p-Value		*p* < 0.001	*p* = 0.12	*p* < 0.001	*p* < 0.001	*p* < 0.001	*p* < 0.001
	Mean MEDs, *n* ± SD	3.0 ± 1.1	0.7 ± 1.2	0.9 ± 1.2	1.3 ± 1.4	1.6 ± 1.4	1.7 ± 1.4	2.0 ± 1.4
	Mean MEDs reduction from BL, *n* (*p*-Value)		2.3 (*p* < 0.001)	2.1 (*p* < 0.001)	1.7 (*p* < 0.001)	1.4 (*p* < 0.001)	1.2 (*p* < 0.001)	1.0 (*p* < 0.001)
Group 2	Eyes, *n*	30	30	30	30	27	26	26
	Mean IOP, mmHg ± SD	21.5 ± 4.7	17.6 ± 7.1	19.4 ± 6.3	16.6 ± 4.5	14.4 ± 2.9	14.5 ± 3.7	14.1 ± 3.3
	Mean IOP reduction from BL, mmHg (%)		3.9 (14.3%)	2.1 (6.2%)	4.9 (19.1%)	7.4 (30.7%)	7.2 (30.3%)	7.6 (32.4%)
	p-Value		*p* = 0.007	*p* < 0.069	*p* < 0.001	*p* < 0.001	*p* < 0.001	*p* < 0.001
	Mean MEDs, *n* ± SD	3.4 ± 0.8	0.7 ± 1.1	1.0 ± 1.4	1.3 ± 1.3	1.6 ± 1.4	1.7 ± 1.3	1.9 ± 1.4
	Mean MEDs reduction from BL, *n* (*p*-Value)		2.8 (*p* < 0.001)	2.5 (*p* < 0.001)	2.1 (*p* < 0.001)	1.9 (*p* < 0.001)	1.8 (*p* < 0.001)	1.6 (*p* < 0.001)

IOP = intraocular pressure; SD = standard deviation; BL = baseline; MEDs = medications.

3.2. Success

Table 3 reports the proportions of complete and qualified success with different levels of IOP target at 12 months over the entire cohort and for Groups 1 and 2. The success was defined as complete if a specific IOP level was reached without antiglaucoma medications, and as qualified, if target IOP was achieved using medications. The IOP endpoints chosen to stratify success results were <16, <18 and <21 mmHg. Moreover, outcomes were more strictly sorted by a 25% reduction in IOP from the baseline value. At 12 months of follow-up, 14.0% of Group 1 eyes reached an IOP of 18 mmHg or lower with no medications and 66.0% achieved success either by the use or without medications. In Group 2, 17.9% of eyes reached an IOP of 18 mmHg or lower with surgery alone and 82.1% achieved a qualified success. Overall, 15.4% of eyes attained an IOP of 18 mmHg or lower with no medications and 71.8% achieved a qualified success.

Considering an additional reduction of IOP higher than 25% to estimate our primary success endpoint, 40.0% and 67.9% of eyes reached an IOP of 18 mmHg or lower with or without medications in Group 1 and in Group 2, respectively.

Figure 3 shows the observations on the preoperative IOP values (horizontal axis) and the postoperative ones (vertical axis). The horizontal lines represent the different IOP endpoints (21, 18 and 16 mmHg), while diagonal lines define null and 25% reduction level of IOP from baseline.

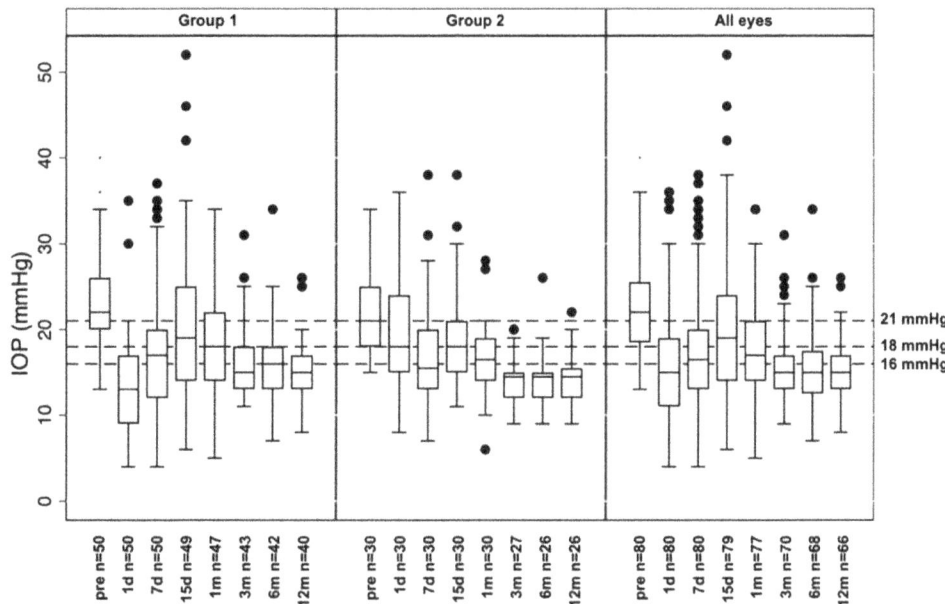

(**A**)

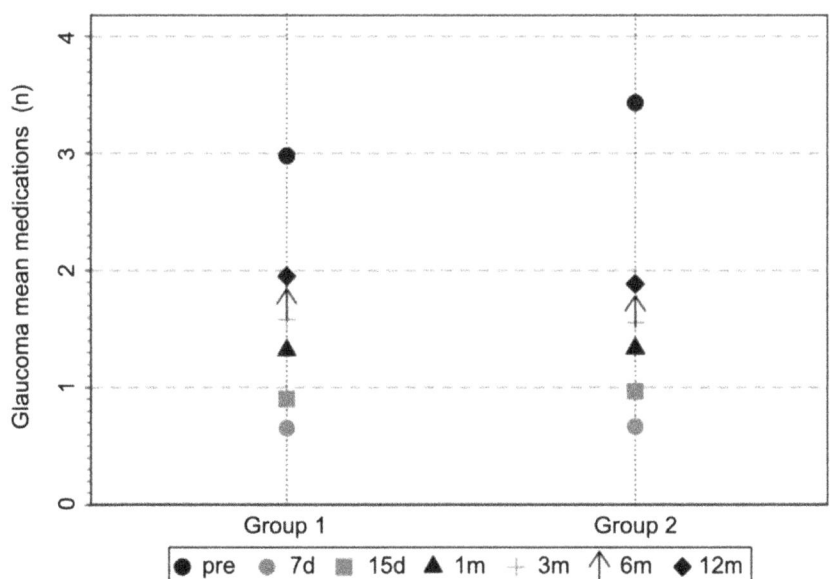

(**B**)

Figure 2. Boxplot of IOP distributions at baseline and at each follow-up visit for Groups 1 and 2 and for all the cohort ((**A**), above). Mean medications at the baseline and at each follow-up visit in Groups 1 and 2 ((**B**), below).

Table 3. Success rates overall and in the groups at 12 months.

		Success Rate (%) at 12 Months		
		All Included Eyes	Group 1	Group 2
≤16 mmHg	Complete	14.1	14.0	14.3
	Qualified	58.9	48.0	78.8
≤18 mmHg	Complete	15.4	14.0	17.9
	Qualified	71.8	66.0	82.1
≤21 mmHg	Complete	17.9	18.0	17.9
	Qualified	80.8	76.0	89.3
≤16 mmHg and ≥25% IOP reduction	Complete	10.3	10.0	10.7
	Qualified	43.6	32.0	64.3
≤18 mmHg and ≥25% IOP reduction	Complete	11.5	10.0	14.0
	Qualified	50.0	40.0	67.9

IOP = intraocular pressure.

Figure 4 reports the Kaplan–Meier survival plots for probability of qualified success in Group 1 and Group 2, using the failure criterion of an IOP value higher than 18 mmHg in three subsequent visits. Log-rank Chi-squared test suggested the acceptance of the hypothesis on the equality of survivor estimates in the two groups ($p = 0.28$).

3.3. Safety

After twelve months of follow up, no significant change in BCVA was observed in Group 1 (from $7.9/10 \pm 2.4$ to $7.7/10 \pm 2.9$, $p = 0.31$). A BCVA gain, after 12 months, resulted statistically significant only in Group 2 (from $6.8/10 \pm 2.1$ to $9.1/10 \pm 2.6$, $p < 0.001$), due to the combination of SC viscodilation with phaco.

Most complications were recorded in the first follow-up week. During the surgical procedure, a mild blood reflux in AC was considered a sign of successful catheterization of SC, occurring in almost 100% of our patients. Cases of micro or mild hyphema on the first postoperative day, defined respectively as circulating red blood cells without a blood level, and as blood layer filling less than 1 mm in the anterior chamber, were not considered as AEs, given the physiological and self-limiting nature of these occurrences. Two eyes (2.5%) developed moderate and severe hyphema and were reported as AEs. The first one showed a 3 mm layer of blood combined with peaks of high IOP 2 days after surgery. The second case reported a sustained hyphema filling more than half of the AC associated with BCVA reduction to hand motion without a rise of IOP. Both cases required a wash of the AC, three and ten days after surgery respectively, with complete recovery.

Four eyes (5.0%) had mild hypotony (4–5 mmHg) within the first month postoperatively. No shallow anterior chamber or choroidal detachment were detected. All cases resolved without any intervention. One eye (1.3%) reached an IOP level >10 mmHg above baseline more than 30 days postoperatively.

Twelve subjects (15.0%) required a secondary intervention due to an unreached IOP target level: trabeculectomy in nine cases (75%), and deep sclerectomy in three cases (25%). The mean IOP and number of medications before these surgical procedures were 26.3 ± 6.5 mmHg and 2.8 ± 1.3, respectively. One phakic eye needed cataract extraction 6 months after surgery. Three eyes developed complications unrelated to glaucoma surgery within 6 and 12 months: hypertensive anterior uveitis successfully treated with topical steroid (one eye), active choroidal neovascularization due to age-related macular degeneration (one eye), posterior capsular opacity needing Nd:YAG laser capsulotomy (one eye).

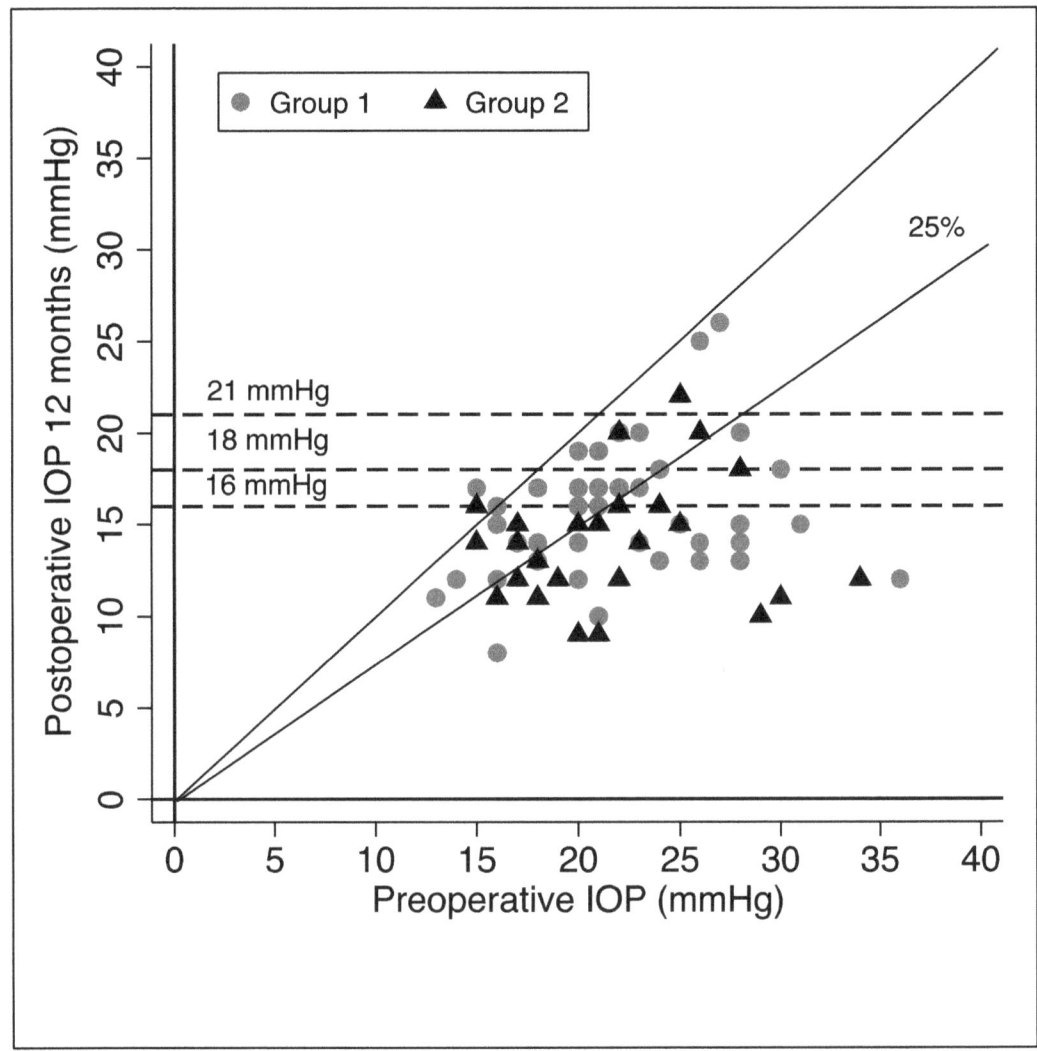

Figure 3. Scatter plot of observations on the pre- and 12-month postoperative IOP values, different IOP endpoints values (horizontal lines) and null or 25% reduction from baseline IOP diagonal lines.

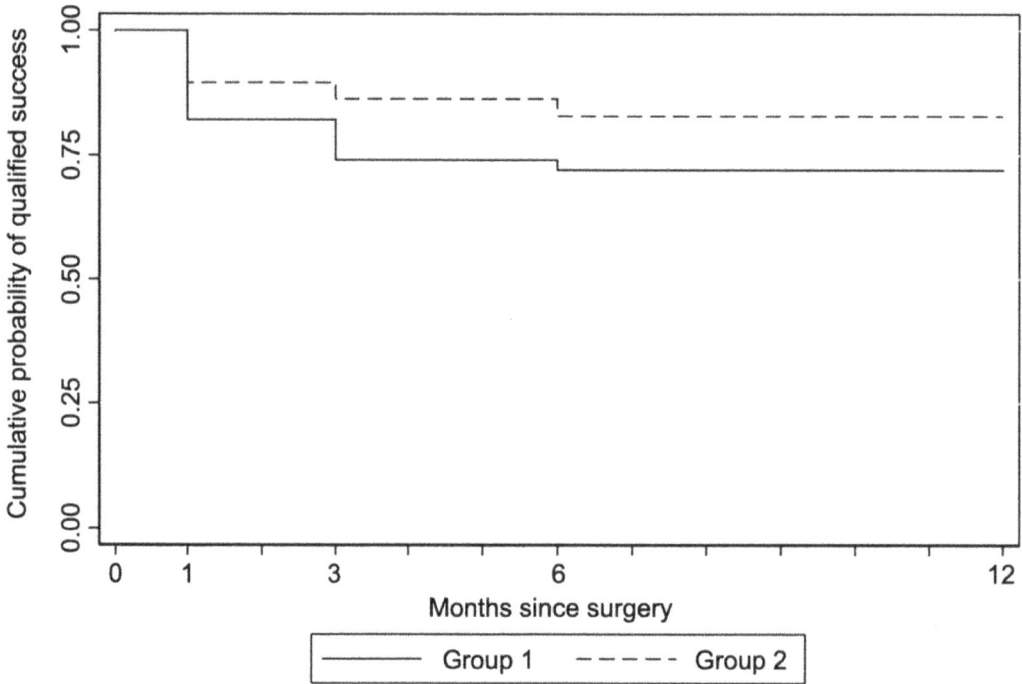

Figure 4. Kaplan–Meier survival estimates for Groups 1 and 2 (failure IOP > 18 mmHg at 3 consecutive follow up visits).

4. Discussion

Trabeculectomy has been the gold standard in glaucoma surgery since 1968 [11]. Although this procedure continues to have a significant role due to the capacity to achieve long-standing significant IOP lowering, non-penetrating filtering surgeries (NPFS) have been proposed to achieve IOP reduction avoiding serious sight threatening complications such as shallow anterior chamber, uncontrolled hypotension, choroidal detachment and macular folds. Outflow resistance can be attributed to three structures: the juxtacanalicular meshwork, SC and collector channels [12]. Non penetrating filtering surgery (NPFS) such as canoloplasty, include techniques focused on the dilation of SC to facilitate aqueous outflow through the physiological route. The aim is to remove mechanical obstructions in the collector channels, by enhancing and providing additional routes for aqueous outflow. Viscodilation separates the trabecular lamellae and creates microperforations within the inner wall of SC, allowing for enhanced diffusion of aqueous through the proximal system into the distal system and thereby countering the pathological changes seen in glaucoma [13].

Preliminary procedures focusing on SC were historically sinusotomy described by Kraznov in 1962, followed by Stegmann's viscocanalostomy [14,15]. Ab externo canaloplasty (ABeC), proposed by Lewis and coworkers in 2007, is a surgical technique that uses a microcatheter to perform a 360° cannulation of SC positioning a tension suture within the canal that provides an inward distension [16]. The aim of this technique is to restore the physiological outflow pathways of the aqueous humor independently of external wound healing. Numerous studies have shown that canaloplasty is a relatively safe and effective surgical technique that lowers IOP with persistent control of pressure during many years of follow-up. Moreover, it implies easier postoperative management and less complications compared with trabeculectomy [17–19].

In the past several years, there has been a gain in popularity of MIGS to address the need of achieving long-term IOP control in the safest possible way. MIGS is characterized by an ab-interno approach, inducing minimal trauma and disruption of eye anatomy with conjunctiva sparing and a rapid recovery [10]. With the advent of MIGS, surgeons have been choosing to perform earlier surgery in patients with mild to moderate glaucoma in order to achieve the target IOP with fewer medications [20].

A minimally invasive technique, called ab-interno canaloplasty (ABiC), has recently been developed to reap the advantages of ABeC, avoiding conjunctival and scleral dissection [21]. Considering that ABeC and ABiC tend to have a rather long and steep learning curve, OMNI viscosurgical system has been refined to allow an easier cannulation of SC and a more standardized viscodilation of outflow pathways. Moreover, ABeC is not always successful in providing a 360° catheterization of SC and failure rates range from 10.1 to 26% [22], which can be due to anatomical anomalies of SC, trabecular meshwork scars, neovascularization of iridocorneal angle, but also lack of surgical experience. In our study, 100% of complete catheterization of SC was achieved due to a good preliminary gonioscopic evaluation of angle structures and to "surgeon friendly" characteristics of the device.

Both ABeC and ABiC utilize an illuminated microcatheter to access, catheterize, and viscodilate the proximal and distal outflow system. The OMNI viscosurgical system is a single-handed device, equipped with a metallic cannula that encases a microcatheter, control wheel for advancing and retracting microcatheter, viscoelastic reservoir/infusion pump and a locking mechanism. These devices facilitate automatic delivery of a predetermined amount of viscoelastic fluid to dilate 360° of SC. Although OMNI has been designed to perform, when desired, a secondary trabeculotomy in addition to viscodilation of SC to treat juxtacanalicular meshwork resistances, we used the device only to viscodilate without unroofing the SC.

Our primary success endpoint at 12-month follow-up visit was defined as the proportion of eyes achieving an IOP value equal or under 18 mmHg with a reduction higher than 25% from baseline, either on the same number or fewer ocular hypotensive medications, and with no additional IOP-lowering surgery or laser. This choice was based on the baseline characteristics of our cohort of patients, including only mild to moderate open angle glaucomas, in which intraocular pressure of 18 mmHg or below was an acceptable criterion for controlling progression. The proportions of success defined with the endpoints of 16 and 21 mmHg, with an IOP reduction higher than 25% from baseline, were also analyzed.

In our study, 40% and 67.9% of eyes reached the primary endpoint at 12 months in Group 1 and Group 2 respectively. These results appeared to be worse than the outcomes of ABeC as a standalone procedure (68.1%) and combined with phaco (77.8%) [17], probably because of the presence of the suture that provides a more durable distension of SC.

In our cohort, the mean IOP reduction at 12 months compared to baseline was of 26.8% in Group 1 (from 23.0 ± 5.7 mmHg to 15.6 ± 3.6 mmHg) and 32.4% in Group 2 (from 21.5 ± 4.7 to 14.1 ± 3.3). The IOP reduction was statistically significant in both groups during the entire follow-up. The difference in IOP reduction at 12 months in Group 2, compared with Group 1, was not statistically significant. The overall reduction in IOP in the entire cohort was 29.0% at 12 months (from 22.5 ± 5.3 mmHg to 15.0 ± 3.6 mmHg). Similar IOP changes have been described for ABeC [17,18] and ABiC [21,23–25] in previous studies. Brusini [19] reported a more favorable reduction in IOP from 29.4 ± 7.9 preoperatively to 16.8 ± 4.2 mmHg at 12 months probably due to the higher IOP level at baseline compared with the other studies.

Our surgical goal was decreasing IOP and/or reducing glaucoma drops. The mean number of medications at 12 months decreased from 3.0 ± 1.1 to 2.0 ± 1.4, in Group 1, and from 3.4 ± 0.8 to 1.9 ± 1.4, in Group 2, and was statistically significant in all groups at all time points. Compared with other clinical studies, our patients tended to be on a higher number of medications before surgery. The mean reduction of antiglaucoma drops of 1.0 and 1.6 respectively for Group 1 and Group 2 after 12 months was similar to ABeC and ABiC [17,18,23].

The results showed that surgery provided effective IOP control and reduction, with few AEs. Self-limiting microhyphema was frequently observed due to the physiological blood reflux from SC, thus not considered as an AE. Only clinically significant hyphemas (i.e., layered and >1 mm and persisting for 1 week or more) were recorded as AEs in this study. One eye reported a 3 mm hyphema associated with an important postoperative IOP elevation, while another case presented with a blood level filling more than half of AC associated with an important decrease of visual acuity. These two eyes (2.5%) underwent a washout of the anterior chamber three and ten days after surgery, respectively, without further postoperative sight threatening complications. These AEs occurred even if the surgeons carefully screened for and avoided patients from taking anticoagulant therapy during the perioperative period, whenever possible, and were careful in maintaining an adequate pressure of the globe at the end of the procedure. Ondrejka et al. [26] reported a 2.8% rate of hyphema between 1 and 3 mm that spontaneously resolved within 7 days, which was similar to the 2.5% rate reported in our results. Vold et al. [27] reported a slightly greater incidence of postoperative clinically significant hyphema >1 mm (4%), in addition to Sarkisian et al. [28] (4.9% of moderate and severe hyphema) and Grabska-Liberek et al. [29] (35%, of which half required AC washout on the first postoperative day due to marked IOP elevation). The higher rate of hyphema could be due to the fact that the surgeons used the OMNI system to perform canaloplasty combined with trabeculotomy. The rates of hyphema for the ABiC procedure reported in literature ranges from 0% to 20% [21,23–25]. The higher rate of 20% was found in the study by Kazerounian [25], which refers to mild hyphema cases with no late sequelae.

In our study, four eyes developed mild postoperative hypotony (IOP 4–5 mmHg) within the first month but resolved without any intervention. No shallow anterior chamber or choroidal detachment were detected. IOP had major fluctuations within the first 30 days postoperative because of antiglaucoma drops discontinuation after surgery and the use of steroids during the first weeks. The incidence of IOP spikes was low after the first month of follow-up with only one eye (1.3%) reaching an IOP > 10 mmHg from baseline at 1 month. The use of the OMNI did not affect visual acuity.

The statistical analysis showed differences between groups at baseline. The mean preoperative BCVA in Group 2 was clearly lower compared to Group 1 due to the fact that Group 2 included only phakic eyes that were scheduled to perform cataract extraction combined to glaucoma surgery, in comparison with the predominately higher number of pseudophakic eyes in the other group. Patients in Group 2 showed a higher number of preoperative medications prior to surgery, however, the reduction of medications at 12 months between the two groups was not significantly different. In Group 1, a total of 10 and 3 eyes underwent previous deep sclerectomy and trabeculectomy respectively, while in Group 2, all eyes were naïve to prior surgery. The previous surgeries did not tend to interfere with the cannulation and viscodilation of SC using the OMNI system. With regards to deep sclerectomy, 4 of 10 eyes reached the primary endpoint at the 12-month follow-up visit, achieving an IOP value less than or equal to 18 mmHg and a reduction higher than 25% from baseline. This value was the same when compared with the results of the entire Group 1. This could probably be due to the fact that deep sclerectomy surgery tends to leave the trabecular meshwork undamaged, thus permitting a good dilation of SC and collectors by viscoelastic pressure during the OMNI system procedure. Due to the limited number of eyes in our cohort, it is difficult to establish the role of previous trabeculectomy when performing the OMNI procedure. Only one eye of three reached the primary success endpoint at 12 months.

Although there are a wide number of studies on ABeC and ABiC, literature is poor regarding outcomes of viscodilation of SC performed with OMNI system without trabeculotomy. Our results are similar to those reported for traditional ABeC and ABiC procedures. Viscodilation combined with trabeculotomy using OMNI viscosurgical system is considered an interesting option by some surgeons probably due to the possibility of treating the juxtacanalicular meshwork resistances as well as to enhance the outflow across SC and collectors [27–30]. Albeit with a similar effectiveness in IOP control and reduction, trabeculotomy seems to result in more AEs in terms of hyphema.

The OMNI system has several advantages compared to other MIGS procedures, which include: (1) unlike XENgel, it is not a filtering procedure, thus it is not mandatory that the conjunctiva is in good condition to obtain a filtering bleb; (2) it is easier to perform when compared to other similar techniques, such as ab-interno canaloplasty (ABiC); (3) it is more respectful of trabecular structures in comparison with trabectome or gonioscopy assisted transluminal trabeculotomy (GATT), which extensively open Schlemm's canal and trabecular meshwork; and, (4) it could theoretically be more effective than i-Stent, however, studies have not been performed to date that compare these two techniques.

The OMNI system, however, has some disadvantages which include: (1) the difficulty to correctly find Schlemm's canal in eyes with little or no pigment in the trabecular meshwork; (2) the impossibility to follow the microcatheter for the entire canal path, which can travel quite a distance far from the entrance; and (3) the possible bleeding into the anterior chamber, which seldom occurs.

The limitations of this study include the retrospective nature of collected data, the relatively low number of subjects included, the short follow-up period, and the enrollment of both eyes of the same patient in some cases. Furthermore, not all eyes were naïve to prior surgery: thirteen had already underwent previous major glaucoma surgery (trabeculectomy and deep sclerectomy). This choice was based on previous studies which have shown that canaloplasty can also be successfully performed in patients with failed trabeculectomy in which SC has been left mostly undamaged from previous filtering surgeries [31,32]. There was no standardized protocol for reducing or increasing medications, but the medical therapy was adjusted to reach the target IOP on a case-by-case basis. Follow-up was limited to 1 year. Due to the limited number of patients included in our cohort, it was difficult to assess the role and influence of glaucoma types on surgery between the groups. Future prospective studies are currently underway to help address this issue. Longer-term studies on a larger group of prospectively enrolled patients are needed to assess the duration of IOP reduction with this surgical technique.

In conclusion, viscodilation of SC using OMNI viscosurgical system, with or without cataract extraction, appears to be a promising surgical procedure to effectively control and reduce IOP with a highly safer profile, even if a high percentage of eyes require a medical treatment. Further studies are needed to report long-term results and complications, and to assess the real advantage of an associated trabeculotomy.

Author Contributions: Conceptualization, G.T., C.S. and P.B.; methodology, G.T., C.S. and P.B.; validation, G.T., C.S. and P.B.; formal analysis, G.T., M.Z., L.R., C.S. and P.B.; investigation, G.T., M.Z., V.P., L.R., C.S., A.G. and P.B.; resources, C.S. and P.B.; writing—original draft preparation, G.T.; writing—review and editing, G.T., M.Z. and P.B.; visualization, G.T., M.Z., L.R., C.S. and P.B.; supervision, C.S. and P.B.; project administration, C.S. and P.B.; All authors have read and agreed to the published version of the manuscript.

Funding: This research received no external funding.

Institutional Review Board Statement: The study was conducted in accordance with the Declaration of Helsinki, and approved by the local Institutional Review Boards and Ethics Committee (considering standardized surgical practices already in routine use).

Informed Consent Statement: Informed consent was obtained from all subjects involved in the study.

Conflicts of Interest: The authors declare no conflict of interest.

References

1. Quigley, H.A.; Broman, A.T. The number of people with glaucoma worldwide in 2010 and 2020. *Br. J. Ophthalmol.* **2006**, *90*, 262–267. [CrossRef] [PubMed]
2. Kim, J.H.; Rabiolo, A.; Morales, E.; Yu, F.; Afifi, A.A.; Nouri-Mahdavi, K.; Caprioli, J. Risk factors for fast visual field progression in glaucoma. *Am. J. Ophthalmol.* **2019**, *207*, 268–278. [CrossRef] [PubMed]

3. Kass, M.A.; Heuer, D.K.; Higginbotham, E.J.; Johnson, C.A.; Keltner, J.L.; Miller, J.P.; Parrish, R.K., II; Wilson, M.R.; Gordon, M.O. The Ocular Hypertension Treatment Study: A randomized trial determines that topical ocular hypotensive medication delays or prevents the onset of primary open-angle glaucoma. *Arch. Ophthalmol.* **2002**, *120*, 701–713. [CrossRef]
4. The Advanced Glaucoma Intervention study (AGIS): 7. the relationship between control of intraocular pressure and visual field deterioration. *Am. J. Ophthalmol.* **2000**, *130*, 429–440. [CrossRef]
5. Newman-Casey, P.A.; Robin, A.L.; Blachley, T.; Farris, K.; Heisler, M.; Resnicow, K.; Lee, P.P. The Most Common Barriers to Glaucoma Medication Adherence: A Cross-Sectional Survey. *Ophthalmology* **2015**, *122*, 1308–1316. [CrossRef] [PubMed]
6. Dreer, L.E.; Girkin, C.; Mansberger, S.L. Determinants of medication adherence to topical glaucoma therapy. *J. Glaucoma* **2012**, *21*, 234–240. [CrossRef]
7. Gedde, S.J.; Singh, K.; Schiffman, J.C.; Feuer, W.J. Tube versus Trabeculectomy Study Group. The Tube Versus Trabeculectomy Study: Interpretation of results and application to clinical practice. *Curr. Opin. Ophthalmol.* **2012**, *23*, 118–126. [CrossRef]
8. Gedde, S.J.; Herndon, L.W.; Brandt, J.D.; Budenz, D.L.; Feuer, W.J.; Schiffman, J.C. Surgical complications in the tube versus trabeculectomy study during the first year of follow-up. *Am. J. Ophthalmol.* **2007**, *143*, 23–31. [CrossRef]
9. Saheb, H.; Ahmed, I.I. Micro-invasive glaucoma surgery: Current perspectives and future directions. *Curr. Opin. Ophthalmol.* **2012**, *23*, 96–104. [CrossRef] [PubMed]
10. Brusini, P.; Filacorda, S. Enhanced glaucoma staging system (GSS 2) for classifying functional damage in glaucoma. *J. Glaucoma* **2006**, *15*, 40–46. [CrossRef]
11. Klink, T.; Sauer, J.; Körber, N.J.; Grehn, F.; Much, M.M.; Thederan, L.; Matlach, J.; Salgado, J.P. Quality of life following glaucoma surgery: Canaloplasty versus trabeculectomy. *Clin. Ophthalmol.* **2015**, *9*, 7–16. [PubMed]
12. Battista, S.A.; Lu, Z.; Hofmann, S.; Freddo, T.; Overby, D.R.; Gong, H. Reduction of the available area for aqueous humor outflow and increase in meshwork herniations into collector channels following acute IOP elevation in bovine eyes. *Investig. Ophthalmol. Vis. Sci.* **2008**, *49*, 5346–5352. [CrossRef] [PubMed]
13. Grieshaber, M.C.; Pienaar, A.; Olivier, J.; Stegmann, R. Comparing two tensioning suture sizes for 360 degrees viscocanalostomy (canaloplasty): A randomised controlled trial. *Eye* **2010**, *24*, 1220–1226. [CrossRef]
14. Krasnov, M.M. Sinusotomy. *Trans. Am. Acad. Ophthalmol. Otolaryngol.* **1972**, *76*, 368–374.
15. Stegmann, R.; Pienaar, A.; Miller, D. Viscocanalostomy for open-angle glaucoma in Black African patients. *J. Cataract Refract. Surg.* **1999**, *25*, 316–322. [CrossRef]
16. Lewis, R.A.; von Wolff, K.; Tetz, M.; Korber, N.; Kearney, J.R.; Shingleton, B.; Samuelson, T.W. Canaloplasty: Circumferential viscodilation and tensioning of Schlemm's canal using a flexible microcatheter for the treatment of open-angle glaucoma in adults. Interim clinical study analysis. *J. Catataract Refract. Surg.* **2007**, *33*, 1217–1226. [CrossRef] [PubMed]
17. Lewis, R.A.; von Wolff, K.; Tetz, M.; Koerber, N.; Kearney, J.R.; Shingleton, B.J.; Samuelson, T.W. Canaloplasty: Three-year results of circumferential viscodilation and tensioning of Schlemm canal using a microcatheter to treat open-angle glaucoma. *J. Cataract Refract. Surg.* **2011**, *37*, 682–690. [CrossRef]
18. Bull, H.; von Wolff, K.; Körber, N.; Tetz, M. Three-year canaloplasty outcomes for the treatment of open-angle glaucoma: European study results. *Graefes Arch. Clin. Exp. Ophthalmol.* **2011**, *245*, 1537–1545. [CrossRef]
19. Brusini, P. Canaloplasty in open-angle glaucoma surgery: A four-year follow-up. *Sci. World J.* **2014**, *2014*, 469609. [CrossRef]
20. Kerr, N.M.; Wang, J.; Barton, K. Minimally invasive glaucoma surgery as primary stand-alone surgery for glaucoma. *Clin. Exp. Ophthalmol.* **2017**, *45*, 393–400. [CrossRef]
21. Davids, A.M.; Pahlitzsch, M.; Boeker, A.; Winterhalter, S.; Maier-Wenzel, A.K.; Klamann, M. Ab interno canaloplasty (ABiC)—12-month results of a new minimally invasive glaucoma surgery (MIGS). *Graefes Arch. Clin. Exp. Ophthalmol.* **2019**, *257*, 1947–1953. [CrossRef]
22. Cagini, C.; Peruzzi, C.; Fiore, T.; Spadea, L.; Lippera, M.; Lippera, S. Canaloplasty: Current value in the management of glaucoma. *J. Ophthalmol.* **2016**, *2016*, 7080475. [CrossRef]
23. Hughes, T.; Traynor, M. Clinical results of ab interno canaloplasty in patients with open-angle glaucoma. *Clin. Ophthalmol.* **2020**, *14*, 3641–3650. [PubMed]
24. Körber, N. Ab interno canaloplasty for the treatment of glaucoma: A case series study. *Spektrum Augenheilkd* **2018**, *32*, 223–227. [CrossRef]
25. Kazerounian, S.; Zimbelmann, M.; Lörtscher, M.; Hommayda, S.; Tsirkinidou, I.; Müller, M. Canaloplasty ab interno (AbiC)—2-Year-Results of a Novel Minimally Invasive Glaucoma Surgery (MIGS) Technique. *Klin. Monbl. Augenheilkd.* **2021**, *238*, 1113–1119. [CrossRef]
26. Ondrejka, S.; Körber, N. 360 ab-interno Schlemm's canal viscodilation in primary open-angle glaucoma. *Clin. Ophthalmol.* **2019**, *13*, 1235–1246. [CrossRef] [PubMed]
27. Vold, S.D.; Williamson, B.K.; Hirsch, L.; Aminlari, A.E.; Cho, A.S.; Nelson, C.; Dickerson, J.E., Jr. Canaloplasty and Trabeculotomy with the OMNI System in Pseudophakic Patients with Open-Angle Glaucoma: The ROMEO Study. *Ophthalmol. Glaucoma* **2020**, *4*, 173–181. [CrossRef]
28. Sarkisian, S.R.; Mathews, B.; Ding, K.; Patel, A.; Nicek, Z. 360° ab-interno trabeculotomy in refractory primary open-angle glaucoma. *Clin. Ophthalmol.* **2019**, *13*, 161–168. [CrossRef] [PubMed]

29. Grabska-Liberek, I.; Duda, P.; Rogowska, M.; Majszyk-Ionescu, J.; Skowyra, A.; Koziorowska, A.; Kane, I.; Chmielewski, J. 12-month interim results of a prospective study of patients with mild to moderate open-angle glaucoma undergoing combined viscodilation of Schlemm's canal and collector channels and 360° trabeculotomy as a standalone procedure or combined with cataract surgery. *Eur. J. Ophthalmol.* **2021**. online ahead of print. [CrossRef]
30. Brown, R.H.; Tsegaw, S.; Dhamdhere, K.; Lynch, M.G. Viscodilation of Schlemm's canal and trabeculotomy combined with cataract surgery for reducing intraocular pressure in open-angle glaucoma. *J. Cataract Refract. Surg.* **2020**, *46*, 644–645. [CrossRef]
31. Brusini, P.; Tosoni, C. Canaloplasty after failed trabeculectomy: A possible option. *J. Glaucoma* **2014**, *23*, 33–34. [CrossRef] [PubMed]
32. Wang, H.; Xin, C.; Han, Y.; Shi, Y.; Ziaei, S.; Wang, N. Intermediate outcomes of ab externo circumferential trabeculotomy and canaloplasty in POAG patients with prior incisional glaucoma surgery. *BMC Ophthalmol.* **2020**, *20*, 389. [CrossRef] [PubMed]

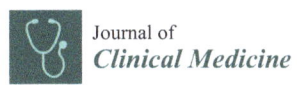

Journal of
Clinical Medicine

MDPI

Article

Different Effects of Aging on Intraocular Pressures Measured by Three Different Tonometers

Kazunobu Sugihara and Masaki Tanito *

Department of Ophthalmology, Shimane University Faculty of Medicine, Izumo 693-8501, Japan;
ksugi@med.shimane-u.ac.jp
* Correspondence: mtanito@med.shimane-u.ac.jp; Tel.: +81-853-20-2284

Abstract: This study aimed to compare intraocular pressures (IOP) using different tonometers, Goldmann applanation (IOP_{GAT}), non-contact (IOP_{NCT}), and rebound (IOP_{RBT}), and to assess the effects of aging and central corneal thickness (CCT) on the measurements. The IOP_{GAT}, IOP_{NCT}, IOP_{RBT}, mean patient age (65.1 ± 16.2 years), and CCT (521.7 ± 39.2 μm) were collected retrospectively from 1054 eyes. The differences among IOPs were compared by the paired t-test. Possible correlations between devices, age, and CCT were assessed by linear regression analyses. The effects of age and CCT on the IOP reading were assessed by mixed-effects regression models. The IOP_{GAT} values were 2.4 and 1.4 mmHg higher than IOP_{NCT} and IOP_{RBT}, respectively; the IOP_{NCT} was 1.0 mmHg lower than IOP_{RBT} ($p < 0.0001$ for all comparisons). The IOPs measured by each tonometer were highly correlated with each other ($r = 0.81–0.90$, $t = 45.2–65.5$). The linear regression analyses showed that age was negatively correlated with IOP_{NCT} ($r = -0.12$, $t = -4.0$) and IOP_{RBT} ($r = -0.14$, $t = -4.5$) but not IOP_{GAT} ($r = 0.00$, $t = -0.2$); the CCT was positively correlated with IOP_{GAT} ($r = 0.13$, $t = 4.3$), IOP_{NCT} ($r = 0.29$, $t = 9.8$), and IOP_{RBT} ($r = 0.22$, $t = 7.2$). The mixed-effect regression models showed significant negative correlations between age and IOP_{NCT} ($t = -2.6$) and IOP_{RBT} ($t = -3.4$), no correlation between age and IOP_{GAT} ($t = 0.2$), and a significant positive correlation between CCT and the tonometers ($t = 3.4–7.3$). No differences between IOP_{GAT} and IOP_{RBT} were seen at the age of 38.8 years. CCT affects IOPs from all tonometers; age affects IOP_{NCT} and IOP_{RBT} in different degrees. IOP_{RBT} tended to be higher than IOP_{GAT} in young subjects, but this stabilized in middle age and became higher in older subjects.

Keywords: age; central corneal thickness; Goldmann Applanation tonometer; non-contact tonometer; rebound tonometer; iCare

Citation: Sugihara, K.; Tanito, M. Different Effects of Aging on Intraocular Pressures Measured by Three Different Tonometers. *J. Clin. Med.* **2021**, *10*, 4202. https://doi.org/10.3390/jcm10184202

Academic Editor: Maria Letizia Salvetat

Received: 31 August 2021
Accepted: 15 September 2021
Published: 17 September 2021

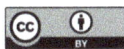
1. Introduction

Intraocular pressure (IOP) is the only known modifiable risk factor relevant to the treatment of glaucoma. Goldmann applanation tonometry (GAT) has been considered the "gold standard" for IOP measurement, although its readings are affected by central corneal thickness (CCT), corneal curvature, the modulus of corneal elasticity, and tear film [1]. Noncontact tonometry (NCT) using air-puff pressure has several favorable characteristics, including no corneal contact and no requirement for local anesthesia, which facilitates convenient use [1]. Rebound tonometry (RBT) uses the impact rebound principle by launching a magnetized probe against the cornea using a solenoid; the speed of deceleration of probe is measured and converted into the IOP [2]. There is no need for an air puff, corneal anesthesia, and slit-lamp mounting, and the measurement skill enables affordable, quick, and repeated IOP measurements even in children and very old patients [3].

Previously, many studies have reported excellent correlations between IOP readings and GAT and NCT or RBT IOPs, although the IOP values themselves varied among the tonometers [4–16]. Most previous studies have assessed the CCT as a surrogate for explaining the measurement difference among tonometers [4–16]; however, other parameters that possibly affect IOP differences among tonometers have not been studied extensively.

During the routine use of the various tonometers in the clinic, we realized that RBT may yield higher IOP readings than GAT in young patients, while this scenario was reversed in older patients. To test our suspicion, we compared the IOP readings of GAT, NCT, and RBT and investigated the effects of age and CCT on the IOP readings in subjects who visited our glaucoma clinic.

2. Subjects and Methods

2.1. Subjects

This retrospective study adhered to the tenets of the Declaration of Helsinki; the institutional review board (IRB) of Shimane University Hospital reviewed and approved the research. Based on the approval, written informed consent from each subject was waived; instead, the study protocol was posted at the study institutions to notify participants about the study. Among the 716 subjects who visited the glaucoma clinic of one author (MT) during April 2018 and March 2019, a review of the medical charts identified 1054 eyes of 544 subjects that fulfilled the inclusion criteria and were included in the analyses. The inclusion criteria were the measurement of IOPs using GAT (IOP_{GAT}), NCT (IOP_{NCT}), and RBT (IOP_{RBT}) on the same day and the recording of the CCT. In our glaucoma clinic, the IOPs obtained using the three different devices and CCT were recorded as routine examinations during the initial patient visit; most data collected were obtained at the initial visit; however, when multiple records of a subject were eligible, the most recent data were collected. No exclusion criterion was set in this real-world data analysis study; accordingly, all subjects who met the inclusion criteria were consecutively included irrespective of glaucoma or non-glaucoma, newly diagnosed or follow-up patients, treated or untreated, and the presence or absence of corneal and other eye diseases. Typically, one glaucoma specialist (MT) used the GAT and RBT (iCARE Rebound Tonometer TA01i, M.E. Technica, Tokyo, Japan) to record the IOPs. One of nine certified orthoptists in our department recorded the IOP using a non-contact air-puff tonometer (TonoRef III, Nidek, Aichi, Japan), and the CCT was recorded using a corneal pachymeter equipped in a specular microscope (EM-3000, Tomey, Nagoya, Japan). No pre-planned calibration of the tonometers was performed for this study.

2.2. Statistical Analysis

The differences among the IOPs assessed using the three tonometers were compared using the paired *t*-test. Possible correlations between three devices, their differences, i.e., NCT minus GAT ($IOP_{NCT-GAT}$), RBT minus GAT ($IOP_{RBT-GAT}$), and RBT minus NCT ($IOP_{RBT-NCT}$), age, and CCT were assessed by linear regression analyses. The effects of age and CCT on each tonometer were further assessed using a mixed-effects regression model in which each patient's identification number was regarded as a random effect, and both age and CCT were regarded as fixed effects. All continuous data were expressed as the mean ± standard deviation (SD). All statistical analyses were performed using the JMP version 11.0 statistical software (SAS Institute, Inc., Cary, NC). $p < 0.05$ was considered statistically significant.

3. Results

The subject ages, CCTs, and IOPs measured using the different tonometers are summarized in Table 1. The IOP_{GAT} was 2.4 and 1.4 mmHg higher than the IOP_{NCT} and IOP_{RBT}, respectively, and the IOP_{NCT} was 1.0 mmHg lower than IOP_{RBT} value (Table 1 and Figure S1A–C).

The IOPs measured by the different tonometers were highly correlated with each other ($r = 0.81–0.90$, $t = 45.2–65.5$) (Table 2 and Figure S2A–C). The linear regression analyses showed that the subjects' ages were negatively correlated with the IOP_{NCT} ($r = -0.12$, $t = -4.0$) and the IOP_{RBT} ($r = -0.14$, $t = -4.5$) but not with the IOP_{GAT} ($r = 0.00$, $t = -0.2$) (Table 2 and Figure S3A–F). Age was also negatively correlated with the CCT ($r = -0.13$, $t = -4.2$) (Table 2 and Figure S4). The linear regression analyses showed that the CCT was positively correlated with the IOP_{GAT} ($r = 0.13$, 4.3), IOP_{NCT} ($r = 0.29$, $t = 9.8$), and IOP_{RBT} ($r = 0.22$, $t = 7.2$) (Table 2 and Figure S5A–F).

Table 1. Age, central corneal thickness (CCT), and intraocular pressures (IOPs) from 1054 eyes of 544 subjects.

Parameters	Mean ± SD	Range	Lower 95% CI	Upper 95% CI	*p* Value
Age, years	65.1 ± 16.2	11–96	63.7	66.4	-
CCT, μm	521.7 ± 39.2	337–675	519.4	524.1	-
IOP_{GAT}, mmHg	16.9 ± 6.9	2–59	16.4	17.3	-
IOP_{NCT}, mmHg	14.4 ± 5.5	2–47	14.1	14.7	-
IOP_{RBT}, mmHg	15.4 ± 6.7	2–53	15.0	15.8	-
Differences in IOP between tonometers					
$IOP_{NCT\text{-}GAT}$, mmHg	−2.4 ± 4.0	−41–+22	−2.7	−2.2	<0.0001
$IOP_{RBT\text{-}GAT}$, mmHg	−1.4 ± 3.1	−15–+22	−1.2	−1.6	<0.0001
$IOP_{RBT\text{-}NCT}$, mmHg	1.0 ± 3.4	−12–+26	0.8	1.2	<0.0001

The *p* values are calculated by using a paired *t*-test between each pair of tonometer groups. SD = standard deviation; CI = confidence interval.

Table 2. Possible correlations among age, CCT, and IOPs measured by each tonometer.

Parameters	Slope	Lower 95% CI	Upper 95% CI	*r*	*t*-Value	*p* Value
Correlation between tonometers (per mmHg)						
IOP_{NCT}: IOP_{GAT}	0.64	0.62	0.68	0.81	45.2	<0.0001
IOP_{RBT}: IOP_{GAT}	0.87	0.85	0.90	0.90	65.5	<0.0001
IOP_{RBT}: IOP_{NCT}	1.05	1.01	1.08	0.86	54.4	<0.0001
Correlation with age (per year)						
IOP_{GAT}, mmHg	0.00	−0.03	0.02	0.00	−0.2	0.8736
IOP_{NCT}, mmHg	−0.04	−0.06	−0.02	−0.12	−4.0	<0.0001
IOP_{RBT}, mmHg	−0.06	−0.08	−0.03	−0.14	−4.5	<0.0001
$IOP_{NCT\text{-}GAT}$, mmHg	−0.04	−0.05	−0.02	−0.16	−5.2	<0.0001
$IOP_{RBT\text{-}GAT}$, mmHg	−0.05	−0.07	−0.04	−0.29	−9.7	<0.0001
$IOP_{RBT\text{-}NCT}$, mmHg	−0.02	−0.03	0.00	−0.07	−2.4	0.0152
CCT, μm	−0.31	−0.45	−0.02	−0.13	−4.2	<0.0001
Correlation with CCT (per μm)						
IOP_{GAT}, mmHg	0.02	0.01	0.03	0.13	4.3	<0.0001
IOP_{NCT}, mmHg	0.04	0.03	0.05	0.29	9.8	<0.0001
IOP_{RBT}, mmHg	0.04	0.03	0.05	0.22	7.2	<0.0001
$IOP_{NCT\text{-}GAT}$, mmHg	0.02	0.01	0.02	0.17	5.6	<0.0001
$IOP_{RBT\text{-}GAT}$, mmHg	0.01	0.01	0.02	0.18	5.8	<0.0001
$IOP_{RBT\text{-}NCT}$, mmHg	0.00	−0.01	0.00	−0.04	−1.3	0.1961

The *t* and *p* values are calculated by linear regression analyses between each pair of indicated parameters. CI = confidence interval; *r* = Pearson's correlation coefficient.

Finally, the effects of age and CCT on the IOPs measured by the three tonometers were assessed by mixed-effects regression models to adjust the interaction between age and CCT and cancel the bias resulting from the inclusion of both eyes of a subject (Table 3). Significant negative correlations were also seen between age and the IOP_{NCT} ($t = -2.6$) and IOP_{RBT} ($t = -3.4$), a non-significant correlation between age and the IOP_{GAT} ($t = 0.2$), and significant positive correlations between the CCT and all three tonometers ($t = 3.4$–7.3) (Table 3).

Table 3. Effects of age and CCT on the IOPs measured by each tonometer.

Parameters	Slope	Lower 95% CI	Upper 95% CI	*t*-Value	*p* Value
IOP$_{GAT}$, mmHg					
Age (per year)	0.00	−0.03	0.03	0.2	0.8109
CCT (per μm)	0.02	0.01	0.03	3.4	0.0008
IOP$_{NCT}$, mmHg					
Age (per year)	−0.03	−0.05	−0.01	−2.6	0.0088
CCT (per μm)	0.01	0.01	0.02	3.9	<0.0001
IOP$_{RBT}$, mmHg					
Age (per year)	−0.05	−0.08	−0.02	−3.4	0.0008
CCT (per μm)	0.03	0.02	0.04	5.2	<0.0001
IOP$_{NCT-GAT}$, mmHg					
Age (per year)	−0.03	−0.05	−0.02	−3.8	0.0002
CCT (per μm)	0.01	0.01	0.02	3.9	<0.0001
IOP$_{RBT-GAT}$, mmHg					
Age (per year)	−0.05	−0.07	−0.04	−7.6	<0.0001
CCT (per μm)	0.01	0.00	0.01	3.3	0.0010
IOP$_{RBT-NCT}$, mmHg					
Age (per year)	−0.02	−0.03	0.00	−2.3	0.0229
CCT (per μm)	0.00	−0.01	0.00	−1.4	0.1520

The *t* and *p* values are calculated by mixed-effect regression models to adjust the interaction between age and CCT and cancel the bias resulting from the inclusion of both eyes of a subject. CI = confidence interval; *r* = Pearson's correlation coefficient.

4. Discussion

As reported previously [4–16], the IOPs measured using the three devices were correlated with each other, and all were affected by the CCT (Table 2). A significant positive association between the CCT and IOP$_{NCT-GAT}$ and IOP$_{RBT-GAT}$ (Table 2) suggested a larger effect of the CCT on the IOPs obtained with NCT or RBT than with GAT, as reported previously [6,15].

We identified a significant negative correlation between age and IOP$_{NCT}$ or IOP$_{RBT}$, while the correlation between age and IOP$_{GAT}$ was not significant (Table 2). Since the IOP$_{RBT-NCT}$ was negatively correlated with age (Table 2), the impact of age is the greatest on the RBT among the tonometers tested. The absolute *t*-value was the largest for age with the IOP$_{RBT-GAT}$ (*t* = −7.6) among the models that included CCT and age (Table 3), suggesting that age determines the difference in IOP readings between GAT and RBT more than CCT. A recent report has found a negative correlation between IOP$_{RBT}$ and age [17], and thus our results are in agreement with the previous report. Subject age and the detected difference between GAT and RBT readings in previous and current studies are summarized in Table 4. Including the current study, some studies have reported minus IOP$_{RBT-GAT}$ values [10,12–14], while others have reported plus IOP$_{RBT-GAT}$ values [4–8,11,15,16]; this discrepancy is not fully explained by the difference in the CCT. Scatterplots of the subjects' ages and IOP$_{RBT-GAT}$ from previous studies (Table 4 and Figure 1) clearly suggest the roles of age and IOP$_{RBT-GAT}$. Previously, 0 IOP$_{RBT-GAT}$ was reported in subjects with a mean age of 59.3 years [9]. In the current subjects, based on linear regression analyses (Figure S3E), the age of subjects with 0 IOP$_{RBT-GAT}$ was calculated to be 38.8 years. Thus, a lower/higher association of IOP readings between GAT and RBT is reversed based on the ages of the subjects. Other than the CCT, it has been proposed that corneal biomechanical properties such as corneal hysteresis (CH) and corneal resistance factors (CRF) affect the RBT and GAT differently [7,9,13]; both the CH and CRF decreased with aging [18]; thus, age-dependent changes in corneal biomechanical properties may be associated with our observation but need to be confirmed.

Table 4. Summary of subjects' age and $IOP_{RBT-GAT}$ in previous studies.

Icare Model	Age, Years	$IOP_{RBT-GAT}$, mmHg	Reference
iCareTa01i	63.8 ± 15.6	1.8 ± 2.8	4
iCareTa01i	61.3 ± 14.4	1.4 ± 2.7	5
iCareTa01i	52.0 ± 20.0	1.40 ± 2.19	6
iCareTa01i	22.3 ± 3.3	1.94 ± 2.75	7
iCarePro	63.7 ± 14.1	1.97 ± 3.29	8
iCarePro	59.3 ± 19.9	0.0	9
iCarePro	47.5 ± 105	−0.38	10
iCarePro	8.89 ± 3.41	2.56 ± 4.62	11
iCareTa01i	71.0 ± 7.5	−2.46 ± 2.10	12
iCarePro	71.0 ± 7.5	−1.42 ± 2.35	12
iCareTa01i	67.5 ± 10.9	−1.67 ± 3.07	13
iCareTa01i	70.95 ± 7.76	−1.71	14
iCarePro	56.9 ± 18.3	0.3	15
iCarePro	11.44 ± 2.31	1.97 ± 0.15	16
iCareTa01i	65.1 ± 16.2	−1.4 ± 3.1	Current study

The data are expressed as mean ± standard deviation.

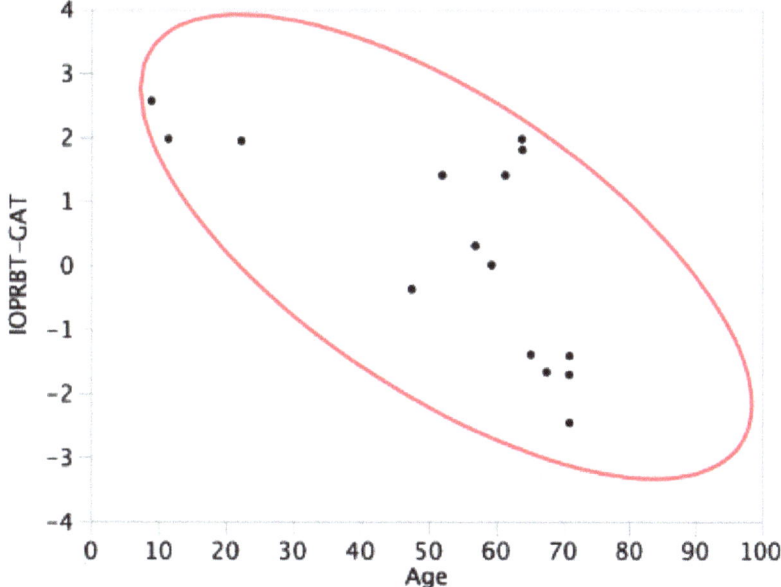

Figure 1. Correlations between subjects' age (years) and intraocular pressure (IOP) (rebound tonometry minus Goldmann applanation tonometry) (RBT-GAT) (mmHg) in the current and previous studies. The scatterplots and a 90% bivariate normal ellipse are shown.

The limitations of the current study included the retrospective design and the inclusion of eyes with various types of glaucoma and glaucoma suspects. Because of the retrospective nature of the study, the methods of tonometry and examiners were not predetermined, although one examiner recorded the GAT and RBT using specific devices. We reviewed all patients who visited during the indicated period and included all patients who fulfilled the inclusion criteria, thus minimizing the selection bias. The inclusion of both eyes of a patient may have introduced bias, although we minimized this by using a mixed-effects regression model. Other than age and CCT, the modules of corneal elasticity [1] should affect the results. When the IOP elevates, the deviation between IOP_{NCT} and IOP_{GAT} becomes larger (Figure S2A); this may be explained by the effect of changes in corneal elasticity. Despite the various backgrounds of subjects included and the retrospective study design, we believe that our real-world data analysis is reasonable to test our suspicion, described in the introduction section.

5. Conclusions

In conclusion, CCT affects the IOP readings of GAT, NCT, and RBT, while age affects the NCT and RBT by different degrees. The RBT readings tended to be higher than the GAT readings in young subjects, but this stabilized in middle age and was reversed in older subjects.

Supplementary Materials: The following are available online at https://www.mdpi.com/article/10.3390/jcm10184202/s1, Figure S1: Differences in the intraocular pressure (IOP) (mmHg) among the tonometers, Figure S2: Correlations between the intraocular pressure (IOP) (mmHg) measured using different tonometers, Figure S3: Correlations between age (years) and intraocular pressure (IOP) (mmHg) measured using different tonometers, Figure S4: Correlations between age (years) and central corneal thickness (CCT) (μm), Figure S5: Correlations between the central corneal thickness (CCT) (μm) and intraocular pressure (IOP) (mmHg) measured using different tonometers.

Author Contributions: Conceptualization, K.S., M.T.; methodology, K.S., M.T.; formal analysis, K.S., M.T.; investigation, K.S., M.T.; data curation, K.S., M.T.; writing—original draft preparation, M.T.; writing—review and editing, K.S. All authors have read and agreed to the published version of the manuscript.

Funding: This research received no external funding.

Institutional Review Board Statement: The study adhered to the tenets of the Declaration of Helsinki; the institutional review board (IRB) of Shimane University Hospital reviewed and approved the research (IRB No. 20080911-1; 9 December 2020).

Informed Consent Statement: The IRB approval did not require each patient to provide written informed consent for publication; instead, the study protocol was posted at the study's institutions to notify participants about the study.

Data Availability Statement: The data are fully available upon reasonable request to the corresponding author.

Conflicts of Interest: The authors report no conflict of interest in this work.

References

1. Chihara, E. Assessment of true intraocular pressure: The gap between theory and practical data. *Surv. Ophthalmol.* **2008**, *53*, 203–218. [CrossRef] [PubMed]
2. Kontiola, A. A new electromechanical method for measuring intraocular pressure. *Doc. Ophthalmol.* **1996**, *93*, 265–276. [CrossRef] [PubMed]
3. Nakakura, S. Icare® rebound tonometers: Review of their characteristics and ease of use. *Clin. Ophthalmol.* **2018**, *12*, 1245–1253. [CrossRef] [PubMed]
4. Martinez-de-la-Casa, J.M.; Garcia-Feijoo, J.; Castillo, A.; Garcia-Sanchez, J. Reproducibility and clinical evaluation of rebound tonometry. *Investig. Ophthalmol. Vis. Sci.* **2005**, *46*, 4578–4580. [CrossRef] [PubMed]
5. Martinez-de-la-Casa, J.M.; Garcia-Feijoo, J.; Vico, E.; Fernandez-Vidal, A.; Benitez del Castillo, J.M.; Wasfi, M.; Garcia-Sanchez, J. Effect of corneal thickness on dynamic contour, rebound, and goldmann tonometry. *Ophthalmology* **2006**, *113*, 2156–2162. [CrossRef] [PubMed]
6. Nakamura, M.; Darhad, U.; Tatsumi, Y.; Fujioka, M.; Kusuhara, A.; Maeda, H.; Negi, A. Agreement of rebound tonometer in measuring intraocular pressure with three types of applanation tonometers. *Am. J. Ophthalmol.* **2006**, *142*, 332–334. [CrossRef] [PubMed]
7. Chui, W.S.; Lam, A.; Chen, D.; Chiu, R. The influence of corneal properties on rebound tonometry. *Ophthalmology* **2008**, *115*, 80–84. [PubMed]
8. Kim, K.N.; Jeoung, J.W.; Park, K.H.; Yang, M.K.; Kim, D.M. Comparison of the new rebound tonometer with Goldmann applanation tonometer in a clinical setting. *Acta Ophthalmol.* **2013**, *91*, e392–e396. [PubMed]
9. Smedowski, A.; Weglarz, B.; Tarnawska, D.; Kaarniranta, K.; Wylegala, E. Comparison of three intraocular pressure measurement methods including biomechanical properties of the cornea. *Investig. Ophthalmol. Vis. Sci.* **2014**, *55*, 666–673. [CrossRef] [PubMed]

10. Güler, M.; Bilak, Ş.; Bilgin, B.; Şimşek, A.; Çapkin, M.; Hakim Reyhan, A. Comparison of Intraocular Pressure Measurements Obtained by Icare PRO Rebound Tonometer, Tomey FT-1000 Noncontact Tonometer, and Goldmann Applanation Tonometer in Healthy Subjects. *J. Glaucoma.* **2015**, *24*, 613–618. [CrossRef] [PubMed]
11. Feng, C.S.; Jin, K.W.; Yi, K.; Choi, D.G. Comparison of Intraocular Pressure Measurements Obtained by Rebound, Noncontact, and Goldmann Applanation Tonometry in Children. *Am. J. Ophthalmol.* **2015**, *160*, 937–943.e1. [CrossRef] [PubMed]
12. Kato, Y.; Nakakura, S.; Matsuo, N.; Yoshitomi, K.; Handa, M.; Tabuchi, H.; Kiuchi, Y. Agreement among Goldmann applanation tonometer, iCare, and Icare PRO rebound tonometers; non-contact tonometer; and Tonopen XL in healthy elderly subjects. *Int. Ophthalmol.* **2018**, *38*, 687–696. [CrossRef] [PubMed]
13. Brown, L.; Foulsham, W.; Pronin, S.; Tatham, A.J. The Influence of Corneal Biomechanical Properties on Intraocular Pressure Measurements Using a Rebound Self-tonometer. *J. Glaucoma.* **2018**, *27*, 511–518. [PubMed]
14. Zakrzewska, A.; Wiącek, M.P.; Machalińska, A. Impact of corneal parameters on intraocular pressure measurements in different tonometry methods. *Int. J. Ophthalmol.* **2019**, *12*, 1853–1858. [CrossRef] [PubMed]
15. Chen, M.; Zhang, L.; Xu, J.; Chen, X.; Gu, Y.; Ren, Y.; Wang, K. Comparability of three intraocular pressure measurement: ICare pro rebound, non-contact and Goldmann applanation tonometry in different IOP group. *BMC Ophthalmol.* **2019**, *19*, 225. [CrossRef] [PubMed]
16. Uzlu, D.; Akyol, N.; Türk, A.; Oruç, Y. A comparison of three different tonometric methods in the measurement of intraocular pressure in the pediatric age group. *Int. Ophthalmol.* **2020**, *40*, 1999–2005. [CrossRef] [PubMed]
17. Nakakura, S.; Mori, E.; Fujio, Y.; Fujisawa, Y.; Matsuya, K.; Kobayashi, Y.; Tabuchi, H.; Asaoka, R.; Kiuchi, Y. Comparison of the Intraocular Pressure Measured Using the New Rebound Tonometer Icare ic100 and Icare TA01i or Goldmann Applanation Tonometer. *J. Glaucoma.* **2019**, *28*, 172–177. [CrossRef] [PubMed]
18. El Massry, A.A.K.; Said, A.A.; Osman, I.M.; Bessa, A.S.; Elmasry, M.A.; Elsayed, E.N.; Bayoumi, N.H.L. Corneal biomechanics in different age groups. *Int. Ophthalmol.* **2020**, *40*, 967–974. [CrossRef] [PubMed]

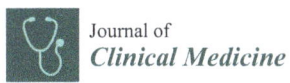

Article

Corneal Higher-Order Aberrations after Microhook ab Interno Trabeculotomy and Goniotomy with the Kahook Dual Blade: Preliminary Early 3-Month Results

Hiromitsu Onoe, Kazuyuki Hirooka *, Hideaki Okumichi ⓘ, Yumiko Murakami and Yoshiaki Kiuchi

Department of Ophthalmology and Visual Science, Hiroshima University, 1-2-3 Kasumi, Minami-Ku, Hiroshima 734-8551, Japan; onoehir@hiroshima-u.ac.jp (H.O.); okumic@hiroshima-u.ac.jp (H.O.); ymiko00@hiroshima-u.ac.jp (Y.M.); ykiuchi@hiroshima-u.ac.jp (Y.K.)
* Correspondence: khirooka9@gmail.com; Tel.: +81-82-257-5247; Fax: 81-82-257-5249

Abstract: We examined postoperative corneal higher-order aberrations (HOAs) present after combined phacoemulsification with either microhook ab interno trabeculotomy (μLOT-Phaco) or goniotomy, using the Kahook Dual Blade (KDB-Phaco). Retrospective study: A total of 45 eyes underwent μLOT-Phaco and KDB-Phaco (LOT-Phaco) procedures, with 21 eyes that underwent cataract surgery alone used as controls. Visual acuity and corneal HOAs, coma-like aberrations, and spherical-like aberrations were analyzed before and at 1, 2, and 3 months after the surgeries. Risk factors that could potentially influence HOAs were evaluated. No significant postoperative changes were noted for corneal HOAs, coma-like aberrations, and spherical-like aberrations after cataract surgery alone. The mean corneal HOAs, coma-like aberrations, and spherical-like aberrations were 0.222 ± 0.115 μm, 0.203 ± 0.113 μm, and 0.084 ± 0.043 μm at baseline and 0.326 ± 0.195 μm ($p < 0.001$), 0.302 ± 0.289 μm ($p = 0.03$), and 0.150 ± 0.115 μm ($p < 0.001$) at 3 months after LOT-Phaco, respectively. Results of the analysis for risk factors suggested that a longer incision in Schlemm's canal could influence corneal HOAs, coma-like aberrations, and spherical-like aberrations after LOT-Phaco. Although no significant postoperative changes were observed in corneal HOAs and coma-like or spherical-like aberrations after cataract surgery alone, a significant increase in corneal HOAs and coma-like or spherical-like aberrations remained after the LOT-Phaco procedure.

Keywords: higher-order aberrations; ab interno trabeculotomy; Kahook Dual Blade; glaucoma

Citation: Onoe, H.; Hirooka, K.; Okumichi, H.; Murakami, Y.; Kiuchi, Y. Corneal Higher-Order Aberrations after Microhook ab Interno Trabeculotomy and Goniotomy with the Kahook Dual Blade: Preliminary Early 3-Month Results. *J. Clin. Med.* **2021**, *10*, 4115. https://doi.org/10.3390/jcm10184115

Academic Editor: Maria Letizia Salvetat

Received: 11 August 2021
Accepted: 10 September 2021
Published: 12 September 2021

Publisher's Note: MDPI stays neutral with regard to jurisdictional claims in published maps and institutional affiliations.

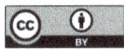
1. Introduction

Glaucoma is the leading the cause of blindness [1]. Although medication and laser therapy alone are used to try to decrease the intraocular pressure (IOP), incisional surgery is performed when these prove to be ineffective. The trabecular meshwork has been shown to be the most resistant part of the aqueous humor outflow, with glaucomatous eyes found to have a greater resistance in this area [2]. Theoretically, when attempting to improve the control of the IOP, incision or removal of the trabecular meshwork should result in a reduction in this resistance [3]. Thus, the use of devices, such as the trabectome, Kahook Dual Blade (KDB; New World Medical, Rancho, Cucamonga, CA, USA), and microhook (Inami & Co., Ltd., Tokyo, Japan), in conjunction with 5-0 nylon sutures has been utilized during attempts designed to reduce the resistance of the trabecular meshwork from within the anterior chamber [4–7]. These techniques all fall within the designation of minimally invasive glaucoma surgery (MIGS) and can be performed by using procedures that utilize the iridocorneal angle from within the anterior chamber.

As compared to other vision threatening complications, corneal topographic changes are often less serious. However, the frequently reported vision complaints made by patients could potentially be related to corneal topographic changes. Due to recent advances in wavefront analysis, it has become possible to more closely evaluate ocular surgeries, such as refractive surgery and cataract surgery. Results have shown that there are changes in the higher-order aberrations (HOAs), which were found to be related to the postoperative visual function [8,9]. Moreover, the effect of trabeculectomy on HOAs in glaucoma patients has also been reported [10–12]. Increases in the HOAs are believed in general to lead to decreases in the functional visual acuity. However, the specific effect associated with MIGS combined with cataract surgery on ocular HOAs has yet to be definitively established.

The purpose of our current study was to examine patients undergoing phacoemulsification cataract extraction in conjunction with the placement of an intraocular lens (IOL) combined with either μLOT (μLOT-Phaco) or goniotomy with KDB (KDB-Phaco) and then investigate the improvement of the HOAs following surgery.

2. Materials and Methods

2.1. Patients

Between December 2019 and September 2020, this retrospective study examined eyes undergoing either μLOT-Phaco in 31 eyes or KDB-Phaco in 14 eyes at Hiroshima University Hospital, Japan. Twenty-one eyes undergoing phacoemulsification cataract extraction in conjunction with the placement of an IOL (Phaco) were additionally examined and used as the controls. All patients were followed for at least 3 months after surgery. The Institutional Review Board of the Hiroshima University approved the study protocol (IRB No. E-2240). In accordance with the principles outlined in the Declaration of Helsinki, all subjects provided written informed consent in addition to the standard consent for surgery prior to their enrollment and participation in the research study.

Patients who had previously undergone intraocular surgery were excluded. Inclusion criteria required patients to be ≥50 years of age and have no history of refractive surgery or other significant ocular diseases.

2.2. Surgical Techniques

Trabeculotomy was performed by using 2 different kinds of trabecular hooks, the microhook or the KDB. Selection of the hooks used in the surgeries was based on the preferences and decisions of the surgeons. The glaucoma procedure was performed under direct gonioscopy after the cataract procedure in both the μLOT-Phaco and KDB-Phaco patient groups. A 2.8 mm corneal incision was created at the temporal position. A standard phacoemulsification technique; Whitestar Signature Pro (Johnson & Johnson, New Brunswick, NJ, USA) was used to remove the nucleus during all procedures. The IOLs (PCB00V, Johnson & Johnson; XY1, HOYA, Tokyo, Japan) were implanted in the capsular bag. After cataract surgery, a microhook was inserted into the anterior chamber. The inner wall of the Schlemm's canal and trabecular meshwork were incised by a microhook at 4 clock hours (nasal quadrant: 120°) or at 6 clock hours (inferior and nasal bisection: 180°). The extent of the incision in the Schlemm's canal in degrees (EIS) was based on decisions of the surgeons. The KDB was introduced into the anterior chamber for the purpose of performing excisional goniotomy, with the pointed chip engaging the trabecular meshwork to the point where its heel was resting within Schlemm's canal. In order to excise a strip of the trabecular meshwork, the KDB was then advanced approximately 4 clock hours (nasal quadrant: 120°). After removal of the ophthalmic viscosurgical device, a 27-gauge cannula was used to hydrate the incisions. There were no sutures placed or used at the end of the surgery. Postoperative anti-inflammatory and anti-infective therapies were administered for 3 to 4 weeks in all patients.

2.3. Wavefront Analysis

A wavefront analyzer (KR-1W, Topcon Co., Tokyo, Japan) was utilized to measure the anterior, posterior, and total corneal wavefront aberrations preoperatively and at 1, 2, and 3 months postoperatively. Aberrometry measurements were performed automatically for a total of three times. Displayed wavefront aberrations included corneal HOAs, trefoil, coma, spherical, third-order, and fourth-order aberrations of the Zernike polynomials, which were calculated as root mean square values.

2.4. Statistical Analysis

A paired *t*-test or chi-square test was used to compare the values for the LOT-Phaco and Phaco alone groups. A multivariable regression model was used to determine the factors that were associated with the increases in the HOAs at 3 months after LOT-Phaco. The independent variables used included the age, EIS (120° or 180°), baseline corneal HOAs, IOP at one day after surgery, IOP at 3 months after surgery, and the device used (KDB or microhook). To ensure that clinically relevant and confounding variables remained, the analysis used backward elimination selection. All data are reported as the mean ± standard deviation (SD). All statistical analyses were conducted by using JMP software version 15 (SAS Inc., Cary, NC, USA). *P*-values less than 0.05 were considered statistically significant.

3. Results

Phacoemulsification cataract extraction was performed in 21 eyes, with combined phacoemulsification with trabeculotomy performed in 31 eyes when using the microhook and in 14 eyes when using the KDB. Table 1 presents the clinical characteristics for the enrolled participants. The mean ages for the μLOT-Phaco and KDB-Phaco (LOT-Phaco) groups and the cataract surgery (Phaco) control group were 73.3 ± 8.8 years and 78.9 ± 6.0 years, respectively.

Table 1. Baseline patient characteristics.

	LOT-Phaco (*n* = 45)	Phaco (*n* = 21)	*p*-Value
Age (years)	73.3 ± 8.8	78.9 ± 6.0	0.001
Gender (M/F)	16/29	9/12	0.57
Visual acuity (logMAR)	0.28 ± 0.27	0.16 ± 0.19	0.09
Baseline IOP (mmHg)	17.8 ± 6.1	12.5 ± 3.1	<0.001
Diagnosis			
POAG	15		
PACG	19		
Exfoliation glaucoma	8		
Secondary glaucoma	3		
Device (microhook/KDB)	31/14		
EIS (120°/180°)	27/18		

M, male; F, female; IOP, intraocular pressure; POAG, primary open-angle glaucoma; PACG, primary angle closure glaucoma; KDB, Kahook Dual Blade; EIS, extent of the incision in the Schlemm canal in degrees.

Figure 1 presents the IOP trends noted between the two groups over the study course. The mean IOP in the LOT-Phaco group was 18.0 ± 6.3 mmHg at baseline, while it was 12.9 ± 3.0, 12.3 ± 2.9, 12.6 ± 2.5 mmHg at 1, 2, and 3 months, respectively. The mean IOP in the Phaco group was 11.7 ± 2.5 mmHg at baseline, while it was 12.2 ± 2.6, 11.4 ± 2.4, 11.7 ± 2.1 mmHg at 1, 2, and 3 months, respectively. At all of the study visits, there was a significant reduction noted in the IOP as compared to baseline in the LOT-Phaco group. Table 2 shows the pre- and postoperative visual acuities in both groups. At all study visits in both groups, there was a significant increase observed in the visual acuity as compared to baseline.

Table 3 shows the pre- and postoperative corneal HOAs, coma-like aberrations, and spherical-like aberrations. No significant postoperative changes were observed in the Phaco group for the corneal HOAs and coma-like or spherical-like aberrations. However, corneal HOAs and coma-like or spherical-like aberrations were significantly increased in the LOT-Phaco group at every visit following the initial surgery. Figure 2 demonstrates baseline versus 3 months after LOT-Phaco corneal HOAs (A) and coma-like (B) or spherical-like aberrations (C).

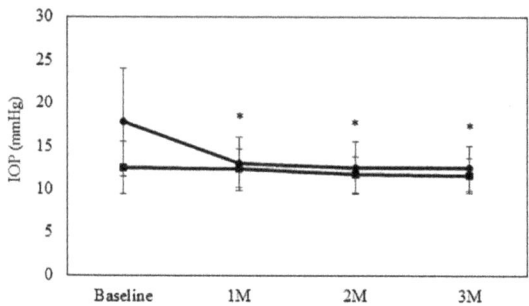

Figure 1. Mean intraocular pressure following Phaco-alone or LOT-Phaco. The intraocular pressure was significantly reduced in LOT-Phaco group compared with baseline. * $p < 0.05$ compared with baseline. Filled circle LOT-Phaco group; filled square Phaco group.

Table 2. Postoperative logMAR visual acuity.

	LOT-Phaco	*p*-Value	Phaco	*p*-Value
Baseline	0.28 ± 0.27		0.16 ± 0.19	
1M	0.10 ± 0.28	<0.001	0.01 ± 0.13	0.004
2M	0.08 ± 0.27	<0.001	−0.003 ± 0.13	0.001
3M	0.06 ± 0.23	<0.001	−0.03 ± 0.14	<0.001

Table 3. Postoperative corneal higher-order, coma-like, and spherical-like aberrations.

	LOT-Phaco	*p*-Value	Phaco	*p*-Value
Corneal higher-order				
Baseline	0.222 ± 0.115		0.230 ± 0.229	
1M	0.297 ± 0.161	<0.001	0.252 ± 0.134	0.44
2M	0.356 ± 0.255	0.002	0.268 ± 0.142	0.21
3M	0.326 ± 0.195	<0.001	0.272 ± 0.137	0.12
Coma-like				
Baseline	0.203 ± 0.113		0.206 ± 0.107	
1M	0.251 ± 0.137	0.004	0.228 ± 0.133	0.44
2M	0.305 ± 0.201	0.003	0.239 ± 0.145	0.26
3M	0.302 ± 0.289	0.03	0.244 ± 0.127	0.14
Spherical-like				
Baseline	0.084 ± 0.043		0.092 ± 0.058	
1M	0.151 ± 0.100	<0.001	0.098 ± 0.050	0.69
2M	0.162 ± 0.174	0.01	0.107 ± 0.050	0.27
3M	0.150 ± 0.115	<0.001	0.113 ± 0.071	0.20

Data shown are mean ± SD (μm).

The risk factor that was identified as being associated with the increased corneal HOAs, coma-like aberrations, and spherical-like aberrations at 3 months after LOT-Phaco was EIS for the 180° Schlemm's canal opening (Table 4).

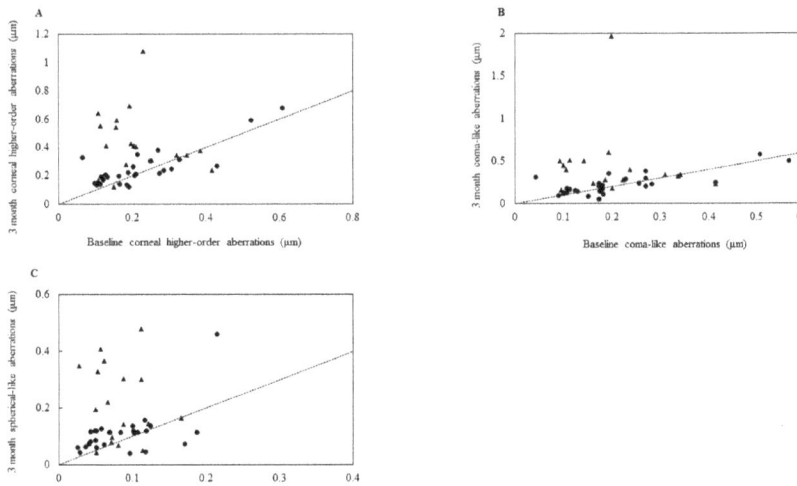

Figure 2. Scatterplot showing baseline versus 3-month corneal higher-order (**A**), coma-like (**B**), or spherical-like aberrations (**C**). Filled circle 120° EIS group; filled triangle 180° EIS group.

Table 4. Stepwise multiple regression analysis for factors associated with postoperative corneal higher-order, coma-like, and spherical-like aberrations' changes.

	Corneal Higher-Order				Coma-like				Spherical-like			
	Univariate		Multivariate		Univariate		Multivariate		Univariate		Multivariate	
Factors	β	*p*-Value	β	*p*-Value	β	*p*-Value	β	*p*-Value	β	*p*-Value	β	*p*-Value
Age	−0.003	0.38			−0.004	0.93			−0.002	0.23		
IOP one day after surgery	0.002	0.54			0.006	0.27			0.001	0.63		
IOP 3 months after surgery	0.009	0.45			0.012	0.49			0.005	0.43	0.013	0.04
Device (KDB)	−0.134	0.03			−0.138	0.14			−0.080	0.02		
Baseline corneal HOAs	−0.558	0.03	−0.526	0.02								
Baseline coma-like aberrations					−0.570	0.14						
Baseline spherical-like aberrations									−0.473	0.23		
EIS (120°)	−0.200	<0.001	−0.098	<0.001	−0.222	<0.001	−0.111	0.01	−0.108	<0.001	−0.064	<0.001

IOP, intraocular pressure; KDB, Kahook Dual Blade; HOAs, higher-order aberrations; EIS, extent of the incision in the Schlemm's canal in degrees.

4. Discussion

Recently, procedures using new microsurgical devices are being developed for MIGS [5,7]. MIGS is commonly defined as a surgical procedure that uses an ab interno approach, results in minimal trauma with very little, minimal or no conjunctival manipulation, and has a good safety profile and rapid recovery [13]. However, at 3 months after the LOT-Phaco procedure in our current study, we found that the there was a continued significant increase in the total HOAs and coma-like or spherical-like aberrations.

Changes in the HOAs following trabeculectomy have been reported in several studies [10–12]. Fukuoka et al. [10] found that there was an increase in the ocular coma-like and total higher-aberrations incidence at 1 month after trabeculectomy, with these changes shown to return to baseline levels by 3 months. In contrast, we previously reported finding corneal HOAs were significantly increased from baseline up until 3 months after trabeculectomy [11]. Moreover, we also found that hypotony could influence corneal HOAs after filtration surgery [11]. However, in our current study, we found that hypotony was not observed in all cases.

In this current study, eyes undergoing Phaco were used as the controls. Although we did not find any significant postoperative changes in the corneal HOAs and coma-like or spherical-like aberrations after undergoing Phaco, results did show that these parameters were significantly increased following LOT-Phaco. However, the only difference noted between these surgeries was for the incision in Schlemm's canal. In addition, the 180° more extensive incision in Schlemm's canal was found to be a risk factor that influenced the corneal HOAs, coma-like aberrations, and spherical-like aberrations. In the 120° Schlemm's canal incision group, corneal HOAs, coma-like aberrations, and spherical-like aberrations were 0.227 ± 0.128 μm, 0.206 ± 0.124 μm, and 0.086 ± 0.050 μm at baseline and 0.251 ± 0.131 μm ($p = 0.12$), 0.217 ± 0.123 μm ($p = 0.47$), and 0.110 ± 0.077 μm ($p = 0.10$) at 3 months after LOT-Phaco, respectively. When compared to the baseline values, there were no significant differences observed. In the 180° Schlemm's canal incision group, however, corneal HOAs, coma-like aberrations, and spherical-like aberrations were 0.216 ± 0.095 μm, 0.198 ± 0.098 μm, and 0.080 ± 0.034 μm at baseline and 0.439 ± 0.223 μm ($p = 0.001$), 0.430 ± 0.406 μm ($p = 0.04$), and 0.211 ± 0.136 μm ($p = 0.002$) at 3 months after LOT-Phaco, respectively. Based on these findings, we assume that Schlemm's canal plays an important role in maintaining corneal formation.

Corneal HOAs and coma-like or spherical-like aberrations were significantly higher than baseline until 2 months (data not shown) and were no longer significantly different from the baseline at 3 months in the 120° Schlemm's canal incision group. Therefore, we assume that those aberrations in the 180° Schlemm's canal incision group may also return to baseline if we extend the follow-up period.

Current study limitations included, first, the effect of the corneal thickness, axial length, type of implanted IOL, and eccentricity in each eye. However, it is our belief that the influence of these factors is probably low. Second, it is known that age has an influence on corneal HOAs [14]. The mean age in our current study was significantly different between the LOT-Phaco and Phaco groups. However, we found no influence of age for HOAs following the surgery in our current study. Third, although increases in HOAs are believed to lead to decreases in functional visual acuity, our current study did not evaluate the functional visual acuity, with only the visual acuity evaluated. However, we are presently undertaking an evaluation of the vision-related quality of life that is present after undergoing the LOT-Phaco procedure. Fourth, the relationship between the EIS and the reduction in IOP remains unclear. The mean IOP reduction in our current study was $21.2 \pm 4.8\%$ and $27.3 \pm 5.8\%$ ($p = 0.42$) at 3 months after surgery in the 120° EIS and 180° EIS groups, respectively. Manabe et al. [15] previously reported that there was no correlation between the EIS (range 150° to 320°) during suture trabeculotomy and the postoperative reduction in the IOP. Thus, a further long-term comparison of the postoperative outcomes of EIS in a larger number of patient cases will need to be undertaken in the future.

In conclusion, even though the corneal HOAs and coma-like or spherical-like aberrations exhibited no significant increase from the baseline in the Phaco group, the corneal HOAs and coma-like or spherical-like aberrations in the LOT-Phaco group remained significantly increased from the baseline for up to 3 months after the procedure. Thus, a more extensive incision in the Schlemm canal should be considered to be a risk factor that can influence corneal HOAs and coma-like or spherical-like aberrations.

Author Contributions: Conceptualization, K.H.; methodology, K.H.; software, H.O. (Hiromitsu Onoe); validation, H.O. (Hiromitsu Onoe), H.O. (Hideaki Okumichi), Y.M., and Y.K.; formal analysis, H.O. (Hiromitsu Onoe); investigation, H.O. (Hiromitsu Onoe); resources, K.H.; data curation, H.O. (Hiromitsu Onoe); writing—original draft preparation, K.H.; writing—review and editing, K.H.; visualization, K.H.; supervision, K.H.; project administration, K.H.; funding acquisition, K.H. All authors have read and agreed to the published version of the manuscript.

Funding: This research was funded by a Grant-in-Aid for Scientific Research from the Ministry of Education, Culture, Sports, Science, and Technology of Japan (20K09827).

Institutional Review Board Statement: The study was conducted according to the guidelines of the Declaration of Helsinki and approved by the Institutional Review Board of the Hiroshima University (protocol code E-2240 and date of approval).

Informed Consent Statement: Informed consent was obtained from all subjects involved in the study.

Data Availability Statement: The data analyzed in this study are available from the corresponding author upon reasonable request.

Conflicts of Interest: The authors declare no conflict of interests.

References

1. Quigley, H.A.; Broman, A.T. The number of people with glaucoma worldwide in 2010 and 2020. *Br. J. Ophthalmol.* **2006**, *90*, 262–267. [CrossRef] [PubMed]
2. Johnson, M. What controls aqueous humor outflow resistance? *Exp. Eye Res.* **2006**, *82*, 545–557. [CrossRef] [PubMed]
3. Cook, C.; Foster, P. Epidemiology of glaucoma: What's new? *Can. J. Ophthalmol.* **2012**, *47*, 223–226. [CrossRef] [PubMed]
4. Minckler, D.S.; Baerveldt, G.; Alfaro, M.R.; Francis, B.A. Clinical results with the Trabecutome for treatment of open-angle glaucoma. *Ophthalmology* **2005**, *112*, 962–967. [CrossRef] [PubMed]
5. Seibold, L.K.; Soohoo, J.R.; Ammar, D.A.; Kahook, M.Y. Preclinical investigation of ab interno trabeculectomy using a novel dual-blade device. *Am. J. Ophthalmol.* **2013**, *155*, 524–529. [CrossRef] [PubMed]
6. Sato, T.; Kawaji, T.; Hirata, A.; Mizoguchi, T. 360-degree suture trabeculotomy ab interno to treat open-angle glaucoma: 2-year outcomes. *Clin. Ophthalmol.* **2018**, *12*, 915–923. [CrossRef] [PubMed]
7. Tanito, M.; Sano, I.; Ikeda, Y.; Fujihara, E. Shore-term results of microhook ab interno trabeculotomy, a novel minimally invasive glaucoma surgery in Japanese eyes: Initial case series. *Acta Ophthalmol.* **2017**, *95*, e354–e360. [CrossRef] [PubMed]
8. Mierdel, P.; Kaemmerer, M.; Krinke, H.E.; Seiler, T. Effects of photorefractive keratectomy and cataract surgery on ocular optical errors of higher order. *Graefes Arch. Clin. Exp. Ophthalmol.* **1999**, *237*, 725–729. [CrossRef] [PubMed]
9. Oshika, T.; Klyce, S.D.; Applegate, R.A.; Howland, H.C.; El Danasoury, M.A. Comparison of corneal wavefront aberrations after photorefractive keratectomy and laser in situ keratomileusis. *Am. J. Ophthalmol.* **1999**, *127*, 1–7. [CrossRef]
10. Fukuoka, S.; Amano, S.; Honda, N.; Mimura, T.; Usui, T.; Araie, M. Effect of trabeculectomy on ocular and corneal higher order aberrations. *Jpn. J. Ophthalmol.* **2011**, *55*, 460–466. [CrossRef] [PubMed]
11. Kobayashi, N.; Hirooka, K.; Nitta, E.; Ukegawa, K.; Tsujikawa, A. Visual acuity and corneal higher-order aberrations after EX-PRESS or trabeculectomy, and the determination of associated factors that influence visual function. *Int. Ophthalmol.* **2018**, *38*, 1969–1976. [CrossRef] [PubMed]
12. Jo, S.H.; Seo, J.H. Short-term change in higher-order aberrations after mitomycin-C-augmented trabeculectomy. *Int. Ophthalmol.* **2019**, *39*, 175–188. [CrossRef] [PubMed]
13. Saheb, H.; Ahmed, I.I. Micro-invasive glaucoma surgery: Current perspectives and future directions. *Curr. Opin. Ophthalmol.* **2012**, *23*, 96–104. [CrossRef] [PubMed]
14. Oshika, T.; Okamoto, C.; Samejima, T.; Tokunaga, T.; Miyata, K. Contrast sensitivity function and ocular higher-order wavefront aberrations in normal human eyes. *Ophthalmol.* **2006**, *113*, 1807–1812. [CrossRef] [PubMed]
15. Manabe, S.; Sawaguchi, S.; Hayashi, K. The effect of the extent of the incision in the Schlemm canal on the surgical outcomes of suture trabeculotomy for open-angle glaucoma. *Jpn. J. Ophthalmol.* **2017**, *61*, 99–104. [CrossRef] [PubMed]

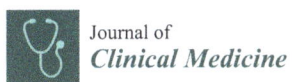

Article

Influence of Chronic Ocular Hypertension on Emmetropia: Refractive, Structural and Functional Study in Two Rat Models

Silvia Mendez-Martinez [1,2,*], Teresa Martínez-Rincón [1,2], Manuel Subias [1,2], Luis E. Pablo [1,2,3], David García-Herranz [4,5,6], Julian García Feijoo [3,7], Irene Bravo-Osuna [3,4,5], Rocío Herrero-Vanrell [3,4,5], Elena Garcia-Martin [1,2,3] and María J. Rodrigo [1,2,3]

[1] Department of Ophthalmology, Miguel Servet University Hospital, 50009 Zaragoza, Spain; teresamrincon@gmail.com (T.M.-R.); manusubias@gmail.com (M.S.); lpablo@unizar.es (L.E.P.); egmvivax@yahoo.com (E.G.-M.); mariajesusrodrigo@hotmail.es (M.J.R.)
[2] Miguel Servet Ophthalmology Research Group (GIMSO), Aragon Health Research Institute (IIS Aragon), 50009 Zaragoza, Spain
[3] National Ocular Pathology Network (OFTARED), Carlos III Health Institute, 28040 Madrid, Spain; jgarciafeijoo@hotmail.com (J.G.F.); ibravo@ucm.es (I.B.-O.); rociohv@farm.ucm.es (R.H.-V.)
[4] Innovation, Therapy and Pharmaceutical Development in Ophthalmology (InnOftal) Research Group, UCM 920415 Department of Pharmaceutics and Food Technology, Faculty of Pharmacy, Complutense University of Madrid, 28040 Madrid, Spain; davgar07@ucm.es
[5] Health Research Institute, San Carlos Clinical Hospital (IdISSC), 28040 Madrid, Spain
[6] University Institute for Industrial Pharmacy (IUFI), School of Pharmacy, Complutense University of Madrid, 28040 Madrid, Spain
[7] Department of Ophthalmology, San Carlos Clinical Hospital (IdISSC), Complutense University of Madrid, 28040 Madrid, Spain
* Correspondence: oftalmosmm@gmail.com; Tel.: +34-9-7676-5558

Citation: Mendez-Martinez, S.; Martínez-Rincón, T.; Subias, M.; Pablo, L.E.; García-Herranz, D.; Feijoo, J.G.; Bravo-Osuna, I.; Herrero-Vanrell, R.; Garcia-Martin, E.; Rodrigo, M.J. Influence of Chronic Ocular Hypertension on Emmetropia: Refractive, Structural and Functional Study in Two Rat Models. *J. Clin. Med.* 2021, 10, 3697. https://doi.org/10.3390/jcm10163697

Academic Editor: Maria Letizia Salvetat

Received: 19 July 2021
Accepted: 17 August 2021
Published: 20 August 2021

Publisher's Note: MDPI stays neutral with regard to jurisdictional claims in published maps and institutional affiliations.

Abstract: Chronic ocular hypertension (OHT) influences on refraction in youth and causes glaucoma in adulthood. However, the origin of the responsible mechanism is unclear. This study analyzes the effect of mild-moderate chronic OHT on refraction and neuroretina (structure and function) in young-adult Long-Evans rats using optical coherence tomography and electroretinography over 24 weeks. Data from 260 eyes were retrospectively analyzed in two cohorts: an ocular normotension (ONT) cohort (<20 mmHg) and an OHT cohort (>20 mmHg), in which OHT was induced either by sclerosing the episcleral veins (ES group) or by injecting microspheres into the anterior chamber. A trend toward emmetropia was found in both cohorts over time, though it was more pronounced in the OHT cohort ($p < 0.001$), especially in the ES group ($p = 0.001$) and males. IOP and refraction were negatively correlated at week 24 ($p = 0.010$). The OHT cohort showed early thickening in outer retinal sectors ($p < 0.050$) and the retinal nerve fiber layer, which later thinned. Electroretinography demonstrated early supranormal amplitudes and faster latencies that later declined. Chronic OHT accelerates emmetropia in Long–Evans rat eyes towards slowly progressive myopia, with an initial increase in structure and function that reversed over time.

Keywords: glaucoma; intraocular pressure; refractive error; neuroretina; myopia

1. Introduction

An increase in intraocular pressure (IOP) is the main factor for developing primary open-angle glaucoma (POAG), which leads to chronic progressive optic neuropathy and is a leading cause of irreversible blindness worldwide [1]. An association between POAG and high myopia was found, as highly myopic patients experience increased risk and earlier onset [2] of this sight-threatening disease [3–6]. The prevalence of myopia and high myopia (spherical equivalent less than −6.00 D) in the global population is currently 28.3%, and this is expected to increase by 2050 [7]. Highly myopic eyes suffer from structural changes such as peripheral retinal atrophic areas, tilted nerve appearance, temporal crescent of the optic disc [8], vitreoretinal traction, retinoschisis, lamellar or complete macular hole, retinal pigment epithelium (RPE) alterations and myopic choroidal neovascularization, lacquer cracks and chorioretinal atrophy, decreased choroidal thickness, scleral thinning with irregular curvature and staphyloma [9], and decreased retinal nerve fiber layer (RNFL) thickness, among others [10]. All these structural differences in myopic eyes are probably related to biomechanical stretching resulting from the imbalance between IOP and the elastic properties of the sclera [11–14]. Several animal and human studies have claimed the baropathic nature of axial myopia [15]. Indeed, several topical ocular hypotensive drugs were used in animal [16,17] and in human [18] studies to demonstrate the influence of IOP on axial length and refractive errors.

Unfortunately, POAG is difficult to diagnose in highly myopic eyes as the structural configuration of the optic nerve acts as a confounder variable in diagnostic tests such as spectral domain optical coherence tomography (SD-OCT), visual fields and electroretinography (ERG) [19–22]. Commercially available OCT devices still do not accurately measure RNFL thickness using automatic segmentation protocols in highly myopic eyes, exhibiting thinner average distributions in the superior, nasal, and inferior sectors, with greater temporal thickness, and a temporal shift in the superior and inferior peak locations [9].

To overcome the difficulties of structural diagnosis, OCT-based ganglion cell layer (GCL) analysis was proposed as a parameter for earlier detection of glaucomatous damage in myopic patients [23]. However, glaucoma is an aging-linked neurodegenerative pathology, so age could be a confounding factor in SD-OCT measurements. Indeed, animal studies showed contradictory results, with no definitive correlation between aging and thinning of the GCL [24–27] as detected in other neurodegenerative diseases [28], especially with the RNFL parameter [29–31]. Electrophysiological tests also showed functional impairment in patients affected by ocular hypertension, glaucoma, demyelinating optic neuropathies and Alzheimer's disease in both human [32] and animal studies [33,34], with a functional electrical deficit followed by structural tomographic thinning [35], even without visual dysfunction [34]. Hence, there is ample scope for studying the physiopathology of neurodegenerative diseases, aging, myopia and glaucoma.

The aim of this study is to analyze the impact of chronic ocular hypertension (OHT) on the refractive error, structure and function of the neuroretina in two different OHT-inducing animal models, comparing it with a control cohort presenting ocular normotension (ONT) over 24 weeks.

2. Materials and Methods

A retrospective study was conducted by collecting data from a proprietary database of animal glaucoma projects (PI17/01946, MAT2017-83858-C2-2). To investigate the impact of IOP on the eye, 260 rat eyes were classified as inclusion criteria into ONT (if IOP was <20 mmHg) or OHT (if IOP was >20 mmHg) cohorts.

2.1. Animals

Long–Evans rats (40% male, 60% female) were used for the study. All animals were four weeks old, their weights ranged from 50–100 g at the start of the study and were similar to that reported by the supplier (Janvier-labs, Le Genest-Saint-Isle, France) over the study. The animal study was carried out in the experimental surgery department of the Biomedical Research Center of Aragon (CIBA). The experiments were previously approved by the Ethics Committee for Animal Research (PI34/17) and were carried out in strict accordance with the Association for Research in Vision and Ophthalmology's Statement for the use of Animals.

The control ONT cohort included non-intervened eyes. The OHT cohort comprised the episcleral sclerosis (ES) group, in which OHT was induced by biweekly sclerosis of the episcleral veins with hypertonic (1.8M) solution as described [36]. The microspheres (MS) group, in which OHT was induced by injecting poly-lactic-acid-glycolic (PLGA) microspheres into the anterior chamber at baseline biweekly for the first month and then once monthly until week 20 as described [35,37]. All OHT injections were performed in the right eye under surgical conditions: controlled temperature, topical tetracaine (1 mg/mL + oxibuprocaine 4 mg/mL) eye drops (Anestesico doble Colirccusi®, Alcon Cusí® SA, Barcelona, Spain) and intraperitoneal (60 mg/kg of Ketamine + 0.25 mg/kg of Dexmedetomidine) anesthetic. Afterwards, the rats were left to recover in an enriched 2.5% oxygen atmosphere and were treated with antibiotic ointment (erythromycin 5 mg/g (Oftalmolosa Cusí® eritromicina, Alcon Cusí® SA, Barcelona, Spain)).

For detailed methodology characteristics, consult the original articles [27,35,37,38].

2.2. Intraocular Pressure

IOP measurements using a Tonolab® tonometer (Tonolab, TiolatOy Helsinki, Helsinki, Finland) were recorded in the morning every week. The IOP value was obtained from the average of 18 rebounds. This procedure was accomplished using a sedative mixture of 3% sevoflurane gas and 1.5% oxygen for less than 3 min in order to avoid hypotension effects [39].

2.3. Optical Coherence Tomography

SD-OCT (Spectralis, Heidelberg® Engineering, Heidelberg, Germany) was used to analyze the refractive status and the structure of the neuroretina over six months. Recordings were performed at the initial (0 weeks), middle (12 weeks) and end time of the study (24 weeks). In addition, an intermediate test was performed at week 8 of the study, which corresponds to 12 weeks of age of the rat. At this age, development and growth of the retina end and the retina reaches maturity [40]. A plane power polymethylmethacrylate (PMMA) contact lens with a thickness of 270 μm and a diameter of 5.2 mm (Cantor+Nissel®, Northamptonshire, UK) was adapted to the cornea to obtain high-quality images [41].

Refractive status was measured in diopters (D). The RNFL protocol was used for imaging acquisition. This protocol explores the optic nerve head, which is the most posterior structure of the rat eye, as the eye is elongated. Retinal images were adjusted and acquired by focusing on the retinal vascular structure. The diopters obtained through focusing were then analyzed as the diopter power of the eyeball.

Structural analysis: The RNFL, retina posterior pole (R) and GCL protocol with automatic segmentation were used to quantify neuroretinal thickness (in micrometers). These protocols analyze an area of 1, 2 and 3 mm around the center of the optic disc using 61 scans. Subsequent follow-up examinations were acquired at the same location using the eye-tracking software and follow-up application. Biased examinations were discarded or manually corrected by a masked, trained technician if the algorithm had obviously erred. The R and GCL analyzed the 9 ETDRS areas (central area and inner or outer sectors divided into inferior, superior, nasal, and temporal sectors) and the total volume. The RNFL protocol analyzed 6 peripapillary sectors (inferotemporal, temporal, superotemporal, superonasal, nasal, and inferonasal).

For ERG and OCT acquisition, the rats were anesthetized by intraperitoneal administration of 60 mg/kg of Ketamine + 0.25 mg/kg of Dexmedetomidine.

2.4. Electroretinography

Electroretinography performed to analyze the outer and inner neuroretinal cells' functionality at weeks 0, 12 and 24. The electroretinography device (Roland consult® RETIanimal ERG, Brandenburg an der Havel, Germany) was used to stimulate simultaneously both eyes and explore them in multisteps using the flash scotopic and the photopic negative response (PhNR) protocols. Scotopic test examined rod response: step 1: −40 dB, 0.0003 cds/m², 0.2 Hz (20 recordings averaged); step 2: −30 dB, 0.003 cds/m², 0.125 Hz (18 recordings averaged); step 3: −20 dB, 0.03 cds/m², 8.929 Hz (14 recordings averaged); step 4: −20 dB, 0.03 cds/m², 0.111 Hz (15 recordings averaged). Photopic test examined retinal ganglion cell functionality: blue background 470 nm, 25 cds/m² and red LED flash

625 nm, 0.30 cds/m^2, 1.199 Hz (20 recordings averaged). For this purpose, the animals were prepared and the ERG tests were performed as [27,35] described.

2.5. Statistical Analysis

Statistical analysis was performed by a blinded researcher. Descriptive analysis of quantitative variables was performed using (mean ± standard deviation [SD]). As the Kolmogorov–Smirnov test showed a no normal distribution of the variables, comparisons between both the ONT and OHT cohorts and ES and MS groups were conducted using the non-parametric Mann–Whitney U test and comparisons among the ONT, ES and MS cohorts were made using the Kruskal–Wallis H test. Eyes in every cohort were divided into two groups: those with a diopter power higher or lower than 17 D for the ONT eyes and 6 D for the OHT eyes. These sub-groups were used to study the logistic regression to the model so that correlations between refraction and OCT parameters or IOP values could be made. Correlations with the refractive status of the eye, age, OCT thicknesses, and ERG parameters were performed using Spearman correlation coefficient and logistic regression analysis. p values < 0.05 were considered statistical significative; the Bonferroni correction for multiple comparisons was also calculated to avoid a high false-positive rate.

3. Results

A total of 260 eyes of Long–Evans rats were analyzed from two different cohorts: 74 eyes with an IOP lower than 20 mmHg (ONT cohort serving as control), and 186 eyes with an IOP higher than 20 mmHg, named the OHT cohort, which in turn was divided into two sub-groups by induced OHT model: 62 eyes based on the ES model and 124 eyes based on the biodegradable MS model.

3.1. IOP Analysis

Comparing ONT and OHT cohorts. ONT eyes (16.09 ± 2.25 mmHg (range: 13.37–17.62 mmHg)) showed statistically significant ($p < 0.05$) lower IOP than OHT eyes (23.66 ± 1.40 mmHg (range 21.44–26.74 mmHg)). **Comparing both OHT groups**. The ES group presented the highest IOP values up to week 12, after which the trend reversed ($p < 0.001$) (Figure 1a). Analyzing by sex, males suffered from slightly higher IOP values in both the ONT and OHT groups, and reached statistical significance at weeks 8, 10 and 16 ($p = 0.022$, $p < 0.001$ and $p = 0.023$, respectively) (Figure 1b).

3.2. Refraction

Comparing ONT and OHT cohorts. Both the ONT and OHT cohorts experienced a physiological trend toward emmetropia throughout the follow-up, especially over the first weeks of the study; from 35.16 ± 6.38 D at baseline (Table S1 Supplementary Materials) to 11.87 ± 3.21 D in the ONT and 11.98 ± 5.21 in the OHT at 8 weeks. However, the OHT cohort exhibited lower refractive power that reached statistical significance at week 24 (+4.54 ± 1.5 D in the ONT cohort vs.+0.88 ± 2.36 D in the OHT cohort, $p < 0.001$) (Figure 2). **Comparing both OHT groups**. A small difference between both OHT groups was also detected ($p = 0.001$), with slightly lower dioptric values for the ES group (+1.66 ± 1.53 D in MS vs. +0.10 ± 2.91 D in ES) (Figure 2a). No statistically significant differences were found in refraction between sexes ($p > 0.05$), although males consistently presented lower dioptric power throughout the follow-up, especially in the OHT cohort (Figure 2b).

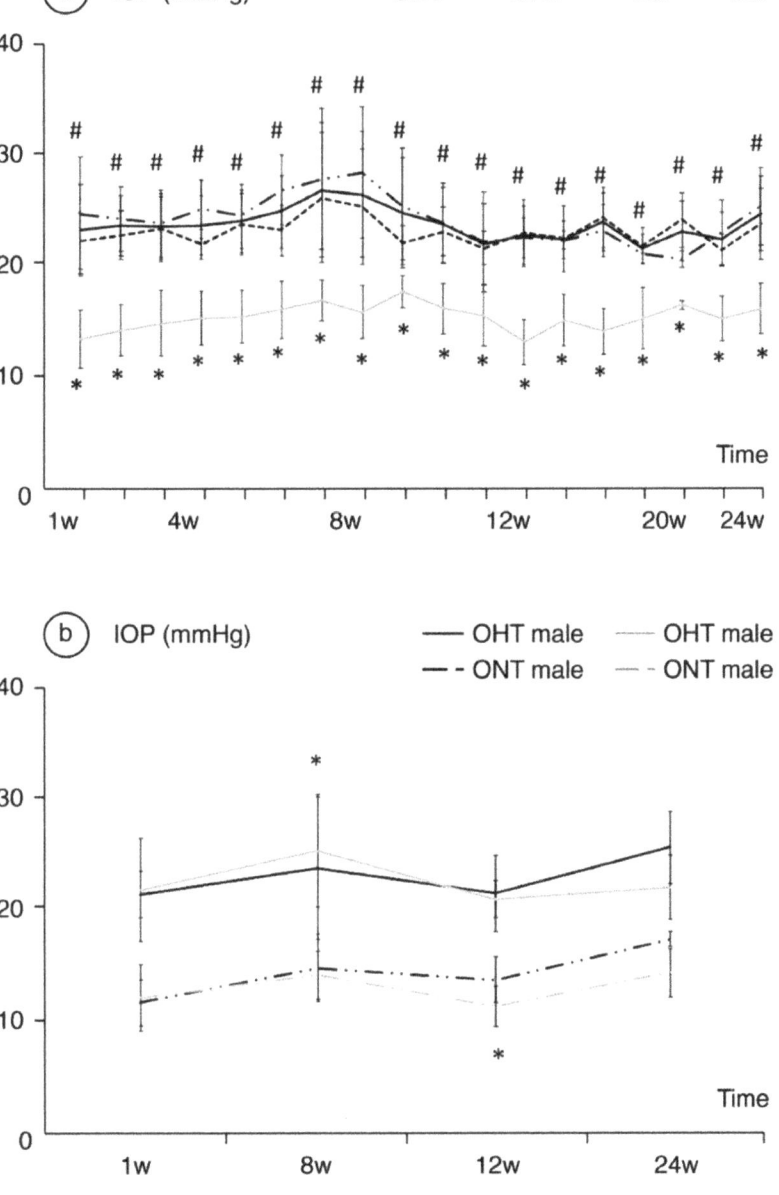

Figure 1. Analysis of intraocular pressure (IOP) in mmHg over the 24-week follow-up comparing the ocular normotension (ONT) and ocular hypertension (OHT) cohorts (**a**) and comparing both sexes (**b**). Abbreviations: w: week; ES: episcleral sclerosis group; MS: microspheres group; * statistical differences between the ONT and the OHT cohorts; #: statistical differences between the ES and MS groups.

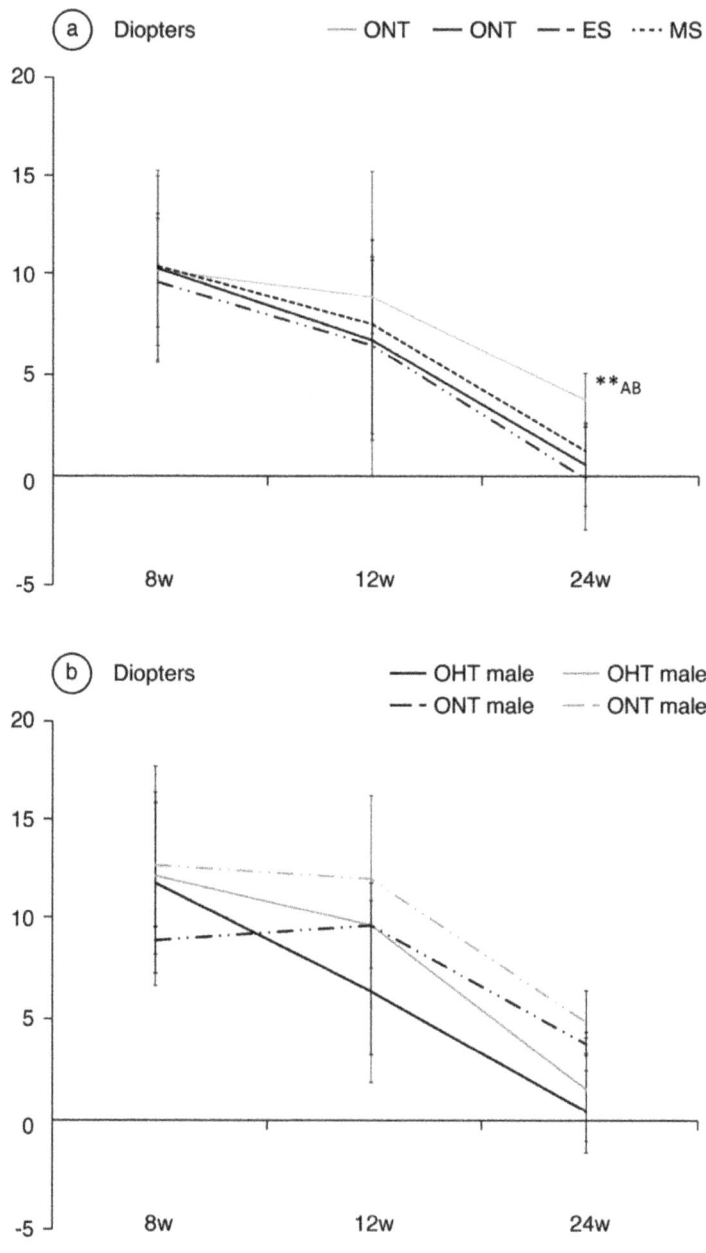

Figure 2. Analysis of refractive power in diopters over the 24-week follow-up, comparing the ocular normotension (ONT) and ocular hypertension (OHT) cohorts (**a**) and comparing both sexes (**b**). Abbreviations: w: week; ES: episcleral sclerosis group; MS: microspheres group; **: statistical differences between groups (ONT vs.ES vs. MS) (Kruskal Wallis); A: statistical differences between ONT and ES; B: statistical differences between ONT and MS.

3.3. Analysis of the Correlation between Refraction, Ocular Hypertension, and OCT Parameters

There were no statistically significant correlations between the OCT values and the refractive status of the eye. IOP > 20 mmHg at week 24 was positively correlated to lower dioptric values with a B coefficient of 4.01 ($p = 0.01$) for the OHT cohort vs. 4.65 ($p = 0.009$) for the ONT cohort.

3.4. OCT Analysis

Comparing ONT and OHT cohorts. The most significant differences were found in week 8, when the OHT cohort exhibited thicker R values in the inner temporal sector and all the outer sectors (Table 1). The highest percentage differences by sector also followed the glaucomatous rule inferior > superior > nasal > temporal until week 12. The ONT cohort experienced a progressive decrease in RNFL thickness over time, and the OHT cohort showed an increase in RNFL thickness at week 12 in both the ES and MS groups (Figure 3). **Comparing both OHT groups**. Differences between the ONT and OHT cohorts were usually related to the values found in the MS group.

Table 1. Statistically significant differences found by optical coherence tomography parameters analyzed at weeks 8, 12 and 24.

Time	OCT Protocol	Sector	ONT (Mean ± SD in μm)	OHT (Mean ± SD in μm)	D%	p *		OHT Groups (Mean ± SD in μm)	p †
8 W	R	Central	277.20 ± 17.86	**263.21 ± 22.03**	−5.05	0.022	MS	263.80 ± 22.89	0.022
							ES	**260.30 ± 17.86**	
		Temporal Inner	**244.70 ± 8.35**	251.90 ± 18.50	+2.86	0.047	MS	**250.78 ± 14.82**	0.047
							ES	257.50 ± 31.74	
		Inferior Outer	**239.90 ± 6.19**	250.50 ± 11.13	+4.23	0.003	MS	251.40 ± 11.34	0.003
							ES	**246.00 ± 9.30**	
		Nasal Outer	**243.30 ± 4.34**	253.60 ± 12.85	+4.06	0.002	MS	253.96 ± 11.84	0.002
							ES	**251.90 ± 17.60**	
		Superior Outer	**246.30 ± 4.19**	256.86 ± 17.28	+4.13	0.017	MS	257.04 ± 16.69	0.017
							ES	**256.00 ± 20.89**	
		Temporal Outer	**245.00 ± 6.48**	254.10 ± 16.10	+3.58	0.013	MS	**253.12 ± 12.17**	0.013
							ES	259.00 ± 29.37	
	GCL	Central	19.80 ± 3.39	**17.03 ± 3.34**	−13.99	0.014	MS	**16.78 ± 3.27**	0.014
							ES	18.30 ± 3.62	
		Superior Inner	24.10 ± 1.85	**20.91 ± 4.03**	−13.24	0.004	MS	**20.53 ± 4.04**	0.004
							ES	22.80 ± 3.61	
12 W	R	Central	285.33 ± 18.90	**266.00 ± 16.73**	−6.76	0.039	MS	267.33 ± 17.21	0.039
							ES	**265.56 ± 17.61**	
24 W	RNFL	Nasal Superior	39.27 ± 7.25	28.88 ± 11.99	−26.46	0.036	MS	31.00 ± 10.66	0.050
							ES	**27.60 ± 13.10**	

OCT: optical coherence tomography; R: retina; GCL: ganglion cell layer complex; RNFL: retinal nerve fiber layer; W: week; ONT: ocular normotension cohort; OHT: ocular hypertension cohort; ES: episcleral sclerosis group; MS: microspheres group; D%: differences in percentage; p: statistical differences (<0.05): * U Mann Whitney; † Kruskal Wallis; the lowest thickness values are highlighted in bold.

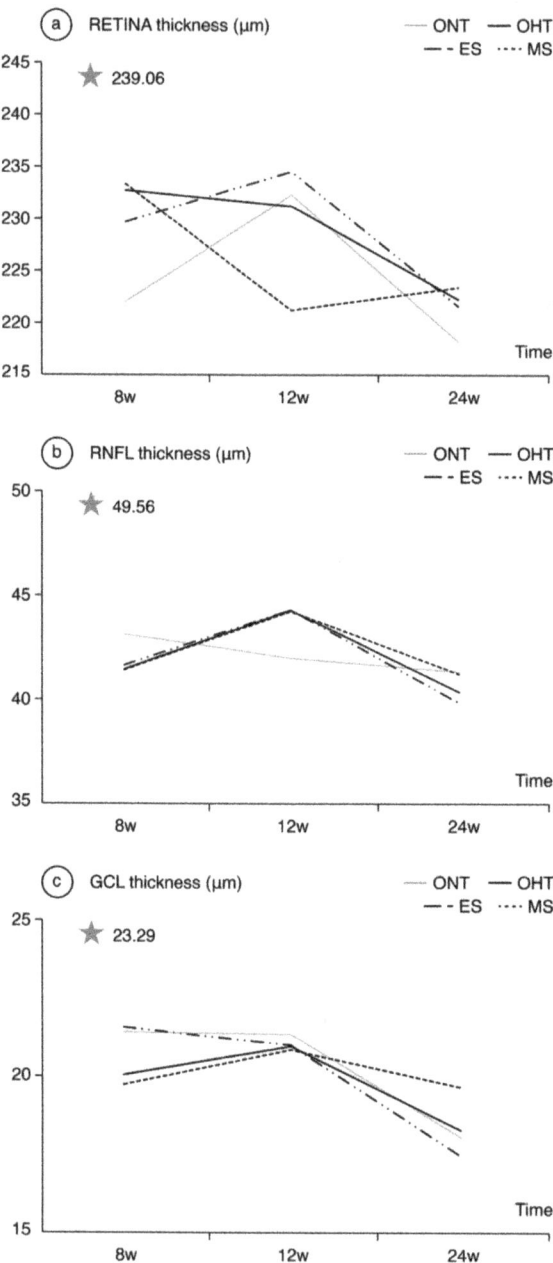

Figure 3. Neuroretinal thickness measured by optical coherence tomography in both the ocular normotension and ocular hypertension cohorts and the ocular hypertension sub-groups at 8, 12, 24 weeks follow-up. (**a**) Retina thickness, (**b**) Retina nerve fiber layer thickness, (**c**) Ganglion cell layer thickness. The analysis is based on the mean values of all the OCT sectors. ONT: ocular normotension cohort; OHT: ocular hypertension cohort; ES: episcleral sclerosis group; MS: microspheres group; RNFL: retinal nerve fiber layer; GCL: ganglion cell layer; μm: thickness in micrometers; W: week; star: baseline thickness.

3.5. ERG Analysis

Comparing ONT and OHT cohorts. The ONT cohort presented wider variability in subject responses compared to the OHT cohort (Figures 4–6). In the OHT cohort, a stronger response was found in scotopic and photopic conditions in week 12, with shorter latencies (Figures 4a, 5a and 6a) and greater amplitudes (Figures 4b, 5b and 6b). However, maintenance of hypertension over time (week 24) decreased the electrical signal in the ERG, which almost matched the ONT values, especially in the later stages. **Comparing both OHT groups.** Generally, the MS groups exhibited faster latency and greater amplitude in week 12 in scotopic and photopic conditions, although this trend reversed in week 24.

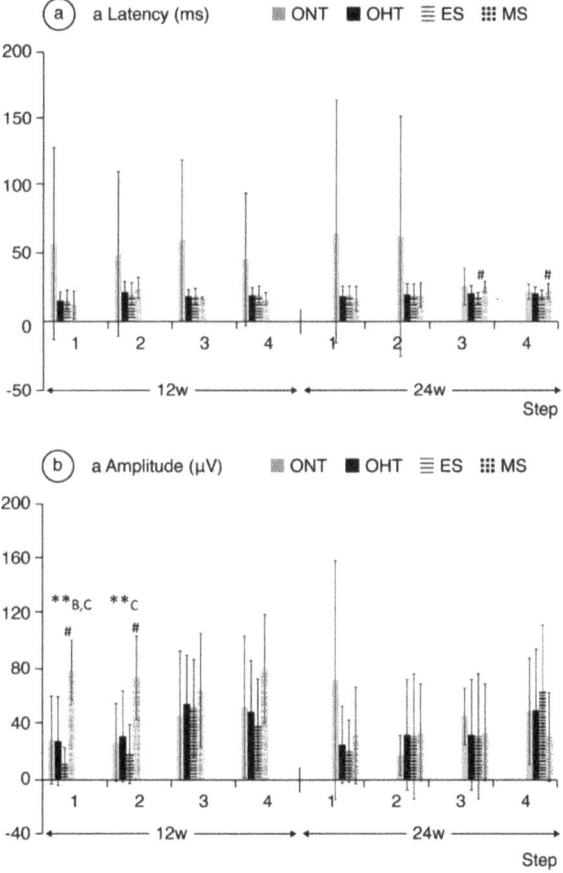

Figure 4. a-wave electroretinographic response in both the ocular normotension and ocular hypertension cohorts and the ocular hypertension sub-groups at weeks 12 and 24. (**a**) a-latency in milliseconds of photoreceptors under scotopic conditions. (**b**) a-amplitude in microvolts of photoreceptors under scotopic conditions. Abbreviations: ONT: ocular normotension group; OHT: ocular hypertension group; ES: episcleral sclerosis group; MS: microspheres group; w: week; ms: milliseconds; μV: microvolts; **: statistical differences between groups (ONT vs. ES vs. MS) (Kruskal–Wallis); #: statistical differences between the ES and MS groups; A: statistical differences between ONT and ES; B: statistical differences between ONT and MS; C: statistical differences between ES and MS. Scotopic test (rod response): step 1: −40 dB, 0.0003 cds/m^2, 0.2 Hz (20 recordings averaged); step 2: −30 dB, 0.003 cds/m^2, 0.125 Hz (18 recordings averaged); step 3: −20 dB, 0.03 cds/m^2, 8.929 Hz (14 recordings averaged); step 4: −20 dB, 0.03 cds/m^2, 0.111 Hz (15 recordings averaged).

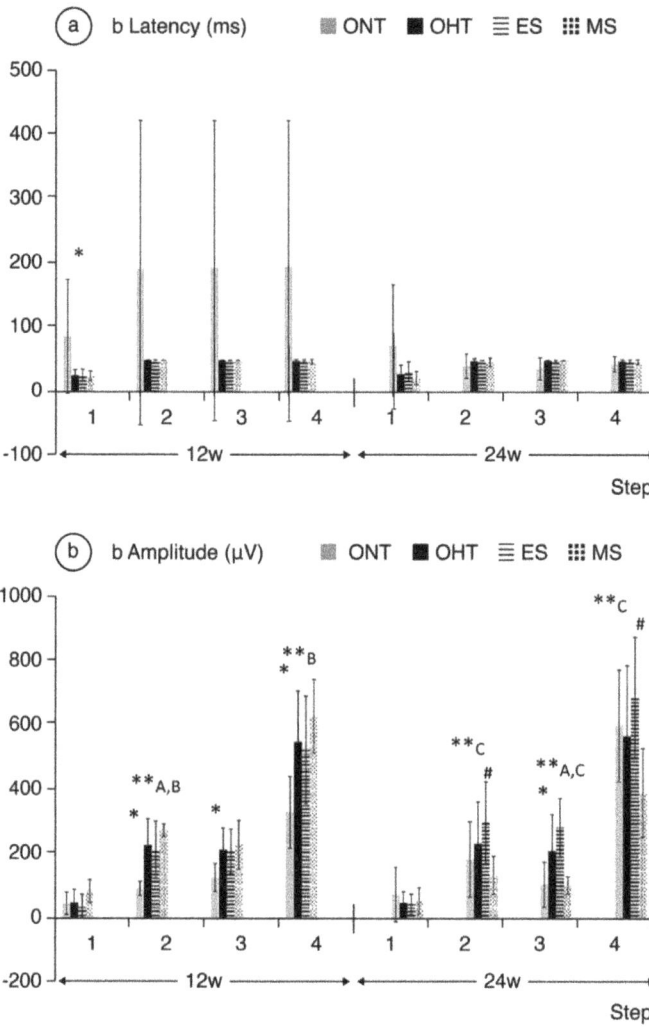

Figure 5. b-wave electroretinographic response in both the ocular normotension and ocular hypertension cohorts and the ocular hypertension sub-groups at weeks 12 and 24. (**a**) b-latency in milliseconds of intermediate cells under scotopic conditions. (**b**) b-amplitude in microvolts of intermediate cells under scotopic conditions. ONT: ocular normotension group; OHT: ocular hypertension group; ES: episcleral sclerosis group; MS: microspheres group; w: week; ms: milliseconds; μV: microvolts; * statistical differences between the ONT and OHT cohorts. **: statistical differences between groups (ONT vs. ES vs. MS) (Kruskal–Wallis); #: statistical differences between the ES and MS groups; A: statistical differences between ONT and ES; B: statistical differences between ONT and MS; C: statistical differences between ES and MS. Scotopic test (rod response): step 1: −40 dB, 0.0003 cds/m², 0.2 Hz (20 recordings averaged); step 2: −30 dB, 0.003 cds/m², 0.125 Hz (18 recordings averaged); step 3: −20 dB, 0.03 cds/m², 8.929 Hz (14 recordings averaged); step 4: −20 dB, 0.03 cds/m², 0.111 Hz (15 recordings averaged).

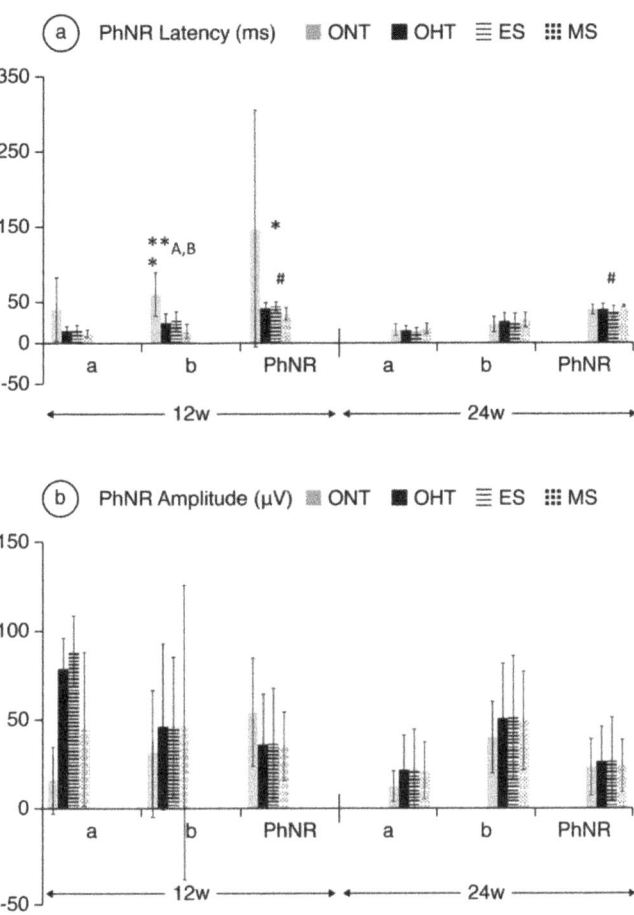

Figure 6. PhNR wave electroretinographic response in both the ocular normotension and ocular hypertension cohorts and the ocular hypertension sub-groups at weeks 12 and 24. (**a**) PhNR latency of in milliseconds under photopic conditions. (**b**) PhRN amplitude in microvolts under photopic conditions. Abbreviations: ONT: ocular normotension group; OHT: ocular hypertension group; ES: episcleral sclerosis group; MS: microspheres group; w: week; ms: milliseconds; μV: microvolts; * statistical differences between the ONT and OHT cohorts. **: statistical differences between groups (ONT vs. ES vs. MS) (Kruskal–Wallis); #: statistical differences between the ES and MS groups; A: Statistical differences between ONT and ES; B: Statistical differences between ONT and MS. Photopic test: blue background 470 nm, 25 cds/m^2 and red LED flash 625 nm, 0.30 cds/m^2, 1.199 Hz (20 recordings averaged). a: photoreceptors response; b: intermediate cells response; PhNR: ganglion cells response.

4. Discussion

The effects of ocular hypertension have been described in a multitude of short-term animal studies, generally up to a maximum of 8 weeks of follow-up [37,42–44]. This study analyzes the effect of chronic OHT maintained over time focusing the study between 8 and 24 weeks of chronicity. To our knowledge, this is the first retrospective longitudinal 24-week study carried out in young-adult Long-Evans rats in vivo using automatically segmented OCT images that analyze the effect of mild-moderate OHT (between 20–30 mmHg) on refraction from the neuroretinal perspective (structure and function) and employs two different OHT-inducing models (ES vs. MS), in comparison to healthy controls. This allows us to analyze the neurodegenerative process in conditions of chronic OHT on myopia.

4.1. Refractive Analysis

The total optic power of the eye depends on factors such as axial length, corneal power and lens power. At birth, human eyes are usually hyperopic, and afterwards there is a trend toward emmetropia as the cornea structure stabilizes, though axial length may continue to grow until the second decade. However, in high myopia there is continuous, progressive axial elongation throughout life, possibly due to genetic, environmental and behavioral factors [45,46]. Although all the mechanisms involved in this progressive enlargement of the eyeball are not completely understood, the effect of IOP on axial elongation of the posterior pole [47,48], the importance of sclera stiffness [49] and the dynamic responses of the sclera after a chronic increase in IOP [50] have been factors involved in the emmetropization process.

Ocular hypertension in congenital glaucoma occurs in developing loose tissue, meaning the sclera still exhibit great plasticity and stretch, increasing axial length [51]. This is similar to what occurs in high myopia [52,53], which supports the incidence of high myopia in adulthood [54]. When ocular hypertension occurs in older ages, scleral tissues are more rigid and stiffen [55], explaining the greater glaucomatous damage (IOP spikes are more poorly mitigated by less elastic sclera), the outward shift of the lamina cribosa and remodeling of connective tissue [56], and the deeper anterior chamber described in both the ES model and DBA/2J glaucomatous mice (not observed in OHT models using cauterization, probably due to the experimental intervention itself) [57,58]. Indeed, there is increasing evidence about the development of delayed and sustained OHT associated with repeated intravitreal anti-vascular endothelial growth factor injections in retinal diseases, such as age-related macular degeneration [59,60]. Several structure optic nerve head manifestations after intravitreal volume injections have been lately described as a mechanical displacement of the optic nerve head and canal expansion, with a widening and deepening of the optic, a prelaminar tissue thinning and a Bruch membrane opening expansion, suggesting structural changes after IOP and volume increase in aged patients, with rigid sclera [61]. Our experiments started when the rats were 4 weeks old, so they should not be considered either adults or newborns, but young rats. The refractive status was likewise not consistent with high myopia (−6 D) so, in our opinion, eye elongation was presumably more similar to what occurs in human POAG. Our OHT models supported the pre-existing evidence, as the ES cohort presented higher IOP, greater axonal damage, and lower dioptric power.

This study demonstrated the influence of sustained mild–moderate IOP on the emmetropization process. The baseline optical power was 35.16 ± 6.28 D (as [62] reported), with a progressive trend toward emmetropia in both ONT and OHT eyes. However, the statistically significant correlations to refraction were found only with mild–moderate OHT at week 24 in both ES and MS models, and were not found with functional or structural alterations. Therefore, a chronic sustained increase in IOP was considered the main risk factor involved in the loss of refractive power in OHT eyes. In this regard, animal and human studies also correlated hypotensive treatments such as trabeculectomy [63] and topical drugs such as latanoprost [16] to a decrease in total axial length, although studies with drugs such as timolol showed inconsistencies in both human [18] and animal models [17]. One of the next steps worth studying in future prospective studies is the influence of prompt normalization of IOP on refraction in these OHT models as a possible treatment for myopia.

Nowadays, high myopia is increasingly prevalent in populations that carry out near-vision activities [64,65]. Sharp focus on a near image requires concomitant activation of both inferior and medial rectus muscles, and the subsequent compression of the eyeball by both muscles may cause an increase in IOP [66], similar to what happens in other compressive pathologies [67,68]. In addition, greatest drainage of aqueous humor occurs mainly via the nasal and lower episcleral veins [69–73], so sustained compression of these muscles at these locations during near-vision activities for extended periods of time would increase IOP. Moreover, in childhood and early adulthood, when eye elongation is easily achieved as it is less rigid, refractive power may consequently decrease [74]. Indeed, lower dioptric power would require higher demand for more synkinesis accommodation/convergence, creating a vicious circle [75]. Current studies with atropine drops are showing promising results in controlling myopia by producing a reversible anti-accommodative effect [76,77], and the dose-dependent anti-muscarinic effect on the smooth muscles of the episcleral veins could also balance the outflow.

In this study, the ES model, in which the outflow of the episcleral veins is limited, induced higher IOP and higher negative dioptric power. MS model produced a progressive alteration of the trabecular meshwork due to the mechanical clogging [78], but in a slower and more progressive structural and functional damage, more similar to that of the human POAG, and a lower negative dioptric power [35]. Moreover, a trend toward higher dioptric power was found in females, as well as lower levels of IOP, attributed to estrogens [79]. Scleral stiffness depends on choroidal vascular factors, among others, so estrogens could contribute to vascular protection against peripapillary rigidity and posterior location of the optic nerve head, which could explain the higher myopia rates found in male rats.

To our knowledge, this is the first study that longitudinally monitors eye growth in vivo (by indirect study of optical power) using non-invasive, simple, objective OCT technology that demonstrates progressive myopization in glaucomatous rats, influenced by sex and the OHT-inducing model. Refractive study in small animals usually requires invasive, expensive or low-reliability techniques such as enucleation, magnetic resonance imaging or ultrasound biomicroscopy, respectively, which makes longitudinal studies with the same animal impracticable. Previous ocular biometric studies using OCT on healthy [80,81] and glaucomatous mice [50,82] have been performed. However, only one study of healthy rats measured biometrics in vivo using high-resolution A-scan ultrasonography [62], and no convincing evidence of emmetropization during normal eye development was detected. Similar results were found in this study, in which the ONT cohort never experienced negative optical power (myopia), unlike rats in the OHT cohort.

Analysis of refractive status constitutes a methodological limitation. As it was a retrospective study, it was not designed to analyze axial length, so the refractive status of the eye was measured with the OCT focuser, which improves image quality when acquiring OCT scans. The value obtained via this method is acceptable, but less accurate than axial length. Moreover, the use of a rigid contact lens for OCT imaging from which the retinal focusing data were obtained, introduces a tear lens, whose power will vary according to the mismatch between the fixed, posterior radius of curvature of the lens and anterior corneal radius, which can be expected to increase with age, and may also be altered in response to intracameral injections of MS. However, the lens was used in each examination, so the induced error would be constant, and the refractive trend found in our results would be constant throughout the study.

4.2. Structural Analysis

A decrease in RNFL thickness is a common feature in both myopic [83] and glaucomatous patients, though RNFL segmentation errors in automated SD-OCT analysis are frequent in myopia [84]. The good correlation observed between GCL and RNFL analysis has surpassed total retinal quantification, and GCL analysis has emerged as a more appropriate imaging tool for detecting early glaucomatous progression in myopic patients [85].

When analyzing the R, RNFL and GCL values, OCT protocols were performed around the optic disc as rats do not have macula, so central values could lead to misinterpretations. This is one of the main reasons why correlations to human retina are limited. As regards general trends, differences in R thickness between the ONT and OHT cohorts were seen up to week 8, although they then decreased through week 24, possibly due to a neurodegenerative process, with an initial inflammatory response that causes an increase in thickness (activated microglia and other inflammatory mediators [31]), and a final atrophic pattern. The greater thickness found in external sectors of peripheral retina could be attributed to peripheral immune infiltration [31]. On the other hand, it is important to highlight that there were no correlations between refraction and R, GCL, and RNFL thicknesses. IOP was therefore the most important factor modifying retinal thickness, meaning that the RNFL thinning observed in the OHT cohorts in week 24 was secondary to neurodegeneration rather than a stretching of the retinal tissue. Hence, OCT has demonstrated its reliability when analyzing retinal structures in neurodegenerative diseases [28], even during the emmetropization process.

Comparing both OHT groups, the ES group exhibited thicker R, RNFL and GCL values at week 8, but the thickness loss rate was also higher over time, reaching the lowest thickness at the end of follow-up. As this cohort suffered from higher IOP levels, these eyes could have suffered intense damage (a more extreme response) at GCL level that explains this drop. Conversely, RNFL analysis of the OHT cohorts showed an initial increase in thickness until week 12, after which the trend reversed in both groups, although it did so more dramatically in the ES group, supporting this theory.

The lack of histological studies is the main handicap of structural analysis, but several studies reflected the good correlation between immunohistochemistry and OCT thicknesses, making SD-OCT reliable for research in retinal degeneration [28]. Another limitation of this study was not having considered the lateral magnification that occurs as the anterior chamber increases, which overstates the retinal thickness. Most myopic eyes may therefore have even smaller retinal thicknesses [86].

4.3. Functional Analysis

ERG showed supranormal responses in the OHT cohorts, especially in the MS group in week 12. These outcomes were also observed in other animal studies with acute [43,47] and chronic [48] non-ischemic increases in IOP. This noxa could lead to initial hyperstimulation of the neuronal structures, especially bipolar and intermediate cells, while the process is neither ischemic nor chronic. In other words, we are possibly witnessing the beginning of the disease in an early or even reversible phase. However, this initially stronger electrical response disappeared at week 24, suggesting the decline of this phenomenon, probably due to ischemia or neurodegenerative damage, as occurs in POAG. It has also been hypothesized that the supranormal ERG responses could be related to the increase in illuminated retinal area during the test (greater axial length means greater retinal area, compared to normal axial length), though this hypothesis could not explain all the ERG findings [44], among them the fact that the supranormal electrical response is not sustained over time, but only when the eye is more hyperopic (in early phases of the study). In contrast, human studies showed a negative correlation between axial length (but not refractive error) and the values of ERG responses in healthy adults [20,87], as occurs here at later stages. This pattern of electrical response was more extreme in the MS group and was consistent throughout the steps, showing a coherent pattern of electrical behavior in photoreceptor and bipolar cells. However, because the ES model is more aggressive, this suprasignal could have occurred before week 12 in the ES model. We may therefore have witnessed an ongoing decay phase.

This functional behavior could be somehow correlated to the structural OCT findings of this study. At week 12, the GCL and RNFL are not as damaged, and their status is reversible, which could be correlated to the ERG hyperresponsive pattern. This could be supported by a previous study (also using Long–Evans rats) with a similar electrical pattern after chronic IOP elevation (by circumlimbal suture) that returned to baseline after suture removal [88]. This functional damage was not correlated with structural damage to GCL density, but with a reduction in the RNFL in week 15 in the post-hoc analysis [88]. Again, it is important to note that the only parameter that was statistically correlated to the refraction was IOP > 20 mmHg, not the ERG parameters. Our results therefore suggest that refractive status also appears to be an independent factor for ERG tests when analyzing POAG.

5. Conclusions

In this article, we pointed out the relationship between ocular hypertension and refraction over time. Visual disturbances in glaucomatous patients could also be associated with a progressive negative refractive error, in addition to the neurodegenerative damage associated with glaucoma, so frequent assessment of refraction may be important in these patients over time. The study of functional and structural tests in early and late stages in two different POAG models produced a deeper understanding of the pathophysiological retinal damage caused by the increase in IOP, with an initial increase in electrical signal associated with a thickening pattern detected using OCT, followed by functional and structural impairment. In addition, the lack of correlation between the refractive status of the eye and the structure and function of the retina provided further insight into the usefulness of OCT and ERG in relation to the emmetropia process.

Supplementary Materials: The following are available online at https://www.mdpi.com/article/10 .3390/jcm10163697/s1, Table S1: Baseline characteristics of the study.

Author Contributions: Conceptualization, M.J.R., L.E.P. and E.G.-M.; methodology, M.J.R., S.M.-M. and E.G.-M.; software, E.G.-M.; validation, M.J.R., and E.G.-M.; formal analysis E.G.-M.; investigation, S.M.-M., T.M.-R., M.S., M.J.R.; resources, L.E.P., J.G.F., I.B.-O., R.H.-V., E.G.-M.; data curation, S.M.-M., T.M.-R., M.S., M.J.R., D.G.-H.; writing—original draft preparation, S.M.-M.; writing—review and editing, S.M.-M. and M.J.R.; visualization, S.M.-M. and M.J.R.; supervision, E.G.-M., M.J.R.; project administration, E.G.-M., L.E.P., M.J.R.; funding acquisition, E.G.-M., L.E.P. All authors have read and agreed to the published version of the manuscript.

Funding: This research was funded by Rio Hortega Research Grants M17/00213, PI17/01726, PI17/01946 and PI20/00437 (Carlos III Health Institute), and by MAT2017-83858-C2-2, MAT2017-83858-C2-1 and PID2020-113281RB-C2-2 MINECO/AEI/ERDF, EU, UCM Research Group 920415, ISCIII-FEDER "Una manera de hacer Europa" RETICS Oftared, RD16/0008/0004, RD16/0008/0009, and RD16/0008/029. D.G.H. acknowledges a UCM-Santander fellowship (CT17/17-CT17-18).

Institutional Review Board Statement: The study was conducted according to the guidelines of the Declaration of Helsinki, and approved by the Ethics Committee for Animal Research (PI34/17) and were carried out in strict accordance with the Association for Research in Vision and Ophthalmology's Statement for the use of Animals.

Informed Consent Statement: Not applicable.

Data Availability Statement: The data are available only upon request to the corresponding author.

Conflicts of Interest: The authors declare no conflict of interest. The funders had no role in the design of the study; in the collection, analyses, or interpretation of data; in the writing of the manuscript, or in the decision to publish the results.

References

1. Agis Investigators. The Advanced Glaucoma Intervention Study (AGIS): 7. The relationship between control of intraocular pressure and visual field deterioration.The AGIS Investigators. *Am. J. Ophthalmol.* **2000**, *130*, 429–440. [CrossRef]
2. Shim, S.H.; Sung, K.R.; Kim, J.M.; Kim, H.T.; Jeong, J.; Kim, C.Y.; Lee, M.Y.; Park, K.H. Korean Ophthalmological Society the Prevalence of Open-Angle Glaucoma by Age in Myopia: The Korea National Health and Nutrition Examination Survey. *Curr. Eye Res.* **2017**, *42*, 65–71. [CrossRef] [PubMed]
3. Wong, T.Y.; Klein, B.E.K.; Klein, R.; Knudtson, M.; Lee, K.E. Refractive errors, intraocular pressure, and glaucoma in a white population. *Ophthalmology* **2003**, *110*, 211–217. [CrossRef]
4. Xu, L.; Wang, Y.; Wang, S.; Wang, Y.; Jonas, J.B. High myopia and glaucoma susceptibility the Beijing Eye Study. *Ophthalmology* **2007**, *114*, 216–220. [CrossRef] [PubMed]
5. Ikuno, Y. Overview of the Complications of High Myopia. *Retina* **2017**, *37*, 2347–2351. [CrossRef]
6. Saw, S.M.; Gazzard, G.; Shin-Yen, E.C.; Chua, W.H. Myopia and associated pathological complications. *Ophthalmic Physiol. Opt.* **2005**, *25*, 381–391. [CrossRef]

7. Holden, B.A.; Fricke, T.R.; Wilson, D.A.; Jong, M.; Naidoo, K.S.; Sankaridurg, P.; Wong, T.Y.; Naduvilath, T.J.; Resnikoff, S. Global Prevalence of Myopia and High Myopia and Temporal Trends from 2000 through 2050. *Ophthalmology* **2016**, *123*, 1036–1042. [CrossRef]

8. Kim, T.-W.; Kim, M.; Weinreb, R.N.; Woo, S.J.; Park, K.H.; Hwang, J.-M. Optic Disc Change with Incipient Myopia of Childhood. *Ophthalmology* **2012**, *119*, 21.e3–26.e3. [CrossRef] [PubMed]

9. Ng, D.S.C.; Cheung, C.Y.L.; Luk, F.O.; Mohamed, S.; Brelen, M.E.; Yam, J.C.S.; Tsang, C.W.; Lai, T.Y.Y. Advances of optical coherence tomography in myopia and pathologic myopia. *Eye* **2016**, *30*, 901–916. [CrossRef]

10. Leung, C.K.S.; Mohamed, S.; Leung, K.S.; Cheung, C.Y.L.; Chan, S.L.W.; Cheng, D.K.Y.; Lee, A.K.C.; Leung, G.Y.O.; Rao, S.K.; Lam, D.S.C. Retinal nerve fiber layer measurements in myopia: An optical coherence tomography study. *Investig. Ophthalmol. Vis. Sci.* **2006**, *47*, 5171–5176. [CrossRef] [PubMed]

11. Schmid, K.L.; Hills, T.; Abbott, M.; Humphries, M.; Pyne, K.; Wildsoet, C.F. Relationship between intraocular pressure and eye growth in chick. *Ophthalmic Physiol. Opt.* **2003**, *23*, 25–33. [CrossRef] [PubMed]

12. Read, S.A.; Collins, M.J.; Annis-Brown, T.; Hayward, N.M.; Lillyman, K.; Sherwin, D.; Stockall, P. The short-term influence of elevated intraocular pressure on axial length. *Ophthalmic Physiol. Opt.* **2011**, *31*, 398–403. [CrossRef] [PubMed]

13. Tokoro, T.; Funata, M.; Akazawa, Y. Influence of intraocular pressure on axial elongation. *J. Ocul. Pharmacol.* **1990**, *6*, 285–291. [CrossRef] [PubMed]

14. McBrien, N.A.; Jobling, A.I.; Gentle, A. Biomechanics of the Sclera in Myopia: Extracellular and Cellular Factors. *Optom. Vis. Sci.* **2009**, *86*, E23–E30. [CrossRef]

15. McMonnies, C.W. An examination of the baropathic nature of axial myopia. *Clin. Exp. Optom.* **2014**, *97*, 116–124. [CrossRef] [PubMed]

16. El-Nimri, N.W.; Wildsoet, C.F. Effects of topical latanoprost on intraocular pressure and myopia progression in young guinea pigs. *Invest. Ophthalmol. Vis. Sci.* **2018**, *59*, 2644–2651. [CrossRef] [PubMed]

17. Schmid, K.L.; Abbott, M.; Humphries, M.; Pyne, K.; Wildsoet, C.F. Timolol lowers intraocular pressure but does not inhibit the development of experimental myopia in chick. *Exp. Eye Res.* **2000**, *70*, 659–666. [CrossRef] [PubMed]

18. Huang, J.; Wen, D.; Wang, Q.; McAlinden, C.; Flitcroft, I.; Chen, H.; Saw, S.M.; Chen, H.; Bao, F.; Zhao, Y.; et al. Efficacy comparison of 16 interventions for myopia control in children: A network meta-analysis. *Ophthalmology* **2016**, *123*, 697–708. [CrossRef]

19. Patel, N.B.; Garcia, B.; Harwerth, R.S. Influence of anterior segment power on the scan path and RNFL thickness using SD-OCT. *Investig. Ophthalmol. Vis. Sci.* **2012**, *53*, 5788–5798. [CrossRef] [PubMed]

20. Sachidanandam, R.; Ravi, P.; Sen, P. Effect of axial length on full-field and multifocal electroretinograms. *Clin. Exp. Optom.* **2017**, *100*, 668–675. [CrossRef] [PubMed]

21. Biswas, S.; Lin, C.; Leung, C.K.S. Evaluation of a myopic normative database for analysis of retinal nerve fiber layer thickness. *JAMA Ophthalmol.* **2016**, *134*, 1032–1039. [CrossRef]

22. Biswas, S.; Jhanji, V.; Leung, C.K.S. Prevalence of glaucoma in myopic corneal refractive surgery candidates in Hong Kong China. *J. Refract. Surg.* **2016**, *32*, 298–304. [CrossRef] [PubMed]

23. Shoji, T.; Nagaoka, Y.; Sato, H.; Chihara, E. Impact of high myopia on the performance of SD-OCT parameters to detect glaucoma. *Graefe's Arch. Clin. Exp. Ophthalmol.* **2012**, *250*, 1843–1849. [CrossRef]

24. Neufeld, A.H.; Gachie, E.N. The inherent, age-dependent loss of retinal ganglion cells is related to the lifespan of the species. *Neurobiol. Aging* **2003**, *24*, 167–172. [CrossRef]

25. Harman, A.M.; MacDonald, A.; Meyer, P.; Ahmat, A. Numbers of neurons in the retinal ganglion cell layer of the rat do not change throughout life. *Gerontology* **2003**, *49*, 350–355. [CrossRef]

26. Levkovitch-Verbin, H.; Vander, S.; Makarovsky, D.; Lavinsky, F. Increase in retinal ganglion cells' susceptibility to elevated intraocular pressure and impairment of their endogenous neuroprotective mechanism by age. *Mol. Vis.* **2013**, *19*, 2011–2022. [PubMed]

27. Rodrigo, M.J.; Martinez-Rincon, T.; Subias, M.; Mendez-Martinez, S.; Luna, C.; Pablo, L.E.; Polo, V.; Garcia-Martin, E. Effect of age and sex on neurodevelopment and neurodegeneration in the healthy eye: Longitudinal functional and structural study in the Long–Evans rat. *Exp. Eye Res.* **2020**, *200*, 108208. [CrossRef] [PubMed]

28. Cuenca, N.; Fernández-Sánchez, L.; Sauvé, Y.; Segura, F.J.; Martínez-Navarrete, G.; Tamarit, J.M.; Fuentes-Broto, L.; Sanchez-Cano, A.; Pinilla, I. Correlation between SD-OCT, immunocytochemistry and functional findings in an animal model of retinal degeneration. *Front. Neuroanat.* **2014**, *8*, 1–20. [CrossRef]

29. Garcia-Martin, E.; Pablo, L.E.; Bambo, M.P.; Alarcia, R.; Polo, V.; Larrosa, J.M.; Vilades, E.; Cameo, B.; Orduna, E.; Ramirez, T.; et al. Comparison of peripapillary choroidal thickness between healthy subjects and patients with Parkinson's disease. *PLoS ONE* **2017**, *12*, e0177163. [CrossRef]

30. Garcia-Martin, E.; Pueyo, V.; Martin, J.; Almarcegui, C.; Ara, J.R.; Dolz, I.; Honrubia, F.M.; Fernandez, F.J. Progressive changes in the retinal nerve fiber layer in patients with multiple sclerosis. *Eur. J. Ophthalmol.* **2010**, *20*, 167–173. [CrossRef]

31. Ramirez, A.I.; de Hoz, R.; Salobrar-Garcia, E.; Salazar, J.J.; Rojas, B.; Ajoy, D.; López-Cuenca, I.; Rojas, P.; Triviño, A.; Ramírez, J.M. The role of microglia in retinal neurodegeneration: Alzheimer's disease, Parkinson, and glaucoma. *Front. Aging Neurosci.* **2017**, *9*, 1–21. [CrossRef] [PubMed]

32. Parisi, V. Correlation between morphological and functional retinal impairment in patients affected by ocular hypertension, glaucoma, demyelinating optic neuritis and Alzheimer's disease. *Semin. Ophthalmol.* **2003**, *18*, 50–57. [CrossRef]
33. Chouhan, A.K.; Guo, C.; Hsieh, Y.-C.; Ye, H.; Senturk, M.; Zuo, Z.; Li, Y.; Chatterjee, S.; Botas, J.; Jackson, G.R.; et al. Uncoupling neuronal death and dysfunction in Drosophila models of neurodegenerative disease. *Acta Neuropathol. Commun.* **2016**, *4*, 62. [CrossRef] [PubMed]
34. Moschos, M.M.; Markopoulos, I.; Chatziralli, I.; Rouvas, A.; Papageorgiou, S.G.; Ladas, I.; Vassilopoulos, D. Structural and Functional Impairment of the Retina and Optic Nerve in Alzheimer's Disease. *Curr. Alzheimer Res.* **2012**, *9*, 782–788. [CrossRef] [PubMed]
35. Rodrigo, M.J.; Garcia-Herranz, D.; Subias, M.; Martinez-Rincón, T.; Mendez-Martínez, S.; Bravo-Osuna, I.; Carretero, A.; Ruberte, J.; Garcia-Feijoo, J.; Pablo, L.E.; et al. Chronic Glaucoma Using Biodegradable Microspheres to Induce Intraocular Pressure Elevation. Six-Month Follow-Up. *Biomedicines* **2021**, *9*, 682. [CrossRef]
36. Morrison, J.C.; Moore, C.G.; Deppmeier, L.M.H.; Gold, B.G.; Meshul, C.K.; Johnson, E.C. A rat model of chronic pressure-induced optic nerve damage. *Exp. Eye Res.* **1997**, *64*, 85–96. [CrossRef]
37. Garcia-Herranz, D.; Rodrigo, M.J.; Subias, M.; Martinez-Rincon, T.; Mendez-Martinez, S.; Bravo-Osuna, I.; Bonet, A.; Ruberte, J.; Garcia-Feijoo, J.; Pablo, L.; et al. Novel Use of PLGA Microspheres to Create an Animal Model of Glaucoma with Progressive Neuroretinal Degeneration. *Pharmaceutics* **2021**, *13*, 237. [CrossRef]
38. Rodrigo, M.J.; Cardiel, M.J.; Fraile, J.M.; Mendez-Martinez, S.; Martinez-Rincon, T.; Subias, M.; Polo, V.; Ruberte, J.; Ramirez, T.; Vispe, E.; et al. Brimonidine-LAPONITE® intravitreal formulation has an ocular hypotensive and neuroprotective effect throughout 6 months of follow-up in a glaucoma animal model. *Biomater. Sci.* **2020**, *8*, 6246–6260. [CrossRef]
39. Ding, C.; Wang, P.; Tian, N. Effect of general anesthetics on IOP in elevated IOP mouse model. *Exp. Eye Res.* **2011**, *92*, 512–520. [CrossRef]
40. Nadal-Nicolás, F.M.; Vidal-Sanz, M.; Agudo-Barriuso, M. The aging rat retina: From function to anatomy. *Neurobiol. Aging* **2018**, *61*, 146–168. [CrossRef]
41. Liu, X.; Wang, C.H.; Dai, C.; Camesa, A.; Zhang, H.F.; Jiao, S. Effect of contact lens on optical coherence tomography imaging of rodent retina. *Curr. Eye Res.* **2013**, *38*, 1235–1240. [CrossRef] [PubMed]
42. Pang, I.H.; Clark, A.F. Inducible rodent models of glaucoma. *Prog. Retin. Eye Res.* **2020**, *75*. [CrossRef]
43. Choh, V.; Gurdita, A.; Tan, B.; Prasad, R.C.; Bizheva, K.; Joos, K.M. Short-term moderately elevated intraocular pressure is associated with elevated scotopic electroretinogram responses. *Investig. Ophthalmol. Vis. Sci.* **2016**, *57*, 2140–2151. [CrossRef] [PubMed]
44. Tan, B.; Gurdita, A.; Choh, V.; Joos, K.M.; Prasad, R.; Bizheva, K. Morphological and functional changes in the rat retina associated with 2 months of intermittent moderate intraocular pressure elevation. *Sci. Rep.* **2018**, *8*, 7727. [CrossRef] [PubMed]
45. Summers Rada, J.A.; Shelton, S.; Norton, T.T. The sclera and myopia. *Exp. Eye Res.* **2006**, *82*, 185–200. [CrossRef] [PubMed]
46. Harper, A.R.; Summers, J.A. The Dynamic Sclera: Extracellular Matrix Remodeling in Normal Ocular Growth and Myopia Development. *Exp. Eye Res.* **2015**, *133*, 100–111. [CrossRef] [PubMed]
47. Tan, B.; MacLellan, B.; Mason, E.; Bizheva, K. Structural, functional and blood perfusion changes in the rat retina associated with elevated intraocular pressure, measured simultaneously with a combined OCT+ERG system. *PLoS ONE* **2018**, *13*, e0193592. [CrossRef]
48. Frankfort, B.J.; Kareem Khan, A.; Tse, D.Y.; Chung, I.; Pang, J.J.; Yang, Z.; Gross, R.L.; Wu, S.M. Elevated intraocular pressure causes inner retinal dysfunction before cell loss in a mouse model of experimental glaucoma. *Investig. Ophthalmol. Vis. Sci.* **2013**, *54*, 762–770. [CrossRef] [PubMed]
49. Campbell, I.C.; Hannon, B.G.; Read, A.T.; Sherwood, J.M.; Schwaner, S.A.; Ethier, C.R. Quantification of the efficacy of collagen cross-linking agents to induce stiffening of rat sclera. *J. R. Soc. Interface* **2017**, *14*, 20170014. [CrossRef]
50. Cone-Kimball, E.; Nguyen, C.; Oglesby, E.N.; Pease, M.E.; Steinhart, M.R.; Quigley, H.A. Scleral structural alterations associated with chronic experimental intraocular pressure elevation in mice. *Mol. Vis.* **2013**, *19*, 2023–2039.
51. Pruett, R.C. Progressive myopia and intraocular pressure: What is the linkage? A literature review. *Acta Ophthalmol. Suppl.* **1988**, *185*, 117–127. [CrossRef]
52. Shen, L.; You, Q.S.; Xu, X.; Gao, F.; Zhang, Z.; Li, B.; Jonas, J.B. Scleral and Choroidal Thickness in Secondary High Axial Myopia. *Retina* **2016**, *36*, 1579–1585. [CrossRef]
53. Jonas, J.B.; Holbach, L.; Panda-Jonas, S. Histologic differences between primary high myopia and secondary high myopia due to congenital glaucoma. *Acta Ophthalmol.* **2016**, *94*, 147–153. [CrossRef]
54. Yassin, S.A. Long-Term Visual Outcomes in Children with Primary Congenital Glaucoma. *Eur. J. Ophthalmol.* **2017**, *27*, 705–710. [CrossRef]
55. Liu, B.; McNally, S.; Kilpatrick, J.I.; Jarvis, S.P.; O'Brien, C.J. Aging and ocular tissue stiffness in glaucoma. *Surv. Ophthalmol.* **2018**, *63*, 56–74. [CrossRef]
56. Downs, J.C. Optic nerve head biomechanics in aging and disease. *Exp. Eye Res.* **2015**, *133*, 19–29. [CrossRef] [PubMed]
57. Nissirios, N.; Chanis, R.; Johnson, E.; Morrison, J.; Cepurna, W.O.; Jia, L.; Mittag, T.; Danias, J. Comparison of anterior segment structures in two rat glaucoma models: An ultrasound biomicroscopic study. *Invest. Ophthalmol. Vis. Sci.* **2008**, *49*, 2478–2482. [CrossRef]

58. Morrison, J.C.; Cepurna, W.O.; Johnson, E.C. Modeling glaucoma in rats by sclerosing aqueous outflow pathways to elevate intraocular pressure. *Exp. Eye Res.* **2015**, *141*, 23–32. [CrossRef]
59. Sudhalkar, A.; Bilgic, A.; Vasavada, S.; Kodjikian, L.; Mathis, T.; De Ribot, F.M.; Papakostas, T.; Vasavada, V.; Vasavada, V.; Srivastava, S.; et al. Current intravitreal therapy and ocular hypertension: A review. *Indian J. Ophthalmol.* **2021**, *69*, 236–243. [CrossRef] [PubMed]
60. Hoguet, A.; Chen, P.P.; Junk, A.K.; Mruthyunjaya, P.; Nouri-Mahdavi, K.; Radhakrishnan, S.; Takusagawa, H.L.; Chen, T.C. The Effect of Anti-Vascular Endothelial Growth Factor Agents on Intraocular Pressure and Glaucoma: A Report by the American Academy of Ophthalmology. *Ophthalmology* **2019**, *126*, 611–622. [CrossRef] [PubMed]
61. Rebolleda, G.; Puerto, B.; De Juan, V.; Gómez-Mariscal, M.; Muñoz-Negrete, F.J.; Casado, A. Optic nerve head biomechanic and IOP changes before and after the injection of aflibercept for neovascular age-related macular degeneration. *Investig. Ophthalmol. Vis. Sci.* **2016**, *57*, 5688–5695. [CrossRef] [PubMed]
62. Guggenheim, J.A.; Creer, R.C.; Qin, X.J. Postnatal refractive development in the Brown Norway rat: Limitations of standard refractive and ocular component dimension measurement techniques. *Curr. Eye Res.* **2004**, *29*, 369–376. [CrossRef]
63. Usui, S.; Ikuno, Y.; Uematsu, S.; Morimoto, Y.; Yasuno, Y.; Otori, Y. Changes in axial length and choroidal thickness after intraocular pressure reduction resulting from trabeculectomy. *Clin. Ophthalmol.* **2013**, *7*, 1155–1161. [CrossRef] [PubMed]
64. Leo, S.W. Scientific Bureau of World Society of Paediatric Ophthalmology and Strabismus (WSPOS) Current approaches to myopia control. *Curr. Opin. Ophthalmol.* **2017**, *28*, 267–275. [CrossRef] [PubMed]
65. Spillmann, L. Stopping the rise of myopia in Asia. *Graefe's Arch. Clin. Exp. Ophthalmol.* **2020**, *258*, 943–959. [CrossRef]
66. De Jong, P.T.V.M. Myopia: Its historical contexts. *Br. J. Ophthalmol.* **2018**, *102*, 1021–1027. [CrossRef]
67. Kalmann, R.; Mourits, M.P. Prevalence and management of elevated intraocular pressure in patients with Graves' orbitopathy. *Br. J. Ophthalmol.* **1998**, *82*, 754–757. [CrossRef]
68. Kim, W.S.; Chun, Y.S.; Cho, B.Y.; Lee, J.K. Biometric and refractive changes after orbital decompression in Korean patients with thyroid-associated orbitopathy. *Eye* **2016**, *30*, 400–405. [CrossRef]
69. Huang, A.S.; Li, M.; Yang, D.; Wang, H.; Wang, N.; Weinreb, R.N. Aqueous Angiography in Living Nonhuman Primates Shows Segmental, Pulsatile, and Dynamic Angiographic Aqueous Humor Outflow. *Ophthalmology* **2017**, *124*, 793–803. [CrossRef] [PubMed]
70. Huang, A.S.; Francis, B.A.; Weinreb, R.N. Structural and functional imaging of aqueous humour outflow: A review. *Clin. Exp. Ophthalmol.* **2018**, *46*, 158–168. [CrossRef] [PubMed]
71. Huang, A.S.; Camp, A.; Xu, B.Y.; Penteado, R.C.; Weinreb, R.N.; Huang, A. Aqueous Angiography: Aqueous Humor Outflow Imaging in Live Human Subjects HHS Public Access. *Ophthalmology* **2017**, *124*, 1249–1251. [CrossRef] [PubMed]
72. Lin, K.Y.; Mosaed, S. Ab externo imaging of human episcleral vessels using fiberoptic confocal laser endomicroscopy. *J. Ophthalmic Vis. Res.* **2019**, *14*, 275–284. [CrossRef]
73. Khatib, T.Z.; Meyer, P.A.R.; Lusthaus, J.; Manyakin, I.; Mushtaq, Y.; Martin, K.R. Hemoglobin Video Imaging Provides Novel In Vivo High-Resolution Imaging and Quantification of Human Aqueous Outflow in Patients with Glaucoma. *Ophthalmol. Glaucoma* **2019**, *2*, 327–335. [CrossRef] [PubMed]
74. Jensen, H. Myopia progression in young school children and intraocular pressure. *Doc. Ophthalmol.* **1992**, *82*, 249–255. [CrossRef] [PubMed]
75. Greene, P.R. Mechanical considerations in myopia: Relative effects of accommodation, convergence, intraocular pressure, and the extraocular muscles. *Am. J. Optom. Physiol. Opt.* **1980**, *57*, 902–914. [CrossRef] [PubMed]
76. Lee, C.-Y.; Sun, C.-C.; Lin, Y.-F.; Lin, K.-K. Effects of topical atropine on intraocular pressure and myopia progression: A prospective comparative study. *BMC Ophthalmol.* **2016**, *16*, 114. [CrossRef]
77. Yam, J.C.; Jiang, Y.; Tang, S.M.; Law, A.K.P.; Chan, J.J.; Wong, E.; Ko, S.T.; Young, A.L.; Tham, C.C.; Chen, L.J.; et al. Low-Concentration Atropine for Myopia Progression (LAMP) Study: A Randomized, Double-Blinded, Placebo-Controlled Trial of 0.05%, 0.025%, and 0.01% Atropine Eye Drops in Myopia Control. *Ophthalmology* **2019**, *126*, 113–124. [CrossRef]
78. Biswas, S.; Wan, K.H. Review of rodent hypertensive glaucoma models. *Acta Ophthalmol.* **2019**, *97*, e331–e340. [CrossRef]
79. Schmidl, D.; Schmetterer, L.; Garhöfer, G.; Popa-Cherecheanu, A. Gender Differences in Ocular Blood Flow. *Curr. Eye Res.* **2015**, *40*, 201–212. [CrossRef]
80. Zhou, X.; Xie, J.; Shen, M.; Wang, J.; Jiang, L.; Qu, J.; Lu, F. Biometric measurement of the mouse eye using optical coherence tomography with focal plane advancement. *Vis. Res.* **2008**, *48*, 1137–1143. [CrossRef]
81. Jiang, M.; Wu, P.C.; Fini, M.E.; Tsai, C.L.; Itakura, T.; Zhang, X.; Jiao, S. Single-shot dimension measurements of the mouse eye using SD-OCT. *Ophthalmic Surg. Lasers Imaging* **2012**, *43*, 252–256. [CrossRef] [PubMed]
82. Chou, T.H.; Kocaoglu, O.P.; Borja, D.; Ruggeri, M.; Uhlhorn, S.R.; Manns, F.; Porciatti, V. Postnatal elongation of eye size in DBA/2J mice compared with C57BL/6J mice: In vivo analysis with whole-eye OCT. *Investig. Ophthalmol. Vis. Sci.* **2011**, *52*, 3604–3612. [CrossRef] [PubMed]
83. Hsu, C.-H.; Chen, R.I.; Lin, S.C. Myopia and glaucoma: Sorting out the difference. *Curr. Opin. Ophthalmol.* **2015**, *26*, 90–95. [CrossRef] [PubMed]
84. Suwan, Y.; Rettig, S.; Park, S.C.; Tantraworasin, A.; Geyman, L.S.; Effert, K.; Silva, L.; Jarukasetphorn, R.; Ritch, R. Effects of Circumpapillary Retinal Nerve Fiber Layer Segmentation Error Correction on Glaucoma Diagnosis in Myopic Eyes. *J. Glaucoma* **2018**, *27*, 1. [CrossRef]

85. Kansal, V.; Armstrong, J.J.; Pintwala, R.; Hutnik, C. Optical coherence tomography for glaucoma diagnosis: An evidence based meta-analysis. *PLoS ONE* **2018**, *13*, e0190621. [CrossRef]
86. Lozano, D.C.; Twa, M.D. Development of a rat schematic eye from in vivo biometry and the correction of lateral magnification in SD-OCT imaging. *Investig. Ophthalmol. Vis. Sci.* **2013**, *54*, 6446–6455. [CrossRef] [PubMed]
87. Westall, C.A.; Dhaliwal, H.S.; Panton, C.M.; Sigesmun, D.; Levin, A.V.; Nischal, K.K.; Héon, E. Values of electroretinogram responses according to axial length. *Doc. Ophthalmol.* **2001**, *102*, 115–130. [CrossRef]
88. Liu, H.-H.; He, Z.; Nguyen, C.T.O.; Vingrys, A.J.; Bui, B.V. Reversal of functional loss in a rat model of chronic intraocular pressure elevation. *Ophthalmic Physiol. Opt.* **2017**, *37*, 71–81. [CrossRef]

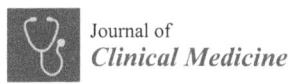

Journal of
Clinical Medicine

Article

Factors Associated with Increased Neuroretinal Rim Thickness Measured Based on Bruch's Membrane Opening-Minimum Rim Width after Trabeculectomy

Do-Young Park and Soon-Cheol Cha *

Department of Ophthalmology, Yeungnam University Hospital, Yeungnam University College of Medicine, Daegu 42415, Korea; dypark@ynu.ac.kr
* Correspondence: sccha@yumail.ac.kr

Abstract: Purpose: To investigate the factors associated with an increase in the neuroretinal rim (NRR) thickness measured based on Bruch's membrane opening-minimum rim width (BMO-MRW) after trabeculectomy in patients with primary open-angle glaucoma (POAG). Methods: We analyzed the BMO-MRW using spectral-domain optical coherence tomography (SD-OCT) of patients with POAG who underwent a trabeculectomy for uncontrolled intraocular pressure (IOP) despite maximal IOP reduction treatment. The BMO-MRW was measured before and after trabeculectomy in patients with POAG. Demographic and systemic factors, ocular factors, pre- and post-operative IOP, and visual field parameters were collected, together with SD-OCT measurements. A regression analysis was performed to investigate the factors that affected the change in the BMO-MRW after the trabeculectomy. Results: Forty-four eyes of 44 patients were included in the analysis. The IOP significantly decreased from a preoperative 27.0 mmHg to a postoperative 10.5 mmHg. The mean interval between the trabeculectomy and the date of post-operative SD-OCT measurement was 3.3 months. The global and sectoral BMO-MRW significantly increased after trabeculectomy, whereas the peripapillary retinal nerve fiber layer thickness did not show a difference between before and after the trabeculectomy. Younger age and a greater reduction in the IOP after the trabeculectomy were significantly associated with the increase in the BMO-MRW after trabeculectomy. Conclusions: The NRR thickness measured based on the BMO-MRW increased with decreasing IOP after trabeculectomy, and the increase in the BMO-MRW was associated with the young age of the patients and greater reduction in the IOP after trabeculectomy. Biomechanically, these suggest that the NRR comprises cells and substances that sensitively respond to changes in the IOP and age.

Keywords: neuroretinal rim reversal; Bruch's membrane opening-minimum rim width; trabeculectomy; intraocular pressure

Citation: Park, D.-Y.; Cha, S.-C. Factors Associated with Increased Neuroretinal Rim Thickness Measured Based on Bruch's Membrane Opening-Minimum Rim Width after Trabeculectomy. *J. Clin. Med.* **2021**, *10*, 3646. https://doi.org/10.3390/jcm10163646

Academic Editors: Maria Letizia Salvetat, Marco Zeppieri, Paolo Brusini and Michele Lanza

Received: 7 July 2021
Accepted: 16 August 2021
Published: 18 August 2021

Publisher's Note: MDPI stays neutral with regard to jurisdictional claims in published maps and institutional affiliations.

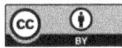
1. Introduction

Reducing intraocular pressure (IOP) from glaucoma filtration surgery is accompanied by dynamic structural changes in the optic nerve head (ONH) [1–12]. These changes are called "reversal of disc cupping" because neuroretinal rim (NRR) tissue thickening is noted in funduscopic imaging and confocal scanning laser ophthalmoscopy [4,5,9,10,12]. Since optical coherence tomography (OCT) became available, several studies have been conducted on the detailed structural changes in the ONH and peripapillary retinal nerve fiber layer (RNFL) thickness after glaucoma filtration surgery [1–3,7,8,11]. Studies using OCT have found that the lamina cribrosa (LC) depth decreased after trabeculectomy, whereas the peripapillary RNFL thickness was unchanged [2,3,7].

More recently, Bruch's membrane opening (BMO)-related OCT parameters have enabled the quantification of the NRR tissue of the ONH [13,14]. As expected, the representative parameters—BMO-MRW and BMO-minimum rim area—were reported to increase after trabeculectomy [3,7,11,15].

The increase in the NRR thickness after trabeculectomy is believed to occur secondary to the relief of compressive and stretch forces on the NRR tissue due to a reduced IOP [3]. Depending on the characteristics of the cells or substances filling the NRR tissue, the degree of the increase in the NRR thickness after trabeculectomy might be different. However, it is not yet known which factors affect the increase in NRR thickness following a postoperative IOP decrease.

In this study, using spectral-domain OCT (SD-OCT) and analyzing the BMO-based parameters of the NRR before and after trabeculectomy, we aimed to determine the factors that affect the changes in NRR thickness due to an IOP decrease after trabeculectomy.

2. Methods

2.1. Participants

For this retrospective, interventional study, all patients who underwent trabeculectomy at Yeungnam University Hospital from March 2020 to December 2020 were reviewed, and patients who met the following inclusion and exclusion criteria were selected. The study was approved by the Yeungnam University Hospital Institutional Review Board (IRB) and followed the tenets of the Declaration of Helsinki (IRB no. 2021-03-066). Considering the nature of the retrospective study, the requirement to obtain informed consent was waived by the IRB of the Yeungnam University Hospital.

The inclusion criteria were as follows: (1) patients aged 20 years or older who were diagnosed with primary open-angle glaucoma (POAG) and underwent trabeculectomy for uncontrolled IOP despite the maximum IOP reduction treatment, (2) patients who underwent at least one disc SD-OCT examination within 1 month prior to the glaucoma surgery, (3) patients who underwent at least one disc SD-OCT examination between 1 and 6 months after glaucoma surgery, and (4) patients whose IOP remained stable below 20 mmHg from immediately after the surgery to the time of the postoperative SD-OCT scan. POAG was diagnosed based on the following criteria: (1) the presence of typical glaucomatous optic disc changes (increased cupping, focal or diffuse loss of the NRR, or an RNFL defect), (2) glaucomatous visual field (VF) defect in at least two consecutive tests, (3) an open angle observed during a gonioscopic examination, and (4) IOP > 21 mmHg with or without the use of an antiglaucomatous medication. All patients underwent limbal- or fornix-based trabeculectomy with mitomycin C, which was performed by a glaucoma specialist (DYP, CSC).

Regarding the exclusion criteria, patients who underwent glaucoma surgery with a diagnosis of angle-closure glaucoma or secondary glaucoma, such as neovascular glaucoma, uveitic glaucoma, or exfoliation glaucoma, were excluded because factors such as sudden fluctuations in the IOP before surgery, ONH ischemia, or ocular inflammation may affect the analysis of changes in the ONH according to the decrease in the IOP after surgery. Cases of a needling procedure or additional surgery due to an increased IOP after surgery, cases requiring additional procedures because of hypotony, or cases with an IOP of less than 6 mmHg were excluded.

The following parameters were collected from the included patients: age, sex, presence of hypertension or diabetes, phakic status, average IOP after maximum medical IOP-lowering treatment within 3 months before surgery, average IOP within 6 months after surgery, axial length, central corneal thickness (CCT), and VF parameters (mean deviation (MD), pattern standard deviation, and VF index). SD-OCT measurements (BMO and RNFL parameters) taken before and after surgery were also collected, together with the period from the surgery to the SD-OCT measurement.

2.2. Measurement of Bruch's Membrane Opening-Minimum Rim Width Using Spectral-Domain Optical Coherence Tomography

A Spectralis SD-OCT (Heidelberg Engineering GmbH, Heidelberg, Germany) was used to measure BMO-related parameters in the ONH. SD-OCT imaging was performed in accordance with the standard operating procedures. The scanning was focused on the center of the BMO, and 24 radial equidistant cross-sectional images were obtained. The BMO-MRW and RNFL thickness values were automatically calculated on a global and sectoral basis using the device's standard operating software. The BMO area was also calculated automatically. If necessary, automated delineation of the internal limiting membrane and BMO were manually corrected.

2.3. Statistical Analyses

A paired *t*-test or a Wilcoxon signed-rank test was performed depending on data normality to compare the variables before and after trabeculectomy. We performed univariable and multivariable regression analyses using a generalized linear model to identify factors associated with an increase in the BMO-MRW after trabeculectomy. Characteristics with a *p*-value < 0.1 in the univariable analysis were included in the multivariable analysis. In the multivariable regression analysis, two models were used to avoid multicollinearity. Beta coefficients were calculated based on a 10 μm increase in the BMO-MRW. A *p*-value < 0.05 was considered statistically significant. Statistical analyses were performed using IBM SPSS software version 24.0 (IBM Corp., Armonk, NY, USA) and R statistical package version 3.5.3 (R Foundation for Statistical Computing, Vienna, Austria).

3. Results

Sixty-six eyes of 66 patients with POAG underwent trabeculectomy from March 2020 to December 2020. Of these, 10 and 6 eyes were excluded from the analysis due to the absence of an OCT examination before and after surgery, respectively. Four eyes were excluded due to the presence of postoperative hypotony. Two eyes were excluded due to poor OCT image quality. Finally, 44 eyes of 44 patients were included in the analysis.

Demographic and baseline information of the patients is summarized in Table 1. The mean age of the 44 patients was 62.5 years (standard deviation (SD), 15.1 years), of whom 33 (75%) were male. The mean interval between trabeculectomy and the postoperative SD-OCT examination was 3.3 months (SD, 1.9 months).

Table 1. Demographic and baseline characteristics of the patients.

Variables	Total Subjects (*n* = 44)
Age, years	62.5 ± 15.1
Gender, male/female	33/11
Diabetes, yes/no	15/29
Hypertension, yes/no	12/32
Phakia/pseudophakia	28/16
Central corneal thickness, μm	548.1 ± 37.4
Axial length, mm	24.2 ± 1.3
Visual field MD, dB	−20 ± 7.5
Visual field PSD, dB	8.4 ± 3.0
Visual field VFI, %	44.7 ± 26.5
Average RNFL thickness, μm	62.5 ± 22.4
BMO-area, μm^2	2.32 ± 0.56
Global BMO-MRW, μm	151.9 ± 45.5

IOP: intraocular pressure; MD: mean deviation; PSD: pattern standard deviation; dB: decibel; VFI: visual field index; RNFL: retinal nerve fiber layer; BMO-MRW: Bruch's membrane opening-minimum rim width. Data are presented as mean ± standard deviation or *n* (frequency).

The IOP significantly decreased from a preoperative 27.0 mmHg (SD, 6.6 mmHg) to a postoperative 10.5 mmHg (SD, 3.3 mmHg). The global BMO-MRW significantly increased from a preoperative value of 151.9 μm to a postoperative value of 181.8 μm (*p* < 0.001). In addition to the global BMO-MRW, the BMO-MRW by sector also significantly increased postoperatively, except for the inferotemporal (TI) sector (Table 2). The BMO area and average peripapillary RNFL thickness did not show a significant difference between preoperatively and postoperatively (Table 2).

Table 2. Intraocular pressure, BMO-MRW, and RNFL thickness at baseline and the postoperative OCT examination.

	Preoperative	Postoperative	*p*-Value
IOP, mmHg	27 ± 6.6	10.5 ± 3.3	**<0.001**
BMO-area, μm^2	2.32 ± 0.56	2.29 ± 0.57	0.52
Global BMO-MRW, μm	151.9 ± 45.5	181.8 ± 84.7	**<0.001**
BMO-MRW_TS, μm	127.3 ± 55.1	143.1 ± 83	**0.007**
BMO-MRW_T, μm	132.4 ± 45	153.8 ± 75.7	**0.002**
BMO-MRW_TI, μm	138.1 ± 78.8	152 ± 108.1	0.06
BMO-MRW_NI, μm	189.3 ± 66.7	212.8 ± 94	**0.004**
BMO-MRW_N, μm	169.7 ± 55.7	195.6 ± 73.6	**<0.001**
BMO-MRW_NS, μm	161.4 ± 61.9	183.7 ± 70.5	**<0.001**
Average RNFL thickness, μm	62.5 ± 22.4	61.6 ± 19.7	0.68
RNFL_TS, μm	79.2 ± 42	71.6 ± 31.9	0.08
RNFL_T, μm	57.4 ± 25.8	57.1 ± 24.8	0.87
RNFL_TI, μm	71.6 ± 33.1	70.3 ± 37.1	0.72
RNFL_NI, μm	66.2 ± 28.2	67.8 ± 24.9	0.37
RNFL_N, μm	53.6 ± 23.6	54.9 ± 20.7	0.45
RNFL_NS, μm	70 ± 35.5	64.9 ± 28.4	0.20

IOP: intraocular pressure; BMO-MRW: Bruch's membrane opening-minimum rim width; RNFL: retinal nerve fiber layer. TS: superotemporal; T: temporal; TI: inferotemporal; NI: inferonasal; N: nasal; NS: superonasal. Data are presented as mean ± standard deviation. Statistically significant *p*-values are shown in bold.

Univariable regression analysis found that the increase in the global BMO-MRW after trabeculectomy was greater when the patient's age was lower, the CCT was thinner, the VF MD was better, the preoperative average RNFL thickness was greater, and the IOP reduction was higher (Table 3). Multivariable regression analyses found that younger age and greater reduction in the IOP after trabeculectomy remained significant factors that affected the increase in the BMO-MRW after trabeculectomy (Table 3, Figure 1). Unlike the BMO-MRW, the change in the average RNFL thickness was not affected by the patients' age or the amount of reduction in IOP after trabeculectomy (Supplementary Table S1).

Table 3. Factors associated with an increase in the global BMO-MRW (per 10 μm) after trabeculectomy.

	Univariable		Multivariable			
			Model 1		Model 2	
Variables	Beta (95% CI)	*p*-Value	Beta (95% CI)	*p*-Value	Beta (95% CI)	*p*-Value
Age, per 1 year older	−0.19 (−0.31 to −0.08)	**0.001**	−0.11 (−0.20 to −0.02)	**0.02**	−0.10 (−0.19 to −0.00)	0.05
Gender, male	−0.96 (−5.38 to 3.46)	0.67				
Diabetes	−1.01 (−5.06 to 3.04)	0.63				
Hypertension	−0.77 (−5.20 to 3.65)	0.73				
Phakia/pseudophakia	−1.80 (−5.76 to 2.16)	0.38				
Duration, months	0.36 (−0.69 to 1.41)	0.51				
Central corneal thickness, 40 μm	−2.04 (−3.98 to −0.09)	**0.04**	−0.55 (−1.97 to 0.86)	0.45	−0.40 (−1.85 to 1.05)	0.59
Axial length, mm	0.78 (−1.31 to 2.87)	0.47				
Visual field MD, dB	0.28 (0.04 to 0.52)	**0.03**			0.09 (−0.09 to 0.28)	0.33
Visual field PSD, dB	0.25 (−0.39 to 0.89)	0.44				
Preoperative average RNFL thickness, 10 μm	0.80 (−0.04 to 1.63)	0.07	0.26 (−0.32 to 0.85)	0.38		
Preoperative global BMO-MRW thickness, 10 μm	0.28 (−0.14 to 0.70)	0.21				
Preoperative IOP, mmHg	0.13 (−0.16 to 0.43)	0.39				
Postoperative IOP, mmHg	−0.63 (−1.03 to −0.24)	**0.003**				
Reduction of IOP, mmHg	0.28 (0.11 to 0.45)	**0.002**	0.19 (0.01 to 0.37)	**0.04**	0.21 (0.04 to 0.38)	**0.02**

IOP: intraocular pressure; MD: mean deviation; PSD: pattern standard deviation; dB: decibel; RNFL: retinal nerve fiber layer; BMO-MRW: Bruch's membrane opening-minimum rim width. Visual field MD and the average preoperative RNFL thickness were strongly associated with each other; thus, each was analyzed separately in the multivariable analysis. Beta coefficients were calculated based on the 10 μm increase in the BMO-MRW. Statistically significant *p*-values are shown in bold.

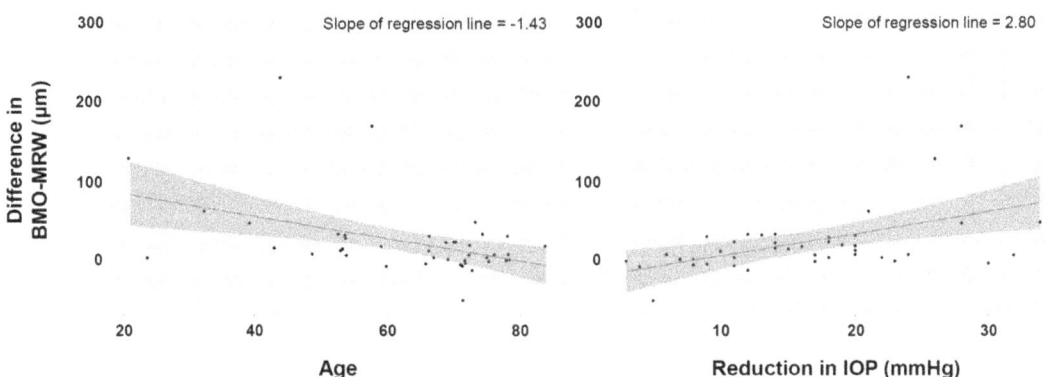

Figure 1. Scatter plot showing the relationship between the increase in the Bruch's membrane opening-minimum rim width (BMO-MRW) after trabeculectomy and the patients' age (left) and the amount of IOP reduction after trabeculectomy (right).

4. Discussion

NRR thinning is a major change that is observed in the disc in glaucoma, and it is important in diagnosing glaucoma and judging the progression of glaucoma. NRR thinning is known to be dynamically reversed after glaucoma surgery [2–12]. Therefore, understanding the factors that are associated with these changes can help to determine the progression of patients with glaucoma after glaucoma surgery. In addition, identifying the factors that are associated with the reversal of NRR thinning has important implications in that it may help to better understand the biomechanical properties of the NRR and infer the pathogenesis of disc cupping. In this study, we found that the BMO-MRW increased significantly after trabeculectomy, whereas there was no significant change in the RNFL. In multivariable regression analysis, changes in BMO-MRW were greater with a greater reduction in the IOP after trabeculectomy, even more so in younger patients.

Several studies reported changes in the structure of the ONH after glaucoma filtration surgery. Previously, it was reported that the NRR became thicker on two-dimensional fundus photographs [4–6,9,10,12]. Subsequently, through cross-sectional ONH analysis using SD-OCT, it was found that the depth of the LC decreased and its thickness increased [8]. Changes in the LC depth after the IOP reduction via glaucoma filtration surgery were also reported to be observed in myopic eyes with a tilted disc [16]. It was also reported that the LC curvature flattened and the LC depth decreased as the IOP decreased after surgery [17,18]. These changes were thought to be the result of connective tissue remodeling and collagen rearrangement occurring in the LC. Previous studies showed that the amount of change in the LC depth or curvature after glaucoma filtration surgery was related to the higher perioperative IOP reduction and younger patients' age [8,17], which were also found in this study to be associated with changes in the BMO-MRW after surgery. These suggest that, similar to the LC, the NRR measured based on the BMO-MRW had a composition that can be reversibly changed following lowering of IOP by filtering surgery, which could be affected by the amount of IOP reduction and young age.

Histologically, it is known that the composition of the NRR and LC differs [19]. In other words, when the nerve fiber axon passes through the NRR-containing prelaminar and LC, the cells and substances that consist of the surrounding structures are changed. In the peripapillary area, thin-bodied glial cells are distributed parallel to the axons [19,20]. In the NRR-containing prelamina, glial cells show a loose arrangement and glial fibers are distributed perpendicular to the nerve fiber bundle [19,21]. In the LC, connective tissue consisting of collagen, elastin, and laminin separates the glial cells and axons as the main components. Different from the LC, the NRR is known to have little connective tissue. Considering these characteristics, the structural changes in the NRR according to the fluctuation in the IOP after surgery might be related to the plasticity of distribution of the glial cells. In fact, in an animal model of glaucoma, it was reported that as the IOP increased, the processes of astrocytes thickened and the distribution of the astrocytes changed from perpendicular to parallel to the axons [22,23]. In addition, there was a study that showed that the population of glial cells in the optic nerve in rodents varies with age [24,25]. Therefore, we assumed that age-dependent changes that occur in glial cells when the IOP increases might be reversed when the IOP decreases after trabeculectomy.

Unlike the BMO-MRW, in this study, the peripapillary RNFL did not show a reversible change according to the postoperative IOP reduction, which is consistent with the results of previous studies [2,3,7]. This implies that it was not the thickness or number of axons, but rather the properties and distribution of glial cells surrounding the axons that were different in the peripapillary RNFL and BMO-MRW according to the decrease in the IOP after trabeculectomy. More studies assessing the characteristics and distributions of the glial cells comprising the ONH in humans or primates, their changes with age and IOP, and plasticity and reversibility of the changes are required.

This study has several limitations. First, in this study, we did not evaluate the change in LC-related parameters after trabeculectomy, such as the LC depth, thickness, or curvature. This was because we analyzed the ONH only with radial scan, which is not appropriate for analyzing the LC. Therefore, we were not able to obtain the results regarding the change in the LC in response to an IOP decrease after trabeculectomy, and it was not possible to interpret the change in the BMO-MRW after surgery in relation to the change in the LC. Further studies assessing the correlation between the changes in the BMO-MRW after trabeculectomy and changes in the LC and whether the factors associated with these changes have an independent effect are needed. Second, we did not observe long-term changes in the BMO-MRW after trabeculectomy. Previously, it was reported that after 6 months of glaucoma drainage device surgery or trabeculectomy, the BMO-MRW was not significantly different from preoperative values [7,26]. Therefore, our results should be interpreted as showing that the transient increase in the BMO-MRW following postoperative IOP decrease was associated with age and the amount of IOP reduction after trabeculectomy. It is not yet known whether age and amount of IOP reduction are also related to the duration for the BMO-MRW to normalize after surgery. Third, this study was not conducted in a prospective manner; thus, we cannot exclude the potential selection bias. However, most of the parameters analyzed in this study, including OCT parameters, were items that are examined in a routine manner in our clinic before surgery and within 6 months after surgery. A prospective study with regular follow-up OCT examinations after trabeculectomy is needed in the future.

In conclusion, by quantitatively analyzing the BMO-MRW measured using SD-OCT, we confirmed that the NRR thickness increased after trabeculectomy. The increase in the BMO-MRW was related to the younger age of the patients and a greater reduction in the IOP after trabeculectomy. Clinically, we should consider these when judging the progression of glaucoma based on changes in the NRR after trabeculectomy. Biomechanically, these suggest that the cells or substances that make up the NRR respond to changes in the IOP after trabeculectomy, which may vary depending on age and the IOP.

Supplementary Materials: The following are available online at https://www.mdpi.com/article/10.3390/jcm10163646/s1, Table S1: Factors associated with increase in the average RNFL thickness (per 10 µm) after trabeculectomy.

Author Contributions: Conceptualization, D.-Y.P.; Data curation, D.-Y.P.; Formal analysis, D.-Y.P.; Funding acquisition, D.-Y.P.; Investigation, D.-Y.P.; Methodology, D.-Y.P.; Resources, S.-C.C.; Supervision, S.-C.C.; Validation, S.-C.C.; Writing—original draft, D.-Y.P.; Writing—review and editing, S.-C.C. All authors have read and agreed to the published version of the manuscript.

Funding: This work was supported by the Basic Science Research Program (2019R1F1A1062796 and 2019M3E5D1A02068088) through the National Research Foundation of Korea funded by the Ministry of Science, ICT and Future Planning. The funders had no role in study design, data collection and analysis, decision to publish, or preparation of the manuscript.

J. Clin. Med. **2021**, *10*, 3646

Institutional Review Board Statement: The study was approved by the Yeungnam University Hospital Institutional Review Board (IRB) and followed the tenets of the Declaration of Helsinki (IRB no. 2021-03-066).

Informed Consent Statement: Informed consent was waived due to the nature of the retrospective study.

Data Availability Statement: The data presented in this study are available from the authors upon reasonable request. The data are not publicly available due to privacy and ethical issue.

Conflicts of Interest: All authors declare no conflict of interest.

References

1. Aydin, A.; Wollstein, G.; Price, L.L.; Fujimoto, J.G.; Schuman, J.S. Optical coherence tomography assessment of retinal nerve fiber layer thickness changes after glaucoma surgery. *Ophthalmology* **2003**, *110*, 1506–1511. [CrossRef]
2. Chang, P.T.; Sekhon, N.; Budenz, D.L.; Feuer, W.J.; Park, P.W.; Anderson, D.R. Effect of Lowering Intraocular Pressure on Optical Coherence Tomography Measurement of Peripapillary Retinal Nerve Fiber Layer Thickness. *Ophthalmology* **2007**, *114*, 2252–2258. [CrossRef] [PubMed]
3. Gietzelt, C.; Lemke, J.; Schaub, F.; Hermann, M.M.; Dietlein, T.S.; Cursiefen, C.; Enders, P.; Heindl, L.M. Structural Reversal of Disc Cupping After Trabeculectomy Alters Bruch Membrane Opening–Based Parameters to Assess Neuroretinal Rim. *Am. J. Ophthalmol.* **2018**, *194*, 143–152. [CrossRef]
4. Greenidge, K.C.; Spaeth, G.L.; Traverso, C.E. Change in Appearance of the Optic Disc Associated with Lowering of intraocular Pressure. *Ophthalmology* **1985**, *92*, 897–903. [CrossRef]
5. Irak, I.; Zangwill, L.; Garden, V.; Shakiba, S.; Weinreb, R.N. Change in Optic Disk Topography After Trabeculectomy. *Am. J. Ophthalmol.* **1996**, *122*, 690–695. [CrossRef]
6. Katz, L.J.; Spaeth, G.L.; Cantor, L.B.; Poryzees, E.M.; Steinmann, W.C. Reversible Optic Disk Cupping and Visual Field Improvement in Adults with Glaucoma. *Am. J. Ophthalmol.* **1989**, *107*, 485–492. [CrossRef]
7. Kiessling, D.; Christ, H.; Gietzelt, C.; Schaub, F.; Dietlein, T.S.; Cursiefen, C.; Heindl, L.M.; Enders, P. Impact of ab-interno trabeculectomy on Bruch's membrane opening-based morphometry of the optic nerve head for glaucoma progression analysis. *Graefe's Arch. Clin. Exp. Ophthalmol.* **2018**, *257*, 339–347. [CrossRef] [PubMed]
8. Lee, E.J.; Kim, T.-W.; Weinreb, R.N. Reversal of Lamina Cribrosa Displacement and Thickness after Trabeculectomy in Glaucoma. *Ophthalmology* **2012**, *119*, 1359–1366. [CrossRef]
9. Lesk, M.R.; Spaeth, G.L.; Azuara-Blanco, A.; Araujo, S.V.; Katz, L.; Terebuh, A.K.; Wilson, R.P.; Moster, M.R.; Schmidt, C.M. Reversal of optic disc cupping after glaucoma surgery analyzed with a scanning laser tomograph. *Ophthalmology* **1999**, *106*, 1013–1018. [CrossRef]
10. Quigley, H.A. The Pathogenesis of Reversible Cupping in Congenital Glaucoma. *Am. J. Ophthalmol.* **1977**, *84*, 358–370. [CrossRef]
11. Sanchez, F.G.; Sanders, D.S.; Moon, J.J.; Gardiner, S.K.; Reynaud, J.; Fortune, B.; Mansberger, S.L. Effect of Trabeculectomy on OCT Measurements of the Optic Nerve Head Neuroretinal Rim Tissue. *Ophthalmol. Glaucoma* **2020**, *3*, 32–39. [CrossRef] [PubMed]
12. Robin, A.; Quigley, H.A. Transient Reversible Cupping in Juvenile-Onset Glaucoma. *Am. J. Ophthalmol.* **1979**, *88*, 580–584. [CrossRef]
13. Chauhan, B.C.; O'Leary, N.; AlMobarak, F.A.; Reis, A.S.; Yang, H.; Sharpe, G.P.; Hutchison, D.M.; Nicolela, M.T.; Burgoyne, C. Enhanced Detection of Open-angle Glaucoma with an Anatomically Accurate Optical Coherence Tomography–Derived Neuroretinal Rim Parameter. *Ophthalmology* **2012**, *120*, 535–543. [CrossRef]
14. Reis, A.S.C.; O'Leary, N.; Yang, H.; Sharpe, G.P.; Nicolela, M.T.; Burgoyne, C.; Chauhan, B.C. Influence of Clinically Invisible, but Optical Coherence Tomography Detected, Optic Disc Margin Anatomy on Neuroretinal Rim Evaluation. *Investig. Opthalmol. Vis. Sci.* **2012**, *53*, 1852–1860. [CrossRef] [PubMed]
15. Koenig, S.F.; Hirneiss, C.W. Changes of Neuroretinal Rim and Retinal Nerve Fiber Layer Thickness Assessed by Optical Coherence Tomography After Filtration Surgery in Glaucomatous Eyes. *Clin. Ophthalmol.* **2021**, *15*, 2335–2344. [CrossRef] [PubMed]
16. Lee, S.H.; Lee, E.J.; Kim, J.M.; Girard, M.J.A.; Mari, J.M.; Kim, T.-W. Lamina Cribrosa Moves Anteriorly After Trabeculectomy in Myopic Eyes. *Investig. Opthalmol. Vis. Sci.* **2020**, *61*. [CrossRef]
17. Lee, S.H.; Yu, D.-A.; Kim, T.-W.; Lee, E.J.; Girard, M.; Mari, J.M. Reduction of the Lamina Cribrosa Curvature After Trabeculectomy in Glaucoma. *Investig. Opthalmol. Vis. Sci.* **2016**, *57*, 5006–5014. [CrossRef] [PubMed]
18. Kadziauskienė, A.; Jašinskienė, E.; Ašoklis, R.; Lesinskas, E.; Rekašius, T.; Chua, J.; Cheng, C.-Y.; Mari, J.M.; Girard, M.J.; Schmetterer, L. Long-Term Shape, Curvature, and Depth Changes of the Lamina Cribrosa after Trabeculectomy. *Ophthalmology* **2018**, *125*, 1729–1740. [CrossRef]
19. Lee, E.J.; Han, J.C.; Park, D.Y.; Kee, C. A neuroglia-based interpretation of glaucomatous neuroretinal rim thinning in the optic nerve head. *Prog. Retin. Eye Res.* **2020**, *77*, 100840. [CrossRef]
20. Hayreh, S.S.; Vrabec, F. The Structure of the Head of the Optic Nerve in Rhesus Monkey. *Am. J. Ophthalmol.* **1966**, *61*, 136–150. [CrossRef]

21. Triviño, A.; Ramírez, J.M.; Salazar, J.J.; Ramírez, A.I.; Garcia-Sánchez, J. Immunohistochemical Study of Human Optic Nerve Head Astroglia. *Vis. Res.* **1996**, *36*, 2015–2028. [CrossRef]
22. Tehrani, S.; Johnson, E.C.; Cepurna, W.O.; Morrison, J.C. Astrocyte Processes Label for Filamentous Actin and Reorient Early Within the Optic Nerve Head in a Rat Glaucoma Model. *Investig. Opthalmol. Vis. Sci.* **2014**, *55*, 6945–6952. [CrossRef] [PubMed]
23. Lye-Barthel, M.; Sun, D.; Jakobs, T.C. Morphology of Astrocytes in a Glaucomatous Optic Nerve. *Investig. Opthalmol. Vis. Sci.* **2013**, *54*, 909–917. [CrossRef]
24. Miller, R.H.; David, S.; Patel, R.; Abney, E.R.; Raff, M.C. A quantitative immunohistochemical study of macroglial cell development in the rat optic nerve: In vivo evidence for two distinct astrocyte lineages. *Dev. Biol.* **1985**, *111*, 35–41. [CrossRef]
25. Cooper, M.; Crish, S.D.; Inman, D.M.; Horner, P.J.; Calkins, D.J. Early astrocyte redistribution in the optic nerve precedes axonopathy in the DBA/2J mouse model of glaucoma. *Exp. Eye Res.* **2015**, *150*, 22–33. [CrossRef]
26. Gietzelt, C.; Von Goscinski, C.; Lemke, J.; Schaub, F.; Hermann, M.M.; Dietlein, T.S.; Cursiefen, C.; Heindl, L.M.; Enders, P. Dynamics of structural reversal in Bruch's membrane opening-based morphometrics after glaucoma drainage device surgery. *Graefe Arch. Clin. Exp. Ophthalmol.* **2020**, *258*, 1227–1236. [CrossRef] [PubMed]

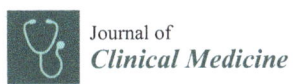

Journal of
Clinical Medicine

Article

Comparison of Efficacy between 120° and 180° Schlemm's Canal Incision Microhook Ab Interno Trabeculotomy

Naoki Okada, Kazuyuki Hirooka *, Hiromitsu Onoe, Yumiko Murakami, Hideaki Okumichi and Yoshiaki Kiuchi

Department of Ophthalmology and Visual Science, Hiroshima University, Hiroshima 734-8551, Japan; naokimed@hiroshima-u.ac.jp (N.O.); onoehir@hiroshima-u.ac.jp (H.O.); yumiko00@hiroshima-u.ac.jp (Y.M.); okumic@hiroshima-u.ac.jp (H.O.); yoshiaki@hiroshima-u.ac.jp (Y.K.)
* Correspondence: khirooka9@gmail.com; Tel.: +81-82-257-5247; Fax: +81-82-257-5249

Citation: Okada, N.; Hirooka, K.; Onoe, H.; Murakami, Y.; Okumichi, H.; Kiuchi, Y. Comparison of Efficacy between 120° and 180° Schlemm's Canal Incision Microhook Ab Interno Trabeculotomy. *J. Clin. Med.* **2021**, *10*, 3181. https://doi.org/10.3390/jcm10143181

Academic Editors: Maria Letizia Salvetat, Marco Zeppieri and Paolo Brusini

Received: 11 June 2021
Accepted: 17 July 2021
Published: 19 July 2021

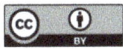
Abstract: We compared surgical outcomes in patients with either primary open-angle glaucoma or exfoliation glaucoma after undergoing combined phacoemulsification with either a 120° or 180° incision during a Schlemm's canal microhook ab interno trabeculotomy (μLOT-Phaco). This retrospective comparative case series examined 52 μLOT-Phaco eyes that underwent surgery between September 2017 and December 2020. Surgical qualified success was defined as an intraocular pressure (IOP) of $\leq$20 mmHg, $\geq$20% IOP reduction with IOP-lowering medications, and no additional glaucoma surgery. Success rates were evaluated by Kaplan-Meier survival analysis. The number of postoperative IOP-lowering medications and occurrence of complications were also assessed. Mean preoperative IOP in the 120° group was 16.9 ± 7.6 mmHg, which significantly decreased to 10.9 ± 2.7 mmHg ($p < 0.01$) and 11.1 ± 3.1 mmHg ($p = 0.01$) at 12 and 24 months, respectively. The mean number of preoperative IOP-lowering medications significantly decreased from 2.8 ± 1.4 to 1.4 ± 1.4 ($p < 0.01$) at 24 months. Mean preoperative IOP in the 180° group was 17.1 ± 7.0 mmHg, which significantly decreased to 12.1 ± 3.2 mmHg ($p = 0.02$) and 12.9 ± 1.4 mmHg ($p = 0.01$) at 12 and 24 months, respectively. The mean number of preoperative IOP-lowering medications significantly decreased from 2.9 ± 1.2 to 1.4 ± 1.5 ($p < 0.01$) at 24 months. The probability of qualified success at 24 months in the 120° and 180° groups was 50.4% and 54.6%, respectively ($p = 0.58$). There was no difference observed for hyphema formation or IOP spikes. Surgical outcomes were not significantly different between the 120° and 180° incisions in Schlemm's canal.

Keywords: ab interno trabeculotomy; intraocular pressure; glaucoma; incision in the Schlemm's canal in degrees; post-surgical complication

1. Introduction

Worldwide, glaucoma is the second most common cause of blindness [1]. Elevated intraocular pressure (IOP) has been reported by several studies to be an important risk factor for glaucoma and disease progression [2,3]. First-line therapy involves topical medications, which have a demonstrated and proven record of efficacy in all adult glaucoma stages. Incisional surgery is often considered when topical medications are not able to adequately reduce the IOP. New devices introduced over the last few years include minimally invasive glaucoma surgery (MIGS), which has generated great interest within the field. The greatest resistance for the aqueous humor outflow has been shown to be within the trabecular meshwork, with glaucomatous eyes exhibiting an even greater resistance in this region [4]. Devices and techniques, such as the trabectome, microhook, and Kahook Dual Blade, have been employed as ways for reducing the resistance of the trabecular meshwork.

While using a gonio lens, Tanito et al. [5] performed an ab interno trabeculotomy procedure, which utilized an original microhook (Inami & Co., Ltd., Tokyo, Japan), in order to incise the internal wall of the trabecular meshwork. In these original studies,

Tanito et al. [5,6] utilized a 240° incision of the trabecular meshwork. In our own recent study, we found that after combined phacoemulsification with either a microhook or a Kahook Dual Blade ab interno trabeculotomy, there was a significant increase in the corneal higher-order aberrations (HOAs) [7]. After examining the extent of the incision in the Schlemm's canal in degrees (EIS) (which included both a 120° and 180° group), we determined that the risk factor associated with the increased corneal HOAs was the EIS in the 180° Schlemm's canal opening group [7]. Based on these previously reported findings, this suggests that both the efficacy and safety of the 120° or 180° of the EIS should be investigated in a microhook ab interno trabeculotomy (μLOT).

Therefore, the purpose of our current study was to examine the efficacy and safety of both the 120° and the 180° incisions in phacoemulsification cataract extraction with μLOT (μLOT-Phaco).

2. Materials and Methods

This study evaluated data obtained from patients who underwent μLOT-Phaco between September 2017 and December 2020 at Hiroshima University Hospital. The study protocol was approved by the Institutional Review Board of Hiroshima University. All subjects provided written informed consent in accordance with the principles outlined in the Declaration of Helsinki, in addition to the standard consent for surgery.

Although patients with primary open-angle glaucoma (POAG) and exfoliation glaucoma were included in the study, any patient with a history of previous ocular surgery was excluded. In addition, all subjects had to have a minimum of 3 months of postoperative follow-up in order to be included in the analysis. When both eyes were treated in the patient, only the first eye treated was used for the analysis.

A 2.8-mm incision was created in the temporal position of the cornea. Removal of the nucleus during all procedures was performed using a standard phacoemulsification technique: Whitestar Signature Pro (Johnson & Johnson, New Brunswick, NJ, USA). All of the intraocular lens (IOLs) (PCB00V, Johnson & Johnson; XY1, HOYA, Tokyo, Japan) were implanted in the capsular bag. The μLOT surgical technique has been previously described [8]. In brief, after the cataract surgery, μLOT was performed under direct gonioscopy, with the microhook inserted into the anterior chamber through the corneal incision. Subsequently, after insertion of the tip of the microhook into Schlemm's canal, it was then moved circumferentially in order to incise the inner wall of the Schlemm's canal and the trabecular meshwork at 4 clock hours (nasal quadrant: 120°) or at 6 clock hours (inferior and nasal bisection: 180°) (Video, Supplemental Digital Content, Video S1). All decisions regarding the degree of the incision in Schlemm's canal were made by the surgeon performing the procedure. A 27-gauge cannula was used to hydrate the incisions after the removal of the ophthalmic viscosurgical device. Each individual surgeon was responsible for the postoperative administration of anti-inflammatory, anti-infective, and miotic therapies. Furthermore, the restarting of the IOP-lowering medications was performed in accordance with the judgment of the surgeon.

All statistical analyses were conducted using JMP software version 15 (SAS Inc., Cary, NC, USA). The Student's t-test for continuous variables and a chi-square test for categorical variables were used to compare the clinical characteristics between the 120° and 180° incision groups. A chi-square test was also used to compare the postoperative complications. In addition, mean IOP and mean number of IOP-lowering medications, along with their reductions from baseline, were determined at each time point by group and compared between groups. When a combination of IOP-lowering medications was used, this was counted as two drugs. This study also performed a Kaplan-Meier survival analysis, with a drop of the IOP of at least 20%, an IOP $\leq$ 20 mmHg with (qualified success) or without (complete success) administration of IOP-lowering medications, and no additional glaucoma surgery all defined as being a success. Surgical success was achieved if, after $\geq$3 months of follow-up because of the occurrence of postoperative IOP fluctuations after trabeculotomy [9]. Continuous data are presented as the mean $\pm$ standard deviation. p values < 0.05 were considered to indicate statistical significance.

3. Results

A total of 52 consecutive eyes from 52 patients with open-angle glaucoma (POAG: 34, exfoliation glaucoma: 18) were included in this study. Table 1 presents the clinical characteristics of the enrolled participants. There were no significant differences observed between the 120° and 180° incision groups in terms of age, gender, glaucoma type, preoperative IOP, and the number of glaucoma eye drops.

Table 1. Clinical characteristics.

	120°	180°	p Value
No. eyes	30	22	
Age (years)	72.3 ± 10.4	75.4 ± 10.8	0.30
Gender (M/F)	18/12	13/9	0.94
Type of glaucoma			0.82
POAG	20	14	
Exfoliation glaucoma	10	8	
Preoperative IOP (mmHg)	16.9 ± 7.6	17.1 ± 7.0	0.94
No. IOP-lowering medications	2.8 ± 1.4	2.9 ± 1.2	0.89
Mean deviation (dB)	-13.9 ± 1.4	-9.2 ± 1.7	0.03

M; male, F; female, POAG; primary open-angle glaucoma; IOP; intraocular pressure.

Table 2 shows the IOP and changes from baseline at each time point for each group. The mean IOP in the 120° incision group was 16.9 ± 7.6 mmHg at baseline, while it was 12.5 ± 2.7 mmHg ($n = 25$; $p = 0.01$), 10.9 ± 2.7 mmHg ($n = 14$; $p < 0.01$), 11.2 ± 3.0 mmHg ($n = 13$; $p < 0.01$), and 11.1 ± 3.1 mmHg ($n = 10$; $p = 0.01$) at 6, 12, 18, and 24 months, respectively. In the 180° incision group, the IOP was 17.1 ± 7.0 mmHg at baseline, while it was 12.9 ± 2.4 mmHg ($n = 22$; $p = 0.045$), 12.1 ± 3.2 mmHg ($n = 21$; $p = 0.02$), 12.6 ± 2.7 mmHg ($n = 16$; $p = 0.02$), and 12.9 ± 1.4 mmHg ($n = 13$: $p = 0.01$) at 6, 12, 18, and 24 months, respectively. Figure 1 shows pre-operative and postoperative (final visit) IOPs for all patients in the study.

Table 2. Differences in preoperative and postoperative IOP.

	120°			180°			
	IOP at Each Time Point (mmHg)	Change from Baseline (%)	p Value *	IOP at Each Time Point (mmHg)	Change from Baseline (%)	p Value *	p Value **
Baseline	16.9 ± 7.6 ($n = 30$)			17.1 ± 7.0 ($n = 22$)			0.94
Month 6	12.5 ± 2.7 ($n = 25$)	18.8 ± 26.6	0.01	12.9 ± 2.4 ($n = 22$)	15.3 ± 28.6	0.045	0.62
Month 12	10.9 ± 2.7 ($n = 14$)	29.5 ± 29.7	<0.01	12.1 ± 3.2 ($n = 21$)	24.1 ± 25.4	0.02	0.27
Month 18	11.2 ± 3.0 ($n = 13$)	26.1 ± 31.2	<0.01	12.6 ± 2.7 ($n = 16$)	22.7 ± 29.3	0.02	0.77
Month 24	11.1 ± 3.1 ($n = 10$)	34.2 ± 27.2	0.01	12.9 ± 1.4 ($n = 13$)	23.1 ± 26.4	0.01	0.07

IOP; intraocular pressure; * Calculated using paired *t*-test for IOP between preoperative and postoperative value; ** Calculated using Student's *t*-test for % changes from baseline between the groups.

Table 3 shows the mean number of IOP-lowering medications at each time point for each group. The mean number of IOP-lowering medications in the 120° incision group was 2.8 ± 1.4 at baseline, while it was 0.9 ± 1.1 ($p < 0.01$), 1.0 ± 1.3 ($p < 0.01$), 1.1 ± 1.3 ($p < 0.01$), and 1.4 ± 1.4 ($p < 0.01$) at 6, 12, 18, and 24 months, respectively. In the 180° incision group, the mean number of IOP-lowering medications was 2.9 ± 1.2 at baseline, while it was 0.9 ± 1.1 ($p < 0.01$), 0.9 ± 1.1 ($p < 0.01$), 1.2 ± 1.3 ($p < 0.01$), and 1.4 ± 1.5 ($p < 0.01$) at 6, 12, 18, and 24 months, respectively. Figure 2 shows the numbers of pre-operative and postoperative IOP-lowering medications.

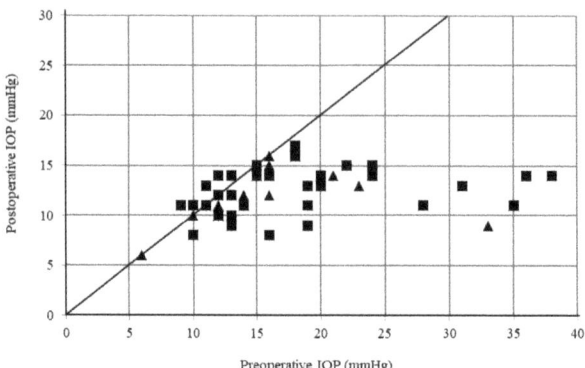

Figure 1. Scattergram of preoperative versus postoperative intraocular pressure (IOP). Triangle: 120° incision group, Square: 180° incision group.

Table 3. Differences in preoperative and postoperative number of IOP-lowering medication.

	120°		180°		
	Number of Medications at Each Time Point	*p* Value *	Number of Medications at Each Time Point	*p* Value *	*p* Value **
Baseline	2.8 ± 1.4 (*n* = 30)		2.9 ± 1.2 (*n* = 22)		0.89
Month 6	0.9 ± 1.1 (*n* = 25)	<0.01	0.9 ± 1.1 (*n* = 22)	<0.01	0.94
Month 12	1.0 ± 1.3 (*n* = 14)	<0.01	0.9 ± 1.1 (*n* = 21)	<0.01	0.86
Month 18	1.1 ± 1.3 (*n* = 13)	<0.01	1.2 ± 1.3 (*n* = 16)	<0.01	0.78
Month 24	1.4 ± 1.4 (*n* = 10)	<0.01	1.4 ± 1.5 (*n* = 13)	<0.01	>0.99

IOP; intraocular pressure; * Calculated using Wilcoxon signed-ranks test for number of IOP-lowering medication between preoperative and postoperative values; ** Calculated using Mann-Whitney's U test for postoperative values between the groups.

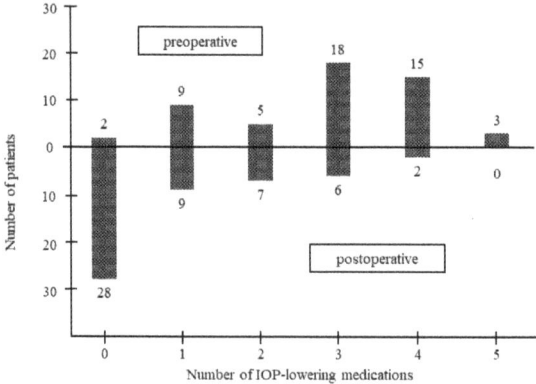

Figure 2. Bar graph showing the number of preoperative and postoperative medications.

Figure 3 shows the Kaplan-Meier survival curves used to compare the surgical outcomes in the 120° and 180° groups. At 12 and 24 months postoperatively, qualified success rates in the 120° and 180° groups were 50.4% and 54.6%, and 50.4% and 54.6%, respectively (*p* = 0.87) (Figure 3A). In contrast, the complete success rates in the 120° and 180° groups were 33.2% and 27.3%, and 33.2% and 27.3%, respectively (*p* = 0.58) (Figure 3B).

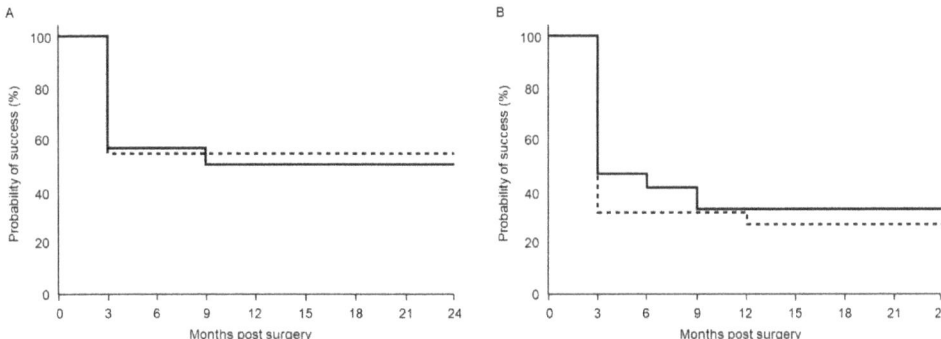

Figure 3. Survival cure analysis success rate of intraocular pressure control after combined phacoemulsification when using either a 120° or 180° incision during Schlemm's canal microhook ab interno trabeculotomy. Surgery failure was defined as an intraocular pressure drop of < 20%, intraocular pressure > 20 mmHg with (**A**) or without (**B**) intraocular pressure-lowering medication, and additional glaucoma surgery. Solid line: 120° group, Dashed line: 180° group.

Within 1 week after the surgery in the 120° and 180° groups, IOP spikes (an IOP increase of > 30 mmHg) occurred in 2 (6.7%) and 1 (4.6%) eyes, respectively ($p = 0.75$). All of these subsided in conjunction with the administration of IOP-lowering medications. Hyphema was defined as red blood cells accumulated in the anterior chamber of the eye [10]. In the 120° and 180° groups, hyphema with niveau formation occurred in 5 (16.7%) and 4 (18.2%) eyes, respectively ($p = 0.89$) (Table 4). In the 120° group, the extent of the niveau formation of hyphema was below 2 mm in 1 eye, while it was below 1 mm in 4 eyes, with a mean time of resolution of the hyphema of 7.2 days. In the 180° group, the extent of the niveau formation of hyphema in all eyes was below 1 mm, with a mean time of resolution of the hyphema of 4.3 days. None of the eyes required any additional glaucoma surgery.

Table 4. Postoperative complications.

	120°	180°	*p* Value
Hyphema with niveau formation	5 (16.7%)	4 (18.2%)	0.89
Transient IOP elevation > 30 mmHg	2 (6.7%)	1 (4.6%)	0.75

IOP; intraocular pressure.

4. Discussion

The results of the current study showed there was a similar efficacy between the 120° and the 180° incision in the Schlemm's canal μLOT-Phaco procedures. In addition, there were no significant difference observed for the surgical success rate, mean IOP, IOP reduction rate, and IOP-lowering medications scores between the 120° and 180° incisions in Schlemm's canal.

Manabe et al. [11] examined increases in the extent of the incision in Schlemm's canal to ≥150° and reported that this did not affect the reduction in the IOP at 1 year postoperatively. Sato et al. [12] also showed that neither the 180° nor the 360° incision in Schlemm's canal affected the IOP reduction. Furthermore, Mori et al. [13] reported that there was no significant difference for the 1-year success rate between the 1- and 2-quadrant incisions in Schlemm's canal when using μLOT. In enucleated human eyes, as compared to results for the 360° incision in the Schlemm's canal LOT, the 30° and 120° incisions resulted in 42% and 85% reductions in outflow resistance, respectively [14]. Therefore, incisions greater than 120° may not be able to further reduce the IOP in the different types of MIGS. In contrast, the 360° suture trabeculotomy achieved lower IOP values as compared to the 120° metal trabeculotomy [15]. However, in that study, the 120° incisions were created with metal probes. It may be difficult to evaluate surgical outcomes according to the extent of the incision because of the different incision approaches.

A previous study reported finding a positive correlation between the extent of the incision in Schlemm's canal (ranging from 150 to 320°) and the hyphema score at 1 day postoperatively [11]. Furthermore, another study found that there was a significant difference between the 180° and 360° Schlemm's canal incisions for the frequency of postoperative hyphema [11]. However, our current study found no significant differences for either the complications noted between the 120° and 180° incisions or for the safety between these two techniques. In addition, Mori et al. [13] recently examined the hyphema formation between 1- and 2-quadrant incisions in Schlemm's canal groups and reported finding there was no difference between the groups. These results suggest that incisions more than 180° in Schlemm's canal are likely to cause greater blood reflux from the collector channels, thereby leading to a higher frequency of postoperative hyphema.

Our recent study additionally showed that a more extensive incision (180° vs. 120°) in Schlemm's canal was a risk factor for potential changes in the corneal HOAs, coma-like, and spherical-like aberrations [7]. Corneal HOAs in the 120° Schlemm's canal incision group were 0.227 ± 0.128 μm at baseline and 0.251 ± 0.131 μm ($p = 0.12$) at 3 months after surgery [7]. However, corneal HOAs in the 180° Schlemm's canal incision group were 0.216 ± 0.095 μm at baseline and 0.439 ± 0.223 μm ($p = 0.001$) at 3 months after surgery [7]. These results suggest that increases in the HOAs can subsequently lead to functional visual acuity decreases. In order to definitively confirm these findings, we are presently evaluating the vision-related quality of life that occurs after patients undergo μLOT-Phaco procedure.

We evaluated data obtained from patients who underwent μLOT-Phaco in the current study. However, Chen et al. [16] previously reported an average 13% reduction in IOP and 12% reduction in IOP-lowering medications 1 year after phacoemulsification in patients with POAG. Therefore, the true effect associated with the μLOT procedure is difficult to determine.

In our current study, there were some limitations. First, this was a retrospective study. As a result, the 120° or 180° incisions in the Schlemm's canal were not randomly assigned to the subjects. Furthermore, outcome data were not specifically collected but rather obtained during our routine clinical practice. Second, this study only evaluated a relatively small number of cases. A small sample size might have led to the non-significant difference between the 120° and 180° incisions in Schlemm's canal. Therefore, in order to obtain better rigorous comparative evidence and data, a multi-center, randomized, prospective study will need to be undertaken. Recent MIGS procedures have been performed in relatively medically controlled glaucoma patients to reduce medication [17]. Such cases were included in the current study and had a relatively low baseline IOP and IOP reduction in each group. In the current study, all cases of failure had a <20% IOP reduction in all patients. To verify the results in eyes with a higher baseline IOP, a subgroup of cases with a baseline IOP $\geq$ 21 mmHg was analyzed. The mean IOP in the 120° incision group was reduced from 31.2 ± 6.3 mmHg ($n = 5$) at baseline to 12.0 ± 2.4 mmHg at the final visit. The mean IOP in the 180° incision group was also reduced from 26.5 ± 5.8 mmHg ($n = 6$) at baseline to 13.8 ± 0.8 mmHg at the final visit. These results were comparable to those of the original study population.

In conclusion, the current findings demonstrate that there was no difference in the surgical success between the 120° and 180° incisions in the Schlemm's canal μLOT-Phaco. However, corneal HOAs, coma-like, and spherical-like aberrations were associated with a more extensive incision in Schlemm's canal, thereby suggesting that extensive incisions are a risk factor in these procedures. Therefore, the authors strongly recommend the use of a 120° incision during Schlemm's canal μLOT-Phaco.

Supplementary Materials: The following are available online at https://www.mdpi.com/article/10.3390/jcm10143181/s1, Video S1: Technique of microhook ab interno trabeculotomy.

Author Contributions: Conceptualization, K.H.; methodology, K.H.; software, N.O.; validation, N.O., K.H., H.O. (Hiromitsu Onoe), Y.M., H.O. (Hideaki Okumichi), and Y.K.; formal analysis, N.O.;

investigation, N.O.; resources, Y.K.; data curation, N.O.; writing—original draft preparation, K.H.; writing—review and editing, K.H.; visualization, K.H.; supervision, K.H.; project administration, K.H.; funding acquisition, K.H. All authors have read and agreed to the published version of the manuscript.

Funding: This research was funded by a Grant-in-Aid for Scientific Research from the Ministry of Education, Culture, Sports, Science, and Technology of Japan (20K09827).

Institutional Review Board Statement: The study was conducted according to the guidelines of the Declaration of Helsinki, and approved by the Institutional Review Board of Hiroshima University (protocol code E-2436 and date of approval).

Informed Consent Statement: Informed consent was obtained from all subjects involved in the study.

Data Availability Statement: The data analysed in this study are available from the corresponding author on reasonable request.

Conflicts of Interest: The authors declare no conflict of interest.

References

1. Quigley, H.A.; Broman, A.T. The number of people with glaucoma worldwide in 2010 and 2020. *Br. J. Ophthalmol.* **2006**, *90*, 262–267. [CrossRef] [PubMed]
2. Chauhan, B.C.; Mikelberg, F.S.; Balaszi, A.G.; LeBlanc, R.P.; Lesk, M.R.; Trope, G.E.; Canadian Glaucoma Study Group. Canadian Glaucoma Study: 2. risk factors for the progression of open-angle glaucoma. *Arch. Ophthalmol.* **2008**, *126*, 1030–1036. [CrossRef] [PubMed]
3. Heijl, A.; Leske, M.C.; Bengtsson, B.; Hyman, L.; Bengtsson, B.; Hussein, M.; Early Manifest Glaucoma Trial Group. Reduction of intraocular pressure and glaucoma progression: Results from the Early Manifest Glaucoma Trial. *Arch. Ophthalmol.* **2002**, *120*, 1268–1279. [CrossRef] [PubMed]
4. Johnson, M. What controls aqueous humor outflow resistance? *Exp. Eye Res.* **2006**, *82*, 545–557. [CrossRef]
5. Tanito, M.; Sano, I.; Ikeda, Y.; Fujihara, E. Shore-term results of microhook ab interno trabeculotomy, a novel minimally invasive glaucoma surgery in Japanese eyes: Initial case series. *Acta. Ophthalmol.* **2017**, *95*, e354–e360. [CrossRef] [PubMed]
6. Tanito, M.; Ikeda, Y.; Fujihara, E. Effectiveness and safety of combined cataract surgery and microhook ab interno trabeculotomy in Japanese eyes with glaucoma: Report of an initial case series. *Jpn. J. Ophthalmol.* **2017**, *61*, 457–464. [CrossRef] [PubMed]
7. Onoe, H.; Hirooka, K.; Okumichi, H.; Sakata, H.; Murakami, Y.; Kiuchi, Y. Corneal higher-order aberrations after microhook ab interno trabeculotomy and goniotomy with the Kahook Dual Blade. Under submission.
8. Aoki, R.; Hirooka, K.; Goda, E.; Yuasa, Y.; Okumichi, H.; Onoe, H.; Kiuchi, Y. Comparison of surgical outcomes between microhook ab interno trabeculotomy and goniotomy with the Kahook Dual Blade in combination with phacoemulsification: A retrospective, comparative case series. *Adv. Ther.* **2021**, *38*, 329–336. [CrossRef] [PubMed]
9. Tanihara, H.; Negi, A.; Akimoto, M.; Terauchi, H.; Okudaira, A.; Kozaki, J.; Takeuchi, A.; Nagata, M. Surgical effects of trabeculotomy ab externo on adult eyes with primary open angle glaucoma and pseudoexfoliation syndrome. *Arch. Ophthalmol.* **1993**, *111*, 1653–1661. [CrossRef] [PubMed]
10. Brandt, M.T.; Haug, R.H. Traumatic hyphema: A comprehensive review. *J. Oral Maxillofac. Surg.* **2001**, *59*, 1462–1470. [CrossRef] [PubMed]
11. Manabe, S.; Sawaguchi, S.; Hayashi, K. The effect of the extent of the incision in the Schlemm canal on the surgical outcomes of suture trabeculotomy for open-angle glaucoma. *Jpn. J. Ophthalmol.* **2017**, *61*, 99–104. [CrossRef] [PubMed]
12. Sato, T.; Kawaji, T. 12-month randomized trial of 360° and 180° Schlemm's canal incisions in suture trabeculotomy ab interno for open-angle glaucoma. *Br. J. Ophthalmol.*. Online ahead of print. [CrossRef] [PubMed]
13. Mori, S.; Murai, Y.; Ueda, K.; Sakamoto, M.; Kurimoto, T.; Yamada-Nakanishi, Y.; Nakamura, M. Comparison of efficacy and early surgery-related complications between one-quadrant and two-quadrant microhook *ab interno* trabeculotomy: A propensity score matched study. *Acta. Ophthalmol.* Online ahead of print. [CrossRef] [PubMed]
14. Rosenquist, R.; Epstein, D.; Melamed, S.; Johnson, M.; Grant, W.M. Outflow resistance of enucleated human eyes at two different perfusion pressures and different extents of trabeculotomy. *Curr. Eye Res.* **1989**, *8*, 1233–1240. [CrossRef] [PubMed]
15. Chin, S.; Nitta, T.; Shinmei, Y.; Aoyagi, M.; Nitta, A.; Ohno, S.; Ishida, S.; Yoshida, K. Reduction of intraocular pressure using a modified 360-degree suture trabeculotomy technique in primary and secondary open-angle glaucoma: A pilot study. *J. Glaucoma.* **2012**, *21*, 401–407. [CrossRef] [PubMed]
16. Chen, P.P.; Lin, S.C.; Junk, A.K.; Radhakrishnan, S.; Singh, K.; Chen, T.C. The effect of phacoemulsification on intraocular pressure in glaucoma patients: A report by the American academy of ophthalmology. *Ophthalmology* **2015**, *122*, 1294–1307. [CrossRef] [PubMed]
17. Bovee, C.E.; Pasquale, L.R. Evolving surgical interventions in the treatment of glaucoma. *Semin. Ophthalmol.* **2017**, *31*, 91–95. [CrossRef] [PubMed]

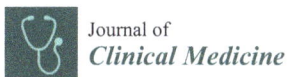

Article

Serum Calcium Level as a Useful Surrogate for Risk of Elevated Intraocular Pressure

Yu-Min Chang [1], Jiann-Torng Chen [1], Ming-Cheng Tai [1], Wei-Liang Chen [2,3] and Ying-Jen Chen [1,*]

[1] Department of Ophthalmology, Tri-Service General Hospital, School of Medicine, National Defense Medical Center, Taipei 114, Taiwan; m7886916@yahoo.com.tw (Y.-M.C.); jt66chen@gmail.com (J.-T.C.); mingtai1966@yahoo.com.tw (M.-C.T.)

[2] Division of Family Medicine, Department of Family and Community Medicine, Tri-Service General Hospital, School of Medicine, National Defense Medical Center, Taipei 114, Taiwan; weiliang0508@gmail.com

[3] Division of Geriatric Medicine, Department of Family and Community Medicine, Tri-Service General Hospital, School of Medicine, National Defense Medical Center, Taipei 114, Taiwan

* Correspondence: yj12664@gmail.com; Tel.: +886-8792-7163

Abstract: Background: Uncontrolled intraocular pressure (IOP) plays a principal role in the deterioration of glaucoma, and the intraocular pressure is also accepted as the most important modifiable factor. Calcium ion has been found to play a vital role in regulating the resistance of the trabecular meshwork in humans. However, the relationship between serum total calcium and IOP has not been well-established. Methods: We investigated the association between serum total calcium and the IOP in a large population (14,037 eligible participants, consisting of 7712 men and 6325 women, were included) at the Tri-Service General Hospital from 2010 to 2016. Several models of covariate adjustments associated with IOP were designed. Univariate and multivariate regression analysis was performed for gender differences in the association between the serum total calcium level and IOP. Results: There was a significant relationship between serum total calcium levels and IOP in women and men with a β coefficient of 0.050 (95% confidence interval (CI), 0.030–0.069) and 0.025 (95%CI, 0.007–0.043). Notably, participants in the highest tertiles of serum total calcium levels had significantly higher IOP, in both the male and female participants. Conclusions: Our study shows that IOP is significantly associated with serum total calcium levels in a large Asian population. This study supports the notion that serum total calcium may play an important role in groups at high risk for elevated IOP.

Keywords: intraocular pressure; serum calcium; female

Citation: Chang, Y.-M.; Chen, J.-T.; Tai, M.-C.; Chen, W.-L.; Chen, Y.-J. Serum Calcium Level as a Useful Surrogate for Risk of Elevated Intraocular Pressure. *J. Clin. Med.* **2021**, *10*, 1839. https://doi.org/10.3390/jcm10091839

Academic Editor: Maria Letizia Salvetat

Received: 6 March 2021
Accepted: 21 April 2021
Published: 23 April 2021

Publisher's Note: MDPI stays neutral with regard to jurisdictional claims in published maps and institutional affiliations.

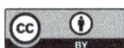
1. Introduction

Glaucoma is a chronic and irreversible disease characterized by progressive loss of retinal ganglion cells [1]; it is a leading cause of permanent blindness in the world. Intraocular pressure (IOP) has been well accepted as the most important modifiable factor for development of glaucoma and the goal of most therapy is to control IOP. Many studies have reported positive associations between IOP and several cardiometabolic conditions, including hypertension, diabetes [2], postprandial glucose [3], coronary atherosclerosis [4], and obesity [5].

The aqueous humor (AH) drainage system in human eyes has two pathways, including conventional or trabecular outflow and uveoscleral outflow. The trabecular outflow is the main drainage route in humans, which is composed of the trabecular meshwork, the juxtacanalicular connective tissue, the endothelial lining of Schlemm's canal, the collecting channels, and the aqueous veins [6]. If any structure in the trabecular outflow pathway is damaged, AH drainage can be impaired, which causes elevation of IOP.

Calcium ion plays an important role in cell signaling and cell contraction; its concentration is modulated by many factors, including the cellular environment. Dysregulation of calcium homeostasis has been found in many neurodegenerative diseases, such as Huntington's disease, Parkinson's disease, Alzheimer's disease, amyotrophic lateral sclerosis, and multiple sclerosis [7,8]. In a primary open angle glaucoma (POAG) model from postmortem donor eyes, one study discovered the mitochondrial function of trabecular meshwork (TM) cells was damaged, which caused the cells to be abnormally vulnerable to calcium ion stress. Hence, the IOP is uncontrolled because of dysfunction in calcium regulation in these cells [9]. Another study reports that transient receptor potential vanilloid 4 (TRPV4) is a central channel for calcium ion and mechanical stretch-sensitivity in human TM cells. Mechanical stress, such as swelling and pressure, can activate TRPV4 and cause extracellular matrix (ECM) remodeling associated with increased TM stiffness and contractility. Finally, when the TM outflow is obstructed, the IOP is elevated [10].

However, serum total calcium is now believed to be associated with metabolic syndrome and other cardiometabolic disease [11,12]. The relationship between metabolic syndrome and high IOP was discovered in previous studies [5,13]. To date, no cross-sectional studies have investigated the association between serum total calcium and IOP in an Asian population with a large sample size. Hence, the aim of our study is to explore the influence of serum total calcium on IOP in an Asian population.

2. Materials and Methods

2.1. Design of the Study

We collected the medical records of healthy examinations including laboratory examinations, ophthalmological examinations, body composition, and self-reported questionnaires between 2010 and 2016 in a medical center, the Tri-Service General Hospital (TSGH) in Taiwan. Only participants over 20 years old were included in this study. This was a retrospective study to determine the association of IOP with serum total calcium levels. Our exclusion criteria were as follows: missing laboratory data; those lacking comprehensive examinations; any systemic disease that could affect the IOP and homeostasis of serum calcium (hypertension, diabetes, chronic kidney disease, coronary atherosclerosis, and obesity); any glaucoma history or having received anti-glaucoma therapy; using any eyedrops in the past month; histories of ocular hypertension, ectatic dystrophies, and contact-lens-related complications; histories of any intraocular surgery; and an inter-eye IOP difference above 3 mmHg [14]. If the participants received more than one healthy examination during this period, we only selected the data at the first visit to analyze. Finally, 14,037 eligible participants, consisting of 7712 men and 6325 women, were included in the analysis (Figure 1). The study was conducted in accordance with the principles of the Declaration of Helsinki, and it received institutional review board approval from TSGH.

2.2. Ophthalmological Examinations

Ophthalmological examinations were performed by professional ophthalmologists in a standard ophthalmological examination room in TSGH, including best-corrected visual acuity (BCVA), IOP, biomicroscopic examinations, and dilated fundus examinations. A CT-80 non-contact computerized tonometer was used to obtain the IOP of both eyes, and the mean IOP values of both eyes were recorded for logistic regression.

2.3. Covariates

Age, gender, and personal history (smoking and drinking) were obtained by a self-assessment questionnaire. Bioelectrical impedance analysis (InBody720, Biospace, Inc., Cerritos, CA, USA) was applied to measure the percentage body fat. Participants must have fasted for at least 8 h before blood draws. Uric acid, serum total cholesterol, aspartate aminotransferase, creatinine, highly sensitive C-reactive protein, thyroid-stimulating hormone, and total calcium were included in laboratory examinations and were analyzed by various methods. A Hitachi 737 automated analyzer was used to measure uric acid. Enzymatic colorimetric methods were applied to detect total cholesterol and aspartate aminotransferase. The Jaffe method using alkaline picrate was used to measure creatinine.

Highly sensitive C-reactive protein was accessed by latex-enhanced nephelometry. An immune-enzymatic assay was applied to detect thyroid-stimulating hormone. Finally, the o-cresolphthalein complexone method was used to measure serum total calcium levels. All methods were executed based on the relevant guidelines and regulations of TSGH.

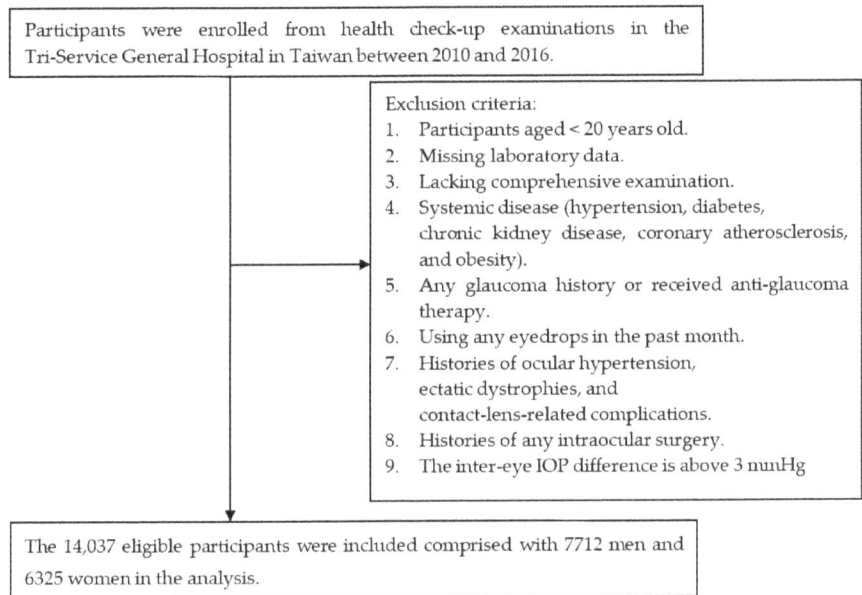

Figure 1. Flowchart of subject selection.

2.4. Statistical Analyses

The differences between men and women with respect to demographic characteristics and laboratory data were analyzed by *t*-test and chi-squared test. Gender difference in IOP was found in many studies. Some studies revealed the IOP was higher in the male group than in the female group [15,16]. However, some studies proposed the opposite view [17,18]. The effect of modification by serum total calcium level and gender was tested by interaction terms in the models for the IOP. There were significant interactions between serum total calcium level and gender. According to the significant findings of the interaction testing, further stratified analyses were performed. Multivariate linear and logistic regression models were used to investigate the association between serum total calcium and IOP. Three models of co-variate adjustments were designed: Model 1 = unadjusted; Model 2 = Model 1 + age, gender, percentage body fat, total cholesterol, uric acid, aspartate aminotransferase, creatinine, highly sensitive C-reactive protein, and thyroid-stimulating hormone, which were recognized as correlated variables with IOP [19–21]; and Model 3 = Model 2 + smoking and drinking, which were also recognized as correlated variables with IOP [22]. Multivariate linear regression analysis was used for gender differences in the association between the serum total calcium level and IOP. In addition, we divided serum total calcium levels into tertiles to perform tertiles-based analysis, and participants in the lowest tertile were regarded as the reference group. The cut-off levels of serum total calcium for the tertiles were as follows: 5 mg/dL < T1 $\leq$ 9.1 mg/dL; 9.1 mg/dL < T2 $\leq$ 9.4 mg/dL; and 9.4 mg/dL < T3 $\leq$ 12 mg/dL. We also used the logistic regression to calculate the odds ratios and to investigate the relationship between serum total calcium and the risk of high IOP. In our study, high IOP was defined as 18 mmHg, according to a previous study [23]. A receiving operating characteristic (ROC) curve plot was used to find the optimal cut-off of serum total calcium. Furthermore, the area under the

ROC (AUROC) and the corresponding 95% confidence intervals (CI) were all calculated. A P value less than 0.05 was defined as statistically significant for all analyses. Data analysis of this study was conducted using IBM Statistical Product and Service Solutions Statistics version 22.0.

3. Results

3.1. Demographics of the Participants

Clinical demographic information including age, IOP, percentage body fat, and biochemical data in men and women are presented in Table 1. The study group comprised 14,037 participants (7712 men and 6325 women; mean age 46.88 ± 13 years and 47.00 ± 12.61 years, respectively). Table 1 shows that the IOP was higher in men (14.80 ± 3.10 mmHg) and that the percentage body fat ($31.94 \pm 6.67\%$) and total cholesterol (191.29 ± 36.66 mg/dL) were higher in women.

Table 1. Characteristics of participants between gender.

Variables	Male (n = 7712)	Female (n = 6325)	p-Value
Continuous Variables, Mean (SD)			
Age (years)	46.88 (13.00)	47.00 (12.61)	0.577
IOP (mmHg)	14.80 (3.10)	14.54 (3.09)	<0.001
Percentage body fat (%)	25.00 (6.33)	31.94 (6.67)	<0.001
Total cholesterol (mg/dL)	189.31 (36.09)	191.29 (36.66)	0.001
Uric acid (mg/dL)	6.49 (1.33)	4.76 (1.10)	<0.001
Aspartate aminotransferase (U/L)	23.01 (13.52)	19.63 (9.31)	<0.001
Creatinine (mg/dL)	0.97 (0.34)	0.68 (0.17)	<0.001
highly sensitive C-reactive protein (mg/dL)	0.25 (0.56)	0.21 (0.42)	<0.001
Thyroid-stimulating hormone (IU/mL)	2.15 (1.54)	2.47 (1.96)	<0.001
Serum total calcium (mg/dL)	9.28 (0.40)	9.21 (0.41)	0.310
Category Variables, (n, %)			
Smoking	3448 (44.7)	515 (8.1)	<0.001
Drinking	4242 (55.0)	1544 (24.1)	<0.001

Abbreviations: SD, standard deviation; IOP, intraocular pressure.

3.2. Association between Serum Total Calcium and Intraocular Pressure

In our study, we found a prominent relationship between serum total calcium levels and IOP. The results were analyzed by linear regression and are shown in Table 2. The β coefficient of the IOP was 0.045 (95% confidence interval, 0.033–0.058, $p < 0.001$), 0.039 (95% confidence interval, 0.026–0.053, $p < 0.001$), and 0.040 (95% confidence interval, 0.027–0.053, $p < 0.001$) in Models 1, 2, and 3, respectively. We further divided the participants into two groups by gender, and there was still a significant association between serum total calcium levels and IOP.

Table 2. Association between serum total calcium and the intraocular pressure.

Variable	Model [a] 1 β (95% CI)	p Value	Model [a] 2 β (95% CI)	p Value	Model [a] 3 β (95% CI)	p Value
Total	0.045 (0.033–0.058)	<0.001	0.039 (0.026–0.053)	<0.001	0.040 (0.027–0.053)	<0.001
Male	0.037 (0.020–0.055)	<0.001	0.024 (0.007–0.042)	0.007	0.025 (0.007–0.043)	0.006
Female	0.051 (0.032–0.070)	<0.001	0.049 (0.030–0.069)	<0.001	0.050 (0.030–0.069)	<0.001

[a] Adjusted covariates: Model 1 = unadjusted; Model 2 = Model 1 + age, gender, percentage body fat, total cholesterol, uric acid, aspartate aminotransferase, creatinine, highly sensitive C-reactive protein and thyroid-stimulating hormone; Model 3 = Model 2 + smoking and drinking. Abbreviations: CI, confidence interval.

As shown in Table 3, serum total calcium levels were divided into tertiles to investigate the association with IOP. Positive associations were found between serum total calcium levels and IOP regardless of gender. In the male group, participants in the highest tertiles of serum total calcium levels had significantly higher IOP with a β coefficient of 0.022 (95% confidence interval, 0.005–0.039, $p < 0.010$) in Model 3 and in the female group, participants in the highest tertiles of serum total calcium levels also had significantly higher IOP with a β coefficient of 0.046 (95% confidence interval, 0.025–0.067, $p < 0.001$) in the same model.

Table 3. Association between tertiles of serum total calcium and intraocular pressure.

Variables	Tertiles	Model [a] 1 β (95% CI)	p Value	Model [a] 2 β (95% CI)	p Value	Model [a] 3 β (95% CI)	p Value
Total	T2 [b] vs. T1 [b]	0.023 (0.011–0.036)	<0.001	0.023 (0.010–0.035)	<0.001	0.023 (0.011–0.035)	<0.001
	T3 [b] vs. T1 [b]	0.039 (0.026–0.052)	<0.001	0.035 (0.022–0.048)	<0.001	0.035 (0.022–0.048)	<0.001
Male	T2 [b] vs. T1 [b]	0.021 (0.005–0.038)	0.012	0.020 (0.004–0.037)	0.016	0.021 (0.004–0.037)	0.013
	T3 [b] vs. T1 [b]	0.031 (0.014–0.047)	<0.001	0.022 (0.005–0.038)	0.012	0.022 (0.005–0.039)	0.010
Female	T2 [b] vs. T1 [b]	0.024 (0.006–0.043)	0.011	0.023 (0.004–0.042)	0.017	0.024 (0.004–0.043)	0.016
	T3 [b] vs. T1 [b]	0.048 (0.028–0.067)	<0.001	0.046 (0.025–0.066)	<0.001	0.046 (0.025–0.067)	<0.001

[a] Adjusted covariates: Model 1 = unadjusted; Model 2 = Model 1 + age, gender, percentage body fat, total cholesterol, uric acid, aspartate aminotransferase, creatinine, highly sensitive C-reactive protein, and thyroid-stimulating hormone; Model 3 = Model 2 + smoking and drinking. [b] Total calcium level: T1: 5–9.1 mg/dL, T2: 9.1–9.4 mg/dL, T3: 9.4–12 mg/dL.

We also performed the logistic regression to examine the association between different serum total calcium tertiles and high IOP and the result is demonstrated in Table 4. In the female population, the risk of high IOP was significantly associated with the higher tertiles of serum total calcium levels in Model 1 (odds ratio = 1.599, 95% confidence interval = 1.171–2.184, $p = 0.003$), Model 2 (odds ratio = 1.522, 95% confidence interval = 1.105–2.097, $p = 0.010$), and Model 3 (odds ratio = 1.539, 95% confidence interval = 1.116–2.122, $p = 0.008$). However, the odds ratios between serum total calcium and high IOP were not significant in the male group. Figure 2 summarizes the optimal cut-off value of serum total calcium by using ROC analysis. The AUROC value was 0.538 (95% confidence interval = 0.515–0.561) in the male group and 0.563 (95% confidence interval = 0.538–0.588) in the female group. The odds ratios for developing high IOP (>18 mmHg) in different models are showed in Table 5. The optimal cut-off value of serum total calcium level was 9.35 mg/dL in the male group by using maximal Youden's index with sensitivity and specificity (50.4/56.5%). Likewise, the optimal cut-off value of serum total calcium level was 9.05 mg/dL in the female group with sensitivity and specificity (76.8/33.0%). We found the significant occurrence of high IOP in the cut-off value in the female group. In contrast, there was no significant difference in the cut-off value in the male group.

Table 4. Gender difference in association between serum total calcium tertiles and the presence of high IOP.

Variables	Tertiles	Model [a] 1 Odds Ratio (95% CI)	p Value	Model [a] 2 Odds Ratio (95% CI)	p Value	Model [a] 3 Odds Ratio (95% CI)	p Value
Female	T2 [b] vs. T1 [b]	1.379 (1.013–1.877)	0.041	1.310 (0.958–1.792)	0.091	1.323 (0.967–1.810)	0.080
	T3 [b] vs. T1 [b]	1.599 (1.171–2.184)	<0.003	1.522 (1.105–2.097)	0.010	1.539 (1.116–2.122)	0.008
Male	T2 [b] vs. T1 [b]	1.232 (0.950–1.598)	0.116	1.192 (0.916–1.550)	0.191	1.208 (0.928–1.572)	0.160
	T3 [b] vs. T1 [b]	1.207 (0.931–1.566)	0.155	1.038 (0.792–1.360)	0.787	1.046 (0.799–1.371)	0.742

[a] Adjusted covariates: Model 1 = unadjusted; Model 2 = Model 1 + age, gender, percentage body fat, total cholesterol, uric acid, aspartate aminotransferase, creatinine, highly sensitive C-reactive protein, and thyroid-stimulating hormone; Model 3 = Model 2 + smoking and drinking. [b] Total calcium level: T1: 5–9.1 mg/dL, T2: 9.1–9.4 mg/dL, T3: 9.4–12 mg/dL.

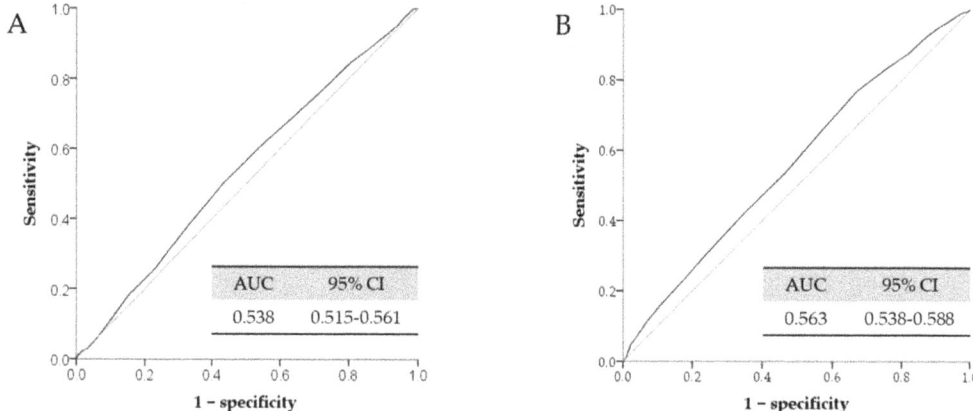

Figure 2. ROCs for serum total calcium and high IOP. (**A**): male group; (**B**): female group. AUC: area under the curve; ROC: receiver operating characteristic. High IOP: > 18 mmHg.

Table 5. Gender difference in association between cut-off points of serum total calcium and the presence of high IOP.

Variables		Male	Female
Cut-off value of serum total calcium (mg/dL)		9.35	9.05
High IOP(>18 mmHg)	Model [a] 1	1.258	1.764
	Odds Ratio (95% CI)	(1.015–1.559)	(1.316–2.366)
	p Value	0.036	<0.001
	Model [a] 2	1.129	1.689
	Odds Ratio (95% CI)	(0.904–1.409)	(1.254–2.275)
	p Value	0.285	0.001
	Model [a] 3	1.136	1.704
	Odds Ratio (95% CI)	(0.910–1.418)	(1.264–2.297)
	p Value	0.261	<0.001

[a] Adjusted covariates: Model 1 = unadjusted; Model 2 = Model 1 + age, gender, percentage body fat, total cholesterol, uric acid, aspartate aminotransferase, creatinine, highly sensitive C-reactive protein, and thyroid-stimulating hormone; Model 3 = Model 2 + smoking and drinking.

4. Discussion

In the current study, we observed an association between serum total calcium and IOP. Regardless of gender, participants with higher serum total calcium levels were associated with higher IOP. Furthermore, in the female population, the risk of high IOP was significantly associated with the higher tertiles of serum total calcium levels. To our best knowledge, our study is the first cross-sectional and retrospective study to evaluate the association between serum total calcium and IOP in an Asian population.

Several lines of evidence suggest that calcium ion is a major cation that triggers a series of cascades and causes an impairment of conventional pathway outflow [9,24]. A study demonstrated that TRPV4 channels serve as important components of the mechanosensitive, calcium ion-initiated pathway within the TM and cause ECM remodeling, which regulates TM stiffness [10]. Furthermore, a study identified a new gene, Cacna2d1, which encodes the voltage-dependent calcium channel complex in the trabecular meshwork and ciliary body, and modulates the IOP [25]. However, these studies were all conducted in in vitro, not in vivo models. On the other hand, our study found positive associations between serum total calcium levels and IOP in an Asian population. This is the first study to demonstrate that serum total calcium could play a critical role in IOP modulation in humans.

Although the possible mechanism of serum total calcium and IOP is unclear, recently, more and more studies have discovered serum total calcium to have some effects on cardiometabolic diseases [11–13]. Disturbance of calcium homeostasis leads to insulin resistance and vascular resistance, which are the crucial factors in cardiometabolic diseases [11]. Previous studies also showed cardiometabolic diseases were associated with IOP [2–5]. Therefore, we propose that the possible mechanism of the association between serum total calcium and IOP may be insulin resistance, or other mechanisms that can cause insulin resistance [11].

IOP can be influenced by many systemic conditions, including blood pressure [26,27], fasting glucose [28], atherosclerotic diseases [26], chronic kidney disease [29], and thyroid hormone [21]. In addition, previous studies also discovered a gender difference of IOP in various populations [15–18]. In our study, the risk of high IOP was significantly associated with the higher tertiles of serum total calcium levels in the female population. The possible reasons for a gender difference might be related to the percentage body fat. Table 1 shows that the percentage body fat is significantly higher in women than in men (p value < 0.001). Published papers also revealed a positive correlation between IOP and obesity [5,30]. The plausible underlying mechanisms have been explained in many studies [31,32]. Excess intraorbital fat tissue can cause episcleral venous pressure increases and ultimately, outflow capability decreases. Furthermore, blood viscosity increases due to obesity and contributes to resistance in episcleral veins. We proposed that the percentage body fat may be a confounding factor regarding the relationship between IOP and serum total calcium levels. Hence, we used three different models to calibrate and reduce the bias. However, the influence of obesity on IOP is far beyond our imagination, and the hormone influence can be considered, so in Tables 4 and 5 the significant association between developing high IOP and serum total calcium levels was only found in women.

Nevertheless, this study has some limitations in spite of our caution. First, this study employed a cross-sectional design that could not reveal causality. Longitudinal analysis is required for future specialists to explore the association between IOP and total calcium levels. Second, the IOP of both eyes was measured only once, and we used the mean IOP of both eyes for analysis. Fluctuations in IOP were ignored in our study, and the mean value of IOP may not reflect the real situation. Third, the study population was recruited from a single center and more large-scale studies from multiple centers should be considered. Fourth, the central corneal thickness (CCT) could influence the IOP measurement reported by many studies [33,34] and this could have caused the IOP measurement bias. However, according to the Singapore Malay Eye Study, Aung et al. discovered age, weight, BMI, presence of diabetes, HbA1C levels, serum glucose levels, metabolic syndrome, and CKD were significantly associated with CCT [35]. In our study, we excluded systemic and ocular diseases (hypertension, diabetes, chronic kidney disease, coronary atherosclerosis, obesity, ocular hypertension, ectatic dystrophies, contact-lens-related complications, and any intraocular surgery) to reduce the influence of CCT on the IOP. Lastly, because the participants' diseases were obtained from self-report histories, we could not exclude the possibility of participants' recall bias.

5. Conclusions

Our study highlights that IOP was significantly associated with serum total calcium levels in a large Asian population. Notably, we also found that a serum total calcium level above 9.05 mg/dL was an important risk factor to predict the high IOP in the female group. Although the exact pathophysiological mechanism underlying the association between serum total calcium and IOP is still not clear, our study provides evidence for future researchers to evaluate it in longitudinal and multi-center trials.

J. Clin. Med. **2021**, *10*, 1839

Author Contributions: Conceptualization, Y.-M.C., W.-L.C. and Y.-J.C.; methodology, Y.-M.C., J.-T.C., M.-C.T., W.-L.C. and Y.-J.C.; software, W.-L.C. and Y.-J.C.; validation, Y.-M.C., J.-T.C., M.-C.T., W.-L.C. and Y.-J.C.; formal analysis, Y.-M.C.; investigation, W.-L.C. and Y.-J.C.; resources, Y.-M.C., W.-L.C. and Y.-J.C.; data curation, Y.-M.C., W.-L.C. and Y.-J.C.; writing—original draft preparation, Y.-M.C.; writing—review and editing, Y.-J.C.; visualization, Y.-M.C.; supervision, J.-T.C., M.-C.T., W.-L.C. and Y.-J.C.; project administration, Y.-M.C., W.-L.C. and Y.-J.C. All authors have read and agreed to the published version of the manuscript.

Funding: This research received no external funding.

Institutional Review Board Statement: The study was approved by the institutional review board of Tri-Service General Hospital, Taipei, Taiwan (TSGHIRB No. 2-107-05-118), which waived the requirement for informed consent from participants and allowed access to the follow-up clinical records. It was conducted in accordance with the requirements of the Declaration of Helsinki.

Informed Consent Statement: Patient consent was waived due to the retrospective nature of this study, and the IRB waived the requirement for obtaining informed consent.

Data Availability Statement: The data presented in this study are available on reasonable request from the corresponding author.

Acknowledgments: We thank for the help of the staff at the Department of Ophthalmology, Tri-Service General Hospital, Division of Family Medicine, Department of Family and Community Medicine, Tri-Service General Hospital and Division of Geriatric Medicine, Department of Family and Community Medicine, Tri-Service General Hospital.

Conflicts of Interest: The authors declare no conflict of interest.

References

1. Quigley, H.A.; Dunkelberger, G.R.; Green, W.R. Retinal Ganglion Cell Atrophy Correlated with Automated Perimetry in Human Eyes with Glaucoma. *Am. J. Ophthalmol.* **1989**, *107*, 453–464. [CrossRef]
2. Hennis, A.; Wu, S.-Y.; Nemesure, B.; Leske, M. Hypertension, diabetes, and longitudinal changes in intraocular pressure. *Ophthalmology* **2003**, *110*, 908–914. [CrossRef]
3. Wu, C.-J.; Fang, W.-H.; Kao, T.-W.; Chen, Y.-J.; Liaw, F.-Y.; Chang, Y.-W.; Wang, G.-C.; Peng, T.-C.; Chen, W.-L. Postprandial Glucose as a Risk Factor for Elevated Intraocular Pressure. *PLoS ONE* **2016**, *11*, e0168142. [CrossRef]
4. Ye, S.; Chang, Y.; Kim, C.-W.; Kwon, M.-J.; Choi, Y.; Ahn, J.; Kim, J.M.; Kim, H.S.; Shin, H.; Ryu, S. Intraocular pressure and coronary artery calcification in asymptomatic men and women. *Br. J. Ophthalmol.* **2015**, *99*, 932–936. [CrossRef] [PubMed]
5. Mori, K.; Ando, F.; Nomura, H.; Sato, Y.; Shimokata, H. Relationship between intraocular pressure and obesity in Japan. *Int. J. Epidemiol.* **2000**, *29*, 661–666. [CrossRef]
6. Tamm, E.R. The trabecular meshwork outflow pathways: Structural and functional aspects. *Exp. Eye Res.* **2009**, *88*, 648–655. [CrossRef] [PubMed]
7. Vosler, P.S.; Brennan, C.S.; Chen, J. Calpain-Mediated Signaling Mechanisms in Neuronal Injury and Neurodegeneration. *Mol. Neurobiol.* **2008**, *38*, 78–100. [CrossRef] [PubMed]
8. Mattson, M.P.; Chan, S.L. Neuronal and glial calcium signaling in Alzheimer's disease. *Cell Calcium* **2003**, *34*, 385–397. [CrossRef]
9. He, Y.; Ge, J.; Tombran-Tink, J. Mitochondrial Defects and Dysfunction in Calcium Regulation in Glaucomatous Trabecular Meshwork Cells. *Investig. Opthalmol. Vis. Sci.* **2008**, *49*, 4912–4922. [CrossRef] [PubMed]
10. Ryskamp, D.A.; Frye, A.M.; Phuong, T.T.T.; Yarishkin, O.; Jo, A.O.; Xu, Y.; Lakk, M.; Iuso, A.; Redmon, S.N.; Ambati, B.; et al. TRPV4 regulates calcium homeostasis, cytoskeletal remodeling, conventional outflow and intraocular pressure in the mammalian eye. *Sci. Rep.* **2016**, *6*, 30583. [CrossRef]
11. Chou, C.-W.; Fang, W.-H.; Chen, Y.-Y.; Wang, C.-C.; Kao, T.-W.; Wu, C.-J.; Chen, W.-L. Association between Serum Calcium and Risk of Cardiometabolic Disease among Community-dwelling Adults in Taiwan. *Sci. Rep.* **2020**, *10*, 3192. [CrossRef]
12. Cho, G.J.; Shin, J.-H.; Yi, K.W.; Park, H.T.; Kim, T.; Hur, J.-Y.; Kim, S.H. Serum calcium level is associated with metabolic syndrome in elderly women. *Maturitas* **2011**, *68*, 382–386. [CrossRef]
13. Oh, S.W.; Lee, S.; Park, C.; Kim, D.J. Elevated intraocular pressure is associated with insulin resistance and metabolic syndrome. *Diabetes Metab. Res. Rev.* **2005**, *21*, 434–440. [CrossRef]
14. Williams, A.L.; Gatla, S.; Leiby, B.E.; Fahmy, I.; Biswas, A.; De Barros, D.M.; Ramakrishnan, R.; Bhardwaj, S.; Wright, C.; Dubey, S.; et al. The Value of Intraocular Pressure Asymmetry in Diagnosing Glaucoma. *J. Glaucoma* **2013**, *22*, 215–218. [CrossRef]
15. Kuo, R.N.; Yang, C.-C.; Yen, A.M.-F.; Liu, T.-Y.; Lin, M.-W.; Chen, S.L.-S. Gender Difference in Intraocular Pressure and Incidence of Metabolic Syndrome: A Community-Based Cohort Study in Matsu, Taiwan. *Metab. Syndr. Relat. Disord.* **2019**, *17*, 334–340. [CrossRef]
16. Imai, K.; Hamaguchi, M.; Mori, K.; Takeda, N.; Fukui, M.; Kato, T.; Kawahito, Y.; Kinoshita, S.; Kojima, T. Metabolic syndrome as a risk factor for high-ocular tension. *Int. J. Obes.* **2010**, *34*, 1209–1217. [CrossRef] [PubMed]

17. Åström, S.; Stenlund, H.; Lindén, C. Intraocular pressure changes over 21 years—A longitudinal age-cohort study in northern Sweden. *Acta Ophthalmol.* **2013**, *92*, 417–420. [CrossRef] [PubMed]
18. Han, X.; Niu, Y.; Guo, X.; Hu, Y.; Yan, W.; He, M. Age-Related Changes of Intraocular Pressure in Elderly People in Southern China: Lingtou Eye Cohort Study. *PLoS ONE* **2016**, *11*, e0151766. [CrossRef]
19. Lee, I.-T.; Wang, J.-S.; Fu, C.-P.; Chang, C.-J.; Lee, W.-J.; Lin, S.-Y.; Sheu, W.H.-H. The synergistic effect of inflammation and metabolic syndrome on intraocular pressure. *Medicine* **2017**, *96*, e7851. [CrossRef] [PubMed]
20. Memarzadeh, F.; Ying-Lai, M.; Azen, S.P.; Varma, R. Associations with Intraocular Pressure in Latinos: The Los Angeles Latino Eye Study. *Am. J. Ophthalmol.* **2008**, *146*, 69–76. [CrossRef]
21. Liu, J.H.; Dacus, A.C.; Bartels, S.P. Thyrotropin releasing hormone increases intraocular pressure. Mechanism of action. *Investig. Ophthalmol. Vis. Sci.* **1989**, *30*, 2200–2208.
22. Chiotoroiu, S.M.; De Popa, D.P.; I Ştefăniu, G.; A Secureanu, F.; Purcărea, V.L. The importance of alcohol abuse and smoking in the evolution of glaucoma disease. *J. Med. Life* **2013**, *6*, 226–229.
23. Tanito, M.; Itai, N.; Dong, J.; Ohira, A.; Chihara, E. Correlation between intraocular pressure level and optic disc changes in high-tension glaucoma suspects. *Ophthalmology* **2003**, *110*, 915–921. [CrossRef]
24. Wiederholt, M.; Thieme, H.; Stumpff, F. The regulation of trabecular meshwork and ciliary muscle contractility. *Prog. Retin. Eye Res.* **2000**, *19*, 271–295. [CrossRef]
25. Chintalapudi, S.R.; Maria, D.; Di Wang, X.; Bailey, J.N.C.; Allingham, R.; Aung, T.; Hysi, P.G.; Wiggs, J.L.; Williams, R.W.; Jablonski, M.M. Systems genetics identifies a role for Cacna2d1 regulation in elevated intraocular pressure and glaucoma susceptibility. *Nat. Commun.* **2017**, *8*, 1755. [CrossRef]
26. Lee, J.S.; Lee, S.H.; Oum, B.S.; Chung, J.S.; Cho, B.M.; Hong, J.W. Relationship between intraocular pressure and systemic health parameters in a Korean population. *Clin. Exp. Ophthalmol.* **2002**, *30*, 237–241. [CrossRef]
27. Wang, Y.X.; Xu, L.; Zhang, X.H.; You, Q.S.; Zhao, L.; Jonas, J.B. Five-Year Change in Intraocular Pressure Associated with Changes in Arterial Blood Pressure and Body Mass Index. The Beijing Eye Study. *PLoS ONE* **2013**, *8*, e77180. [CrossRef] [PubMed]
28. Pimentel, L.G.M.; Gracitelli, C.P.B.; Da Silva, L.S.C.; Souza, A.K.S.; Prata, T.S. Association between Glucose Levels and Intraocular Pressure: Pre-and Postprandial Analysis in Diabetic and Nondiabetic Patients. *J. Ophthalmol.* **2015**, *2015*, 832058. [CrossRef]
29. Nongpiur, M.E.; Wong, T.Y.; Sabanayagam, C.; Lim, S.-C.; Tai, E.-S.; Aung, T. Chronic Kidney Disease and Intraocular Pressure. *Ophthalmology* **2010**, *117*, 477–483. [CrossRef] [PubMed]
30. Klein, B.E.; Klein, R.; Linton, K.L. Intraocular pressure in an American community. The Beaver Dam Eye Study. *Investig. Ophthalmol. Vis. Sci.* **1992**, *33*, 2224–2228.
31. Wu, S.Y.; Leske, M.C. Associations with intraocular pressure in the Barbados Eye Study. *Arch. Ophthalmol.* **1997**, *115*, 1572–1576. [CrossRef] [PubMed]
32. Bulpitt, C.J.; Hodes, C.; Everitt, M.G. Intraocular pressure and systemic blood pressure in the elderly. *Br. J. Ophthalmol.* **1975**, *59*, 717–720. [CrossRef] [PubMed]
33. Doughty, M.J.; Zaman, M.L. Human corneal thickness and its impact on intraocular pressure measures: A review and meta-analysis approach. *Surv. Ophthalmol.* **2000**, *44*, 367–408. [CrossRef]
34. Mansoori, T.; Balakrishna, N. Effect of central corneal thickness on intraocular pressure and comparison of Topcon CT-80 non-contact tonometry with Goldmann applanation tonometry. *Clin. Exp. Optom.* **2018**, *101*, 206–212. [CrossRef] [PubMed]
35. Su, D.H.; Wong, T.Y.; Foster, P.J.; Tay, W.-T.; Saw, S.-M.; Aung, T. Central Corneal Thickness and its Associations with Ocular and Systemic Factors: The Singapore Malay Eye Study. *Am. J. Ophthalmol.* **2009**, *147*, 709–716.e1. [CrossRef]

MDPI

St. Alban-Anlage 66

4052 Basel

Switzerland

Tel. +41 61 683 77 34

Fax +41 61 302 89 18

www.mdpi.com

Journal of Clinical Medicine Editorial Office

E-mail: jcm@mdpi.com

www.mdpi.com/journal/jcm

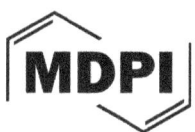

www.ingramcontent.com/pod-product-compliance
Lightning Source LLC
Chambersburg PA
CBHW040249090526
44654CB00118B/215